Practical Guide to Infertility Management and IVF

Practical Guide to Infertility Management and IVF

Editors

Chaitanya Nagori MD DGO
Director
Dr Nagori's Institute for Infertility and IVF
Ahmedabad, Gujarat, India

Sonal Panchal MD
Ultrasound Consultant
Dr Nagori's Institute for Infertility and IVF
Ahmedabad, Gujarat, India

JAYPEE

JAYPEE BROTHERS MEDICAL PUBLISHERS

The Health Sciences Publisher

New Delhi | London

Jaypee Brothers Medical Publishers (P) Ltd

Headquarters
EMCA House
23/23-B, Ansari Road, Daryaganj
New Delhi 110 002, India
Landline: +91-11-23272143, +91-11-23272703
+91-11-23282021, +91-11-23245672
E-mail: jaypee@jaypeebrothers.com

Corporate Office
Jaypee Brothers Medical Publishers (P) Ltd.
4838/24, Ansari Road, Daryaganj
New Delhi 110 002, India
Phone: +91-11-43574357
Fax: +91-11-43574314
E-mail: jaypee@jaypeebrothers.com

Overseas Office
JP Medical Ltd.
83, Victoria Street, London
SW1H 0HW (UK)
Phone: +44-20 3170 8910
E-mail: info@jpmedpub.com

EU GPSR Authorised Representative
Logos Europe, 9 rue Nicolas Poussin
17000, La Rochelle, France
Phone: +33 (0) 6 67 93 73 78
E-mail: Contact@logoseurope.eu

Website: www.jaypeebrothers.com
Website: www.jaypeedigital.com

Practical Guide to Infertility Management and IVF

First Edition: **2021,** Reprint: 2025

ISBN: 978-93-90595-91-4

Printed in India

Preface

Infertility is one of the most frustrating medical and social problems for the couples facing it and being able to treat these patients successfully is one of the most satisfying achievements for the treating personnel. Decades of active researches in the field have unrevealed a huge amount of know-how into the field. But this has led to more complexity and confusion in treating infertile couples.

In this book, we have tried to compile vast amount of information and knowledge with all latest researches included in it. It includes everything from basic knowledge of female and male fertility, investigations, and conventional treatments to the most advanced ART techniques. We have also conveyed clear-cut messages on Do's and Don'ts based on evidences. Practical approach with scientifically-based explanations and to-the-point information is the highlight of this book. We are confident that the book will prove to be an "under the desk, immediate reference book" for every infertility consultant.

Chaitanya Nagori
Sonal Panchal

Contents

1
Chapter
Counseling of an Infertile Couple

INTRODUCTION

Counseling is the backbone of infertility management. The correct explanation about reproduction and dialog with the patients help them conceive. Insler has mentioned in his book that "many patients conceive when they are sitting outside the consulting room." This means that there should be informative literature placed in the waiting room, handouts given to patients, and elaborative explanatory displays placed in the waiting room that patients can read and would help them clear a lot of their misconceptions about reproduction, which they might be reluctant to clear in person.

In the busy outpatient department (OPD), it is very difficult for a practicing gynecologist to spend time with the patients for counseling. I shall put forward a few suggestions from my side:

- There should be informative and illustrative posters placed in the waiting room explaining the physiology of conception.
- Attractive and interesting literature regarding reproductive physiology, causes of infertility, and outline of management should be placed in the waiting room, which should be easily accessible to them.
- We have prepared a small booklet regarding the same, which is given to every patient once detailed consultation has been done about their problems. This booklet helps the patient to go through the things that are already discussed and take a correct decision about the management of their problem.

Such an explanation or literature allows the patients to know what would be the management strategy for their problem and therefore they appreciate the treatment that is given. This transparency also builds the patient's confidence in the treating doctor. It also answers several questions which the couple might be hesistant to ask.

Moreover, it also would be a great means of propagating the correct knowledge about infertility through patients as they would discuss whatever they have read and understood by reading the book with their friends.

One very important suggestion that I would like to give to very busy practitioners is: please allot a specific and separate time slot for patients with fertility problems, so that you can patiently listen to them and discuss the solutions or treatment strategy with them. Remember that the initial counseling and the time spent with them play a very vital role in management of the patient.

Let us now discuss in detail about the different aspects of infertility and its management as these need to be discussed with the patients.

As infertility is a social stigma in our culture, not only the couple (I mean the husband also) but also concerned relatives should be involved in counseling, so that they would allow and co-operate with the couple to take the correct treatment. The refusal of treatment in majority of cases is by in-laws or parents. Therefore, it is very vital that all the people concerned and all those who are going to play a role in decision-making as to whether to continue the treatment or not should know about infertility and the correct treatment option for that particular couple.

WHEN TO START THE TREATMENT?

About 85% of the couples conceive within 1 year of unprotected intercourse and 95% in 2 years. Therefore, if a patient comes for treatment, earlier than a year and a half of continuous unprotected intercourse (active married life), which is very common in rural areas of India and in lower socioeconomic class of people, explaining the above-mentioned fact will increase their faith in you and your treatment and will also prevent unnecessary investigations, anxiety, and frustrations for the patient.

No invasive investigations such as laparoscopy should be done within these 2 years and nature should be given enough time to work for the couple to achieve pregnancy.

Among noninvasive investigations, semen analysis and midcycle/preovulatory scan are the two investigations that may be done. These will more or less prove the normalcy of the couple and then counseling only can help them conceive.

It is commonly observed that couples do conceive very often after the treatment is stopped. This is because the stress and anxiety of treatment are removed and the patient is relaxed. Moreover, when a specialist is treating these couples. They become very enthusiastic about doing some invasive investigation/procedure in every cycle, one after the other such as Rubin's test (RT), hysterosalpingography (HSG), dilatation and curettage (D&C), and laparoscopy, and do not allow an opportunity for conception. Therefore, when this patient is exhausted and abandons treatment, she conceives spontaneously.

Therefore, remember that counseling is more important than overenthusiastic invasive investigations.

COUNSELING FOR SEMEN ANALYSIS

In 40–50% of couples presenting with fertility problems, the male factor is responsible either partially or completely. In our social setup even today, males do not accept this fact and therefore they do not agree for examination or investigations. This problem is more prevalent in people who are less educated. Proper counseling is a must with the male partner before subjecting the female partner to treatment of infertility.

The couple must be explained that according to the recent World Health Organization (WHO) criteria 2010,[1] 15 million sperms/mL, 30% motility, and 4% sperms with normal morphology are considered normal physiological semen criteria. In spite of this even today, we read several laboratories quoting 60 million counts as normal in their reports. Because of this wrong information and ignorance of laboratory officials and clinicians, several patients unnecessarily have to take medicines for long periods to increase their sperm count. Remember that when the sperm count is 15 million/mL or more, no treatment is required. Up to 86% of abnormal sperms is normal and physiological and even patients with 4–14% normal sperms can conceive either naturally or by intrauterine insemination (IUI). It is only when <4% of sperms are normal that in vitro fertilization/intracytoplasmic sperm injection (IVF/ICSI) may be required.

When the sperm count is <15 million/mL, semen analysis must be done at least three times—2 weeks apart and 2 months apart to confirm the diagnosis. These patients should directly not be subjected to IVF or ICSI. Instead, we must try medical treatment for these males to improve the sperm count so that they can conceive naturally or with IUI. The whole moto of medical management of a subfertile male is not to increase the sperm count 5–10 times or to achieve excellent semen parameters. It is to increase the count by a few million so that ICSI can be converted to IVF, IVF to IUI, and perhaps IUI into natural conception. Medical management has been discussed in the chapter on male infertility of this book.

COUNSELING FOR CERVICAL FACTOR

The cervical factor of infertility is rare at present, as surgeries on cervix are not often done. Frequent D&Cs may damage endocervical glands and epithelium. Cauterization of the cervix should be discouraged.

I believe that even today, postcoital test (PCT) is very useful in infertility management. When more than seven sperms are seen per high-power field of microscope, 10–12 hours after intercourse, it is considered an excellent PCT according to the WHO standards.[2]

Majority of assisted reproductive technology (ART) textbooks opine that PCT has no significance. I have found it very useful for counseling the husband. He gets assured that he is normal when PCT is normal, so he does not feel guilty and becomes more cooperative for the treatment. It may not have much role for ART, but it is helpful in cases for regular infertility treatment. These are the patients for whom even timed intercourse can be an option. Many a times when the couple changes the gynecologist, semen analysis is asked for. If the patient already has a few semen analysis reports, I will depend on PCT. The satisfaction of the couple is of the highest level and the confidence increases when the couple sees the moving spermatozoa in cervical secretions under the microscope after 10–12 hours of intercourse. Before doing the test it must be confirmed that it is preovulatory period for the female, considering the cycle length and also that the intercourse was done the previous night.

WHAT INFORMATION DO WE GET FROM A NORMAL POSTCOITAL TEST?

- Preovulatory cervical mucus is normal.
- Sperm count is normal.

Moreover, when the patient (the couple) is shown these moving sperms under microscope even after 12 hours of intercourse, it gives them confidence that both the partners are normal and that helps them conceive.

The patient is explained that these sperms may remain alive for 48–72 hours in the cervix in most patients and in a few, these have also been seen till 7 days. There is a misconception in majority of the couples that intercourse must be done when ovulation occurs. Showing PCT to patients removes this misconception. The cervix acts as a reservoir for sperms, so after the intercourse even if ovulation occurs in 2–3 days, conception can occur. We can explain to the patient that if for conception, the intercourse was needed exactly when ovulation occurs, hardly any raped girl would conceive. The couple should therefore be advised intercourse at least once in 2–3 days during 10–20 days of a 28–30-day cycle. The couple should be clearly told that abstinence of more than 3 days is not advisable during this period, in natural cycle as well as in stimulated cycles for IUI.

Majority of the couples believe that if IUI is done, it is better to have abstinence before to get a good sperm count. But this is not true. An abstinence of more than 3–4 days does not increase the count; instead the percentage of dead sperms in this semen increases. Therefore, intercourse should not be planned; it should be absolutely voluntary and can be done irrespective of the day of IUI.

Abstinence is one of the causes for failed IUI. In majority of gynecology clinics, where there is no IVF setup, the semen preparation laboratory is not adequately equipped, and so the semen preparation is suboptimal and thus chances of conception are less. Moreover, the patient observes abstinence before IUI, so the chance of natural conception also is denied. As a result, the patient does not conceive when she is on treatment but conceives spontaneously when she abandons treatment. Therefore, remember that intercourse at regular intervals in the fertile period is absolutely essential.

Majority of couples with long-term infertility have lost the charm of their marital relations. Their sexual relations are only planned and compulsory, only targeted for childbearing. They must be explained that a child is only a byproduct. The main thing is the love and affection; intercourse is just an expression of this feeling and results in conception. Counseling can help them regain the charm of their marriage. All myths regarding intercourse must be discussed and sorted out, e.g., posture, position, timing, and washing.

Nothing including diet can give gender selection or increase in pregnancy rate.

COUNSELING FOR UTERINE FACTOR

This is to be discussed with the patient after a three-dimensional (3D) ultrasound as 3D ultrasound is now a gold standard for congenital uterine malformations and endometrial pathologies. The patient also can see and understand these 3D pictures and the optimum management then can be easily explained. Fibroids <4–5 cm in size and not touching the endometrium do not require removal. The patient can also be convinced by explaining to them how the embryo comes from the tube to the uterus and implants in the endometrium.

Majority of the patients have a wrong concept that dilatation and curettage (D&C) helps conception. This is a myth and should be clarified. D&C should not be done in modern infertility practice. The only role today of D&C is to exclude endometrial tuberculosis (TB) by either histopathology or TB polymerase chain reaction (PCR) of the endometrial sample along with culture. D&C must not be done to diagnose luteal phase defect or to check whether the endometrium is in the proliferative phase or the secretory phase. It has a higher chance of damaging the endometrium and resulting in infertility.

COUNSELING FOR TUBAL FACTOR

The patient must be explained that fertilization occurs in the fallopian tube and after 4–5 days, the embryo comes to settle in the uterus. This explanation is also useful to counsel if the patient gets an ectopic pregnancy. Tubal evaluation is very important in infertility practice. RT for tubal evaluation should be discarded. Laparoscopy is the gold standard for evaluation of the tubes.

The patient should be explained that at the time of ovulation, the fimbrial end of the tube covers the ovary and a negative pressure of –1 mm Hg (mercury) develops due to movements of the cilia, which sucks the ovum from the follicle into the tubal lumen. So the ovum does not separate and release from the follicle to roll into the tubal lumen, but the tube is vital and instrumental. Therefore, it is important that the tubo-ovarian relation should be healthy; a patent tube is not sufficient. HSG gives us only incomplete information about the patency of the tube. This can be replaced by sonosalpingography (SSG).

Now microsurgery is almost replaced by ART for pathological tubes. The results of microsurgery are very good in tubotubal anastomosis in patients with tubal ligation (TL), especially laparoscopic TL. Therefore, in young patients where TL is done microsurgery should be offered as an alternative to ART as it is a one-time procedure and the patient gets a breathing time for up to 2 years and also has a chance to conceive more than once if the couple wishes so.

COUNSELING FOR OVARIAN CAUSES

The patient should be counseled that ovum is released from the ovary only once in a month and survives for 6–8 hours. Sperms that are stored in the cervix can reach the ova and conception can occur. Ovulation can be confirmed by serum progesterone levels assessed on Day 21–22. Daily sonography is not required just to confirm whether the ovulation has occurred or not if no active treatment or intervention is planned. Basal body temperature record and cervical mucus assessment do not help much in management.

UNEXPLAINED INFERTILITY

About 5–10% of patients are infertile in spite of everything being normal. They have normal semen analysis, normal endoscopy, normal luteal phase, and normal endocrinological reports. These are the patients with unexplained infertility and are the ideal patients for IUI. Six cycles of superovulation with IUI must be tried for these couples before subjecting them to ART. The IUI is the choice of treatment for idiopathic infertility rather than IVF.

COUNSELING FOR INTRAUTERINE INSEMINATION

Intrauterine insemination is a very effective method for fertility treatment. But the couple must be explained that it is not the IUI procedure alone that gives pregnancy; selection of the patient, correct stimulation protocol, precise ultrasound monitoring, and optimum luteal support are all equally important to get pregnancy. So six cycles of properly and dedicatedly done IUI must be tried in patients of <35 years of age and at least three to four cycles in patients up to 40 years of age. It gives an excellent pregnancy rate provided all the steps mentioned earlier are done correctly.

There should not be any abstinence of >48 hours before IUI; otherwise, it decreases the pregnancy rate. Gynecologists should have a good setup for IUI to get excellent results. In-house laboratory should be established in a gynecologist's setup.

COUNSELING FOR DONOR INSEMINATION

Counseling for donor insemination should be done to all the patients who have very low count or azoospermia before proceeding to ICSI. Many patients who cannot afford ART may opt for artificial insemination by donor (AID).

The donor must be unknown. At times, patients may ask to use semen sample from a known donor and that must be discouraged.

The sample must be ordered from a registered semen bank. The donor and couple's identity must not be revealed to each other in any case. The child has a right to ask about his/her genetic prints after 18 years and so the records should be maintained. But when that information is given, the donor's identity must not be revealed.

COUNSELING FOR IN VITRO FERTILIZATION

There are many misconceptions prevailing for IVF treatment regarding three aspects:
1. Indications
2. Results
3. Cost

Indications

It must be clearly understood that IVF is the first choice in only those patients who have bilateral tubal block, severe endometriosis, or severe male factor infertility. IVF may be done in patients with unexplained infertility only when six well-tried superovulation with IUI cycles have failed to give pregnancy. Dysovulatory infertility like polycystic ovaries (PCO) is not an indication of IVF.

Results

Patients believe that IVF is a sure-shot solution to infertility. They have been misled about the same. They must be explained that the results of IVF in the best centers of the world are:
- 30% in the first cycle
- 40–45% in the second cycle
- 50–55% in three cycles
- 60–65% in four cycles
- 65–70% in five cycles
- 70–73% in six cycles

Therefore, patients who do not have absolute indications for IVF should be given a chance of IUI instead of taking them for IVF because about six superovulation with IUI cycles cost the same as one IVF cycle, with more chances of success.

Cost

The IVF is a very expensive procedure. Its cost includes charges for gonadotropins and medicines, which comprises the largest amount, nearing ₹ 60,000–80,000 depending on the requirement of the patient. The second highest cost is of disposables and media. This is also about ₹ 10,000–15,000. Over and above this, the cost also includes consulting fees of the IVF consultant, embryologist, anesthetist, etc. Therefore, it must be understood that when we try to cut-off the cost, one has to compromise on drug quality and disposables. This would definitely compromise with the results also.

With fixed packages, it is likely to do compromise with the quality of treatment.

POINTS TO BE EMPHASIZED (AMERICAN SOCIETY FOR REPRODUCTIVE MEDICINE RECOMMENDATIONS, 2017)

Chances of conception decrease after 35 years and so evaluation must be done after 6 months of marriage in elder age group only.

Intercourse every 1–2 days minimum during the fertile period gives a comparable pregnancy rate. The fertile window starts 6 days prior to ovulation. Smoking, alcohol (>2 pegs), coffee, recreational drugs, and commercially available vaginal lubricants should be discouraged.

CARRY HOME MESSAGE

- Counseling plays a very important role in infertility management.
- About 15 million counts with 30% motility and 4% normal sperms are new WHO 2010 criteria.
- Seven motile sperms/high-power field (HPF) are excellent PCT.
- Dilatation and curettage is done only to rule out tuberculosis.
- Laparoscopy is the gold standard for tubal evaluation.
- Serum progesterone 3 ng/mL on Day 21 indicates ovulation.
- Six cycles of IUI should be tried in unexplained infertility before ART.
- When taking patients for ART, results and cost must be discussed with the patient.

REFERENCES

1. Morshedi M (2010). New 2010 WHO standards (5th edition) for the evaluation of human semen. WHO Guidelines for Semen Analysis. [online] Available from: https://www.aab.org/images/aab/pdf/2014/CRBPPT14/NotesMM%20WHO.pdf [Last accessed March, 2021].
2. Moghissi KS. Postcoital test: physiologic basis, technique and interpretation. Fertil Steril. 1976;27(2):117-29.

2 Chapter

Hormonal Assessment of an Infertile Couple

INTRODUCTION

It is extremely important to ask for precise investigations. Otherwise, it may cause more confusion and a patient has to spend unnecessarily for investigations. This chapter will tell us exactly which investigation should be requested for and when. It is unfortunate that investigations are given more preference than clinical acumen. Clinical acumen is vanishing because of easily available investigations. If I remember days on undergraduate studies, there was a popular book of Clinical Surgery, which had mentioned the sequence as: Provisional diagnosis → Investigations → Final diagnosis. But the sequence followed today is Investigations → Provisional diagnosis → Final diagnosis. This should be strongly discouraged. Provisional diagnosis must be written when an investigation is asked for. Clinicians should never diagnose a condition based on investigations alone.

We have seen patients taking tablet bromocriptine for months or years at a stretch for borderline high prolactin levels. The patient should be treated and not the reports. Remember that the clinician should be the ultimate person to make the diagnosis and decide the treatment. I would humbly request and strongly recommend pathologists not to comment on further investigations, diagnosis, or management. Profiles and packages offered by laboratories are of no use. The clinician must evaluate the requirement of each investigation individually. Moreover, as far as infertility is concerned, any hormonal assessment has clinical value only if done at a particular time of the cycle, and therefore packages and profiles are absolutely meaningless for infertility management. Moreover, it is also essential to understand the physiology of the hypothalamopituitary ovarian axis **(Fig. 1)**. Here, we have emphasized the need for investigations for routine infertility practice, and investigations especially required for in vitro fertilization (IVF) are separately discussed.

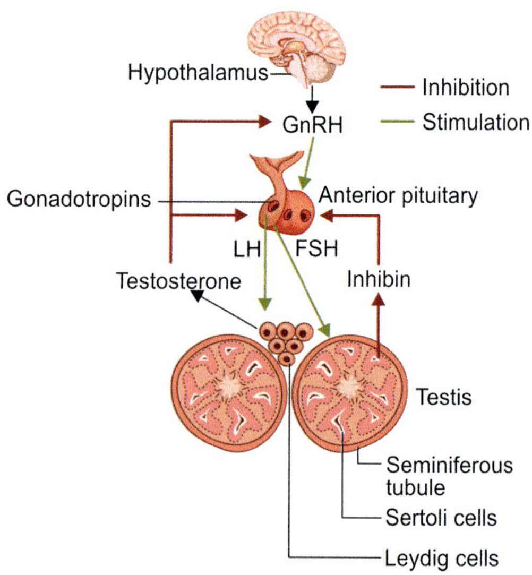

Fig. 1: Hypothalamo-pituitary-testicular axis. (FSH: follicle-stimulating hormone; GnRH: gonadotropin-releasing hormone; LH: luteinizing hormone)

INVESTIGATIONS FOR THE INFERTILE WOMEN

Serum Follicle-stimulating Hormone

- Day 2–3 follicle-stimulating hormone (FSH) is done along with luteinizing hormone (LH) for diagnosis of polycystic ovarian syndrome (PCOS).
  This should not be done as it does not change the line of treatment. PCOS can be diagnosed by history, clinical examination, and ultrasound (US). US diagnosis of polycystic ovaries (PCO) has been discussed in Chapter 12 of this book. We have never used the FSH/LH ratio for the diagnosis of PCOS because an abnormal value of this ratio only indicates anovulation, which is otherwise also evident by history.
- Day 2–3 FSH is done before IVF. Higher FSH indicates lower chances of pregnancy.[1,2] Serum FSH levels up to 10–12 IU/L are considered normal. We do not get Day 2–3 serum FSH done because age + antral follicle count (AFC) gives a better idea for assessing the ovarian reserve. However, systematic reviews from most studies have failed to define a single threshold or cutoff value of serum FSH to describe poor ovarian function.[3]
- Occasionally for diagnosis of menopause, when progesterone withdrawal bleeding is absent, serum FSH can be used to confirm the diagnosis.
- Earlier, serum FSH was assessed in several cycles to decide which cycle can be used for fertility treatment but raised serum FSH in any one cycle can be an indicator of extremely low or no possibility of ongoing pregnancy.[4] Treatment should not be started in selected cycles also when serum FSH is found to be normal.

Basal FSH provides a predictive value for pregnancy which can be judged by baseline scan. High FSH suggests poor ovarian reserve and that can be diagnosed by baseline scan. High FSH is a direct pituitary compensation for the older and less responsive ovary, where reduced oocyte numbers and reduced ovarian hormone production are present and lead to attenuated negative feedback on the hypothalamic/pituitary secretion of FSH. High basal FSH levels should be used for counseling women as regards their outcome rather than exclude them from IVF cycles. FSH above 15 IU/L in young women still show fair pregnancy rates, indicating that quality can compensate for the quantity of oocytes.[5] Cycling women with high FSH should be offered treatment without further delay.[6] We, therefore, routinely do not recommend serum FSH assessment but rely more on baseline scan.

Serum Luteinizing Hormone

- Day 2–3 LH along with serum FSH is done to diagnose PCOS. But high LH indicates only anovulation which can be judged by history. So routine LH is not done.
- *Day 8–9 LH in clomiphene citrate (CC) cycles*: CC stimulates hypothalamus to secrete both FSH and LH. High LH is detrimental to ova and gives a poor pregnancy rate with CC in spite of good ovulation rates. So, when LH is >10–12 IU/L, CC should not be given for the second cycle and patients should be switched over to gonadotropins.

Serum Estradiol Level

- *Follicular maturity*: Serum estradiol (E2) helps to decide the maturity and quality of the follicle. In cases where the follicle looks mature but the endometrium appears thin, it is the E2 level that can decide whether it is the follicular immaturity or a local endometrial cause for the same. A normal E2 level for a mature follicle is 150 pg/mL/follicle. A serum level of E2 less than this indicates a bad quality or immature follicle. A normal serum E2 level with a thin endometrium indicates a local cause. However, in today's practice, if color Doppler is used for assessment of follicular and endometrial quality, the E2 level is not required to assess the physiological maturity of the follicle.

- *For poor responder*: For IVF cycles, E2 is done on Day 2. If E2 is > 80 pg/mL, it indicates a poor IVF outcome as it indicates early follicular recruitment due to high FSH and poor ovarian reserve.[7,8] This is not required for intrauterine insemination (IUI) cycles and in majority of assisted reproductive technology (ART) cycles.
- *To assess ovarian suppression*: In IVF cycles with a long agonist protocol, gonadotropin-releasing hormone agonist (GnRHa) is started from Day 21 of the previous cycle. This downregulates pituitary and FSH; LH levels are therefore very low. In turn, it also brings E2 to baseline levels. To assess downregulation, therefore, E2 is done on Day 2 of the cycle and stimulation may be started if E2 <30 pg/mL, or some may also allow <50 pg/mL. In patients who are on downregulation with oral contraceptive pills, E2 levels are checked after 12 days of oral contraceptive pills to start stimulation.
- *For suspected risk of hyperstimulation*: After superovulation in IUI cycles or when gonadotropins are used for ovulation induction, ovaries may develop multiple follicles. Ovarian hyperstimulation syndrome (OHSS) is feared in such patients. The E2 level can be measured for these patients. In non-IVF cycles, E2 > 1,600 pg/mL and in IVF cycles E2 > 4,000 pg/mL on the day of ovulation trigger can cause OHSS. But the risk of OHSS can also be judged by three-dimensional (3D) US and has been discussed at length in the US section of the book. We, therefore, do not get E2 levels done to assess the risk of OHSS.

We always prefer a chronic low-dose protocol for superovulation with IUI in PCOS patients. In spite of that, if we get four to five follicles in each ovary, we would use GnRHa for ovulation trigger to avoid OHSS. E2 level assessment is not required to decide the ovulation trigger if proper US assessment with Doppler is done.

In IVF/intracytoplasmic sperm injection (ICSI) cycles, OHSS is common for PCOS patients. In these patients, therefore, the antagonist protocol is preferred to the long agonist protocol and agonist is used for ovulation trigger in these patients. This protocol is almost 100% OHSS proof. If we get multiple follicles unexpectedly in an agonist downregulated cycle, the ovarian volume on US can give a clue to the risk of OHSS. This is if the total ovarian volume (of both ovaries) is more than approximately 180 cc.[9] In these cases hCG is withheld. Therefore to avoid OHSS:

- Use a chronic low-dose protocol in PCOS patients.
- Use an antagonist protocol instead of a long agonist protocol for downregulation and agonist as ovulation trigger.
- In doubtful cases, ovarian volume is calculated by 3D US and when ovarian volume is huge, hCG is withheld. The author uses US to assess the risk of OHSS, but E2 can be used by a gynecologist, if the facility of 3D US is not available.

Serum Progesterone

Most of the progesterone is secreted by corpus luteum in the second half of the cycle. Otherwise, it is an intermediate hormone for other steroid hormones.

Normal values are:
- *Follicular phase*: 1 ng/mL
- *LH surge*: 1–2 ng/mL
- *Ovulation*: 3 ng/mL

Midluteal serum progesterone, i.e., a week before menses, is approximately 10 ng/mL. A level of >3 ng/mL indicates ovulation. Therefore, if only ovulation is to be documented and no intervention is planned, repeated US scans are not required. In the same way, endometrial biopsy is not required to confirm secretory changes in the endometrium and serum progesterone estimation suffices for the same.

Ultrasound with color Doppler is a better modality to assess the secretory phase of the cycle. It can define all luteal phase problems—luteal phase defect (LPD)/ luteinized unruptured follicle. This has been discussed in detail in Chapter 23 of this book. Hence, it is the inevitable conclusion that random serum progesterone has little value beyond documenting ovulation.

Serum Prolactin

Prolactin is the hormone secreted by the anterior pituitary and is regulated by the prolactin inhibitory factor, which is secreted from the hypothalamus.
- The normal level of prolactin is 10–25 ng/mL.
- In microadenoma, it is between 100 and 200 ng/mL.
- In macroadenoma, it is >200 ng/mL.
- Immunoassay for prolactin does not reflect the bioassay always.
- Many times, patients have no symptoms in spite of a high prolactin level because of the presence of macromolecules which are big prolactin molecules that account for 10–12% of a normal patient otherwise but showing hyperprolactinemia on laboratory investigation.

Galactorrhea with Normal Prolactin Levels

Patients may come with complaint of galactorrhea and may present with normal serum prolactin levels. This may be mucoid discharge and not actual galactorrhea. Any discharge therefore from the breast should be checked under a microscope. If it contains fat globules, only then it is galactorrhea.

When ovulation induction is done, in many patients, E2 leads to a rise in prolactin levels in the first half of the menstrual cycle. These patients are known as spikers. This is transient hyperprolactinemia. The clinical presentation is poor endometrium in spite of good follicles. This condition is difficult to diagnose, but bromocriptine can be given in a dose of 1.25 mg/BD in these patients in the first half of the cycle. It is a therapeutic test. If endometrium improves, it is continued in the subsequent cycle, otherwise it is stopped. If the patient is a spiker, she needs treatment; otherwise, this condition also deteriorates oocyte quality and causes LPD as a certain amount of prolactin is essential for the development of good follicle and also for corpus luteal function.

Marginally high prolactin levels are also found in PCOS patients due to high E2 and high dehydroepiandrosterone sulfate (DHEAS). In these cases, bromocriptine or cabergoline is not the treatment, and only PCOS is to be treated.

17-OH-Progesterone

This investigation is done in all patients with hirsutism. It is increased due to

21-hydroxylase deficiency. Due to the 21-hydroxylase deficiency in patients of the heterogeneous carrier, late onset of congenital adrenal hyperplasia is observed. 17-OH-progesterone (17-OH-P) is a weak androgen and manifests as hirsutism, acne, clitoral enlargement, and menstrual irregularity at puberty.

The normal level of 17-OH-P is <200 ng/dL. Whenever the level is between 200 and 800 ng/dL, it requires adrenocorticotropic hormone (ACTH) testing. A level of >800 ng/dL is diagnostic of 21-hydroxylase deficiency.[10] These patients are treated with dexamethasone 0.5 mg daily at bedtime.

Serum Testosterone

The normal value of serum testosterone is 20–80 ng/dL. Its normal production is 0.2–0.3 mg/day. Out of this, 80% binds to sex hormone–binding globulin (SHBG) and 19% to albumin. Only 1% is free testosterone.

Testosterone may rise in PCOS and tumors. Tumor is suspected if there is a sudden onset of symptoms due to increased testosterone. PCOS patients show a gradual rise in testosterone levels.[11] Routine estimation of serum testosterone is not required as it does not change the line of treatment.

Serum Dehydroepiandrosterone Sulfate

Dehydroepiandrosterone sulfate is exclusively secreted from adrenal glands **(Table 1)**. The normal value is 350 ng/dL. It increases with hyperprolactinemia. Therefore in patients with PCOS, prolactin and DHEAS are slightly on the higher side which do not require any specific treatment except the treatment of PCOS. This rise is secondary to E2 because of anovulation.

TABLE 1: Sources of testosterone.

Hormone	*Source*
Testosterone	• 50% peripheral conversion • 25% ovary • 25% adrenal
Androstenedione	• 50% ovary • 50% adrenal
Dehydroepiandrosterone (DHEA)	• 90% adrenal • 10% ovary
Dehydroandrosterone (DHA)	• 100% adrenal

Whenever DHEAS is very high, it is due to adrenal tumor. So US is a better guide to diagnose adrenal tumor. Serum testosterone and US suffices to rule out adrenal tumors.

If there is a moderate rise in PCOS, it does not require any treatment. If 17-OH-P is normal, there is no need to search for an adrenal enzyme defect. DHEAS > 700 μg/dL is accepted as a marker for adrenal dysfunction. This is rarely found and does not change the management. Therefore, routine testing of DHEAS is not required.

Inhibin A and B

Inhibin B is predominantly secreted by antral follicles. Low, Day 3 inhibin B level of <45 pg/mL has poor response to superovulation and the patient is less likely to conceive. The same thing can be judged by raised serum FSH, raised serum anti-Müllerian hormone (AMH), or low AFC and so routine use of inhibin B estimation is not justified.

Inhibin A is secreted from preovulatory follicles. Both inhibin A and B are secreted from granulosa cells and regulate FSH by a negative feedback mechanism. Routine estimation of inhibin A does not add any information that may change the management of the patient.

Serum Anti-Müllerian Hormone

It is a member of transforming growth factor (TGF). It is produced from granulosa cells. The expression of AMH is localized in granulosa cells of primary preantral and small antral follicles and has an important role in human folliculogenesis. AMH expression in the follicle decreases when the antral follicle size is >8 mm. In follicles undergoing atresia and in corpus lutea also, the AMH expression is completely lost.[12]

AMH levels in women are low until the age of 8 years, rise rapidly until puberty, and decline steadily from the age of 25 years until menopause, when AMH production ceases.

It is now well established that serum AMH concentrations reflect the number of preantral and small antral follicles in the ovary. This would account for raised AMH levels found in both polycystic ovarian morphology (PCOM) and PCOS.[13]

Physiology

Anti-Müllerian hormone has an inhibiting role in the ovary, contributing to follicular arrest.[14] It lowers the sensitivity of follicles to FSH that is required for normal folliculogenesis. In vitro studies have shown that the action of FSH in promoting follicular growth is counteracted by AMH.[15] It has a steady level throughout the cycle except for a slight dip just after LH peak.[16] However, some investigators have recorded cyclical fluctuations in AMH with a rapid decrease in the early luteal phase.[17]

Anti-Müllerian Hormone and Polycystic Ovary

The reported property of AMH to counteract the actions of FSH implies that the high production of AMH by PCO may have an important role in the pathophysiology of the syndrome.[14] In anovulatory PCOS, the failure of follicle development is due to an intrinsic inhibition of FSH action and this inhibition is due to the high concentration of AMH.[18] Increased ovarian stromal blood flow in PCOS may be because of overexpression of the vascular endothelial growth factor (VEGF), which modulates the permeability of theca cells and increases insulin-like growth factor 1 (IGF-1).[19,20] This, in turn, enhances gonadotropin-stimulated steroid production in granulosa cells and theca cells resulting in increased ovarian androgen production and subsequently increased AMH production.[21] AMH levels are two to three times higher in PCOS than in healthy controls.[22] This has been attributed not only to increased number of antral follicles, but also to higher production of AMH per follicle in patients with PCOS as compared to size-matched counterparts from normal ovary.[23]

In addition, a positive correlation between AMH and serum concentration of both LH and testosterone in PCOS has been reported.[24]

Each individual follicle in a PCO in women with PCOS produces significantly more AMH than its sized-matched counterpart from a normal ovary.[23] Moreover, it has also been shown that metformin administration in PCOS patients is associated with reduction in AMH concentration in follicle and serum, suggesting that the measurement of AMH can be used to evaluate the treatment efficacy with insulin sensitizers.[25]

It can predict ovarian response and menopause by low levels. If AMH is very high in PCOS, it predicts OHSS.

Anti-Müllerian Hormone and In Vitro Fertilization

In IVF patients, the serum AMH value can predict the response of ovary and hence it is useful for counseling the patient.

When calculated optimal AMH cutoff of <1.26 ng/mL was used to predict responses to controlled ovarian stimulation (COS), it was found to have a 97% sensitivity for predicting poor responses (<4 oocytes retrieved) and 98% accuracy in predicting a normal COS response.[26] Nelson et al. suggested AMH-based strategy for deciding the COS protocol **(Table 2)**.[27]

However, we have found AFC equally effective and more precise for prediction of ovarian response. We routinely do not assess AMH levels either in IVF or non-IVF cycles. With extremely low serum AMH levels, moderate, but reasonable pregnancy and live birth rates are still observed in our practice. An extremely low AMH level does not seem to represent an appropriate marker for withholding fertility treatment. Younger women are likely to have better pregnancy rates than their older counterparts with equally low AMH.[28]

Constant AMH and inhibin B levels suggest that neither AMH nor inhibin B is an accurate marker of ovarian response after low-dose gonadotropin ovulation induction in patients with PCOS.[29] Mashiach et al. have also shown a relationship between follicular fluid AMH concentrations and the quality of embryos in patients with PCOS.[30]

Routine use of AMH does not help in managing non-ART patients. We require one to two follicles for superovulation with IUI, and AMH will not help us in changing the line of treatment. A poor responding ovary or low reserve ovary can be very well judged by US.

Serum AMH estimation is indicated in:[31]

- Predicting both over- and under-response in controlled ovarian hyperstimulation (COH) **(Table 3)**
- Determining the most appropriate treatment regimen
- Pretreatment counseling for couples to make an appropriate and informed choice
- Predicting long-term fertility
- Predicting the age of menopause
- Predicting ovarian aging prior to or following chemotherapy/surgery
- Screening for polycystic ovaries

TABLE 2: Anti-Müllerian hormone (AMH) group (pmol/L) and COS protocol.

AMH group (pmol/L)	*GnRH analog*	
<1.0	375 antagonist	(Modified natural cycle)
1.0 to <5	375 agonist	300 antagonist
5.0 to <15	225 agonist	225 agonist
≥25	150 agonist	150 antagonist

TABLE 3: Anti-Müllerian hormone: Values and implications.

Ovarian fertility potential	*pmol/L*	*ng/mL*
Optimal fertility	28.6	4.06
Satisfactory fertility	15.7	2.27
Low fertility	2.2	0.3
Very low/undetectable	0.0	0.0
High level	>48.5	>6.8

The inhibitory effect of AMH on folliculogenesis may, in future, be used for hormonal contraception.

Clinical applications of AMH apart from fertility assessment are as follows:

- To confirm the presence of testicular tissue in children with low testosterone levels
- Differential diagnosis of intersex disorders
- In patients with bilateral nonpalpable gonads
- In females with granulosa cell tumors

Insulin Resistance

Now it has been proved that in patients with PCOS, there is high androgen because of an increased insulin level and its sensitivity. It indicates the severity of PCOS. Clinically, a waist circumference of 35 inches or 90 cm is predictive of abnormal endocrinology and metabolic function.

There are various methods to diagnose insulin resistance. But 2-hour glucose and insulin response is the most reliable one.

Two-hour glucose tolerance test (after 75 g of glucose):

- *Normal*: <140 mg/dL
- *Impaired*: 140–190 mg/dL
- *Noninsulin-dependent diabetes mellitus (DM)*: ≥200 mg/dL

Two-hour insulin response (after 75 g of glucose):

- *Insulin resistance very likely*: 100 150 μU/mL
- *Insulin resistance*: 151–300 μU/mL
- *Severe insulin resistance*: >300 μU/mL

In clinical practice, patients with high insulin resistance are the ones who require ovarian drilling. They have tonically high LH levels and therefore drilling helps. Alternatively, they may also be benefitted by GnRH antagonist.

Antagonist decreases LH levels, prevents premature luteinization, and improves oocyte quality.

Patients with insulin resistance who do not want immediate pregnancy are the patients for metformin therapy. 3D US is a novel way to diagnose insulin resistance, based on the assessment of stromal volume.[32] But for all those who do not have volume US, 2-hour glucose and insulin test are the best alternative. Hence, for chronic anovulation, only three investigations are required:

1. Serum prolactin
2. Serum thyroid-stimulation hormone (TSH)
3. Insulin resistance

Thyroid Function Tests

- The normal level is 0.5–2.5 mIU/mL.
- If TSH is high, measure free T4.
- Any woman after the age of 35 years should be assessed for thyroid function.
- Presence of antithyroid antibodies indicates future hypothyroidism.
- During pregnancy or in recurrent pregnancy loss, it is done every 2 months.
- Requirement of thyroxine decreases with age.
- For hyperthyroidism, T4 is measured and if it is normal, T3 is measured.

Laboratory Investigations for Male Infertility

In patients with male infertility, there are three important hormonal investigations: (1) serum TSH, (2) serum LH, and (3) serum testosterone, used for diagnosis and treatment plan. There are various permutation combinations of these hormones:

- *High FSH, high LH, and low/normal testosterone*: This indicates primary testicular failure, due to spermatogenic and Leydig cell damage. The treatment option for these patients will be only donor insemination or adoption. These patients cannot even provide a sufficient number of sperms for ICSI. However, microdissection testicular sperm extraction (micro-TESE) may help.

- *High FSH, normal LH, and normal testosterone*: This combination indicates primary spermatogenic failure. As LH is normal, there is no Leydig cell damage. This is due to inhibin deficiency. The treatment option for these patients is again donor insemination or adoption. Micro-TESE may be tried.

  In both these groups, the FSH is high. Therefore, instead of assessing these three hormones, one can assess only serum FSH and if that is high evaluation of other two hormones is not required. But if serum FSH is normal, LH and testosterone levels need to be assessed.

  In patients with high FSH, with normal LH and testosterone, the possible diagnosis is varicocele. In grade 3 varicocele, because of testicular damage, FSH is borderline high. In these patients, varicocele ligation + gonadotropins + antioxidants can improve spermatogenesis in many cases.
- *Normal FSH, high LH, and high testosterone*: Normally, LH and testosterone are regulated by the negative feedback mechanism. But in this case, both LH and testosterone are high, as testosterone is not perceived by receptors. This is known as partial androgen resistance. High androgen will be converted into E2 and so the E2/testosterone ratio will be high. This high E2 will cause gynecomastia that is a diagnostic criterion. It also causes oligoasthenoteratozoospermia, which does not respond to drugs. ART is advised in these patients or adoption if the patient cannot afford, after proper counseling.
- *Normal FSH, normal LH, and normal testosterone*: This is a very common finding in our patients. It may be due to organic causes such as obstruction in ductal system, retrograde ejaculation, varicocele, or germ cell failure. The treatment is according to the cause.
  - *Obstruction*: Surgery or ICSI after percutaneous epididymal sperm aspiration/testicular sperm aspiration (PESA/TESA)
  - *Retrograde ejaculation*: α adrenergic blocking drugs + IUI or ART
  - *Varicocele*: Surgery + gonadotropins + antioxidants
  - *Germ cell failure*:
    - *Spermatogonia arrest*: Donor insemination
    - *Spermatid arrest*: FSH + ICSI

  But most commonly, patients having azoospermia with normal FSH, LH, and testosterone do not have any pathological cause. These patients have qualitative failure causing azoospermia or severe oligozoospermia.

  As discussed in the chapter on medical management of male infertility, these patients can be treated with FSH or human menopausal gonadotropin (hMG) 75–150 international units (IU) thrice a week and hCG 5,000 IU twice a week. It has given excellent results in many cases. In these cases, endogenous bioactivity is poor in spite of normal immunological levels [radioimmunoassay (RIA) test]. This is why exogenous FSH, LH, and hCG are useful.
- *Low FSH, low LH, and low testosterone*: These are found in patients who have hypogonadotropic hypogonadism. These patients can be treated with hCG

5,000 IU every fifth day for 5–7 weeks till testosterone becomes normal as it is required for initiation of spermatogenesis. After testosterone becomes normal, FSH 75 IU is added thrice a week for maturation of sperms. This is given for 3–6 months. But results are excellent and it initiates spermatogenesis.

There may be panhypopituitarism which require replacement of thyroid, corticotrophin, and growth hormone (GH).

There may be Kallmann syndrome which is congenital. Prolactinoma is normally macro type that requires surgery.

Hyperprolactinemia

The most diagnostic symptom of hyperprolactinemia is the loss of libido. There is no galactorrhea or gynecomastia. The cause of low testosterone is macroadenoma leading to hyperprolactinemia, and this macroadenoma must be removed surgically. If there is no macroadenoma, oligospermia is because of androgen resistance. The therapy of choice for these patients is long-term bromocriptine or cabergoline.

Thyroid Dysfunction

Autoimmune thyroiditis is the most common condition. Hypothyroidism can cause oligospermia and hyperprolactinemia because of high TSH. Hyperthyroidism also causes oligospermia. Therefore, thyroid function assessment is required in patients with oligospermia.

Adrenal Dysfunction

Infertility may be the only manifestation of adrenal dysfunction. It leads to feminization and softening of the testis. Raised DHEAS also leads to increased prolactin levels. These are also associated with signs and symptoms of adrenal insufficiency. The risk is high in patients with a family history of congenital adrenal hyperplasia.

Endocrine Workup

- Serum FSH
- Serum LH
- Serum testosterone
- Serum prolactin
- Serum TSH and T4
- Serum DHEAS
- Serum E2
- Serum 17-OH-progesterone
- Serum cortisol
- SHBG

CARRY HOME MESSAGE

- Investigation is requested for confirmation of provisional diagnosis.
- FSH > 15 IU/L indicates poor quality and quantity of ova.
- In CC cycle, Day 8 10 FSH should be <10 IU/L.
- E2 > 1,600 pg/mL in an IUI cycle may lead to OHSS.
- Serum progesterone > 3 ng/mL documents ovulation.
- Serum prolactin > 100 IU indicates adenoma.
- Prolactin is high in PCOS patients.
- 17-OH-P is recommended in all patients with hirsutism.
- Low AMH indicates poor ovarian reserve.
- High FSH in males indicates testicular failure.
- Hypogonadotropic hypogonadism has a good fertility prognosis after treatment in both the partners.
- When FSH, LH, and testosterone are normal in men, it is mostly qualitative failure.

REFERENCES

1. Muasher SJ, Oehniger S, Simonetti S, Matta J, Ellis LM, Liu HC, et al. The value of basal and/or stimulated serum gonadotropin levels in prediction of stimulation response and in vitro fertilization outcome. Fertil Steril. 1988;50:298–307.

2. Scott RT, Toner JP, Muasher SJ, Oehninger S, Robinson S, Rosenwaks Z. Follicle-stimulating hormone levels on cycle day 3 are predictive of in vitro fertilization outcome. Fertil Steril. 1989;51:651.
3. Bancsi LF, Broekman FJ, Mol BW, Habbema JD, te Valde ER. Performance of basal follicle stimulating hormone in prediction of poor response and failure to become pregnant after in vitro fertilization: a meta-analysis. Fertil Steril. 2003;79:1091-100.
4. Pearlstone AC, Fournet N, Gambone JC, Pang SC, Buyalos RP. Ovulation induction in women age 40 and older: The importance of basal follicle stimulating hormone level and chronological age. Fertil Steril. 1992;58:674-79.
5. van Rooji IAJ, de Jong E, Broekmans FJM, Looman CWN, Habbema JDF, te Velde E. High follicle stimulating hormone levels should not necessarily lead to the exclusion of subfertile patients from treatment. Fertil Steril. 2004;81:1478-85.
6. Abdalla H, Thum MY. Repeated testing of basal FSH levels has no predictive value for outcome in women with elevated basal FSH. Hum Reprod. 2006;21(1):171-4.
7. Smotrich DB, Widra EA, Gindoff PR, Levy MJ, Hall JL, Stillman RJ. Prognostic value of day 3 estradiol on in vitro fertilization outcome. Fertil Steril. 1995;64:1136-40.
8. Licciardi FL, Lui HC, Rosenwaks Z. Day 3 estradiol serum concentrations as prognosticators of ovarian stimulation response and pregnancy outcome in patients undergoing in vitro fertilization. Fertil Steril. 1995;64:991-4.
9. Oyesanya OA, Parsons JH, Collins WP, Campbell S. Total ovarian volume before human chorionic gonadotrophin administration for ovulation induction may predict the hyperstimulation. Hum Reprod. 1995;10:3211-12.
10. Kuttenn F, Couillin P, Girard F, Billaud L, Vincens M, Boucekkine C, et al. Late onset adrenal hyperplasia in hirsutism. New Engl J Med. 1985;313:224-31.
11. Easterling Jr WE, Talbert LM, Potter HD. Serum testosterone levels in the polycystic ovary syndrome. Am J Obstet Gynecol. 1974;120:385.
12. Elvin JA, Clark AT, Wang P, Wolfman NM, Matzuk MM. Paracrine actions of growth differentiation factor-9 in the mammalian ovary. Mol Endocrinol. 1999;13(6):1035-48.
13. Fanchin R, Maria SL, Righini C, Guibourdenche J, Frydman R, Taieb J. Serum AMH is more strongly related to ovarian follicle status that serum inhibin B, oestradiol, FSH and LH on the day 3. Hum Reprod. 2003;18:323-7.
14. Pellat L, Rice S, Mason HD. Anti-Müllerian hormone and polycystic ovarian syndrome: a mountain too high. Reproduction. 2010;139:825-33.
15. Durlinger AL, Gruijters MJ, Kramer P, Karels B, Kumar TR, Matzik MM. Anti-Müllerian hormone attenuates the effect of FSH on follicle development in the mouse ovary. Endocrinology. 2001;142:4891-9.
16. La Marca A, Stabile G, Artenisio AC, Volpe A. Serum anti-Müllerian hormone throughout the human menstrual cycle. Hum Reprod. 2006;21(12):3103-7.
17. Streuli J, Fraisse T, Chapron C, Bijaoui G, Bischof P, de Ziegler D. Clinical uses of anti-Müllerian hormone assays: pitfalls and promises. Fertil Steril. 2009;91(1):226-30.
18. Pellat L, Rice S, Dilaver N, Heshri A, Galea R, Brincat M, et al. Anti-Müllerian hormone reduces follicle sensitivity to follicle-stimulating hormone in human granulosa cells. Fertile Steril. 2011;96:1246-51.
19. El Behery MM, Diab AE, Mowafy H, Ebrahiem MA, Shehata AE. Effect of laparoscopic ovarian drilling on vascular endothelial growth factor and ovarian stromal blood flow using three dimensional power Doppler. Intern J Gynecol Obstet. 2011;112:119-21.
20. Abd El, Aal DE, Mohamed SA, Amine AF, Meki AR. Vascular endothelial growth factor and insulin-like growth factor 1 in polycystic ovary syndrome and their relation to ovarian blood flow. Eur J Obstet Gynecol reprod Biol. 2005;118:219-24.

21. Willis D, Mason H. Gilling-Smith C, Franks S. Modulation by insulin of follicle stimulating hormone and luteinizing hormone actions in human granulosa cells of normal and polycystic ovaries. J Clin Endocrinol Metab. 1996;81:302-9.
22. Pigny P, Merlen E, Robert Y, Cortet-Rudelli C, Decanter C, Jonard S, et al. Elevated serum level of anti-Müllerian hormone in patients with polycystic ovary syndrome: relationship to the ovarian follicle excess and to the follicular arrest. J Clin Endocrinol Metab. 2003;88:5957-62.
23. Pellat L, Hanna L, Brincat M, Galea R, Brain H, Whitehead S, et al. Granulosa cell production of anti-Müllerian hormone is increased in polycystic ovaries. J Clin Endocrinol Metab. 2007;92:240-5.
24. Carlsen SH, Vanky E, Fleming R. Anti-Müllerian hormone concentrations in androgen suppressed women with polycystic ovary syndrome. Hum Reprod. 2009; 24:1732-8.
25. Piltonen T, Morin Papunen L, Koivunen R, Perheentupa A, Ruokonen A, Tapanainen JS. Serum anti-Müllerian hormone levels remain high until late reproductive age and decrease during metformin therapy in women with polycystic ovary syndrome. Hum Reprod. 2005;20(7):1820-6.
26. Gnoth C, Schuring AN, Friol K, Tigges J, Mallmann P, Godehardt E. Relevance of anti-Müllerian hormone measurement in a routine IVF program. Hum Reprod. 2008;23: 1359-65.
27. Nelson SM, Yates RW, Lyall H, Jamieson M, Traynor I, Gaudoin M, et al. Anti-Müllerian hormone-based approach to controlled ovarian stimulation for assisted conception. Hum Reprod. 2009;24:867-75.
28. Weghofer A, Dietrich W, Barad DH, Gleicher N. Live birth chances in women with extremely low serum anti-Müllerian hormone levels. Hum Reprod. 2011;26(70): 1905-9.
29. Fong SL, Schippe I, de Jong FH, Themmen APN, Visser JA, Laven JSP. Serum anti-Müllerian hormone and inhibin B concentrations are not useful predictors of ovarian response during ovulation induction treatment with rFSH in women with polycystic ovary syndrome. Fertil Steril. 2011;96(2):459-63.
30. Mashiach R, Amit A, Hasson J, Amzalzg S, Almog B, Ben-Yosef D, et al. Follicular fluid levels of anti-Müllerian hormone as a predictor of oocyte maturation, fertilization rate, and embryonic development in patients with polycystic ovarian syndrome. Fertil Steril. 2010;93(7):2299-302.
31. Loh JS, Maheshwari A. Anti-Müllerian hormone—is it a crystal ball for predicting ovarian ageing? Human Reprod. 2011; 26(11):2925-32.
32. Panchal S, Nagori CB. Correlation of ovarian and stromal volumes to fasting and postprandial insulin levels in polycystic ovarian syndrome patients. Int J Infertil Fetal Med. 2014;5(1):12-4.

3 Chapter

Assessing Ovarian Reserve

INTRODUCTION

Assessment of the ovarian reserve is necessary to decide the line of treatment amongst various assisted reproductive technologies (ART) available. Late marriages, career-oriented women, and delay in obstetric career are the factors responsible for the decrease in ovarian reserve in the fertility-desiring females. Knowledge regarding ovarian reserve can change the management of individual patient, as in stimulation protocols can be adjusted or treatments may be refused, advanced, or postponed accordingly.[1]

PHYSIOLOGY

The number of ova in the female fetus at 20 weeks of intrauterine age is 6-7 million and is decreased to approximately 2 million at birth. At puberty, the number decreases to approximately 3-4 lacs. Fertility decreases after the age of 30 years when the numbers of follicles are as low as approximately 25,000 only. After the age of 35 years, the prevalence of infertility sharply increases and when the woman reaches the age of 40 years, approximately only 8,000 ova are available for recruitment **(Box 1)**. After the age of 45 years, 99% of women are expected to be infertile.[2] Antral follicle count (AFC) showed the best correlation with women's age and declined linearly at a rate of 3.8% per year.[3]

Another study has indicated a biphasic pattern of AFC decline. It was documented as 4.8% per year before the age of 37 years compared with 11.7% per annum thereafter.[4]

Box 1: Number of ova available.

- *At 20 weeks*: 6–7 million
- *At birth*: 2 million
- *At puberty*: 3–4 lacs
- *After 30 years*: 25,000
- *After 40 years*: 8,000
- *At menopause*: <1,000

The number of quantity and quality of the follicles in the ovary thus remaining determine the ovarian reserve.[5]

When the number of ova drops to <1,000, menopause occurs. The age of menopause varies between 40 and 60 years with an average age of 51 years. But after the age of 42 years, the fertility of the female decreases drastically.[6]

DEFINITION

The ovarian reserve is the capacity of the ovaries to produce fertilizable ova. This depends on the quality and quantity of ovarian antral and preantral follicles.[5]

OVARIAN RESERVE NEEDS TO BE ASSESSED[7]

- Females of >35 years of age
- Females with unexplained infertility and in females who have had a previous cycle of ovulation induction with gonadotropins and had a poor response

- Females who have a history of an ovarian surgery in the past
- Smokers
- Females who have maternal relations with early menopause. In these females, the ovarian reserve assessment needs to be done at an age much earlier than 35 years as they may be genetically predisposed to low ovarian reserve and early ovarian failure. These females need special advice for the advancement of fertility treatment.
- However, it should be emphasized that a decrease in ovarian reserve does not mean inability to conceive.[7]

It is important to mention here that at this stage, the pattern of reproductive aging as assessed by hormonal and ultrasonographic ovarian reserve tests does not appear to show an abrupt change at a certain age, but follows a continuously increasing rate of decline in the third decade of life. The changes in serum follicle-stimulating hormone (FSH) levels and ultrasonographic ovarian reserve tests follow a quadratic model in regularly menstruating women.[8]

As no test is perfect to comment on fertility potential and plan of treatment, evaluation by the combination of tests may be required for the assessment of ovarian reserve.[8] All the ovarian reserve tests are considered as screening tests, and abnormal tests should be confirmed by other tests.[7]

OVARIAN RESERVE TESTS

Ovarian reserve can be assessed by various clinical, biochemical, or ultrasound features and these are known as markers of ovarian reserve. These can be divided into three heads:

1. Clinical markers
2. Endocrinal markers
3. Ultrasound markers

Clinical Markers

- Age
- Menstrual pattern

Age

It has been already discussed earlier in this chapter that advancing age decreases the ovarian reserve due to apoptosis. This means that age is the most consistent factor that decides the quantity of the ova in the ovary. Moreover, the quality of the ova available has also been negatively correlated with the increasing age.

However, chronological age and ovarian age are not always correlating. A young woman may have low ovarian reserve and a woman of 40 years may also have several antral follicles in her ovaries. Therefore, other tests of ovarian reserve are required for the assessment of ovarian reserve and deciding the line of treatment.

The monthly fecundity rate is about 20% in young couples desiring pregnancy but not undergoing treatment. With increasing age, fecundity decreases and may take a longer time to achieve conception. The Society of Assisted Reproductive Treatment (SART) and Centers for Disease Control and Prevention (CDC) have constantly demonstrated that age is the single most important factor affecting the probability of success of in vitro fertilization (IVF).

This is because 24% of oocytes in a woman of <35 years will be chromosomally abnormal, but this number reaches 52% at the age of 35 years. After 40 years, >90% of the oocytes are abnormal.[9] At the age of 30 years, 75% of the women are expected to conceive naturally within a year, while only 66% will do so at the age of 35 years. So age is an important criterion to decide the fertility potential of a woman.[10]

Chronological age is more related to the quality of the ova rather than increased FSH. Young women with high FSH may give good ova, but old women with low FSH have a high chance of aneuploidy in the ova. This means that the abnormal tests in younger patients have a poor prognosis, but normal tests do not improve the age-related poor prognosis in older patients.

Menstrual Pattern

The length of the menstrual cycle depends on the length of the follicular phase. The length of the normal cycle is 21–35 days (28 days—mean) of which the length of the luteal phase is constant (14 days). There will be high FSH and low serum inhibin B level in these patients. This is common as age advances.[11] This may be responsible for faster follicular growth and short cycles but may also be the cause of more aneuploid ova.

Endocrinal Tests

Endocrinal tests may be divided under two heads:

1. *Static tests*:
    - Day 2 or 3 serum FSH (S FSH)
    - Day 2 or 3 serum estradiol (S E2)
    - Day 3 S FSH and serum luteinizing hormone (S LH)
    - Inhibin B
    - Anti-Müllerian hormone (AMH)
2. *Dynamic tests*:
    - Clomiphene citrate challenge test (CCCT)
    - Gonadotropin-releasing hormone analog stimulation test (GAST)
    - Exogenous FSH ovarian reserve test (EFORT)

Day 2 or 3 Follicle-stimulating Hormone

Follicle-stimulating hormone level in serum, when assessed, must be combined and correlated with estrogen. This is because there is a negative feedback system between FSH and estrogen. On Day 2–3, all follicles in the ovary are small (antral) so the estrogen level is low and FSH levels at this stage are at their baseline levels. Normal FSH with low E2 indicates a normal hypothalamo-pituitary-gonadal axis. The level of FSH increases with increasing age due to falling basal estrogen levels and indicates low ovarian reserve. Fluctuations in the serum FSH levels in different cycles also indicate diminished ovarian reserve.[12]

Normal basal FSH is <10 mIU/mL **(Table 1)**. Levels between 10 and 15 mIU/mL are considered borderline. The ovarian reserve is predicted as very low when the level of FSH is >15 mIU/mL. But it has a poor predictive value for nonpregnancy. No single cutoff of S FSH has been established to predict nonpregnancy. Therefore, cycle cancellation should not be advised only on the ground of high serum FSH levels.

A recent study has demonstrated 100% specificity for failure to achieve a live birth at FSH values above 18 mIU/mL.[13]

Follicle-stimulating hormone is released from the anterior pituitary in a pulsatile manner and also has circadian variations. Moreover, isoforms of FSH are also known and there may be fluctuations in these also. This may lead to variable results when

TABLE 1: Correlation of FSH level and response to ovulation induction drugs.

FSH level	*Response*
<8 mIU/mL	Reassure
8–12 mIU/mL	Average reserve
12–17 mIU/mL	Decreased ovarian reserve
>17 mIU/mL	Extremely poor pregnancy rates

(FSH: follicle-stimulating hormone)

serum FSH levels are assessed at different times in the same patient. Single nucleotide polymorphism (SNP) in FSH-receptive gene may have normal FSH with a poor response. SNPs at 307 and 680 are common.[14]

In this case, it is best to consider the highest value of S FSH (when FSH is assessed several times in a single female) for decision-making and counseling with the patient for fertility treatment planning. Whatever is the ovarian response, the pregnancy rates are poor with high serum FSH levels.

Day 2 or 3 Serum Estradiol

Estradiol is secreted from granulosa cells and reflects follicular activity.

A high E2 level on Day 2–3 of the menstrual cycle indicates early follicular recruitment. This is reflected on ultrasound as a follicle of 10 mm or larger on Day 2–3 of the cycle. This is because of high basal FSH. Cycle cancellation is much higher in IVF cycles when E2 is 80 pg/mL or more or 20 pg/mL or less on Day 2–3 of the menstrual cycle.[15] Day 2 FSH and E2 have a high predictive value for ovarian reserve, and when both are high it indicates poor ovarian reserve.[16] But it must be remembered here that high E2 may mask an abnormal FSH concentration in a patient with diminished ovarian reserve due to a negative feedback mechanism.

In patients with polycystic ovarian syndrome (PCOS), E2 level on Day 2 is high because of cumulative E2 produced from granulosa cells of multiple small follicles. E2 level alone, therefore, is never used as a sole marker for ovarian reserve.

Follicle-stimulating Hormone/Luteinizing Hormone Ratio

The high FSH/LH ratio indicates poor ovarian reserve. FSH rises earlier than LH and frequent measurements may diagnose this rise earlier. The FSH/LH ratio is an early indicator of ovarian aging and a rising FSH/LH ratio could be the first marker of ovarian aging and decreased ovarian reserve.[17]

Inhibin B

Inhibin B is secreted from small antral follicles and selectively inhibits FSH release. As the number of eggs decreases with advancing age, it will lower inhibin B level which in turn gives a higher FSH value because of the negative feedback mechanism. Decrease in Inhibin B occurs earlier than the rise in FSH with decreasing ovarian reserve, but inhibin B assays are variable, require validation, and there is cycle-to-cycle variability.[18] This is why it is not used as a routine investigation for the evaluation of ovarian reserve.

However, inhibin B measurement in the early stages of the ovarian stimulation provides useful information in making a decision to cancel the cycle or to modulate the doses of gonadotropin. A level >45 pg/mL on Day 2–3 is indicative of hyper-response to ovulation induction.

Anti-Müllerian Hormone

It is known as anti-Müllerian hormone because it prevents the development of the Müllerian duct when expressed in males from the testis. In females, AMH is produced by granulosa cells of primordial, preantral, and small antral follicles[19] to inhibit the early stages of follicular development. Its expression is maintained till the follicle is 6 mm in diameter, beyond which follicles grow under the effect of FSH. It is not expressed in atretic follicles, dominant follicles, or corpus lutea. Therefore, AMH is considered to be reflective of FSH-independent follicular growth.

Physiology of anti-Müllerian hormone: The function of AMH is to modulate primordial follicle recruitment. It inhibits the action of FSH on the follicular growth and selection of dominance of the follicles. The function of AMH is inhibition of initial recruitment of primordial follicles and inhibits the activity of granulosa cells and decreases if follicular growth starts with FSH stimulation.[20-22] Hence, AMH is a negative regulator of follicular growth and reduces follicular sensitivity to FSH. FSH exerts negative influence on AMH secretion in small follicles.[23] AMH reflects the quantitative and qualitative assessment of ovarian reserve. The AMH level helps in counseling the woman before chemotherapy as it can predict menopause. Its level becomes negligible, 5 years before actual menopause. It is undetectable before puberty and when the primordial follicle enters the preantral stage, production of AMH starts (follicle size of 2–6 mm). When the follicle starts growing, AMH decreases because of a decrease in the primordial pool. High androgen causes anovulation and anovulatory ovary produces more AMH. Hyperinsulinemia also increases androgen secretion which in turn increases serum AMH and anovulation as is observed in patients with PCOS. Metformin (insulin sensitizer) decreases AMH concentration.[24] There is an inverse correlation between E2 and AMH in follicular fluid of small antral follicle, so AMH and FSH activities are interdependent. A AML level of >3.5 ng/mL predicts excessive response in those three studies.[25]

The AMH level is constant throughout the menstrual cycle, except that it has lower thresholds in the late luteal phase. In poor reserve patients, the AMH level varies from 0.5 to 1.1 ng/mL (ng/mL × 7.14 = pmol/mL), but a low level of AMH alone cannot be used as a single parameter to deny fertility treatment for the patient. Higher doses of gonadotropins are not much useful in decreased ovarian response but flare-up protocol and addition of LH can improve the results. These protocols will be discussed later in this book. Normal AMH has a good prognosis and they are normal responders. High AMH indicates an exaggerated response after gonadotropin stimulation. So a low-dose protocol will be useful in these patients to avoid ovarian hyperstimulation syndrome (OHSS) as well as to improve implantation rates because of lower steroids.

In hypogonadotropic hypogonadism patients, the AMH concentration increases in consecutive cycles after human menopausal gonadotropin (HMG) stimulation because of stimulation of FSH-dependent follicles. So AMH has a limitation that it only reflects the growing follicular pool, responsive to gonadotropin, and may not be reflecting the underlying primordial pool **(Box 2)**.

Normal values of AMH and its interpretation **(Table 2)**:

- *Extremely low levels*: <1 pmol/L [diagnostic systems laboratory (DSL)] or <1.1 pmol/L (Gen II assay). These patients are poor responders and cycle cancellation rates are very high. These patients may be offered ovum donation.

Box 2: Actions of AMH.

- Inhibition of follicular activation and growth
- Inhibition of FSH dependent growth
- Inhibition of granulosa cell growth
- Inhibition of aromatase
- Inhibition of recruitment of primordial follicles in pool of growing follicle
- Decreases follicular sensitivity to gonadotropin stimulation to control follicular growth

(AMH: anti-Müllerian hormone; FSH: follicle-stimulating hormone)

TABLE 2: Normal values of anti-Müllerian hormone (AMH) and its interpretation.

Gen II	*DSL-AMH in pmol/L*	*Interpretation*
<1.1	<1	Cancel cycle-ovum donation
1.1–6.9	1–5	Poor response
7.0–20	5–15	Adequate response
>20	>15	Chances of hyperstimulation

(DSL: diagnostic systems laboratory)

- *Low levels*: 1–5 pmol/L (DSL) or between 1.1 and 6.9 pmol/L in Gen II assay. These patients are poor responders and have decreased ovarian reserve, and less number of ova can be retrieved when they are stimulated for IVF. In these cases, high doses of FSH should be used, maybe maximum permissible maximum, and antagonist protocol should be used.
- *Normal levels*: 5–15 pmol/L (DSL) and it is 7–20 pmol/L by Gen II assay. These are normal responders. In these cases, an agonist protocol is used and the maximum dose of FSH required is 225 IU/day for IVF patients.
- *High level*: AMH is >15 pmol/L (DSL) or >20 pmol/L (gen II assay). These patients are hyper-responders. According to Faddy et al. and Nelson et al., the maximum dose used in these patients is 150 IU daily. But even lower doses and antagonist protocols are preferred.[26,27]

Anti-Müllerian hormone assays: Formerly, two companies having different immunoassays were marketing the kits for AMH assessment. One was DSL and the other one was IOT (Immunotech branded as Beckman Coulter). IOT had four to five times higher values than DSL. This is why there was a confusion and low reliability of the results for AMH assessment numbers and units. Fortunately, the two companies have consolidated now and a single new commercially available assay, the Gen II enzyme-linked immune-absorbent assay, is made available and that has replaced DSL and IOT. Now the new assay is reported as ng/mL like IOT.

Anti-Müllerian Hormone Immunoassays

- *DSL*: pmol/mL
- *IOT*: (ng/mL) × 7.14 = pmol/mL
- *Combination of both Gen II Eliza* (ng/mL)

Though AMH assessment done during ovarian stimulation gives erroneous results, it must always be assessed only before ovulation induction is started. With a chronic low-dose protocol, FSH administration mimics the natural cycle and a significant decrease in AMH is observed till the day of follicular dominance.[28] In IVF cycles with multifollicular development, there is decreased AMH because of a decrease in the number of small follicles.[27] Assessing AMH during ovarian stimulation is not useful. It is also not justified[7] as a routine screening test for decreased ovarian reserve in low-risk population.

The AMH is a negative regulator of follicular growth and reduces follicular sensitivity to FSH. FSH exerts a negative influence on AMH secretion in small follicles.[23] There is no significant difference between the performance of AMH and AFC in predicting the oocyte yield; however, both have a false positive rate of 10–20%.[29]

Clinical Uses of anti-Müllerian Hormone

- To confirm the presence of testicular tissue in children
- Differential diagnosis of patients with intersex disorders
- In patients with nonpalpable gonads
- In granulosa cell tumors, it is elevated.

- For diagnosis of PCOS. AMH is increased due to hyperandrogenism and hyperinsulinemia. But according to the new amendments in the Rotterdam criteria, done in July 2018, AMH cannot be used as the only criteria to diagnose PCOS.
- Metformin reduces AMH concentration and so treatment efficacy can be evaluated for insulin sensitizers.
- High AMH in older patients indicates sustained reproductive lifespan.
  - It helps in deciding stimulation protocol.
  - It can be used as hormone contraception.
  - The AMH antagonist can be used in PCOS.

Endocrine Dynamic Tests

Clomiphene citrate challenge test: The test is based on the fact that clomiphene citrate, when given for ovulation induction, will stimulate the follicle to produce more inhibin and E2 that will in turn lower FSH on Day 10.

The basal level of serum FSH is assessed on Day 3 and then repeated on Day 10 after clomiphene citrate challenge (CC) stimulation. A higher value of FSH (>10 mIU/mL) either on Day 3 or on Day 10 indicates diminished ovarian reserve. The total of both values >26 IU indicates poor reserve.[30,31] Normally, LH rises more than FSH after clomiphene stimulation. But in patients with low reserve, FSH rises more than LH. The speculated mechanism is that smaller follicles produce less inhibin B and less E2, resulting in less negative feedback to FSH that is released due to clomiphene stimulation.[32,33]

This test does not have a high prognostic value as there is no standardized definition of an abnormal test. Because of the availability of better tests such as AFC and AMH, this test is not used routinely.[34]

Gonadotropin-releasing hormone analog stimulation test: In this test, gonadotropin-releasing hormone (GnRh) agonist (leuprolide acetate 1 mg) is given subcutaneously. This causes a massive release of FSH and LH from the pituitary which in turn increases the production of E2 from the follicles within a time frame of 24 hours. This increase in E2 level (twice the baseline level) or flare-up of E2 level in response to stimulation indicates early development of follicles, indicating good ovarian reserve.[34,35] But it lacks standardization in terms of the type of the drug, dose, timing, etc. Therefore, this test is not used routinely in clinical practice.

Exogenous FSH ovarian reserve test: 300 IU of recombinant FSH (rFSH) is given to a patient on Day 3 of the cycle. After 24 hours, E2 and inhibin levels are assessed. An increase in E2, >30 pg/mL, is predictive of a good response.[26,36]

This test, like CCCT and GAST, is far from uniform and not used in clinical practice.

This means that no dynamic tests can be used at present in routine practice. These are not better than basal tests and these cannot predict nonpregnancy in any patient.

Ultrasound Markers

- Ovarian volume
- AFC
- Ovarian blood flow

Ovarian Volume

Ovarian volume can be measured by B mode or by three-dimensional (3D) ultrasound. To assess it on B mode, the ovary is located first.

The probe is rotated to find the long axis of the ovary. The probe is then spanned across the long axis of the ovary to find the longest section of the ovary. Now, the probe is rotated 90° to get a true transverse section of the ovary. On the long axis section measure the largest longitudinal diameter, and AP diameter of the ovary as the largest diameter perpendicular to the longitudinal diameter and measure the transverse diameter on the transverse section. The volume is calculated as D1 × D2 × D3 × 0.523.[37,38] Three-dimensional ultrasound is recommended for more accurate volume calculation. It has low interobserver and intraobserver variability. Ovarian volume of 3 cc is taken as a lower cutoff for a normal reserve ovary. Ovarian volume of <3 cc was significantly predictive of >50% cancellation rates in IVF cycles.[39] But this has a poor predictive value for response to ovulation induction and possibility of pregnancy.[40]

Ovarian volume of >10 cc indicates a possibility of PCOS and may require a lower stimulating dose for ovulation induction. But ovarian volume alone is not predictive of ovarian reserve.

Antral Follicle Count

Antral follicle count is defined as the total number of follicles seen in both ovaries, up to 9 mm in diameter, detected by transvaginal ultrasound (TVS) in the early follicular phase (Day 2–3 of the menstrual cycle). AFC can predict hyperstimulation as well as poor response after gonadotropin stimulation. Low AFC predicts poor response. AFC is also used to predict hyper-response and thus using safe and successful stimulation regimes and to prevent OHSS.[41]

Antral follicle count is found to be as effective as AMH in determining ovarian response.[30,42] Smaller follicles (between 2 and 6 mm) decline in number with age, and these indicate real ovarian reserve.[43]

Antral follicle count is a better marker than Day 3 FSH, E2, and inhibin.[44] Another study concludes that both AFC and AMH correlate with each other, but have independent significance for estimating follicles larger than 12 mm on the day of ovulation trigger. For ova retrieved on ovum pickup (OPU), in the PCOS group both AMH and AFC have similar significance.[45] AFC can be correlated with the quality as well as quantity of the oocytes.[46]

Anti-Müllerian hormone and antral follicle count: Receiver operating characteristic curves showed high accuracy for AMH and AFC for the prediction of poor ovarian response but limited accuracy for nonpregnancy prediction. These data do not show a better predictive ability than AFC.[42,47,48] For the prediction of poor ovarian response a model including AFC + AMH was found to be almost similar to that of (p-value 0.001) using AFC alone.[38] Our study on comparison of AFC and AMH for assessment of ovarian reserve also concluded that AFC alone may suffice as a test for assessing the ovarian reserve.[46]

Antral follicle count has low intercycle as well as interobserver variability. Though, intercycle variability is more significant in young women when AFC is high. Low AFC with ovulatory cycle does not indicate poor reserve. 3D ultrasound is extremely useful for counting antral follicles and sono automated volume calculation (AVC) is the most convenient and accurate amongst all. A more exact value of AFC was acquired when counted by 3D ultrasound. The number of follicles >12 mm on the day of oocyte retrieval correlated significantly with AFC counted by 3D ultrasound rather than 2D ultrasound. Inversion mode with sono AVC is the most convenient method for counting antral follicles when they are multiple.[49]

Ovarian Blood Flow

Ovarian blood flow as a predictor of IVF outcome was assessed by many workers.

However, another study shows ovarian stromal peak systolic velocity (PSV) after pituitary suppression is predictive of ovarian responsiveness and outcome of IVF treatment.[50] Kupesic et al. have shown a correlation between the ovarian stromal flow index (FI) and the number of mature oocytes retrieved in an IVF cycle and pregnancy rates. [Stromal FI (<11 low responder, 11–14 good, >15 risk of OHSS)].[51] *The total number of antral follicles achieved the best predictive value for a favorable IVF outcome, followed by ovarian stromal FI, total ovarian stromal area, and total ovarian volume.*[5]

Measurement of ovarian stromal flow in the early follicular phase is related to subsequent ovarian response in IVF treatment.[52] *Total ovarian vascularization index (VI) and vascularization flow index (VFI) were significantly lower in women aged ≥ 41 years.*[49]

However, it was not found to be accurate and it cannot predict future fertility. It can only predict response to IVF treatment.

The ovarian volume, AFC and VI, FI and VFI determined by 3D power Doppler (PD), all have excellent intraobserver and interobserver reproducibility.[53]

Table 3 presents the finding of our unpublished study.

It is essential to mention here that AFC, ovarian volume, and ovarian 3D-PD flow indices did not significantly change after a short-term treatment of GnRH agonist for pituitary downregulation[54] and can therefore be reliably used for downregulated as well as non-downregulated cycles for assessment of ovarian response.

TABLE 3: 3D-PD indices in PCOS, normal, and poor response ovaries.

Index	*PCOS*	*Normal*	*Poor responding*
VI	5–10	2–5	<2
VFI	2–3	1–2	<0.5

(PCOS: polycystic ovarian syndrome; PD: power Doppler; VFI: vascularization flow index; VI: vascularization index)

CLINICAL APPLICATIONS

Anti-Müllerian hormone and AFC are the most widely used tests. These can assess the ovarian reserve quantitatively and qualitatively. No significant difference is observed between the two in terms of accuracy. Both may contribute and act synergistically.[55]

The new ovarian response predictive index (ORPI) has been presented based on age, AMH, and AFC.[56] It is calculated as AMH × AFC/patient's age. This can be positively correlated with the number of oocytes retrieved and metaphase II stage (MII) oocytes collected.

We decide the stimulation protocol based on parameters such as AFC, ovarian volume, ovarian stromal resistance index (RI), ovarian stromal PSV, stromal FI, age, and body mass index (BMI). The calculation can be simplified as given in **Table 4**.[57]

TABLE 4: Parameter values that indicate when higher dose or lower dose of gonadotropins are required.

	Increase the dose when	*Decrease the dose when*
Age	>35 years	<25 years
BMI	>28 kg/m^2	<20 kg/m^2
AFC	<3 (FNPO)	>12 (FNPO)
Stromal RI	>0.7	<0.5
Stromal PSV	<5 cm/s	>10 cm/s
Stromal FI	<11	>15
Ovarian volume	<3 cc	>10 cc

(AFC: antral follicle count; BMI: body mass index; FI: flow index; FNPO: follicle number per ovary; PSV: peak systolic blood flow velocity; RI: resistance index)

To select the correct stimulation protocol, doses are titrated depending on findings present in a particular patient from a high-dose table or a low-dose table.

INTEGRATED PREDICTORS

La Marca et al. developed an ORPI. This is based on age, AMH, and AFC. ORPI < 0.2 has 86% sensitivity and 89% specificity in predicting poor ovarian response (<3 oocytes), with 88% efficacy. ORPI > 0.9 has the same sensitivity, specificity, and 82% efficacy in the prediction of high response (>15 follicles).[58]

Another study has recently been published in which a scoring system has been devised based on the ultrasound parameters, ovarian volume, AFC, ovarian stromal RI, and ovarian stromal PSV with age and BMI[59] and has shown zero severe ovarian hyperstimulation (OHSS) rate, very low incidence of mild OHSS, and acceptable multiple pregnancy rates **(Tables 5 and 6)**.

TABLE 5: A scoring system based on clinical and ultrasound.

Score	*1*	*2*	*3*	*4*	*5*
Age	>40	35.1–40	30.1–35	25.1–30	<25
BMI	>30	30–28.1	28–25.1	25–22.1	< 22
AFC	< 5	5–10	10–15	15–20	>20
Ovarian volume	< 3	3.1–5	5.1–7	7.1–10	>10
Stromal RI	>0.75	0.75–0.66	0.65–0.56	0.55–0.45	<0.45
Stromal PSV	<3	3.1–5	5.1–7	7.1–10	>10

(AFC: antral follicle count; BMI: body mass index; PSV: peak systolic velocity; RI: resistance index)

Sources: Panchal S, Nagori CB. Ultrasound based decision making on stimulation protocol for superovulated IUI cycles. IJIFM. 2016;7(1):7-13; Nagori C. Ultrasound-based decision making on stimulation protocol for IVF cycles. DSJUOG. 2016;10(3):330-7.

TABLE 6: Dose of rFSH calculated for IUI, IVF (fresh transfer) and IVF for embryo freezing cycle, depending on the baseline score.

	Starting dose of rFSH		
Score	*IUI*	*IVF*	*IVF-Fr*
≥25	25 IU	75 IU	150 IU
21–24	37.5 IU	150 IU	225 IU
16–20	75 IU	]]225 IU	300 IU
11–15	112.5 IU	300 IU	375 IU (LH added)
6–10	150 IU	375 IU	450 IU (LH added)

(rFSH: recombinant follicle-stimulating hormone; IUI: intrauterine insemination; IVF: in vitro fertilization; LH: luteinizing hormone)

BOLOGNA CRITERIA[60]

The European Society of Human Reproduction and Embryology (ESHRE) group has come to the consensus that out of three, two criteria should be present to define poor ovarian reserve for future research:

1. Maternal age > 40 years or other risk factors for poor ovarian reserve (genetic or acquired conditions)
2. Previous history of less than three oocytes with a conventional stimulation protocol
3. Abnormal ovarian reserve test, i.e., AFC < 5–7 or AMH < 0.5–1.1 ng/mL. Two episodes of poor response after maximum stimulation is sufficient to define a patient "poor responder" in absence of advanced maternal age or abnormal ovarian reserve tests.[61]

Many patients, >40 years of age, maybe infertile, though the menstrual cycles are normal. So a patient with good reserve benefits better with IVF and should be offered IVF if AFC is good.[62] Ovarian reserve tests should not be used to promote planned oocyte cryopreservation, but it should be based on a woman's reproductive plans and age.

GENETIC PREDICTORS

Single nucleotide polymorphism in gonadotropins and gonadotropin receptors is not associated with change in ovarian reserve. But some polymorphisms in FSH receptors (FSHR), particularly Ser680 genotype, are related to resistance to FSH stimulation. These patients require high doses of FSH in spite of other ovarian reserve markers being normal.[45,63] These observations require further validation by larger studies.

Facts about ovarian reserve test. (ASRM practice committee opinion):

1. *Ovarian reserve tests to predict reproduction potential among women with unproven fertility*: EAGER (Effect of Aspirin in Gestation and Reproduction) trial showed same pregnancy rate as with low AMH (<1 ng/mL).[64] In patients with AMH < 0.7 or FSH > 10 IU and normal levels, similar cumulative pregnancy rates after 6 and 12 cycles of attempting pregnancy was found as in women with normal levels.[65] So, ovarian reserve markers do not predict the reproductive potential in patients of unproven or proven fertility.
2. *Ovarian reserve tests (ORT) to predict success after controlled ovarian hyperstimulation (COH) and IUI*: Markers of ORT do not predict the likelihood of success following ovarian stimulation and IUI.[66]
3. *ORT to predict oocyte yeild after COH for IVF*: With low AMH (<0.16 ng/mL) 54% cycles were cancelled, 50.7% cycles gave three or less oocytes, 25% had no embryo transfers and live birth rate was 20.5% per transfer, (9.5% per cycle).[67] So low AMH is for counseling the women regarding suboptimal response and yeild of oocytes but should not be used to refuse treatment.[68]
4. Ovarian reserve tests do not predict pregnancy and live birth rates and there are many other variables that play important role.
5. AFC and AMH give the same information aboit ovarian reserve and dose of gonadotropins required for IVF.[69]

SUMMARY OF OVARIAN RESERVE TESTS

Ovarian reserve test	*Favorable results*	*Unfavorable results*
Age (in years)	<35	>35
FSH (IU/L)	<10	>10
Day 3 E2 (pg/mL)	<75	>75
Day 10 progesterone	<0.9	>1.1
AMH (p/mol/L)	15.7–48.5	<15.7
Day 3 inhibin B (pg/ mL)	>45	<45
AFC	>5	<5
Ovarian vascularity	Lower PI	Higher PI
Ovarian volume (cc)	>3	<3
CCCT (FSH only—IU/L)	<12	>12
GAST	Early E2 flare	Persistent high E2/no response

(AFC: antral follicle count; AMH: anti-Müllerian hormone; CCCT: clomiphene citrate challenge test; E2: estradiol; FSH: follicle-stimulating hormone; GAST: gonadotropin-releasing hormone analogue stimulation test; PI: predictive index)

CARRY HOME MESSAGE

- All ovarian reserve tests are considered screening tests and abnormal test results should be confirmed by another test.
- No test or combined test can predict non-pregnancy.
- Age is the single reliable factor.
- The short follicular phase indicates diminishing ovarian reserve (DOR).
- On Day 2–3, FSH > 12–15 indicates DOR.
- On Day 2, E2 > 80 pg/mL indicates DOR.
- The FSH/LH ratio, if high, indicates DOR.
- Inhibin B > 45 pg/mL indicates good reserve.
- CCCT, GAST, and EFORT are not used in clinical practice.
- AMH is extremely reliable for counseling (5–15 pmol/L indicates good reserve).
- Ovarian volume is as reliable as AMH, and AFC > 5 indicates normal reserve.
- Stromal flow decides the doses required and response to stimulation.
- Both AMH and AFC are equally reliable, synergistic, and show no difference between the performances.

REFERENCES

1. Ventura SJ, Mosher WD, Curtin SC, Abma JC. Trends in pregnancy rates for the United States 1976-97: an update. Nat Vital Stat Rep. 2001;49:1-9.
2. Menken J, Trusell J, Larsen U. Age and Infertility. Science. 1986;233(4771):1389-94.
3. Ng EHY, Yeung WSB, Fong DYT, Ho PC. Effects of age on hormonal and ultrasound markers of ovarian reserve in Chinese women with proven fertility. Hum Reprod. 2003;18(10):2169-74.
4. Scheffer GJ, Broekmans FJM, Dorland M, Habbema JD, Looman CW, te Velde ER. Antral follicle counts by transvaginal ultrasonography are related to age in women with proven natural fertility. Fertil Steril. 1999;72:845-51.
5. Broekmans FJ, Kwee J, Hendriks DJ, Mol BW, Lambalk CB. A systematic review of tests predicting ovarian reserve and IVF outcome. Hum Reprod Update. 2006;12:685-718.
6. Van Noord-Zaadstra BM, Looman CW, Alsbach H, Habbema JD, te Velde ER, Karbaat J. Delaying childbearing: effect of age on fecundity and outcome of pregnancy. BMJ. 1991;302:1361-5.
7. Practice committee of American Society for Reproductive Medicine. Testing and interpreting measures of ovarian reserve: a committee opinion. Fertil Steril. 2012; 98:1407-15.
8. Tufan E, Elter K, Durmusoglu F. Assessment of reproductive ageing patterns by hormonal and ultrasonographic ovarian reserve tests. Hum Reprod. 2004;19(11):2484-9.
9. Lim AST, Tsakok MFH. Age related decline in fertility: a link to degenerative oocytes? Fertil Steril. 1997;68:265-71.
10. Leridon H. Can assisted reproduction technology compensate for natural decline in fertility with age? A model assessment. Hum Reprod. 2004;19:1548-53.
11. Van Zonneveld P, Scheffer GJ, Broekmans FJ, Blankenstein MA, de Jong FH, Looman CWN, et al. Do cycle disturbances explain the age related decline of female fertility? Cycle characteristics of women aged

over 40 years compared with a reference population of young women. Hum Reprod. 2003;18(3):495-501.

12. Perloe M, Levy DP, Sills ES. Strategies for ascertaining ovarian reserve among women suspected of subfertility. Int J Fertil Womens Med. 2000;45:215-24.
13. Scott RT Jr, Elkind-Hirch KE, Styne Gross A, Miller KA, Frattarelli JL. The predictive value for in vitro fertility delivery rates is greatly impacted by the method used to select the threshold between normal and elevated basal FSH. Fertil Steril. 2008;89:868-78.
14. Oschsenkuhn R, von Schonfeldt V, Simoni M. FSH receptor polymorphisms and ovarian function. Gynécol Endocrinol. 2009;11(4):265-70.
15. Frattarelli JL, Bergh PA, Drews MR, Sharara FI, Scott RT. Evaluation of basal oestradiol levels in assisted reproductive technology cycles. Fertil Steril. 2000;74(3):518-24.
16. de Carvalho BR, de Rosa-e-Silva ACJ, Rosa-e-Silva JC, dos Reis RM. Use of ovarian reserve markers and variables of response to gonadotropic stimulus as predictors of embryo implantation in ICSI cycles. J Brasileiro de Reproducao Assistida. 2009;13(3):26-9.
17. Mukherjee T, Copperman AB, Lapinski R, Sandler B, Bustillo M, Grunfeld L. An elevated day three follicle-stimulating hormone: luteinizing hormone ratio (FSH:LH) in the presence of a normal day 3 FSH predicts a poor response to controlled ovarian hyperstimulation. Fertil Steril. 1996;65:588-93.
18. Al-Azemi M, Killick SR, Duffy S, Pye C, Refaat B, Hill N, et al. Multi-marker assessment of ovarian reserve predicts oocyte yield after ovulation induction. Hum Reprod. 2011;26(2):414-22.
19. Visser JA, de Jong FH, Laven JS, Themmen APN. Anti-Müllerian hormone: a new marker for ovarian function. Reproduction. 2006;131:1-9.
20. Durlinger AL, Visser JA, Themmen AP. Regulation of ovarian function: the role of anti-Müllerian hormone. Reproduction. 2002;124:601-9.
21. Di Clemente N, Goxe B, Remy JJ, Cate R. Inhibitory effect of AMH upon aromatase activity and LH receptors of granulosa cells of rat and porcine immature ovaries. Endocrine. 1994;2:553-8.
22. Josso N, di Clemente N, Gouedard L. Anti-Müllerian hormone and its receptors. Mol Cell Endocrinol. 2001;179:25-32.
23. Anderson CY, Byskov AG. Estradiol and regulation of anti-Müllerian hormone, inhibin A and inhibin B secretion: analysis of small antral and preovulatory human follicles' fluid. J Clin Endocrinol Metab. 2006;91:4064-9.
24. Piltonen T, Morin Papunen L, Koivunen R, Perheentupa A, Ruokonen A, Tapanainen JS. Serum anti-Müllerian hormone levels remain high until late reproductive age and decrease during metformin therapy in women with polycystic ovary syndrome. Hum Reprod. 2005;20(7):1820-6.
25. La Marca A, Sighinolfi G, Radi D, Argento C, Baraldi E, Artenisio AC, et al. Anti-Müllerian hormone (AMH) as a predictive marker in assisted reproductive technique (ART). Hum Reprod Update. 2010;16:113-30.
26. Faddy MJ, Gosden RG, Gougeon A, Richardson SJ, Nelson JF. Accelerated disappearance of ovarian follicles in mid-life: implications for forecasting menopause. Hum Reprod. 1992;7(10):1342-6.
27. Nelson SM, Yates RW, Fleming R. Serum anti-Müllerian hormone and FSH: prediction of live birth and extremes of response in stimulated cycles-implications for individualization of therapy. Hum Reprod. 2007;22:2414-21.
28. Catteau-Jonard S, Pigny P, Reyss AC, Decanter C, Poncelet E, Dewailly D. Changes in serum anti-Müllerian hormone level during low dose recombinant follicle-stimulating hormone therapy for anovulation in polycystic ovary syndrome. J Clin Endocrinol Metab. 2007;92:4138-43.
29. Broer SL, Dolleman M, Opmeer BC, Fauser BC, Mol BW, Broekmans FJM. AMH and AFC as predictors of excessive response in controlled ovarian hyperstimulation: a meta-analysis. Hum Reprod Update. 2011;17:46-54.

30. La Marca A, Malmusi S, Giulini S, Tamaro LF, Orvieto R, Levratti P, et al. Anti-Müllerian hormone plasma levels in spontaneous menstrual cycle and during treatment with FSH to induce ovulation. Hum Reprod. 2004;19:2738-41.
31. Maheshwari A, Gibreel A, Bhattacharya S, Johnson NP. Dynamic tests of ovarian reserve: a systematic review of diagnostic accuracy. Reprod Bio Med Online. 2009;18(5);717-34.
32. Kwee J, Schats R, McDonnell J, Schoemaker J, Lambalk CB. The Clomiphene citrate challenge test versus the exogenous follicle stimulating hormone ovarian reserve test as a single test for identification of low responders and hyperresponders to in vitro fertilization. Fertil Steril. 2006;85(6):1714-22.
33. Hofmann GE, Danforth DR, Seifer DB. Inhibin-B: the physiologic basis of the clomiphene citrate challenge test for ovarian reserve screening. Fertil Steril. 1998;69(3):474-7.
34. Hendricks DJ, Mol BW, Bansci LF, Bancsi LFJMM, te Velde ER, Broekmans FJM. The CCCT for the prediction of poor ovarian response and nonpregnancy in patients undergoing IVF. Fertil Steril. 2006;86:807-18.
35. Yong PYK, Baird DT, Thong KJ, McNeilly AS, Anderson RA. Prospective analysis of the relationships between the ovarian follicle cohort and basal FSH concentration, the inhibin response to exogenous FSH and ovarian follicle number at different stages of the normal menstrual cycle and after pituitary downregulation. Hum Reprod. 2003;18:35-44.
36. Ravhon A, Lavery S, Micheal S, Donaldson M, Margara R, Trew G, et al. Dynamic assays of inhibin B and oestradiol following buserelin acetate administration as predictors of ovarian response in IVF. Hum Reprod. 2000;15(11):2297-301.
37. Hendriks DJ, Broekmans FJM, Bancsi LFJMM, de Jong FH, Looman CWN, Te Velde ER. Repeated clomiphene citrate challenge testing in the prediction of outcome in IVF: a comparison with basal markers for ovarian reserve. Hum Reprod. 2005;20(1):163-9.
38. Kwee J, Etling MW, Schats R, Bezemer PD, Lambalk CB, Schoemaker J. Comparison of endocrine tests with respect to their predictive value on the outcome of ovarian hyperstimulation in IVF treatment: results of a prospective randomized study. Hum Reprod. 2003;18(7):1422-7.
39. Gibreel A, Maheshwari A, Bhattacharya S, et al. Ultrasound tests of ovarian reserve: a systematic review of accuracy in predicting, fertility outcomes. Hum Fertil. 2009;12(2): 95-106.
40. Syrop CH, Dawson JD, Husman KJ, Sparks AE, Van Voorhis BJ. Ovarian volume may predict assisted reproductive outcomes better than follicle stimulating hormone concentration on day 3. Hum Reprod. 1999;14(7):1752-6.
41. Lass A, Skull J, McVeigh E, Winston RM. Measurement of ovarian volume by transvaginal sonography before ovulation induction with human menopausal gonadotrophin for in-vitro fertilization can predict poor response. Hum Reprod. 1997; 12(2):294-97.
42. Hendriks DJ, Kwee J, Mol BW, te Velde ER, Broekmans FJM. Ultrasonography as a tool for the prediction of outcome in IVF patients: a comparative meta-analysis of ovarian volume and antral follicle count. Fertil Steril. 2007;87:764-75.
43. Muttukrishna S, McGarrigle H, Wakim R, Khadum I, Ranieri DM, Serhal P. Antral follicle count, anti-Müllerian hormone and inhibin B: predictors of ovarian response in assisted reproductive technology? BJOG. 2005;112:1384-90.
44. Nardo LG, Christodoulou D, Gould D, Roberts SA, Fitzgerald CT, Laing I. Anti-Müllerian hormone levels and antral follicle count in women enrolled in in vitro fertilization cycles: relationship to life-style factors, chronological age and reproductive history. Gynecol Endocrinol. 2007;3:1-8.
45. Haadsma ML, Bukman A, Greon H, Roeloffzen EMA, Groenewoud ER, Heineman MJ, et al. The number of small antral follicles (2–6 mm) determines the outcome of endocrine ovarian reserve tests

in subfertile population. Hum Reprod. 2007;22:1925-31.
46. Klinkert ER, Broekmans FJ, Looman CV, Habbema JDF, te Velde ER. The antral follicle count is a better marker than basal follicle-stimulating hormone for the selection of older patients with acceptable pregnancy prospects after in vitro fertilization. Fertil Steril. 2005;83:811-4.
47. Panchal S, Nagori C. Comparison of anti-Müllerian hormone and antral follicle count for assessment of ovarian reserve. J Hum Reprod Sci. 2012;5(3):274-8.
48. Johnstone EB, Rosen MP, Addauan-Andersen C, Cedars MI. Is AFC a marker of oocyte quality? Fertile women have higher AFCs than infertile women. Fertil Steril. 2010;94(4):S63.
49. Gruijters MJ, Visser JA, Durlinger AL, Themmen APN. Anti-Mullerian hormone and its role in ovarian function. Mol Cell Endocrinol. 2003;211:85-90.
50. Ng EH, Chan CC, Yeung WS, Ho PC. Effect of age on ovarian stromal flow measured by three-dimensional ultrasound with power Doppler in Chinese women with proven fertility. Hum Reprod. 2004;19:2132-7.
51. Krishnakumar J, Agarwal A, Nambiar D, Radhakrishnan S. Comparison of antral follicle count, antimullerian hormone and day 2 follicle stimulating hormone as predictor of ovarian response and clinical pregnancy rate in patient with an abnormal ovarian reserve test. Int J Reprod Contracept Obstet Gynecol. 2016;5(8):2762-7.
52. Engmann L, Sladkevicius P, Agrawal R, Bekir JS, Campbell S, Tan SL. Value of ovarian stromal blood flow velocity measurement after pituitary suppression in the prediction of ovarian responsiveness and outcome of in vitro fertilization treatment. Fertil Steril. 1999;71(1):22-9.
53. Kupesic S, Kurjak A. Predictors of in vitro fertilization outcome by three dimensional ultrasound. Hum Reprod. 2002;17(4):950-55.
54. Zaidi J, Barber J, Kyei-Mensah A, Bekir J, Campbell S, Tan SL. Relationship of ovarian stromal blood flow at baseline ultrasound to subsequent follicular response in an in vitro fertilization program. Obstet Gynecol. 1996;88:779-84.
55. Merce LT, Gomez B, Engels V, Bau S, Bajo JM. Intraobserver and interobserver reproducibility ovarian volume, antral follicle count and vascularity indices obtained with transvaginal 3-dimensional ultrasonography, power Doppler angiography and virtual computer aided analysis imaging program. J Ultrasound Med. 2005;24:1279-87.
56. Ng EHY, Chan CCW, Tang OS, Yeung WSB, Ho PC. Effect of pituitary downregulation on antral follicle count, ovarian volume and stromal blood flow measured by three-dimensional ultrasound with power Doppler prior to ovarian stimulation. Hum Reprod. 2004;19(12):2811-5.
57. Oliveira JB, Baruffi RL, Petersen CG, Mauri AL, Nascimento AM, Laura Vagnini L, et al. A new ovarian response prediction index (ORPI): implications for individualized controlled ovarian stimulation. Reprod Biol Endocrinol. 2012;10:94.
58. Broer SL, Mol BW, Hendriks D, Broekmans FJM. The role of anti-Mullerian hormone in prediction of outcome after IVF: comparison with the antral follicle count. Fertil Steril. 2009;91:705-14.
59. Panchal S, Nagori CB. Baseline scan and ultrasound diagnosis of PCOS. Donald School J Ultrasound Obstet Gynecol. 2012;6(3):290-9.
60. La Marca A, Grisendi V, Guilini S, Argento C, Tirelli A, Dondi G, et al. Individualization of FSH dose in IVF/ICSI cycles using the antral follicle count. J Ovarian Res. 2013;6:11.
61. Practice Committee of ASRM. Testing and interpreting measures of ovarian reserve: a committee opinion. Fertil Steril. 2020;114:1151-7.
62. Panchal S, Nagori C. Ultrasound-based decision-making on stimulation protocol for superovulated intrauterine insemination cycles. Int J Infertil Fetal Med. 2016;7(1):7-13.

63. Ferraretti AP, Gianaroli L. The Bologna criteria for the definition of poor ovarian responders: is there a need for revision? Hum Reprod. 2014;29(9):1842-45.
64. Zarek SM, Mitchell EM, Sjaarda LA, Mumford SL, Silver RM, Stanford JB, et al. Antimullerian hormone and pregnancy loss from the effects of aspirin in gestation and reproduction trial. Fertil Steril. 2016;105: 946-52.
65. Steiner AZ, Pritchard D, Stanczyk FZ, Kesner JS, Meadows JW, Herring AH, et al. Association between biomarkers of ovarian reserve and infertility among older women of reproductive age. JAMA. 2017;318:1367-76.
66. van der Steeg JW, Steures P, Eijkemans MJ et al. Predictive value and clinical impact of basal follicle stimulating hormone in subfertile, ovulatory women. J Clin Endocrinol Metab. 2007;92:2163-8.
67. Fleming R, Seifer DB, Frattarelli JL, Ruman J. Assessing ovarian response: antral follicle count versus anti-mullerian hormone. Reprod Biomed Online. 2015;31:486-96.
68. Seifer DB, Tal O, Wantman E, Edul P, Baker VL. Prognostic indicators of assisted reproduction technology outcomes of cycles with ultralow serum antimüllerian hormone: a multivariate analysis of over 5,000 autologus cycles from the Society for Assisted Reproductive Technology Clinic Outcome Reporting System database for 2012–23. Fertil Steril. 2016;105:385-93.
69. Magnussan A, Nilson L, Olerod G, Thurin-Kjelberg A, Bergh C. The addition of anti-müllerian hormone in an algorithm for individualized hormone dosage did not improve the predicition of ovarian response-a randomized controlled trial. Hum Reprod. 2017;32:811-9.

4 Chapter

Baseline Scan

INTRODUCTION

The success of any assisted reproductive technology is chiefly dependent on two decisions: (1) selection of a correct stimulation protocol and (2) correct timing of human chorionic gonadotropin (hCG). The stimulation protocol is to be so designed that there is no ovarian hyperstimulation and the cycle does not need to be canceled because of poor response. This means that it should ideally be tailor-made for each patient.

Selection of a correct stimulation protocol is based on the prestimulation assessment of females to assess ovarian response and reserve. This is done by a baseline ultrasound scan on the 2nd–3rd day of the menstrual cycle. Ovaries must have no active follicle or corpus luteum which confirms that estrogen and progesterone are at their low levels and therefore it is a baseline scan.

The route of the scan has to be transvaginal always. Using a transabdominal approach for ovarian assessment may miss at least 42% of the ovarian anatomical details.[1]

All the scans are done using B-mode ultrasound with color Doppler, pulse Doppler, 3D ultrasound, and 3D power Doppler. Use of color Doppler in this assessment is mandatory because a large number of biochemical or hormonal changes occur during the menstrual cycle, which reflect as vascular and morphological changes in the ovaries and uterus and vascular changes can be assessed by Doppler. 3D ultrasound is especially useful for volume measurements.

TECHNIQUE FOR BASELINE SCAN OF OVARIES

The B-mode ultrasound assessment of the ovaries consists of the assessment of ovarian diameters and volume and counting of antral follicles as quantitative assessment and qualitative assessment of stromal density.

Once the ovary is located, the probe is rotated to find out the longest diameter of the ovary and is stored as one frame on a dual screen. Then the probe is rotated 90° anticlockwise, without any other probe movement to get a true transverse axis of the ovary. Measure the largest longitudinal, transverse, and anteroposterior (AP) diameters of the ovary in centimeters (cm), and ovarian volume can be calculated by the formula ($x \times y \times z \times 0.523$) **(Fig. 1)**.

The number of antral follicles is counted in the whole ovary by taking a 2D sweep across the whole ovary and eyeballing. When counting antral follicles, do not ever rotate the probe. This method is feasible and very reliable when the number of antral follicles is approximately 10–15. But when the number of follicles is much more as in polycystic ovaries, the calculation using B-mode scroll may be inaccurate. In these cases 3D ultrasound with sophisticated software like SonoAVC is used.

Doppler is used to see the presence of vessels in the ovarian stroma **(Fig. 2)**.

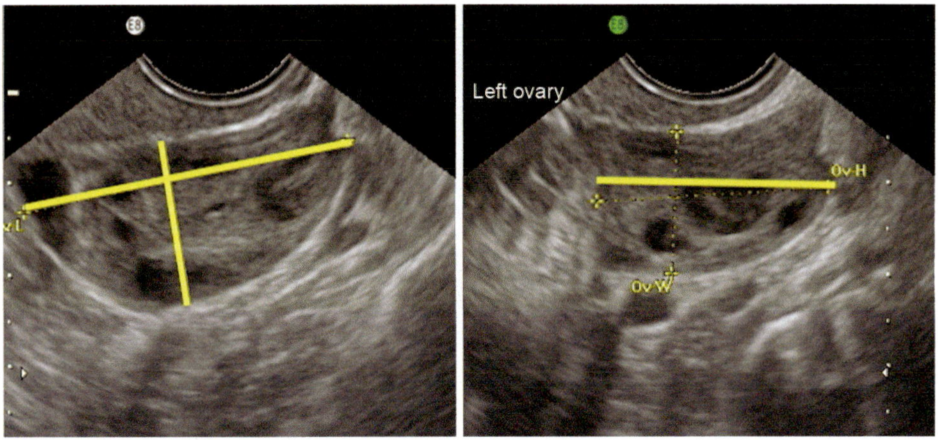

Fig. 1: Measuring ovarian volume on B-mode ultrasound.

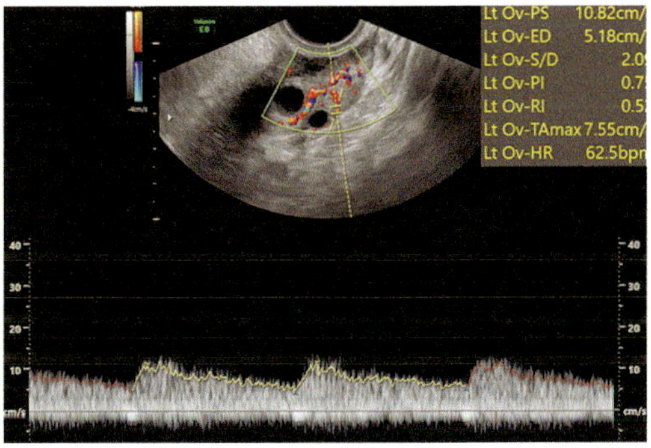

Fig. 2: Ovarian stromal flow assessment on color and spectral Doppler.

Color or power Doppler box is placed on the ovary, so that the whole ovary is included in the color box. The vessel that is close to any of the follicles is not a stromal vessel. The vessel selected for interrogation is a vessel that shows the brightest color on the color Doppler. Rotation of the probe confirms that the vessel is not the main stem of the ovarian artery and is only its branch. Pulse Doppler is used for quantitative assessment of the flows—intraovarian resistance index (RI) and peak systolic velocity (PSV). For color Doppler pulse repetition frequency (PRF) of 0.3, wall filters lowest with optimum gains and balance settings are essential. For pulse Doppler also, the lowest PRF and wall filters are used as stromal flows at the baseline scan are low-velocity flows.

Based on the above-described assessment of the ovaries, these are categorized into normal, low reserve, poorly responding, or polycystic ovaries.

Normal Ovaries

Normal ovaries are the ones that have the largest diameter of 2–3 cm, ovarian volume of 3–6.6 cc, antral follicle count (AFC) per ovary of 4–19, isoechoic stroma **(Fig. 3)**, stromal RI of 0.6–0.7, and stromal PSV of 5–10 cm/s. Ovaries with these features are categorized as normal ovaries because they respond to standard stimulation protocols and produce adequate follicles for the concerned assisted reproduction technology. These standard protocols are 75 IU of recombinant follicle stimulation hormone (rFSH) for intrauterine insemination (IUI) cycles and 150–225 IU of rFSH for in vitro fertilization (IVF) cycles.

Low Reserve Ovaries

Low reserve ovaries are the ones that have fewer than four follicles per ovary. As these have less number of antral follicles, these are also small in size **(Fig. 4)**. The largest diameter

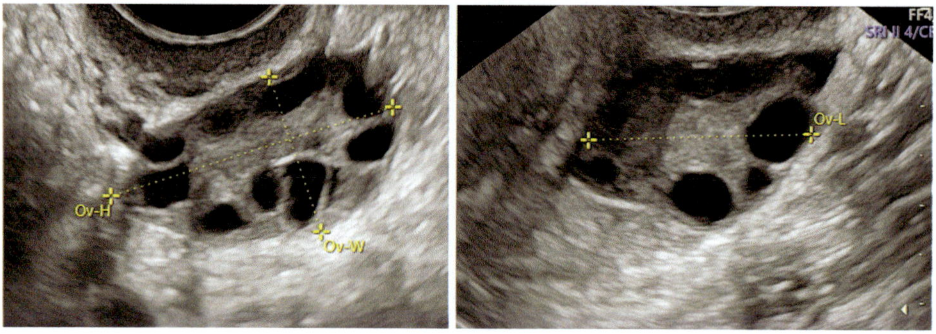

Fig. 3: Normal ovary on B-mode ultrasound.

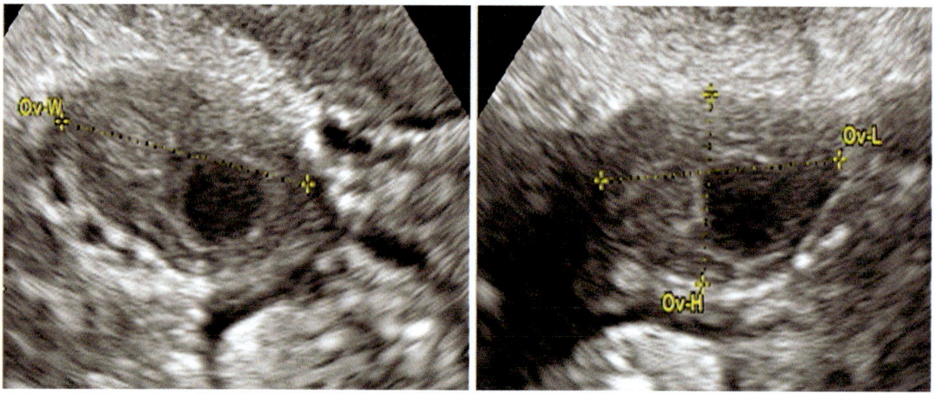

Fig. 4: Low reserve ovary.

of <2 cm and volume <3 cc is a low-reserve ovary. These ovaries produce less number of follicles at the end of stimulation.

Although the AFC is reduced in ovaries with an endometrioma, the number of oocytes retrieved is similar, suggesting that the AFC is underestimated in such ovaries. This is a consequence of an impaired ability to detect small follicles in the presence of an endometrioma.[2]

Anti-Müllerian hormone (AMH) showed a positive linear correlation with AFC in all groups.[3]

Poorly Responding Ovaries

Poorly responding ovaries are the ones that respond poorly to any stimulation. This means that these ovaries require larger doses of gonadotropins for stimulation. This poor response can be attributed to the poor blood flow to these ovaries. The measurement of ovarian stromal flow in the early follicular phase is related to subsequent ovarian response in IVF treatment.[4] Ovarian stromal PSV after pituitary suppression is predictive of ovarian responsiveness and outcome of IVF treatment.[5]

These ovaries show high resistance (RI > 0.7) and low velocity (PSV < 5 cm/s) flow **(Fig. 5)**.

Low reserve and poorly responding ovaries are often used as synonyms, but these are different entities. Reserve relates to AFC or ultimate yield of follicles/ova at the end of stimulation, whereas response relates to the sensitivity of ovary to ovulation-stimulating

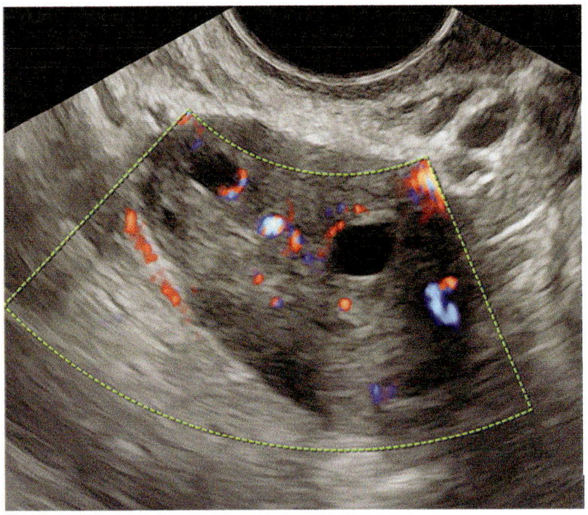

Fig. 5: Poor responding ovary with scanty ovarian stromal flow.

agents to produce those follicles. This means that any ovary would be a permutation-combination of one of the characteristics from each of these two groups. One group has normal response, poor response, and hyper-response and the other group has normal reserve, low reserve, and high reserve or polycystic ovaries. It is a combination of findings such as AFC and stromal flow, RI and PSV that would ultimately decide the optimum stimulation protocol.

DECIDING THE STIMULATION PROTOCOL

Tailor-designing the stimulation protocol is quite a complicated and difficult task for infertility experts, and different workers have tried to simplify this by using ovarian reserve markers such as AFC, AMH, follicle-stimulating hormone (FSH), age. However, a method that uses combination of parameters that assess reserve and response of the ovary has not been established so far. Though according to a study, predictors of ovarian response in order of importance are:[6]

- Number of antral follicles
- Ovarian stromal FI
- Total ovarian stromal area
- Total ovarian volume

How to Decide a Stimulation Protocol?

Antral Follicle Count and Ovarian Volume

To assess the ovarian reserve, AFC is the most useful marker in predicting the ovarian response. Doing AFC assessment alone would be more cost-effective for predicting the ovarian response in patients undergoing controlled ovarian stimulation with gonadotropin-releasing hormone (GnRH) antagonists. AFC had the highest accuracy for predicting ovarian response in patients with an abnormal ovarian reserve test and was statistically significant (number of oocyte aspirated p-value < 0.001) than AMH (p-value 0.06) and FSH (p-value 0.212) in predicting the ovarian response. For the prediction of poor ovarian response, a model including AFC + AMH was found to be almost similar to that of (p-value 0.001) using AFC alone.[7] Precise calculation of AFC, therefore, can help in predicting the ovarian response.

How to count antral follicles?

- By 2D ultrasound, as described earlier, scroll across the ovary and eyeball to count is the easiest method.
- 3D with inversion mode rendering and sono automated volume count (AVC) a specialized 3D ultrasound software for calculation of antral follicle number and volumes. This method is more precise when follicles are multiple [>15 FNPO (follicle number per ovary)]. But postprocessing is required for accurate calculations. Region of interest (ROI) and volume angle are selected to include the whole ovary in all three orthogonal planes on acquired ovarian volume. Sono-AVC

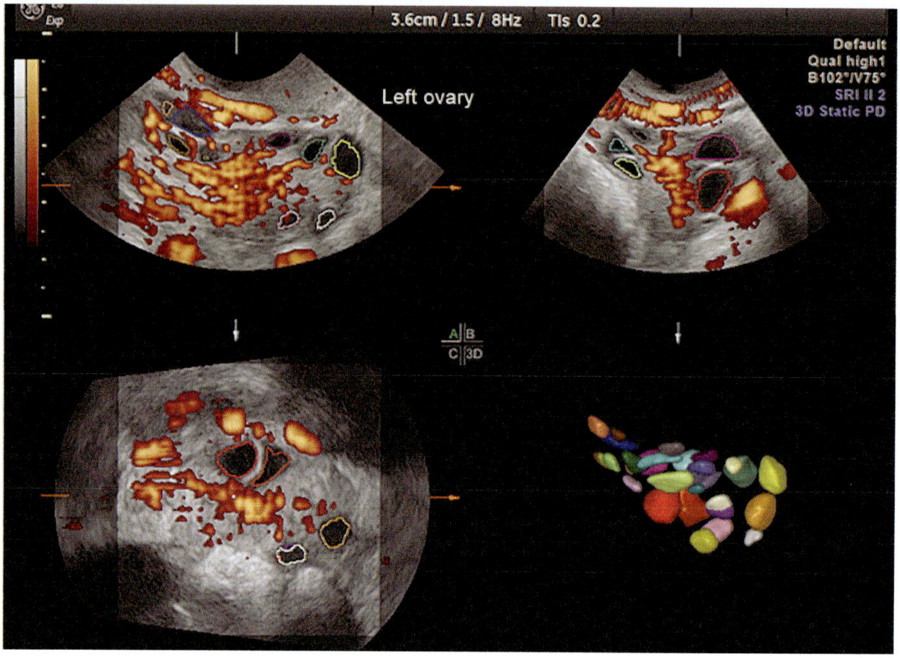

Fig. 6: 3D ultrasound image of the ovary with sono-AVC for calculating antral follicle counts.

is based on inversion-mode rendering. It further color codes each follicle and also shows x, y, and z diameters; mean diameter; and volume of each follicle on the result sheet **(Fig. 6)**.

Ovarian Volume

Ovarian volume correlates with oocytes retrieved.[8] Ovarian volume < 3 cc was significantly predictive of higher IVF cancellation rates > 50%[9] **(Fig. 2)** and ovarian volume was also used in decision-making for the stimulation protocol for ovarian induction. A software called VOCAL (i.e., volume calculation by computer) is used to calculate the ovarian volume **(Fig. 7)**. VOCAL calculates the volume of any structure by rotating it 180°. A step of rotation of 6–30° can be selected. A circumference is drawn around the structure of interest at every step of rotation and at the end of 180° total volume is calculated.

Ovarian volume and AFC correlate with the number of follicles matured and oocytes retrieved. AFC and ovarian volume provide direct measurements of ovarian reserve.[10]

Ovarian Stromal Flow

It is used to assess ovarian response to the dose of gonadotropins. Measurement of ovarian stromal flow in the early follicular phase is related to subsequent ovarian response in IVF treatment.[4] Ovarian stromal PSV after pituitary suppression is predictive of ovarian responsiveness and outcome of IVF treatment.[5] Ovarian blood flow predicts ovarian responsiveness and hence provides a noninvasive and cost-effective prognostic factor of IVF outcome.[11]

The ovarian stromal blood flow was found to be negatively correlated with age. Ovarian blood flow predicts ovarian responsiveness and hence provides a noninvasive and cost-effective prognostic factor of IVF outcome.[5]

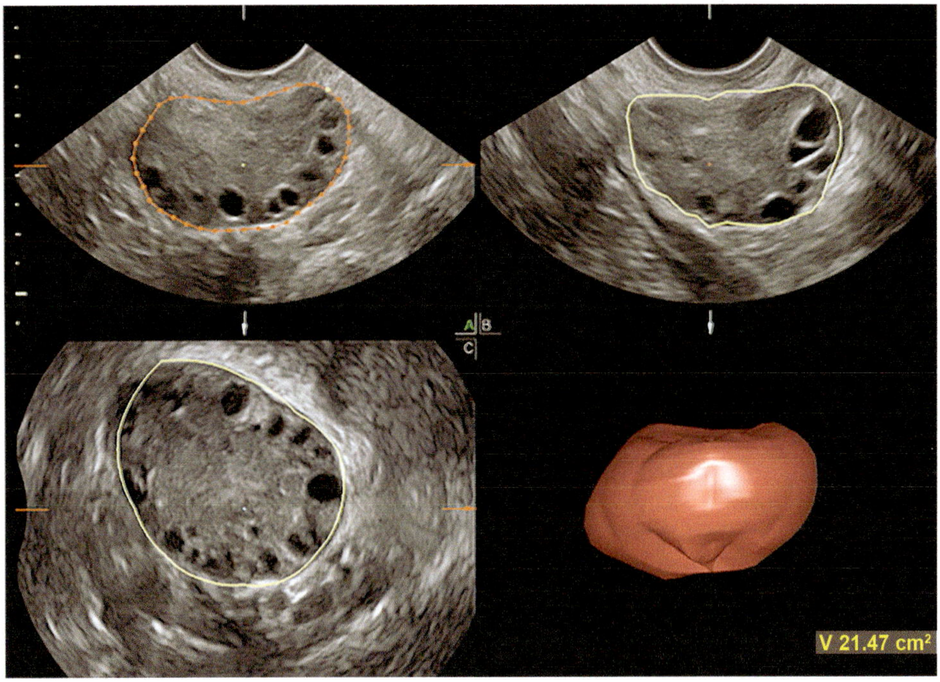

Fig. 7: 3D ultrasound calculated ovarian volume by software called VOCAL.

Kupesic has shown a correlation in the ovarian stromal flow index and the number of mature oocytes retrieved in IVF cycles and pregnancy rates.[6] Stromal FI [<11 low responder, 11–14 good, >15 risk of ovarian hyperstimulation syndrome (OHSS)]. On VOCAL calculated ovarian volume with power Doppler, applying volume histogram gives values of 3D power Doppler indices, vascularity index (VI), flow index (FI), and vascularity flow index (VFI) **(Fig. 8)**. VI is an index for the abundance of flow in the selected volume, FI is an index for the average intensity of flow in a selected volume, and VFI is a perfusion index. Applying threshold volume on the same VOCAL calculated volume will define stromal volume when the threshold is set to differentiate follicles from the rest of the ovarian tissue **(Fig. 9)**. This may aid in recognizing the stromal abundance of polycystic ovary.

Based on all these facts and findings, we understand that ovaries that have high resistance and low-velocity flow require higher doses of gonadotropins for stimulation whereas those with low resistance, high-velocity flow require lower doses of gonadotropins for stimulation.

The total number of antral follicles and ovarian stromal blood flow were the two most significant predictors of response of the ovary to ovulation induction, and ovarian volume was a highly significant predictor of the number of follicles.[2]

Consider the age and BMI also to calculate the stimulation dose. Freiesleben et al.[12] concluded that body weight and AFC may be used to achieve an appropriate ovarian response for IUI in ovulatory patients. Age is known to be one of the most important factors that reduce not only the ovarian reserve but also the oocyte quality.

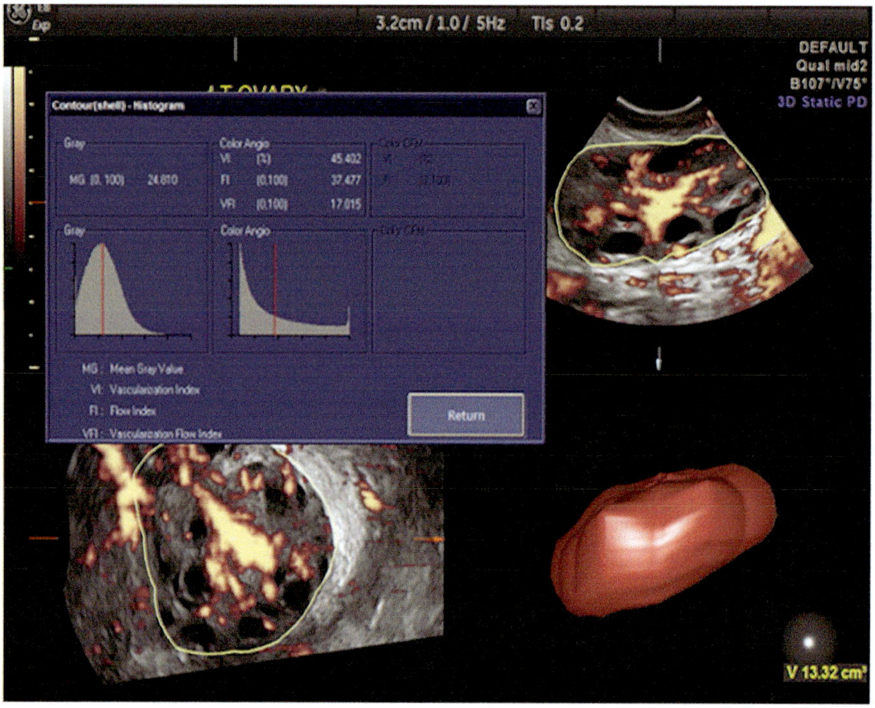

Fig. 8: 3D power Doppler ultrasound image of the ovary with VOCAL calculated volume with volume histogram (blue box) showing VI, FI, and VFI parameters.

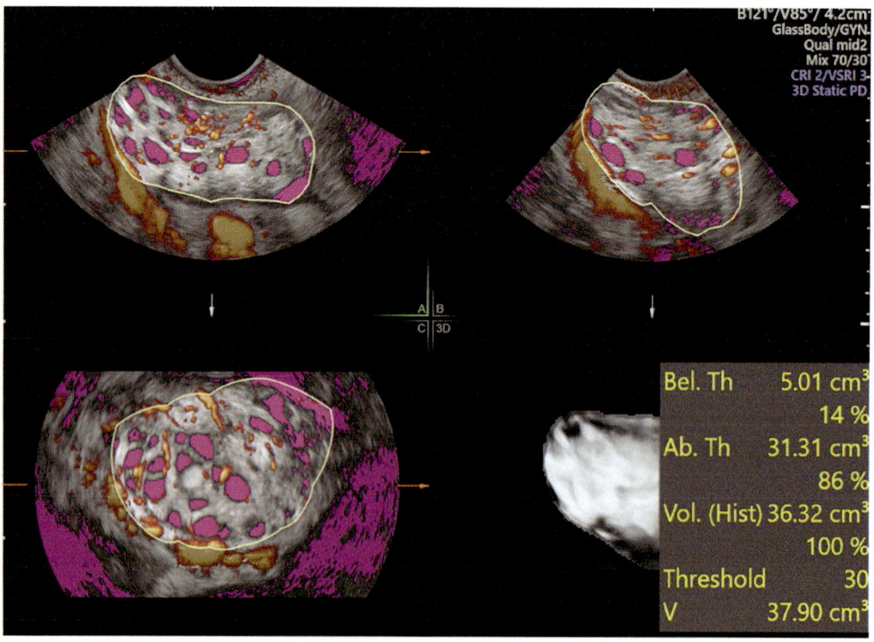

Fig. 9: 3D ultrasound acquired volume of the ovary with VOCAL calculated volume processed by threshold volume to calculate the stromal volume.

Ultrasound parameters and age and BMI are reliable parameters for the decision on stimulation doses.[13] AFC is predictive of the number of follicles (serum estradiol level) on the day of hCG and BMI was predictive of gonadotropins dosage.[14]

As a result of several pilot studies since 2004–2012, we concluded that the final dose calculation can be based on certain factors[15] given in **Table 1**.

Based on the parameters that demand a higher dose or lower dose in a particular patient on the baseline scan, the doses of gonadotropins for ovulation induction are modified.

Depending on the values of age, BMI, AFC, ovarian volume, ovarian stromal RI and PSV, in a particular patient on the baseline scan, the final starting dose for IUI or IVF is calculated. A baseline scoring system has been developed based on the above-mentioned evidences[16,17] **(Table 2)**.

Depending on the baseline score, the doses of rFSH for ovulation induction are as given in **Table 3**.

A transvaginal scan confirms that on the day when gonadotropins are started, all the follicles are smaller than 10 mm. A follicle larger than 10 mm is the dominant follicle. Follicular dominance is confirmed on Day 5 of stimulation.

If on Day 5, the follicle has not grown to dominance and the endometrium is also not growing, then it is considered nonresponse

TABLE 1: Age, BMI, and ultrasound parameter values that may require increase or decrease in the doses of gonadotropins for ovulation induction.

	Increase the dose when	*Decrease the dose when*
Age	>35 years	<25 years
BMI	>28 kg/m^2	<20 kg/m^2
AFC	<3 (FNPO)	>12 (FNPO)
Stromal RI	>0.7	<0.5
Stromal PSV	<5 cm/s	>10 cm/s
Stromal FI	<11	>15
Ovarian volume	<3 cc	>10 cc

(AFC: antral follicle count; BMI: body mass index; FNPO: follicle number per ovary; PSV: peak systolic velocity; RI: resistance index).

TABLE 2: Baseline scoring system, indicating score for a particular value of different parameters used for deciding the dose of gonadotropin for ovulation induction.

Score	*1*	*2*	*3*	*4*	*5*
Age	>40	35.1–40	30.1–35	25.1–30	<25
BMI	>30	30–28.1	28–25.1	25–22.1	<22
AFC	<5	5–10	11–15	16–20	>20
OV	<3	3.1–5	5.1–7	7.1–10	>10
Stromal RI	>0.75	0.75–0.66	0.65–0.56	0.55–0.45	<0.45
Stromal PSV	<3	3.1–5	5.1–7	7.1–10	>10

(AFC: antral follicle count; BMI: body mass index; OV: ovarian volume; PSV: peak systolic velocity; RI: resistance index)

TABLE 3: Doses of rFSH for IUI, IVF (fresh), and IVF (FET) cycles.

Score	*IUI*	*IVF(Fresh)*	*IVF FET*
≥25	25 IU	75 IU	150 IU
21–25	37.5 IU	150 IU	225 IU
16–20	75 IU	225 IU	300 IU
11–15	112.5 IU	300 IU	375 IU
6–10	150 IU	375 IU	450 IU

(FET: frozen embryo transfer; IUI: intrauterine insemination; IVF: in vitro fertilization; rFSH: recombinant follicle-stimulation hormone)

Flowchart 1: Intrauterine insemination (IUI) cycles dose modification depending upon the baseline score in case of nonresponse.

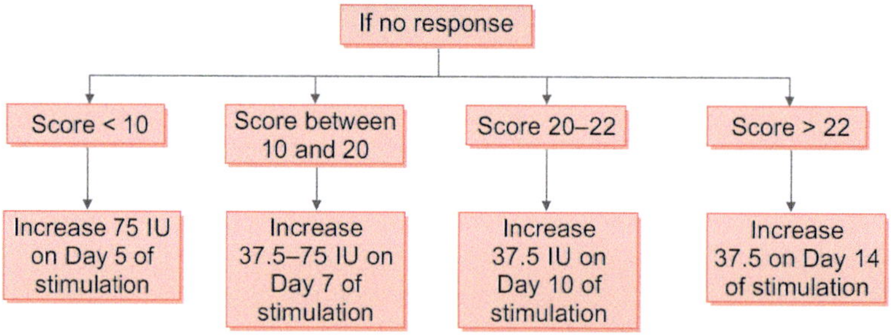

Flowchart 2: IVF cycles, dose modification depending on the baseline score in case of nonresponse.

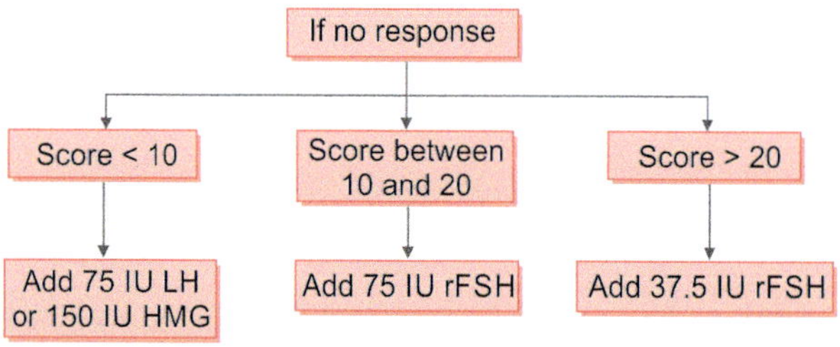

and in these cases, the dose of gonadotropin needs to be modified as shown in **Flowchart 1** for the IUI cycles and as shown in **Flowchart 2** for IVF cycles depending on what was the baseline score.

As per the results of our study, we believe that the scoring system devised in this study for deciding the stimulation protocol is highly reliable for safe planning of stimulation protocols in IUI cycles as the OHSS rates and cycle cancellation rates due to poor response are negligible. Multiple pregnancy rates are also acceptable. This study, we believe may prove to be an important guide for the safe use of gonadotropins for ovulation induction in IUI cycles.

REFERENCES

1. Hull MGR. Polycystic ovarian disease: clinical aspects and prevalence. Res Clin Forums. 1989;11:21-34.
2. Lima ML, Martins WP, Coelho Neto MA, Nastri CO, Ferriani RA, Navarro PA. Assessment of ovarian reserve by antral

follicle count in ovaries with endometrioma. Ultrasound Obstet Gynecol. 2015;46:239-42.
3. Christiansen SC, Eilertsen TB, Eszter V, Carlsen SM. Does AMH reflect follicle number similarly in women with and without PCOS? PLoS One. 2016;11(1):e0146739.
4. Zaidi J, Barber J, Kyei-Mensah A, Bekir J, Campbell S, Tan SL. Relationship of ovarian stromal blood flow at baseline ultrasound to subsequent follicular response in an in vitro fertilization program. Obstet Gynecol. 1996;88:779-84.
5. Engmann L, Sladkevicius P, Agrawal R, Bekin JS, Campbell S, Tan SL. Value of ovarian stromal blood flow velocity measurement after pituitary suppression in the prediction of ovarian responsiveness and outcome of in vitro fertilization treatment. Fertil Steril. 1999;71(1):22-9.
6. Kupesic S, Kurjak A. Predictors of in vitro fertilization outcome by three dimensional ultrasound. Hum Reprod. 2002;17(4):950-5.
7. Krishnakumar J, Agarwal A, Nambiar D, Radhakrishnan S. Comparison of antral follicle count, antimullerian hormone and day 2 follicle stimulating hormone as predictor of ovarian response and clinical pregnancy rate in patient with an abnormal ovarian reserve test. Int J Reprod Contracept Obstet Gynecol. 2016;5(8):2762-7.
8. Popovic-Todorovic B, Loft A, Lindhard A, Bangsbøll S, Andersson AM, Nyboe Andersen A. A prospective study of predictive factors of ovarian response in 'standard' IVF/ICSI patients treated with recombinant FSH. A suggestion for recombinant FSH dosage normogram. Hum Reprod. 2003;18:781-7.
9. Lass A, Skull J, McVeigh E, Margara R, Winston RML. Measurement of ovarian volume by transvaginal sonography before ovulation induction with human menopausal gonadotrophin for in-vitro fertilization can predict poor response. Hum Reprod. 1992;12(2):294-7.
10. te Velde ER. Advances in fertility studies and reproductive medicine [thesis]. Durban: IFFS; 2007. p. 306.
11. Arora A, Gainder S, Dhaliwal L, Suri V. Clinical significance of ovarian stromal blood flow in assessment of ovarian response in stimulated cycle for in vitro fertilization. Int J Reprod Contracept Obstet Gynecol. 2015;4(5):1380-3.
12. Freiesleben NLC, Lossl K, Bogstad J, Bredkjaer HE, Toft B, Loft A, et al. Predictors of ovarian response in intrauterine insemination patients and development of a dosage nomogram. Reprod Biomed Online. 2008;17:632-41.
13. Olivennes F, Howles CM, Borini A, Germond M, Trew G, Wikland M, et al. Individualizing FSH dose for assisted reproduction using a novel algorithm: the CONSORT study. Reprod Biomed Online. 2009;18:195-204.
14. Ng EHY, Tang OS, Chan CC, Ho PC. Ovarian stromal blood flow in the prediction of ovarian response during in vitro fertilization treatment. Hum Reprod. 2005;20:3147-51.
15. Panchal S, Nagori C. Baseline scan and ultrasound diagnosis of PCOS. Donald School J Ultrasound Obstet Gynecol. 2012; 6(3):290-9.
16. Panchal S, Nagori C. Ultrasound based decision making on stimulation protocol for superovulated IUI cycles. IJIFM. 2016;7(1): 7-13.
17. Panchal S, Nagori CB. Ultrasound based decision making on stimulation protocol in IVF. DSJUOG. 2016;10(3):330-7.

5

Chapter

Clomiphene Citrate

INTRODUCTION

Clomiphene citrate (CC) is a mixture of two isomers: enclomiphene (trans) (62%) and zuclomiphene (cis) (38%). Enclomiphene is more potent, more estrogenic, and responsible for ovulation-inducing actions. Enclomiphene has a shorter duration of action and disappears within few days while zuclomiphene is detected over a month because of its slow clearance rate. It accumulates cycle after cycle. Enclomiphene is antiestrogenic centrally and estrogenic peripherally and zuclomiphene is the other way round (estrogenic centrally and antiestrogenic peripherally). CC is in clinical use since 1967 for dysovulatory infertility. The efficacy of the drug varies in clinical practice if the proportions of enclomiphene and zuclomiphene are not maintained.

MECHANISM OF ACTION

Clomiphene citrate acts purely as an antagonist or antiestrogenic agent. It binds with estrogen receptors at hypothalamus, signaling lack of estrogen to the hypothalamus. This, in turn, releases gonadotropin-releasing hormone (GnRH) which causes the pituitary to secrete more follicle-stimulating hormone (FSH) and luteinizing hormone (LH). This stimulates ovarian follicular development. As the estrogen level rises, it does not decrease FSH and LH secretion due to negative feedback mechanism because estrogen receptors are occupied by CC. So there are more FSH and LH in spite of high estrogen. As the duration of action is longer, it allows FSH and LH secretion for a longer period and so causes multifollicular development. Clomiphene has a direct effect on the ovary to stimulate follicular estradiol (E2) synthesis. It increases the GnRH pulse frequency in ovulatory patients[1] and pulse amplitude in anovulatory patients like polycystic ovary syndrome (PCOS).[2] Clomiphene does not display progestational, corticotropic, androgenic, or antiandrogenic properties.

INDICATIONS

WHO Group II Patients

Clomiphene citrate is extremely effective in anovulatory patients in whom the hypothalamo-pituitary-ovarian axis is normal. Normal thyroid function tests and prolactin should be confirmed before starting the treatment. It is not effective in hypogonadotropic hypogonadism, i.e., World Health Organization (WHO) group I as there is no negative feedback mechanism of estrogen.

Luteal Phase Defect

The short luteal phase is associated with low levels of FSH in the follicular phase causing luteal phase defect (LPD). CC will increase FSH and LH in the follicular phase, develop a good follicle, and correct the abnormality in the luteal phase. So, CC is the drug of choice for LPD due to the short luteal phase.[3]

Unexplained Infertility

The rationale of using CC in unexplained infertility is that it corrects subtle hormonal defects due to deficiency of FSH and LH. It increases the number of follicles available for fertilization and corrects LPD. The Cochrane database supports the use of CC in unexplained subfertility. The former belief of cervical dysmenorrhea and decreasing endometrial receptivity in unexplained infertility is not accepted and instead of contraindication, it is now considered the indication for CC in modern era for unexplained infertility. CC with intrauterine insemination (IUI) is beneficial as compared to expectant management.[4] Though there are some studies in which CC has not been found to increase pregnancy rates in ovulatory patients.[5]

CONTRAINDICATIONS

- Large ovarian cyst > 5 cm in diameter. The cycle can be started when the size of the cyst is <5 cm on Day 5 of the cycle.
- Liver disease
- Hypogonadotropic hypogonadism—as the hypothalamic-pituitary-ovarian axis is highly dysfunctional.
- Hypergonadotropic hypogonadism.

BEFORE STARTING CLOMIPHENE CITRATE

- Thyroid function tests should be normal.
- Serum prolactin should be normal.
- Male partner should be evaluated.
- Progesterone withdrawal bleeding should be present in otherwise amenorrhoic patients.
- Adrenal function should be normal.
- Tubal factors should be normal.

TREATMENT REGIMES

Clomiphene citrate is given as a 50-mg dose daily between Day 2 and 5 (both inclusive) for 5 days after spontaneous or induced bleeding. Ovulation, conception, and pregnancy rates are the same independent of the day when CC is started. But Day 5 is the most accepted day for starting the treatment. On Day 5 of the cycle, there is a physiological decrease in serum FSH concentration, which provides the means for selection of the dominant follicle.

Most women (up to 74%)[6] respond to clomiphene with a maximum of 100 mg daily dose. Higher doses have a very poor pregnancy rate. Professor Bruno Lunenfeld and Professor Roy Homburg have recommended only one dose to start with and a maximum of 100 mg daily. The advantage of using this dose is that it can diagnose clomiphene-resistant cases earlier and will cut down superfluous cycles of treatment till ovulation occurs. Dose > 100 mg is not approved by the US Food and Drug Administration (FDA) and adds only a little to pregnancy rates. Higher doses do not increase the ovulation rate or follicular recruitment.[7] **Table 1** shows the ovulation rates with different doses of CC. Even though clomiphene is not deposited in adipose tissues, the dose required for an obese patient is higher. This is due to a high androgen level which inhibits ovulation in obese patients.

The Royal College of Obstetricians and Gynaecologists (RCOG) guidelines with

TABLE 1: Dose of clomiphene citrate and ovulation rate.

Dose	*Ovulation rate*
50 mg	52%
100 mg	22%
150 mg	12%
200 mg	7%

American College of Obstetricians and Gynecologists (ACOG) recommendation depict that CC can be used maximum for 12 months in lifetime and maximum for 6 months continuously. Therefore, monitoring for evidence of ovulation is a must when the patient is on CC.[8,9]

MONITORING

- Serum progesterone in the mid-luteal phase if >3 ng/mL is an evidence of ovulation. It is done to confirm ovulation with CC.
- LH detection kit can help to know the LH surge. Normally, LH surge occurs after 7 days of the last dose of CC.
- Serial sonography just for documenting ovulation is not justified. It does not help to change the line of treatment. It is very inconvenient for the patient as compared to serum progesterone levels' assessment done a week before the expected date of menstruation.
- If LH on Day 8–9 is >10 IU/mL, the success rate is very low because of the poor quality of ova and embryo.
- Endometrial biopsy (EB) should not be done to know the proliferative or secretory phase as it is an invasive test.
- Monitoring during CC treatment is a must because it can be used only for 3–6 months. The majority of conceptions occur within the first 3 months.[10-12]

RESULTS

- CC will induce ovulation in approximately 75–80% of cases.
- Up to 70–75% of the cumulative pregnancy rate can be achieved in 6–9 months.[6]
- In many series, only up to 40% pregnancy rates have been achieved because of antiestrogenic effect on cervical mucus, endometrium, ova, and embryo causing thick cervical mucus, thin endometrium, and the antiestrogenic effect itself that causes high LH and is detrimental to ova and embryo also.[13]
- About 75% of conceptions occur in the first 3 months. So in clinical practice, many consultants use it only for 3 months. After 6 months of therapy, only a few pregnancies are recorded in the literature.
- So, if the patient has not conceived within 3–6 months with CC, re-evaluation of the patient and switching over to further management are required.

High ovulation rate and low pregnancy rate[14] with CC are because of:

- Its antiestrogenic effect on cervix
- Its antiestrogenic effect on endometrium
- High LH, which deteriorates the ovum quality
- Decreased uterine blood flow and decreased PP14, which are required for implantation
- Direct effect on oocytes.

SIDE EFFECTS

- Serious side-effects are extremely rare.
- Transient hot flushes, mood swings, breast tenderness, nausea, and pelvic pain may occur.
- Visual disturbances may occur which are reversible after cessation of treatment.

Alternative treatment is tried if the patient complains of visual disturbances. These side effects are due to the accumulation of Zuclomiphene.

Antiestrogenic Effects of Clomiphene Citrate

Antiestrogenic effects on cervix, endometrium,[15] ovary, ovum, and embryo have been described, but there is no objective evidence that these effects occur or have clinical consequences. Enclomiphene is a more potent antiestrogenic isomer and has a half-life of few days.[16] Though endometrial thickness is within the normal range in majority of cases. This is because clomiphene is a selective estrogen receptor modulator and has a negative effect only on few patients. Very rarely, endometrium suppression is observed which is <6 mm in spite of a good mature follicle. In this case, CC is not given; instead, the patient is to be shifted over to other therapies because endometrial suppression is usually repeated in subsequent cycles. This is because the zuclomiphene component of CC has a very long half-life and its accumulation from cycle to cycle leads to depletion of estrogen receptors, so much so that it may also cause hot flushes, postmenopausal syndrome-like symptoms, visual scotomata, and also cervical dysmenorrhea.[17] CC can be stored in body fat and accumulated in the body around crucial times of implantation, organogenesis, and embryogenesis.[18] Cervical dysmenorrhea can be overcome by IUI. In these patients having antiestrogenic effect, even though the ovulation rate is 80%, the conception rate is only 40%. Exogenous estrogen supplementation has no effect. Exogenous estrogen should not be used to correct cervical dysmenorrhea or increase endometrial thickness as receptors are already occupied by CC and exogenous estrogen will also not be perceived. Tamoxifen and letrozole can be used instead of CC to overcome these side effects. No significant difference in ovulation rates was found with raloxifene and CC.[19] It has been found that the endometrium continues to grow till the size of the follicle reaches 24 mm. It is therefore recommended to wait for the endometrium to grow till that size of the follicle, if at 18–19 mm size of follicle the endometrium is thin. This means that when the follicle actually attains functional maturity, it produces sufficient estrogen, which is when the endometrium grows. This can also be confirmed by Doppler studies. In CC cycles, therefore, a late trigger may be beneficial. The LH surge that occurs prematurely due to rising estrogen may be prevented in these cases because of blocked estrogen receptors by CC.

The argument against delaying trigger is that even though the endometrium is 6 mm, it continues to grow and implantation will occur 7 days after the trigger, by which time the endometrium might attain the required thickness. Moreover, it has also been argued that if the trigger is delayed the estrogen will keep on rising which might be detrimental to implantation.

Risks of Clomiphene Citrate

- Multiple pregnancies (5–8%)—but most are twins or triplets—higher order pregnancies are rare (0.08–1.1%).[20]
- *Miscarriage*: It does not increase the spontaneous miscarriage rate.[21]
- *Congenital anomalies*: There is no substantial evidence that CC causes any particular birth defects or increases the incidence of birth defects.[22] Neural tube defects and hypospadias are the ones most often found in babies of CC-treated mothers. Other defects that were found to be associated with CC were Dandy–Walker malformation, muscular ventricular septal defect (VSD), cloacal exstrophy, anencephaly, all septal heart defects combined, coarctation of aorta, esophageal atresia, craniosynostosis, and omphalocele. Another study though shows that CC is not associated with an increased incidence of craniosynostosis.[23] Fetal malformations may be due to Zuclomiphene that remains in circulation for longer time.
- *Ovarian hyperstimulation syndrome (OHSS)*: Mild OHSS may occur in a few

cases of PCOS, which requires only conservative management. Severe OHSS is rare and I have not seen any in my practice of 30 years.
- *Breast and ovarian cancer*: Previous studies suggested that if CC is used for >12 months, it can increase the incidence of ovarian malignancy. But subsequent studies have proved that fertility drugs are not associated with any invasive cancers. CC does not increase the risk of breast cancer.

Women on clomiphene therapy must be counseled that no causal relationship has been established between ovulation-inducing drugs and breast or ovarian cancer. However, prolonged treatment with CC is futile and should be avoided because it has little success.

TREATMENT ALTERNATIVES

Clomiphene-resistant cases can be treated with:
- Extended CC regime
- Glucocorticoids
- Estrogen
- Bromocriptine
- Human chorionic gonadotropin (hCG)
- Gonadotropins
- GnRh agonist
- GnRh antagonist
- Insulin sensitizers
- Ovarian drilling

Extended Clomiphene Citrate Treatment

- CC is given for 7–10 days.[24]
- 150 mg of CC is given for 8 days.
- 50 mg/day is given for 5 days and an increment of 50 mg/day is done every 5 days to reach 250 mg/day.
- *Stair step protocol*: When there is no follicle development after 14 days of 5 days course of CC, higher dose is given without withdrawal bleed. This reduces the duration of total treatment. But the efficacy of this protocol is controversial.

No factors have been identified that can predict which patient will respond to the extended regime. Such extended regimes have extremely poor pregnancy rates and are not much helpful in clinical practice.

Clomiphene Citrate + Glucocorticoids

This combination is very useful in chronic anovulatory patients. It is also given to those patients who have high dehydroepiandrosterone sulfate (DHEAS). It can be given to all the patients who show an increase in adrenal androgen production. It has given good results even with normal DHEAS and unselected population having clomiphene resistance due to increased androgen. Two large trials evaluated CC-resistant anovulatory patients with normal DHEAS levels. Those treated with dexamethasone on cycle days 3–12 and CC showed 75–88% ovulation rates and 40% conception rates as compared to 15–20% and 5%, respectively, without dexamethasone.[25] Those patients who are resistant to 100–150 mg of CC start ovulating when glucocorticoids are added. Glucocorticoids are given in the form of dexamethasone 0.5 mg daily or prednisolone 5 mg daily continuously for 30 days at bed time. They can be given continuously for 3–6 months. When given at night, they reduce the night peak of adrenocorticotropic hormone (ACTH) and reduces the level of androgens.[26] No serious side effects are seen, though water logging and weight gain have been documented. The dose can be reduced to 0.25 mg/day or can be stopped in the secretory phase of the cycle. As the drug is very cheap and effective and does not have any major disadvantage, it should be tried in chronic anovulatory patients. Glucocorticoids improve response of follicles to stimulation and the health of developing oocytes.[27]

Cochrane review 2009 shows that sequential use of dexamethasone in resistant PCOS patients increase the pregnancy rate five times more.[28]

Clomiphene Citrate + Estrogen

Estrogen was tried to improve cervical mucus and endometrial thickness. But these effects are not due to the dosage and duration of treatment of CC.

It is an idiosyncratic response in the subgroup of CC which may reduce the conception rate. So combination with estrogen is not of any help and should not be used in clinical practice. Empirical treatment with estrogen has no role.

Clomiphene Citrate + Bromocriptine

Bromocriptine is given to the patients of hyperprolactinemia. But there are two definite indications even with a normal prolactin level:

1. *Galactorrhea with a normal prolactin level*: In these cases, galactorrhea must be confirmed by the presence of fat globules under the microscope in the secretions expressed from the breast. It must be differentiated from simple mucoid discharge that does not have fat globules.[29]
2. There are patients who are known as spikers. In these patients, prolactin is increased in the first half of the cycle as nocturnal spikes when CC is used for ovulation induction. These patients are given bromocriptine in the first half of the cycle. It is not to be continued in the second half of the cycle as a normal level of prolactin is required for maintenance of corpus luteum. Clinically, these patients show poor endometrium even though there is no local cause and follicle is very good and meets all parameters on B-mode and color Doppler for optimum maturity. Bromocriptine can be tried in these patients and if endometrium improves, it can be continued for 3–6 months.

Clomiphene Citrate + Human Chorionic Gonadotropin

Routine use of hCG for rupture of the follicle is not justified. If the follicle is mature, it will reflect as serum E2 level of 150 pg/mL or more. This will initiate the LH surge which in turn will cause rupture of the follicle and exogenous hCG is not required. But if the follicle is not mature and if hCG is given as a trigger for ovulation, it will lead to premature luteinization or atresia. Therefore, hCG must not be given just for follicular rupture.[30]

Human chorionic gonadotropin must be combined with clomiphene when IUI is to be done. hCG in these cases is given to time IUI as follicle ruptures at 34–36 hours after hCG injection. A meta-analysis of seven studies comparing triggering ovulation with hCG (1,461 patients) with urinary LH testing to identify endogenous LH surge (1,162 patients) for timing IUI for women with unexplained infertility treated with CC reported lower odds of pregnancy when hCG trigger was used as compared to endogenous LH surge.[31] hCG can also be given in patients proved to have absent, inadequate, or delayed LH surge. This is a common occurrence in endometriosis. hCG, therefore, must be used for timed intercourse, to time IUI, and in cases of delayed LH surge.

Clomiphene Citrate + Gonadotropin

Gonadotropins are often combined with clomiphene with the idea that these would decrease the requirement of gonadotropins. CC, by its direct effect on ovary, increases the sensitivity of ovary to gonadotropins. This combination has a risk of ovarian hyperstimulation and multiple pregnancies. Increased LH secretion induced by CC may also reduce the likelihood of conception.[32]

I am personally never convinced by this combination and would never use it. It does not increase the pregnancy rate. The argument is that CC increases both FSH and LH. The poor pregnancy rate with CC is because of high LH which will remain in spite of adding gonadotropins. The effect of high LH will decrease the implantation and pregnancy rate. So even though we get a follicle after adding gonadotropins, in many of these patients, the follicular quality is not good and pregnancy rates are only comparable to CC alone and much less than gonadotropins alone. Instead, letrozole is a better drug to be combined with gonadotropins. This has been discussed in Chapter 7. A low-dose FSH protocol is recommended by Professor Roy Homburg as a first line of treatment for ovulation induction instead of CC.[33] The study has shown to double the pregnancy rates, with reduced treatment pregnancy interval and more singleton pregnancies.[33]

Gonadotropin-releasing Hormone Agonist

Gonadotropin-releasing hormone agonists are not used routinely in IUI cycles and are reserved only for in vitro fertilization (IVF) cycles. Agonists are used for downregulation and this in IUI cycles only increases the requirement of gonadotropins, without increasing the pregnancy rate.

Clomiphene Citrate + Antagonist

This makes a good combination in thin, lean PCOS patients where LH is tonically raised. It improves the quality of ovum and also the conception rates. For patients on clomiphene therapy, serum LH levels are checked on Day 8–9 of the cycle. If it is >10 IU/mL, it is an indicator of poor pregnancy rates. These are the ideal patients to start antagonist. Regular use of antagonist with CC is not justified because it sharply decreases LH and the quality of the follicle is changed, and it causes regression of the follicle as well as LPDs. Antagonist is started when the size of the follicle is 14 mm and is continued till the day of trigger.

Clomiphene Citrate + Metformin

Several workers have shown that metformin is inferior to CC for ovulation induction, and metformin alone should not be used for ovulation induction.[34]

However, in CC-resistant cases of PCOS, when metformin is combined with CC, it increases ovulation four to nine times than clomiphene alone. Metformin is a very useful drug when the patient does not want to conceive immediately. If metformin is taken for 6 months, it will normalize hormonal milieu. It will decrease LH and androgen. So if CC is given when the patient wants to conceive, ovulation will occur and will decrease the incidence of multiple pregnancies also. Pretreatment with metformin for patients to be treated with CC has been shown to improve ovulation rates[35] and conception rates[36] in several studies. Though another study has clearly shown that metformin pretreatment does not improve the pregnancy rates or extended metformin therapy does not reduce the required dose of CC.[37,38] A meta-analysis of 17 randomized controlled trials (RCTs) in PCOS women has shown both increased ovulation and pregnancy when metformin was added to CC. This effect was found to be statistically significant in obese women with

PCOS, whereas it failed to reach significance in nonobese women with this condition. It is therefore logical to routinely use metformin with CC in obese women with PCOS and glucocorticoid as the first adjunct of choice for nonobese PCOS women failing to respond to CC.[39]

Clomiphene Citrate + Drilling

It is done in CC-resistant PCOS cases. Drilling is also done before switching over to gonadotropins.

Clomiphene + Low-dose Aspirin

Aspirin may be used to increase the blood flow by vasodilatation which may counter the effect of stress in reducing pelvic blood flow.[40] Though in a meta-analysis, this benefit has not been established.[41]

Prior Treatments

- *Clomiphene after prior treatment with oral contraceptive (OC) pills*: The mechanism of action of OC pills is to decrease LH. High LH will cause high androgen, which in turn will cause an ovulation. So OC pills when given for 2–3 months will decrease the LH and in turn androgen improves the sensitivity to clomiphene with the same dose. Therefore, in PCOS patients, prior treatment with OC pills was given routinely in CC-resistant cases and did show good results.
- *Micronized progesterone*: If it is given for 5 days, it modulates LH pulsatility, reducing LH concentration, and induces more favorable environment for CC.

CARRY HOME MESSAGE

- CC should be used for 3–6 months, 100 mg/day starting from Day 5, when LH < 10 IU/mL on Day 10 of cycle.
- Clomiphene citrate + estrogen has no role.

Contd...

Contd...

- Clomiphene citrate + dexamethasone is useful in chronic anovulatory patient and when DHEAS is high.
- Clomiphene citrate + bromocriptine is used in patients with normal prolactin levels with galactorrhea and spikers when prolactin is high in the first half of the cycle.
- Routine use of hCG is not justified.
- Clomiphene citrate + GnRH agonist for downregulation has no role in IUI cycles.
- Clomiphene citrate + antagonist must be used in thin, lean PCOS patients.
- Clomiphene citrate + gonadotropins do not improve pregnancy rates.
- Clomiphene citrate + metformin can be used in CC-resistant PCOS patients.
- Metformin, OC pills, and progesterone are useful prior to CC.
- CC without IUI does not increase the fecundity rates in patients with unexplained infertility but definitely increases the fecundity rates with IUI.[42]
- Ovarian drilling is offered to CC-resistant PCOS.

REFERENCES

1. Kerin JF, Liu JH, Phillipou G, Yen SS. Evidence for a hypothalamic site of action of clomiphene citrate in women. J Clin Endocrinol Metab. 1985;61:265-8.
2. Kettel LM, Roseff SJ, Berga SL, Mortala JF, Yen SS. Hypothalamic-pituitary-ovarian response to clomiphene citrate in women with polycystic ovary syndrome. Fertil Steril. 1993;59:532-8.
3. The Practice Committee of American Society for Reproductive Medicine. The clinical relevance of luteal phase deficiency. Fertil Steril. 2012;98:112-7.
4. Deaton JL, Gibson M, Blackmer KM, Nakajima ST, Badger GJ, Brumsted JR. A randomised controlled trial of clomiphene citrate and intrauterine insemination in couples with explained infertility or surgically corrected endometriosis. Fertil Steril. 1990;54:1083-8.
5. Guzick DS, Carson SA, Coutifaris C, Oversheet JW, Factor-Litvak P, Steinkampf MP, et al. Efficacy of superovulation and intrauterine insemination in the treatment of infertility. N Engl J Med. 1999;340(3):177-83.

6. Thessaloniki ESHRE/ASRM-Sponsored PCOS Consensus Workshop Group. Consensus on infertility treatment related to polycystic ovary syndrome. Fertil Steril. 2008;89:505-22.
7. Dickey RP, Taylor SN, Curole DN, Rye PH, Lu PY, Pyrzak R. Relationship of clomiphene dose and patient weight to successful treatment. Hum Reprod. 1997;12:449-53.
8. Gysler M, March CM, Mishell DR Jr, Bailey EJ. A decade's experience with an individualized clomiphene treatment regimen including its effect on the post-coital test. Fertil Steril. 1982;37:161.
9. Gorlitsky GA, Kase NG, Speroff L. Ovulation and pregnancy rates with clomiphene citrate. Obstet Gynecol. 1978;51:265.
10. Shoham Z, Borenstein R, Lunenfeld B, Pariente C. Hormonal profiles following clomiphene citrate therapy in conception and non-conception cycles. Clin Endocrinol. 1990;33:271-8.
11. Venn A, Lumley J. Clomiphene citrate and pregnancy outcome. Aust NZ J Obstetr Gynecol. 1994;34:56-66.
12. Vandenberg G, Ten SS. Effect of anti-oestrogenic action of clomiphene during the menstrual cycle: evidence for a change in feedback sensitivity. J Clin Endocrinol Metab. 1973;37:356-65.
13. Homburg R. Clomiphene citrate-end of an era? Hum Reprod. 2005;20:2043-51.
14. Out HJ, Coelingh Bennink HJ. Clomiphene citrate or gonadotrophins for induction of ovulation? Hum Reprod. 1998;13:2358-61.
15. Gonen Y, Casper RF. Sonographic demonstration of an adverse effect of clomiphene citrate on endometrial growth. Hum Reprod. 1990;5:670-4.
16. Young SL, Opsahl MS, Fritz A. Serum concentration of enclomiphene and zuclomiphene across consecutive cycles of clomiphene citrate therapy in an ovulatory infertile women. Fertil Steril. 1999;71:639-44.
17. Ghobadi C, Mirhosseini N, Shiran MR, Moghadamnia A, Lennard MS, Ledger WL, et al. Single dose pharmacokinetic study of clomiphene citrate isomers in an ovular patients with polycystic ovary disease. J Clin Pharacol. 2009;49:147-54.
18. Mikkelson TJ, Kroboth PD, Cameron WJ, Dittert LW, Chungi V, Manberg PJ. Single-dose pharmacokinetics of clomiphene citrate in normal volunteers. Fertil Steril. 1986;46:392-6.
19. de Paula Guedes Neto E, Savaris RF, von Eye Corleta H, de Moraes GS, do Amaral Cristovam R, Lessey BA. Prospective, randomized comparison between raloxifene and clomiphene citrate for ovulation induction in polycystic ovary syndrome. Fertil Steril. 2011;96(3):769-73.
20. Reefhuis J, Honein MA, Schieve LA, Rasmussen SA. National birth defects prevention study. Use of clomiphene citrate and birth defects. National birth defects prevention study, 1997-2005. Hum Reprod. 2011;26:451-7.
21. Badawy A, Shokeir T, Allam AF, Abdelhady H. Pregnancy outcome after ovulation induction with aromatase inhibitors or clomiphene citrate in unexplained infertility. Acta Obstet Gynecol Scand. 2009;88:187-91.
22. Correy JF, Marsden De, Schokman FC. The outcome of pregnancy resulting from clomiphene-induced ovulation. Aust N Z J Obstet Gynaecol. 1982;22:18-21.
23. Reefhuis J, Honein MA, Show GM, Romitti PA. Fertility treatments and craniosynostosis: California, Georgia and Iowa, 1993-1997. Pediatrics. 2003;111:1163-6.
24. Flukar MR, Wang IY, Rowe TC. An extended 10-day course of clomiphene citrate in women with CC resistant ovulatory disorder. Fertil Steril. 1996;66:761-4.
25. Elnashar A, Abdelageed E, Fayed M, Sharaf M. Clomiphene citrate and dexamethasone in treatment of clomiphene citrate resistant polycystic ovary syndrome: a prospective placebo-controlled study. Hum Reprod. 2006;21:1805-8.
26. Keay SD, Jenkins JM. Adjunctive use of dexamethasone in Clomid resistant patients. Fertil Steril. 2003;80:230
27. Thurston LM, Norgate DP, Jonas KC, Gregory L, Wood PJ, Cooke BA, et al. Ovarian modulators of type 1 11β-hydroxysteroid

dehydrogenase (11βHSD) activity and intrafollicular cortisol: Cortisone ratios correlate with the clinical outcome of IVF. Hum Reprod. 2003;18:1603-12.
28. Parsanezhad ME, Alborzi S, Motazedian S, Ormani G. Use of dexamethazone and clomiphene citrate in the treatment of clomiphene citrate resistant patient with polycystic ovarian syndrome and normal dehydroepiandrosterone sulphate levels: a prospective double blind, placebo-controlled trial. Fertil Steril. 2002;78:1001-4.
29. Padilla SL, Person GK, McDonough PG, Reindollar RH. The efficacy of bromocriptine in patients with ovulatory dysfunction and normoprolactinemic galactorrhoea. Fertil Steril. 1985;44:695-8.
30. Agrawal SK, Buyalos RP. Corpus luteum function and pregnancy rates with clomiphene citrate therapy: comparison of human chorionic gonadotrophin induced versus spontaneous ovulation. Hum Reprod. 1995;10:328-31.
31. George K, Nair R, Tharyan P. Ovulation triggers in anovulatory women undergoing ovulation induction. Cochrane Database Syst Rev. 2008;3:CD006900.
32. Sagle MA, Hamilton-Fairley D, Kiddy DS. A comparative, randomized study of low dose human menopausal gonadotropin and follicle-stimulating hormone in women with polycystic ovarian syndrome. Fertil Steril. 1990;53:792-7.
33. Homburg R, Hendriks ML, Konig TE, Anderson RA, Balen AH, Brincat M, et al. Clomiphene citrate of low dose FSH for the first-line treatment of infertile women with anovulation associated with polycystic ovary syndrome: a prospective randomized multinational study. Hum Reprod. 2012;27(2):468-73.
34. De Leo V, la Marca A, Ditto A, Morgante G, Cianci A. Effects of metformin on gonadotropin-induced ovulation in women with polycystic ovary syndrome. Fertil Steril. 1999;72:282-3.
35. Kocak M, Caliskan E, Simsir C, Haberal A. Metformin therapy improves ovulation rates, cervical scores and pregnancy rates in clomiphene citrate resistant women with polycystic ovary syndrome. Fertil Steril. 2002;77:101-6.
36. Khorram O, Helliwell JP, Katz S, Bonpane CM, Jaramillo L. Two weeks of metformin improves clomiphene citrate induced ovulation and metabolic profiles in women with polycystic ovary syndrome. Fertil Steril. 2006;85:1448-51.
37. Silbert TI, Kruger TF, Lombard C. Evaluating the equivalence of clomiphene citrate with and without metformin in ovulation induction in PCOS patients. J Assist Reprod Genet. 2009;26:165-71.
38. Cataldo NA, Barnhart HX, Legro RS, Myers ER, Schlaff WD, Carr BR, et al. Extended-release metformin does not reduce the clomiphene citrate dose required to induce ovulation in polycystic ovary syndrome. J Clin Endocrinol Metab. 2008;93:3124-7.
39. Creanga AA, Bradley HM, McCormick C, Witkop CT, et al. Use of metformin in polycystic ovary syndrome: a meta-analysis. Obstet Gynecol. 2008;111:959-68.
40. Ebbesen SMS, Zachariae R, Mehlsen MY, Thomsen D, Højgaard A, Ottosen L, et al. Stressful life events are associated with poor in vitro fertilization (IVF) outcome: a prospective study. Hum Reprod. 2009;24:2173-82.
41. Khairy M, Banerjee K, El-Toukhy T, Coomarasamy A, Khalaf Y. Aspirin in women undergoing in vitro fertilization treatment: a systematic review and meta-analysis. Fertil Steril. 2007;88:822-31.
42. Practice committee of American Society of Reproductive Medicine. Use of clomiphene citrate in infertile women: a committee opinion. Fertil Steril. 2013;100(2):341-8.

6

Chapter

Letrozole

INTRODUCTION

Letrozole is an aromatase inhibitor used for ovulation induction. It is the third generation of aromatase inhibitor. The first and second generations of aromatase inhibitors are not used in clinical practice. The main advantage of letrozole is that it is a reversible enzyme inhibitor. It was for the first time used in 2001 for ovulation induction.[1]

MECHANISM OF INDUCTION OF OVULATION

- *Central mechanism*: Estrogen withdrawal centrally causes an increase in activins produced from the pituitary and several other tissues.[2] This stimulates the synthesis of follicle-stimulating hormone (FSH) by a direct action on gonadotropes.[3]
- *Peripheral mechanism*: Androgens have a stimulatory role in early follicular growth[4] mediated directly through testosterone augmentation of follicular FSH receptor expression[5,6] and directly through androgen stimulation by insulin-like growth factor 1 (IGF-1), which may synergize with FSH to promote folliculogenesis.[7,8]

Aromatase, a cytochrome P450-dependent enzyme, acts as the ultimate step in the synthesis of estrogen, catalyzing the conversion of androgen to estrogen. This conversion occurs at peripheral sites such as muscle, fat, and liver. Letrozole inhibits aromatase enzyme by completely binding to the heme of cytochrome P450 subunits of enzyme so that androgen is not converted to estrogen.

The end result is low estrogen causing negative feedback at hypothalamus and pituitary releasing FSH and luteinizing hormone (LH) releasing factors resulting in high FSH and LH causing folliculogenesis.

As androgen is not converted into estrogen, there is a slightly higher level of androgen which also helps folliculogenesis. Letrozole has no effect on estrogen receptors and acts on hypothalamus. So, it has no deleterious effect on LH surge, cervical mucus, and endometrium.

As FSH and LH stimulate folliculogenesis, estrogen will rise and will cause negative feedback on FSH release so that FSH will decrease. This decrease in FSH is responsible for monofollicular development as other follicles will not grow. This is not the case with clomiphene citrate (CC), which binds to estrogen receptors and FSH will go on rising in spite of high estrogen, leading to multifollicular development. Another important advantage is that along with FSH, LH will not increase and so the quality of ova is not disturbed and does not affect implantation. This is another advantage over CC which causes persistent high LH along with FSH.

INDICATIONS

- *CC-resistant cases*: When 100–150 mg of CC fails to induce ovulation, letrozole should be tried.

- *Polycystic ovary syndrome (PCOS)*: In these patients, baseline estradiol (E2) is elevated which blocks the hypothalamus causing anovulation. Letrozole will reduce estrogen and stimulate hypothalamus to release luteinizing hormone-releasing hormone (LHRH) to secrete more FSH and induce folliculogenesis.
- It is useful in cases where CC induces cervical dysmenorrhea and poor endometrium. Letrozole is devoid of antiestrogenic effect as it does not bind to estrogen receptors.
- When LH is elevated on Day 8 or 9 after CC, letrozole should be tried.
- It is useful in poor responders along with gonadotropins.
- Endometriosis.
- Breast carcinoma.

CHARACTERISTICS

- It causes total suppression of estrogen (up to 97–99%) with doses up to 5 mg/day. Maximum suppression occurs between Day 5 and 7.
- After Day 7, the estrogen level will rise due to folliculogenesis because of increasing FSH after negative feedback of estrogen due to letrozole.
- This rise of estrogen will continue for 5–7 days. This E2 peak will cause LH surge for ovulation. So LH surge occurs after 2 days unlike CC when it occurs early.
- High estrogen rise after 7 days will decrease FSH, which is responsible for monofollicular development.
- It has no antiestrogenic effect on cervical mucus or endometrium.
- Temporary rise of androgen improves the sensitivity of follicle to gonadotropin. The patient, therefore, requires a lower dose of gonadotropins when it is combined with letrozole.
- The half-life of letrozole is 48 hours. So it requires a once daily dose.
- It improves endometrial receptivity.

ADVANTAGES

These may be divided under the following heads:

A. Ovulation
B. Implantation
C. Fetal outcome
D. Maternal complications.

A. Ovulation

- It is almost free from side effects and is well-tolerated.
- Monofollicular development.
- No antiestrogenic effect leading to higher pregnancy rates.
- Low multiple pregnancy rate due to monofollicular development.
- Higher androgen stimulates follicle and so lower doses of gonadotropins are required.
  There is a transient accumulation of androgens in the ovary when letrozole is given for ovulation induction. This creates an androgenic microenvironment in the maturing follicle that enhances the follicular sensitivity to FSH for a short duration (half-life of letrozole is approximately 45 hours). This action is of help to poor responders in whom ovarian aging has already reduced ovarian androgens. It is useful in patients with a high body mass index (BMI).[9]

B. Implantation

- It has a low abortion rate because of no effect on endometrium.
- It improves the level of a marker of endometrial receptivity better than CC.[10]
- Aromatase inhibition may potentially improve endometrial receptivity, especially in patients with endometriosis.[11]

- Concomitant use of aromatase inhibitors with gonadotropins reduces the doses of gonadotropins required[12] and improves the response of gonadotropins in poor responders.[13] It also reduces the supraphysiological levels of estrogen seen with the development of multiple ovarian follicles and improves treatment outcome. Low estrogen levels decrease ubiquitination to allow upregulation of estrogen receptors and increase sensitivity to subsequent estrogen rise.[14] This, in turn, leads to improved endometrial blood flow and faster proliferation of the endometrium, which might have a positive impact on implantation.[15]
- The endometrium of PCOS females is dysfunctional.[16] Estrogen receptors in the endometrium, which should normally reduce in the midsecretory phase,[17] are not reduced, with the altered status of other receptors also. This functional derangement leads to progesterone resistance. This is why antiestrogenic agents for ovulation induction may be beneficial in PCOS patients. Moreover, these agents would also improve endometrial receptivity by suppressing the action of ERα and also has a positive impact on the endometrial expression of αvβ3.[18]

C. Fetal Outcome

The incidence of cardiac anomalies in the letrozole group was slightly lower than the 1 in 400 rates quoted in the general population,[19] whereas the cardiac anomaly rate in fetuses of mothers with CC stimulation was about seven times higher.

D. Maternal Complications

Letrozole also leads to the reduction in the secretion of estrogen from granulosa cells leading to less circulating estrogens; therefore, there are less chances of thrombosis in hyperestrogenic states during controlled ovarian hyperstimulation (COH) and also an additional safety for women with hormone-dependent cancers undergoing fertility therapy.[11]

DOSES

- The recommended dose is 2.5 mg from Day 3 to 7.
- Some workers suggest a 5-mg dose. The disadvantage of a 5-mg dose routinely is not justified as 2.5 mg can suppress 97–99% of the estrogen. A 5-mg dose may suppress more estrogen causing more FSH to be secreted. So, it may not cause monofollicular development. As it is a chemotherapeutic agent, it may be toxic to the ovum and embryo. High doses have no advantage in terms of pregnancy rate.[20]
- *20 mg on Day 3*: It has the advantage of having a short half-life and reduces the embryotoxic effect. But symptoms of hypoestrogenism may develop.
- Anastrozole 1 mg from Day 3 to 7 or anastrozole 5-mg single dose may give poorer results. Anastrozole is weak and less effective for follicular growth.[21]

New Regimes

- *Extended letrozole therapy*: 2.5 mg letrozole is given from Day 1 for 10 days in CC-resistant PCOS patients. It may produce more follicles and may give better pregnancy rates.[22]
- *Letrozole step-up protocol*: One, two, three, and four tablets of 2.5 mg of letrozole are given, respectively, on Day 2, 3, 4, and 5. This gives multifollicular development and a higher pregnancy rate. The mechanism of action in this regime is a longer duration of FSH exposure and

prevention of estrogen secretion from granulosa cells, so estrogen does not rise and FSH does not get suppressed.[23] But in both these cases, the actual advantages of letrozole, unnecessary exposure of ovum to LH, and monofollicular development are lost as both lead to a longer duration of FSH and LH secretion and also lead to multifollicular development. Therefore, larger and more robust studies are required to accept these protocols in routine practice.

SIDE EFFECTS (DRAWBACKS)

- It increases intrafollicular androgen which may arrest the growth of the follicle. But the optimum level of androgen is not yet decided.
- As it is a chemotherapeutic agent for carcinoma of breast, it may be teratogenic to ovum and embryo. But it is not proved.
- A multicentric study of 911 newborns conceived after CC27 and letrozole and another recent study[24] have shown that there was no increase in congenital malformations following the use of letrozole. In a recent randomized control study of letrozole for ovulation induction in 900 patients with unexplained infertility, no increase was found in congenital malformations than CC or gonadotropins.[25]

FUTURE USES

- Letrozole helps to improve implantation in IVF (in vitro fertilization). Some women have high levels of aromatase P450 in the endometrium and are related to poor IVF results. It can be useful to them.
- Decreased supraphysiological estrogen and decreased aromatase will improve implantation.
- It stimulates follicles for in vitro maturation (IVM) in PCOS.
- Letrozole may reduce the chronic pelvic pain of endometriosis.[26]
- Letrozole may be used to reduce the risk of ovarian hyperstimulation syndrome (OHSS) and thrombosis due to hyperestrogenism—when given on Day 4–7 and 10 after human chorionic gonadotropin (hCG) trigger in an IVF patient, it reduces estrogen levels and thus reduce the risk of OHSS.[27]
- Letrozole challenge test may be used for predicting the ovarian response to gonadotropin stimulation. This test is done by evaluating FSH on Day 3 and 7 of a letrozole cycle. The ratio of Day 7 and 3 FSH is >1.5 which predicts poor response to gonadotropins.[28] Aromatase inhibitors are also used to treat male subfertility.
- Anastrozole 1 mg/day or letrozole 2.5 mg/day is the recommended dose for patients with high aromatase activity and increased testosterone to estrogen ratio in nonobstructive azoospermic patients. Therefore, in patients with low testosterone levels, the use of aromatase inhibitors is justified.[29]
- Letrozole can be used for treatment of pregnancy of unknown location (PUL) or ectopic pregnancy. Dose is 5 mg every day for 10 days. As it decreases estrogen, it disturbs progesterone receptors and pregnancy does not proceed further.[30]

AUTHOR'S VIEW

Should letrozole replace CC: I strongly believe that letrozole should be used as the first line of the drug. The argument is that it has a comparable pregnancy rate with CC and it does not increase congenital malformations. The main advantage is that it has no antiestrogenic effect on cervical mucus and endometrium and so it will cut down superfluous cycles of treatment. No antiestrogenic effect is the single most important benefit of letrozole that prevents the use of CC. Efficacy-wise, letrozole gives better ovulation and pregnancy rate compared to CC. The results of the trial by Amer et al. are consistent with the recent Cochrane review indicating that letrozole is better as a primary ovulating agent in PCOS with a 40% increase in pregnancy rates and with a shorter time to pregnancy.[31]

LETROZOLE + GONADOTROPINS

We have found letrozole + recombinant FSH (rFSH), a very useful combination for giving equivalent pregnancy rates like gonadotropins with the advantage that a lower number of ampoules are required. Apart from this, it gives a lower rate of multiple births. It sensitizes the ovary by rise in androgen level, which is an added advantage that reduces the number of gonadotropin ampoules. We have used this combination routinely in superovulation with intrauterine insemination (IUI).

Hence, letrozole is superior to CC in PCOS and poor responders.

Other aromatase inhibitors, especially anastrozole, were also tried for ovulation induction. It appears from clinical studies that anastrozole is less effective than letrozole for ovulation induction.[32,33]

LETROZOLE + CLOMIPHENE CITRATE

As letrozole and CC have different mechanisms of action, the combination of both may improve the ovulation rate than letrozole alone. Mejia et al. gave letrozole 2.5 mg and CC 50 mg from Day 3 to 7 in PCOS patients. Patients who received both the drugs had a higher ovulation rate. But there was no difference in pregnancy rate, multiple pregnancy rate, or abortion rate.

Patients who ovulated showed no difference in endometrial thickness, size of the follicle, or serum progesterone levels. But an absolute difference of 34% in ovulation was noted.[34]

Hajisafi et al. used 100 mg of CC and 5 mg of letrozole in resistant cases of CC and letrozole.[35] This observation requires further studies. LH, which is already high in PCOS, will be increased further when both the drugs are used. This LH will not come down because of receptors occupied by CC even after high estrogen after follicular development. This may reach the "ceiling level of LH." This is the only reason that like CC, the ovulation rate is high with this combination but the pregnancy rate is not increased and perhaps it may decrease instead than when giving only letrozole. Instead, letrozole + FSH is a better combination.

For Ovulation Induction in IVF (Low Responders)

With aging, significant androgen reduction is observed. Letrozole improves intraovarian androgen and sensitizes the follicle to FSH with a relatively short duration of action of 45 hours. Patients treated with letrozole + gonadotropins, both started from Day 2, and letrozole given for 5 days got a higher number of oocytes and higher implantation rates in low responders.[11]

Risk of Ovarian Hyperstimulation Syndrome

Whenever a long protocol is used, there is no option to hCG trigger. E2 reduction by letrozole after ovum pick up is tried by Fatemi et al. as 5 mg dose. They did not observe any change in progesterone and LH in 10 days.[27,36]

But we must keep in mind that E2 reduction does not necessarily mean that the risk of severe OHSS is lessened. However, it definitely reduces the risk of thromboembolism.

Endometriosis

Aromatase is expressed in women with endometriosis. Letrozole will prevent the production of E2. When letrozole or anastrozole is given with GnRHa depot preparation, there is a marked reduction in endometrioma volume and also in CA-125 levels.

Miller et al. confirmed that the use of aromatase inhibitors might improve the IVF success rate in a subset of women with endometriosis and implantation failure.[37]

CARRY HOME MESSAGE

- Letrozole causes monofollicular development.
- It has no antiestrogenic effect.
- It is a drug of choice in PCOS and poor responders.
- Letrozole + gonadotropins is an excellent combination.
- Letrozole may replace CC as the first line of treatment in the future.

REFERENCES

1. Mitwally MFM, Casper RF. Use of aromatase inhibitor for ovulation induction in patients with an inadequate response to clomiphene citrate. Fertil Steril. 2001;75:2-8.
2. Roberts V, Meunier H, Vaughan J, Rivier J, Rivier C, Vale W, et al. Production and regulation of inhibin subunits in pituitary gonadotropes. Endocrinology. 1989;124:552-4.
3. Weil SJ, Vendola K, Zhou J, Adesanya OO, Wang J, Okafor J, et al. Androgen receptor gene expression in the primate ovary: cellular localization, regulation and functional correlations. J Clin Endocrinol Metab. 1989; 837:2479-85.
4. Mason AJ, Berkemeier LM, Schmelzer CH, Schwall RH. Activin B: precursor sequences, genomic structure and in vitro activities. Mol Endocrinol. 1989;3:1352-8.
5. Weil S, Vendola K, Zhou J, Bondy CA. Androgen and follicle-stimulating hormone interactions in primate ovarian follicle development. J Clin Endocrinol Metab. 1999;84:2951-6.
6. Vendola KA, Zhou J, Adesanya OO, Weil SJ, Bondy CA. Androgens stimulate early stages of follicular growth in the primate ovary. J Clin Invest. 1998;101:2622-9.
7. Vendola K, Zhou J, Wang J, Famuyiwa OA, Bievre M, Bondy CA, et al. Androgens promote oocyte insulin-like growth factor I expression and initiation of follicle development in the primate ovary. Biol Reprod. 1999;61:353-7.
8. Giudice LC. Insulin like growth factors and ovarian follicular development. Endocr Rev. 1992;13:641-69.
9. McKnight KK, Nodler JL, Cooper JA, Chapman VR, Cliver SP, Bates GW Jr. Body mass index-associated differences in response to ovulation induction with letrozole. Fertil Steril. 2011;96(5):1206-8.
10. Wallace KL, Johnson V, Sopelak V, Hines R. Clomiphene citrate versus letrozole: molecular analysis of the endometrium in women with polycystic ovary syndrome. Fertil Steril. 2011;96(4):1051-6.
11. Garcia-Valesco JA. The use of aromatase inhibitors in in vitro fertilization. Fertil Steril. 2012;98(6):1356-8.
12. Mitwally MF, Casper RF. Aromatase inhibition reduces the dose of gonadotropin required for controlled ovarian hyperstimulation. J Soc Gynecol Investig. 2004;11:406-15.
13. Mitwally MF, Casper RF. Aromatase inhibition improves ovarian response to follicle stimulating hormone in poor responders. Fertile Steril. 2002;77:776-80.
14. Mitwally MF, Witchel SF, Casper RF. Troglitazone: a possible modulator of ovarian steroidogenesis. J Soc Gynecol Investig. 2002;9:163-7.
15. Nirmala PB, Thampan RV. Ubiquitination of the rat uterine oestrogen receptor: dependence on oestradiol. Biochem Biophys Res Commun. 1995;213:24-31.
16. Giudicel C. Endometrium in PCOS: implantation and predisposition to endocrine CA.

Best Pract Res Clin Endocrinol Metab. 2006;20:235-44.
17. Lessey BA, Killam AP, Metzger DA, Haney AF, Greene GL, McCarty KS Jr. Immunohistochemical analysis of human uterine estrogen and progesterone receptors through the menstrual cycle. J Clin Endocrinol Metab. 1988;67:334-40.
18. Lessey BA, Palomino WA, Apparao KBC, Young SL, Lininger RA. Estrogen receptor-alpha (ER-alpha) and defects in uterine receptivity in women. Repro Biol Endocrinol. 2006;4(1):S9.
19. Hoffman JI. Incidence of congenital heart disease: I. Postnatal incidence. Pediatr Cardiol. 1995;16:103-13.
20. Badawy A, Metwally M, Fawzy M. Randomised controlled trial of three doses of letrozole for ovulation induction in patients with unexplained infertility. Reprod Biomed Online. 2007;14:559-62.
21. Griesinger G, von Otte S, Schultze-Mosgau A, Diedrich K, Schröer A. Follicular and endocrine response to anastrozole versus clomiphene citrate administered in follicular phase to normo-ovulatory women: a randomised comparison. Fertil Steril. 2009;91:1831-6.
22. Badawy A, Mosbah A, Tharwat A, Eid M. Extended letrozole therapy for induction of ovulation in CC resistant PCOS patients: a novel protocol. Fertil Steril. 2009;92:236-9.
23. Mitwally MF, Said T, Galal A. Letrozole step-up protocol: a successful superovulation protocol. Fertil Steril. 2008;89:523-4.
24. Hull MGR. The causes of infertility and relative effectiveness of treatment. In: Templeton AA, Drife JO (Eds). Infertility. London: Springer-Verlag; 1992. pp. 33-62.
25. Legro DM, Raivero CC, Robinson R, Zhung H. Letrozole, clomiphene or gonadotropin for unexplained infertility. N Engl J Med. 2015;373:1230-40.
26. Pavone ME, Bulun SE. Aromatase inhibitors for treatment of endometriosis. Fertil Steril. 2012;98(6):1370-9.
27. Fatemi HM, Popovic-Todorovic B, Donoso P, Papanikolau E, Smitz J, Devreoy P. Luteal phase oestradiol suppression by letrozole: a pilot study in oocyte donors. Reprod Biomed Online. 2008;17:307-11.
28. Bentov Y, Burstein E, Esfandiari N, Casper R. Use of letrozole challenge test to adjust gonadotropin dose in non-downregulated cycles. Fertil Steril. 2011;95(8):2492-3.
29. Schlegel PN. Aromatase inhibitors for male infertility. Fertil Steril. 2012;98(6):1359-62.
30. Mitwally MF, Hozayen WG, Hassanin KMA, Abdalla KA, Abdalla NK. The aromatase inhibitor, letrozole: a novel treatment for ectopic pregnancy. Fertil Steril. 2020;114:361-5.
31. Amer SA, Smith J, Mahran A, Fox P, Fakis A. Double blind randomised controlled trial of letrozole versus clomiphene citrate in subfertile women with PCOS. Hum Reprod. 2017;32:1631-8.
32. Tredway D, Schettz JC, Bock D, Hemsey G, Diamond MP. Anastrozole vs. clomiphene citrate in infertile women with ovulatory dysfunction: a phase II randomized, dose-finding study. Fertil Steril. 2011;95:1720-4.
33. Tredway D, Schettz JC, Bock D, Hemsey G, Diamond MP. Anastrozole single dose protocol in women with oligo- or anovulatory infertility: results of a randomized phase II dose-response study. Fertil Steril. 2011;95:1724-8.
34. Mejia RB, Summers KM, Kresowik JD, Van Voorhis BJ. A randomized controlled trial of combination of letrozole and clomiphene citrate or letrozole alone for ovulation induction in women with PCOS. Fertil Steril. 2019;111(3):571-8.
35. Hajisafi M, Dehgan M, Kiarang N, Sadegh-Asadi N, Shayegh SN, Ghasemi-Rad M. Combined letrozole and clomiphene versus letrozole and clomiphene alone in infertile patients with polycystic ovary syndrome. Drug Des Devel Ther. 2013;7:1427-31.
36. Gracia-Valesco JA, Oyea G, Piro M, Mayoral M, Ruiz M, Toribio M, et al. Letrozole administration during the luteal phase after ovarian stimulation impacts corpus luteum function: a randomized, placebo controlled trial. Fertil Steril. 2009;92:222-5.
37. Miller PB, Parnell BA, Bushnell G, Talliman N, Forstein DA, Higdon HL 3rd, et al. Endometrial receptivity defects during IVF cycles with and without letrozole. Hum Reprod. 2012;27:881-8.

7 Chapter

Gonadotropins

INTRODUCTION

Gonadotropins are direct stimulation to ovaries in contrast to clomiphene citrate and letrozole, which stimulate the hypothalamus and indirectly increase the follicle-stimulating hormone (FSH) and luteinizing hormone (LH) simultaneously. Professor Bruno Lunenfeld first reported the use of human menopausal gonadotropin (HMG) followed by pregnancy in 1963. Now purified preparations of gonadotropins are also available. The availability of recombinant FSH (rFSH) has changed the picture for the demand of gonadotropins.

PHYSIOLOGY

- Primordial follicles are independent of gonadotropin stimulation and they take 10 weeks to develop into antral follicles.
- Antral follicles can respond to gonadotropin stimulation.
- Under the influence of FSH and LH, the antral follicle grows, matures, and ovulates in 2 weeks.
- FSH rise in the late luteal phase of the previous cycle decides the dominant follicle.
- For the follicular cohort, a minimum level of FSH is required and this is called the FSH threshold.
- FSH window means the number of days the FSH levels are above threshold.
- As the sensitivity of follicle to FSH increases with development, a lower amount of FSH is required for further growth of the follicle.
- As the amount of FSH decreases, it stops the growth of other follicles except the dominant follicle. The process of selection of follicle is completed in 7 days. But when gonadotropins are given from outside, we do not decrease the dose of FSH and so there will be a larger number of follicles to grow and ovulate in controlled ovarian stimulation (COS).
- All oocytes are arrested in the prophase stage in meiosis in preantral follicles. This inhibition is removed by LH surge and the first meiotic division will be complete with extrusion of the first polar body. Oocytes should be fertilized within 48–72 hours of the second meiotic division; otherwise the oocyte dies.

FOLLICLE-STIMULATING HORMONE PREPARATIONS AVAILABLE

- *Human menopausal gonadotropin*: 75 IU of FSH and 75 IU of LH activity with human chorionic gonadotropin (hCG) which acts as LH surrogate.
- *Human menopausal gonadotropin-HP (highly purified)*: 75 IU of FSH and 75 IU of LH with <5% of urinary proteins.
- *Urinary FSH (uFSH)*: 75 IU of FSH and 1 IU of LH.
- *FSH-HP*: 75 IU of FSH with <0.1 IU of LH and <1% of urinary proteins.

- *rFSH*: 75 IU of FSH and no LH activity.
- rFSH + recombinant LH (rLH) combination.

PRINCIPLES OF GONADOTROPIN THERAPY

The basic principles were suggested by Insler and Lunenfeld in 1974:[1]

- *Effective dose*: Ovarian response is seen when a certain dose of FSH is given. Below this dose, the ovaries do not respond.
- *Latent phase*: This phase lasts for 3–7 days. It starts with the onset of stimulation, but there is no estrogen rise or ultrasound-demonstrable follicular growth during this phase.
- *Active phase*: This phase starts with ultrasound-demonstrable follicle growth to ovulation and it lasts for 4–6 days.

PHYSIOLOGY OF OVULATION

- FSH stimulates the follicle to growbut. However, continuous stimulation is required for the follicle to grow.
- Follicle secretes estrogen that has a negative feedback on hypothalamus to secrete less FSH and LH.
- When the follicle is mature and estrogen secretion is at its peak, the pituitary receives a positive feedback for LH surge by the short loop.
- LH surge causes ovulation to occur.
- The mature follicle is 16–18 mm and estrogen secretion from such a follicle is 150 pg/mL/follicle.

DIFFERENT REGIMES OF GONADOTROPIN THERAPY

- Step-up protocol
- Step-down protocol
- Chronic low-dose protocol

When to use which protocol depends on the baseline scan and has been discussed in the Chapter 4.

Indications of Gonadotropins Therapy

- Hypogonadotropic hypogonadism (substitutional therapy)
- Hypothalamo-pituitary dysfunction:
  - Clomiphene-resistant patients
  - Clomiphene failure patients
  - Superovulation combined with intrauterine insemination (IUI)
  - Gonadotropin as the first line of treatment
  - Controlled ovarian hyperstimulation (COH) in assisted reproductive technique (ART) cycles.

Step-up Protocol

Baseline scan guides to decide the stimulating dose. Conventionally in a normal responding ovary, 1 amp, i.e., 75 IU of FSH, is started from Day 5 for 5 days. An ultrasound scan is done on Day 6 of stimulation. If this scan shows a follicle of 10–12 mm and/or there is a 2–3-mm increase in endometrial thickness, the same dose is continued till the follicle and endometrium become mature. If there is no increase in the size of the follicle or not much change in the endometrial thickness, the dose is doubled and the scan is repeated after 3 days. If the follicle or endometrium grows, the same dose is continued till the follicle and endometrium are mature; otherwise, the dose is further increased by 75 IU/day. But this is rarely the case now as each patient is assessed on Day 2–3 of period (baseline scan), and if this scan diagnoses poorly responding ovaries, in these patients stimulation is to be started with higher doses.

This protocol has been blamed for higher rates of multiple pregnancies and ovarian hyperstimulation syndrome (OHSS).[2] But I personally do not agree with the statement of higher risk of OHSS as the step-up protocol is never used in polycystic ovary syndrome

(PCOS) patients. The conventional protocol gives excellent pregnancy rates in the normal responding ovary **(Fig. 1)**. We never do estradiol (E2) level before increasing the dose though some centers do. Good ultrasound monitoring can replace hormonal estimations.

Step-down Protocol (Fig. 2)

The step-down protocol is very useful for the poor responding ovaries or low reserve ovaries. According to this protocol, stimulation is started with a higher dose, i.e., 150–225 IU FSH from Day 5 for 5 days. Once the follicle grows to 10–12 mm, the dose is reduced to 75–150 IU FSH; once the follicle size reaches 14 mm, the dose is further reduced, if it was 150 IU, or is continued with 75 IU FSH till follicle and endometrium mature.

Chronic Low-dose Protocol (Fig. 3)

The chronic low-dose protocol is very useful in PCOS patients. Polycystic ovary (PCO) contains almost twice the number of available FSH-sensitive antral follicles in cohort as compared to normal ovaries. This protocol gives good pregnancy rates with very

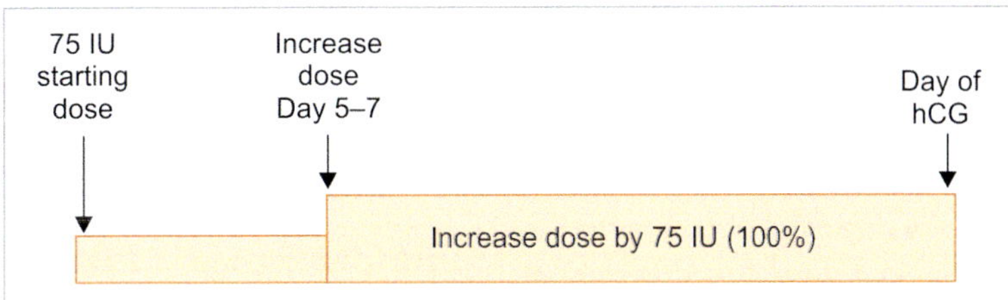

Fig. 1: Conventional protocol. (hCG: human chorionic gonadotropin)

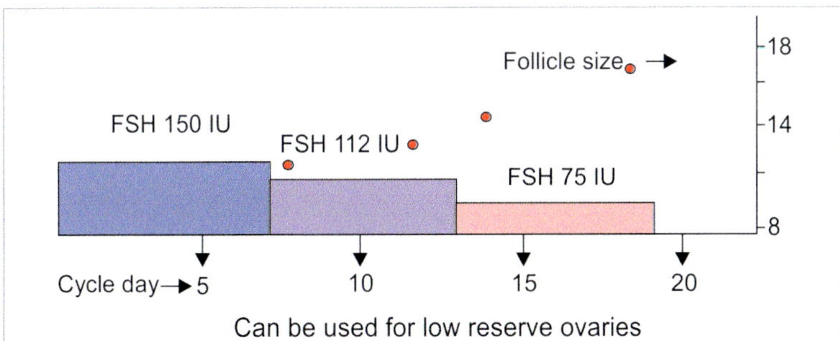

Fig. 2: Step-down protocol. (FSH: follicle-stimulating hormone)

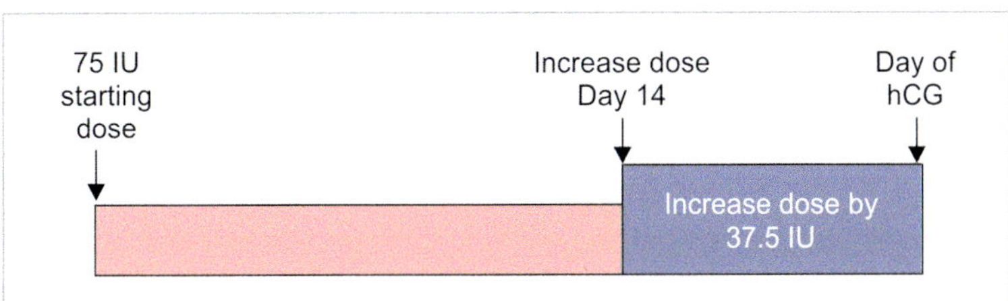

Fig. 3: Chronic low-dose protocol. (hCG: human chorionic gonadotropin)

little risk of OHSS or multiple pregnancies. But it is essential that PCOS is confirmed on a baseline ultrasound scan. In this protocol, stimulation is started with 75 IU of FSH and the same dose is continued for 14 days. If the follicle or endometrium grows, the same dose is continued till mature follicle and endometrium are achieved, otherwise the dose is increased by 37.5 IU for another 7 days. Almost all the patients develop good follicle and endometrium and the incidence of multiple pregnancy and OHSS is extremely low.[3] Majority of the patients develop good follicle within 14 days and we should strongly resist ourselves to increase the dose till then. There may be spotting or some bleeding during this period, which should be ignored. With the chronic low-dose protocol, there is monofollicular development in 70% of cycles, OHSS can be almost totally eliminated, and multiple pregnancy rate can be reduced to 6% with same pregnancy rate as in conventional protocol.[4]

Though the stimulation protocols can be tailor-made for individual patients, depending on the antral follicle count (AFC), ovarian volume, ovarian stromal resistance index (RI), and peak systolic velocity (PSV). This reduces the risk of OHSS to <1%. According to this study, depending on the above-described ultrasound parameters, age, and body mass index (BMI), the scoring system is devised and depending on the initial score of the patient on the baseline scan the starting dose of rFSH can be decided **(Table 1).**[5,6]

For IUI:

Score of ≥ 25	25 IU
20–24	37.5 IU
15–20	75 IU
10–15	112.5 IU
6–10	150 IU

For in vitro fertilization (IVF):

Score of ≥23	75 IU
20–22	150 IU
16–20	225 IU
11–15	300 IU
6–10	375 IU

RECOMBINANT FOLLICLE-STIMULATING HORMONE

The invent of rFSH has changed the management of infertile patients. In 1990, six lakh urine donors were required for 120 million liters of urine for urinary gonadotropin production. This was becoming extremely difficult as with developing techniques in ART, the need for gonadotropins was further increasing. Therefore, there was an urgent

TABLE 1: Scoring system depending on the initial score of the patient on the baseline scan.[5]

Score	*1*	*2*	*3*	*4*	*5*
Age	>40	35.1–40	30.1–35	25.1–30	<25
BMI	>30	30–28.1	28–25.1	25–22.1	<22
AFC	<5	5–10	10–15	15–20	>20
Ovarian volume	<3	3.1–5	5.1–7	7.1–10	>10
Stromal RI	>0.75	0.75–0.66	0.65–0.56	0.55–0.45	<0.45
Stromal PSV	<3	3.1–5	5.1–7	7.1–10	>10

(AFC: antral follicle count; BMI: body mass index; RI: resistance index; PSV: peak systolic velocity)

need for FSH production by an alternate route. The first rFSH was introduced in 1995. But it was in 1992 that Professor Paul Devroey and Germond reported the clinical utility of rFSH.

How is Recombinant FSH Produced?

The objective of recombinant deoxyribonucleic acid (rDNA) technology is to insert genes in the cell to produce desired proteins. The gene that is coded for desired protein is isolated enzymatically from DNA chain. The isolated gene is put in vector (a large segment of DNA).

This is known as rDNA in the host cell. This rDNA produces desired proteins—rFSH. Therefore, human DNA genes into a mammalian cell line produce rFSH, which is 99.9% pure without LH activity. rFSH has a bioactivity of 10,000 IU/mg of protein **(Table 2)**.

Preparation

Follitropin alpha is produced by transfecting Chinese hamster ovary cells with genes for the α and β subunits of human FSH.

The secretory products of these cells undergo a six-step purification process to get a final preparation, which is highly pure biochemically (>99% FSH).

Properties

- It has the highest bioactivity.
- It has no LH or hCG-like activity.
- It has no protein.
- It has a high batch-to-batch consistency.
- It does not produce FSH antibodies in patients.
- It has a low level of oxidation and/or degradation, i.e., 10% as compared to 40% with uFSH.
- Bioactivity mimics the preovulation FSH in normal cycles.

Comparison of rFSH with uFSH

The study conducted by Hedan B clearly indicates the superiority of rFSH **(Table 3)**.[7]

The meta-analysis conducted by Salim Daya and Gunby of 12 randomized controlled trials has proved that rFSH is 20% more likely to achieve pregnancy than uFSH. The amount of FSH used was 400 IU less.[8]

The meta-analysis data was summarized by the author as "The overall conclusion from this meta-analysis is that rFSH is more effective than uFSH because of the higher rates of clinical pregnancy per cycle started and is more efficient because the total dose of gonadotropin required was lower",[8] i.e., 400 IU less.

Prospective meta-analysis has proved that the clinical pregnancy rate is 5% higher

TABLE 2: Product with their specific bioactivity.

Product	*Specific bioactivity*
HMG (1950)	8 IU/mg protein
uFSH (1980)	100–150 IU/mg protein
uHMG-HP	2,000 IU/mg protein
uFSH-HP (1990)	9,000 IU/mg protein
rFSH (1995)	10,000 IU/mg protein

(HP: highly purified; HMG: human menopausal gonadotropin; rFSH: recombinant follicle-stimulating hormone; uFSH: urinary follicle-stimulating hormone)

TABLE 3: Comparison of rFSH with uFSH.

	rFSH	*uFSH*
Higher number of oocytes	10.8	8.9
Lower dose of FSH	2,138 IU	2,385 IU
Shorter period	10.7	11.3
High-quality embryos	3.1	2.6
Pregnancy rate with cryopreservation	25.5%	20.4%

(rFSH: recombinant follicle-stimulating hormone; uFSH: urinary follicle-stimulating hormone)

in rFSH and if cryopreserved embryos are taken into account, the pregnancy rate is 6.4% higher.[9]

Though a recently published Cochrane review has shown no difference in pregnancy outcomes with fresh embryo transfers when rFSH and uFSH were compared. It was concluded that "all available gonadotropins in clinical practice are equally effective and safe" and the choice is based on availability, convenience, and cost.[10]

In MEGASET (Menopur in GnRH Antagonist Cycles with Single Embryo Transfer) trial also it was concluded that HMG-HP and rFSH have the same results.[11]

Comparison of rFSH with uFSH-HP

Recombinant follicle-stimulating hormone is more effective than highly purified FSH in multiple follicular development **(Table 4)**.[12]

Frydman and associates also published the data that rFSH gives more number of oocytes and more embryos with lesser number of injections.[13]

Gearon and Abdalla from Lister hospital, London, in an unpublished study have reported, for the first time, improvement in the quality of oocytes in older women treated with rFSH instead of uFSH-HP. Another randomized single-blind, multicentric multinational study by Schats et al. also confirmed the same findings.

The rFSH gives more embryos with lesser ampoules. More than four embryos in culture have a higher chance of achieving pregnancy.[14] The chances of blastocyst transfer is increased if more than four oocytes are retrieved.[15] But some randomized trials have failed to show the difference in terms of pregnancy rate or miscarriage rate in normal as well as PCOS.[16,17]

The rFSH was associated with a higher per cycle pregnancy rate than uFSH-HP, when used at the same dose, whereas the pregnancy rates were similar when the dose of rFSH was 50% lower.[18]

Recombinant Follicle-stimulating Hormone versus Human Menopausal Gonadotropin

A meta-analysis of eight randomized controlled trials comparing rFSH with HMG has shown that rFSH has 50% higher pregnancy rates.[19]

The FIVNAT (French National Register on in vitro fertilization) report of 1999 showed that the pregnancy rates were higher with rFSH than HMG.

Prospective analysis of 24,000 ART cycles from Germany also showed a higher birth rate and lower dosage with rFSh than HMG.[20] In patients where LH and FSH ratio is high in PCOS, only FSH rather than HMG will improve the results.[21] There is a subgroup of patients

TABLE 4: Comparison of rFSH with uFSH-HP.[12]

	rFSH	*uFSH*	*p value*
Number of ampoules	21.9 ± 5.1	31.9 ± 13.4	<0.0001
FSH days	11 ± 1.6	13.5 ± 3.7	<0.001
Oocytes retrieved	12.2 ± 5.5	7.6 ± 4.4	<0.0001
Embryos transferred	2 ± 0.19	1.9 ± 0.4	NS
Pregnancy rates	53/119 (45%)	42/114 (37%)	NS
Implantation	32	31	NS

(rFSH: recombinant follicle-stimulating hormone; uFSH-HP: highly purified urinary follicle-stimulating hormone)

such as poor responders and elderly patients when HMG-HP is given. It has given higher pregnancy rates, so either rLH or HMG-HP is useful in a subgroup of patients.[22,23]

A meta-analysis including 400,000 IVF cycles showed that compared to rFSH, HMG resulted in fewer oocytes and higher doses.[24]

Facts about Highly Purified Human Menopausal Gonadotropin

- The process is partially successful with specific activity of 2,000 IU/mg of protein.
- In many cases, LH activity has to be added using hCG which has a longer half-life.
- The presence of a variable amount of hCG may further increase variation between different batches of product and result in follicular atresia.[25]
- The HMG-HP contains 30% extraneous proteins including leukocyte elastase inhibitor protein C inhibitor and Zn-α2 glycoprotein apart from hCG.

Different Types of Recombinant Follicle-stimulating Hormone

- Follitropin α; 1995.
- Follitropin β; 1996.
- Follitropin ε: This is a new fully human rFSH (phase i) and has same efficacy.[26,27]
- Immunopotency, biopotency, and internal carbohydrate complexity are same for both but follitropin α contains higher proportion of acidic glycoforms.
- Follitropin α has a specific activity of 13,645 IU/mg whereas that for follitropin β is 9,396 IU/mg.

There is a difference in tolerability between rFSH preparations favoring follitropin α over β.[28] Though follitropin has a higher incidence of OHSS as compared to follitropin β (4.1% as compared to 2.7%).[29]

Fill by Mass Concept

The dose of gonadotropin is expressed in international units (IU). But recent fill by mass (FbM) technique reflects a constant relationship between mass and bioactivity and guarantees consistency of dose from batch to batch. So, the drawbacks of in vivo bioassay can be avoided. Bioassay of FSH preparation is 50 years old. Steelman–Pohley bioassay, which is cumbersome, requires a large number of animals and variation can be 10–20%. But FbM is, through liquid chromatography, supported by glycine mapping isoelectric focusing that demonstrates physicochemical consistency of the product.

The duration of stimulation was significantly shorter in the FbM group, and embryo quality and implantation rates were significantly higher (28.6% in FbM vs. 18.6% in FbIU).[30,31]

Clinical Benefits of Recombinant Follicle-stimulating Hormone[32]

- Improved logistics of pharmaceutical process
- Controlled manufacturing
- Reduced batch-to-batch variability
- Potentially unlimited supply—no shortage
- Not reliant on the urine supply
- No risk of infection
- No risk of contamination with drugs or metabolites
- No seroconversion to antigonadotropin antibodies
- Effective, safe, and less traumatic subcutaneous administration
- Greater purity and specific activity
- Smaller doses required
- More predictable response
- Cost benefit

There are also reports that there is no difference in pregnancy rate when rFSH was compared with uFSH or urinary gonadotropins[33] and no difference in OHSS as well.

PROTOCOLS FOR ASSISTED REPRODUCTIVE TECHNIQUE

Gonadotropins in Assisted Reproductive Technique

In ART cycles also, the stimulation protocol is decided by the baseline scan.

Long-agonist Protocol

Downregulation starts from the 21st day of the previous cycle as nasal spray or subcutaneous injections of GnRH agonist (leuprolide acetate 0.5 mg or decapeptyl 0.1 mg) and is continued till periods. The dose is halved from the day of the period. Depot preparations of agonist can be used instead of daily agonist injections on Day 21 of the previous cycle. The most common starting dose for COS with rFSH is 150–225/day. Increasing the dosage in elderly women does not result in increased oocyte yield.[34] It has been found that 150 IU of rFSH is equivalent to 225 IU of uFSH for follicular growth. The dose of 150 IU is optimum[31] rather than 100 IU that has been mentioned in a comparative study for IVF patients.

Short Protocol

This protocol exploits the flare-up effect of agonist during the ovarian stimulation. Agonist is started with the beginning of the menstrual cycle and flare-up provides the surge of gonadotropins' secretion. A few days later, exogenous gonadotropins are administrated to supplement the flare. Both agonist and gonadotropins are continued till the day of trigger. This protocol is preferred for poor responders.

Ultrashort Protocol

Agonist is given on Days 2, 3, and 4 of the stimulation cycle in the dose of 500–1,000 μg/day and then gonadotropins are given subsequently till the day of hCG.

Antagonist Protocol

High resistance, low-velocity stromal flow, fewer antral follicles, smaller ovarian volume, high BMI, and age > 35 years are the parameters which decide higher doses for stimulation with antagonist protocol whereas low resistance, high-velocity stromal flow, polycystic ovaries, low BMI, and age < 24 years are the parameters which would be in favor of lower doses with the antagonist protocol. Antagonist is started from Day 6 and continued till the day of trigger. In these patients, the GnRh agonist can be used for ovulation trigger, instead of hCG. This protocol reduces the incidence of OHSS significantly. This is known as fixed antagonist protocol. Antagonist can also be used as flexible protocol, when antagonist is started when at least one follicle is 14 mm in diameter.[35] Antagonist protocol has a high cumulative pregnancy rate in both groups, high anti-Müllerian hormone (AMH; 40.1–63.6%), and low AMH (11.1–18.7%).[36] A meta-analysis of 45 randomized controlled trials involving 7,511 women comparing GnRH antagonist protocol and long-agonist protocol for COS in ART has found no significant differences in live birth or ongoing pregnancy rates, but a marked decrease in OHSS with antagonist protocols.[37] Another meta-analysis comparing agonist and antagonist protocols for poor responders has shown an advantage in terms of FSH stimulation, but no statistically significant difference in terms of oocytes retrieved or clinical pregnancy rates.[38]

Antagonist-agonist Protocol

This protocol is especially used for PCOS patients. It is known as OHSS-free protocol. The fixed antagonist protocol is used for downregulation and then agonist is used for ovulation trigger.

Antagonist-agonist Protocol with Human Chorionic Gonadotropin as Luteal Support

The above-mentioned protocol is very likely to lead to luteal phase defect. It is therefore recommended to supplement the luteal phase with 1,500 IU of hCG on Day 3–7–10 of ovum pick-up.[39]

PREDICTORS OF OVARIAN RESPONSE

The predictors of ovarian response are as follows:
- Age
- Body mass index
- Baseline FSH
- AMH (not mentioned in Collin-Howles study)
- AFC

A nomogram can be prepared using these predictors. *Howles and colleagues have prepared a manuscript on the same.*[40] The cost effectivity has been mentioned in the results presented in **Table 5**. These are the results of a computer modeling study.

Individualized dose calculation for COS[36] is presented in **Table 6**.

TABLE 5: Cost effectivity of predictors of ovarian response.

	rFSH	*uFSH*
UK	5,906£	6,060£
USA (social)	40,688$	47,096$
USA (insurance)	28,481$	32,967$
Spain (public insurance)	12,791€	13,007€
Spain (private)	19,739€	20,467€
Germany	21,686€	22,189€

(rFSH: recombinant follicle-stimulating hormone; uFSH: urinary follicle-stimulating hormone)

TABLE 6: Individualized dose calculation for COS.

AMH level	*Predicted response to COS*	*Treatment strategies*
15 pmol/L	High responders (150 IU)	*GnRH antagonist protocol*: Normal oocyte yield, very low excess response, low embryo cryopreservation, high/maintained fresh CPR
5–15 pmol/L	Normal responders (225–300 IU)	*GnRH agonist protocol*: Very low cancellation of oocyte pick-up and OHSS
<5 pmol/L	Poor responders (375 IU)	*High dose FSH*: Long stimulation, high cancellation antagonist strategy; Short stimulation, moderate cancellation

(AMH: anti-Müllerian hormone; COS: controlled ovarian stimulation; CPR: clinical pregnancy rate; OHSS: ovarian hyperstimulation syndrome)

Newer Developments

- *Long-acting FSH*: Long-acting FSH is corifollitropin alpha. It keeps the FSH above the threshold level for multifollicular growth. It is convenient for the patients as they have to take less number of injections. There is no difference in live births and OHSS rate.[41]
- Sustained-release rFSH.[42]
- Oral FSH.

LUTEINIZING HORMONE SUPPLEMENTATION: FOR WHOM, WHEN, AND WHY?

Two-cell–two-gonadotropins Theory

- Both FSH and LH are required for E2 synthesis. LH binds to theca cells to induce androgen synthesis. Androgen diffuses into granulosa cells, where FSH-stimulated aromatization leads to estrogen synthesis.[43]
- LH in the follicular phase helps conversion of progesterone to androgen to reduce follicular phase progesterone, which is detrimental to endometrial receptivity.[44] A combination of rFSH and rLH in a ratio of 2:1 is indicated for women with severe gonadotropin deficiency—hypogonadotropic hypogonadism.[45]

Luteinizing Hormone Threshold

Luteinizing hormone is required for terminal stages of follicular maturation, for meiosis, and for ovulation.

Luteinizing Hormone Ceiling Effect

High LH causes follicular atresia and premature luteinization, and oocyte quality may be compromised.[46]

In patients overresponding to FSH, adding 30 mg rLH leads to monofollicular development.[47] This indicates the LH ceiling effect.

Current Opinion

- The current opinion is that there is no absolute requirement for LH supplementation in unselected patient population.[48]
- However, LH may have benefits in women aged >35 years and those who are poor responders to COS.[49] Though Cochrane review[39] and studies subsequently published have shown that LH supplementation, including for women with advanced age, has no benefit on ongoing pregnancy, with an adjusted odds ratio (OR) of 0.99 [confidence interval (CI) 0.76–1.29].[48]

- LH supplementation may improve outcomes in patients with suboptimal response to FSH stimulation.[50]
- No LH cutoff value is known to identify a female requiring LH supplementation, and LH assessment is therefore of no use.[51]
- In the antagonist cycle, LH supplementation is controversial. Though some studies have shown that it improves results in selected groups.
- LH estimation may not be a reliable guide to decide for LH supplementation because of variable bioactivity and polymorphism.

Summary

Adding LH increases the number of developmentally competent oocytes in a woman with endogenous LH suppressed below 1 IU/L at the start of stimulation. However, with LH > 1 IU/L, adding LH is associated with significantly lower embryo quality and implantation rate compared with rFSH alone.[52] Recombinant human LH (r-hLH) alone can trigger follicular growth arrest in a significant number of patients supporting the existence of LH ceiling during late follicular maturation.[53] rFSH with r-hLH 150 IU from Day 6 might be beneficial in subgroup women in the older reproductive age, having LH polymorphism and less sensitivity to LH.

The results of analysis by age showed a trend toward a higher implantation rate with rFSH alone in patients aged < 35 years. In contrast, the group aged > 35 years had a numerically higher implantation rate in the rFSH plus r-hLH group.[54,55]

Recombinant human LH supplementation on Day 8 in patients having E2 <180 pg/mL and no follicles > 10 mm significantly increases the number of oocytes retrieved, and the requirement of rFSH was also decreased.[56]

But if hCG is added to FSH from the very first day of stimulation, it increases live birth rates.[57]

In Summary

Recombinant human LH supplementation when:

- Age is >35 years.
- Poor initial response to rFSH.

CARRY HOME MESSAGE

- Gonadotropins give better pregnancy rates than clomiphene citrate.
- Step-up protocol is used for normal responding ovaries.
- Chronic low-dose protocol is best for PCOS.
- Recombinant FSH requires lower dosage with better efficacy.
- Recombinant FSH is better than all urinary preparation.
- Recombinant LH is used in poor responders and patients of age > 35 years.

REFERENCES

1. Lunenfeld B, Insler V, Rabau E. The principles of gonadotrophin therapy. Acta Endocrinol Suppl (Copenh). 1970;148:52-101.
2. Westergard LG, Erb K, Laursen SB, Rex S, Rasmussen PE. HMG versus rFSH in normogonadotrophic women down regulated with gonadotrophic releasing hormone agonist who were undergoing IVF and ICSI, a prospective randomised study. Fertil Steril. 2001;76(3):543-9.
3. Homburg R, Levy T, Ben-Rafael Z. A comparative prospective study of conventional regimen with chronic low dos administration of follicle stimulating hormone for anovulation associated with polycystic ovary syndrome. Fertil Steril. 1995;63(4):729-33.
4. Driebergen R, Baer G. Quantification of follicle stimulating hormone (follitropin alpha): is in vivo bioassay still relevant in recombinant age? Curr Med Res Opin. 2003;19:41-6.

5. Panchal S, Nagori C. Ultrasound based decision making on stimulation protocol for superovulated intrauterine insemination cycles. Int J Infertil Fetal Med. 2016;7(1):7-13.
6. Panchal S, Nagori CB. Ultrasound based decision making on stimulation protocol in IVF. Donald School J Ultrasound Obstet Gynecol. 2016;10(3):330-7.
7. Hedon B, Out HJ, Hugues JN, Camier B, Cohen J, Lopes P, et al. Efficacy and safety of recombinant follicle stimulating hormone (Puregon) in infertile women pituitary suppressed with triptorelin undergoing in-vitro fertilization: a prospective randomized, assessor-blind, multicentre trial. Hum Reprod. 1995;10:3102-6.
8. Daya S. Updated meta-analysis of recombinant follicle-stimulating hormone (FSH) versus urinary FSH for ovarian stimulation in assisted reproduction. Fertil Steril. 2002;77(4):711-4.
9. Out HJ, Driessen SG, Mannaerts BM, Coelingh Bennink HJ. Recombinant follicle-stimulating hormone (follitropin beta, Puregon) yields higher pregnancy rates in in vitro fertilization than urinary gonadotropins. Fertil Steril. 1997;68:138-42.
10. van Wely M, Kwan I, Burt AL, Thomas J, Vail A, Van der Veen F, et al. Recombinant versus urinary gonadotrophin for ovarian stimulation in assisted reproductive technology cycles. Cochrane Database Syst Rev. 2011;(2):CD005354.
11. Devroey P, Pellicer A, Andersen AN, Arce JC. A Randomized assessor-blind trial comparing highly purified hMG and recombinant FSH in a GnRh antagonist cycle with compulsory single-blastocyst transfer. Fertil Steril. 2012;97(3):561-71.
12. Bergh C, Howles CM, Borg K, Hamberger L, Josefsson B, Nilsson L, et al. Recombinant follicle stimulating hormone (r-h-FSH; Gonal-F) versus highly purified urinary FSH (Metrodin HP): results of a randomized comparative study in women undergoing assisted reproductive techniques. Hum Reprod. 1997;12:2133-9.
13. Frydman R, Haverell C, Camier B. A double blind randomized study comparing the efficacy of recombinant human (FSH: Gonal-F) versus highly purified urinary FSH (Metrodin-HP) in inducing superovulation in women undergoing assisted reproductive techniques. Hum Reprod. 1998;13:180-5.
14. XV FIGO World Congress of Gynecology and Obstetrics. Copenhagen, Denmark, 3-8 August 1997. Abstracts. Part 1. Acta Obstet Gynecol Scand Suppl. 1997;167(Pt 1):1-119.
15. Scholtes MC, Zeilmaker GH. Blastocyst transfer in day-5 embryo transfer depends primarily on the number of oocytes retrieved and not on age. Fertil Steril. 1998;69:78-83.
16. Yaralli H, Bukulmez O, Gurgan T. Urinary follicle stimulating hormone (FSH) versus recombinant FSH in clomiphene citrate resistant, normogonadotrophic, chronic anovulation: a prospective randomized study. Fertil Steril. 1999;72:276-81.
17. Bayram N, van Wely M, van der Veen F. Recombinant FSH versus urinary gonadotrophins or recombinant FSH for ovulation induction in subfertility associated with polycystic ovary syndrome. Cochrane Database Syst Rev. 2002;(1):CD002121.
18. Matorras R, Osuna C, Exposito A, Crisol L, Pijoan JL. Recombinant FSH versus highly purified FSH in intrauterine insemination: systematic review and meta-analysis. Fertil Steril. 2011;95:1937-42.
19. Daya S, Gunby J, Hughes EG, Collins JA, Sagle MA. Follicle stimulating hormone versus human menopausal gonadotrophins for in-vitro fertilization cycles: a meta-analysis. Fertil Steril. 1995;27:347-54.
20. Ludwig M, Rabe T, Buhler K, Diedrich K, Felberbaum R. Wirksamkeit von recombinanten humane FSH in Vergleich zu urinärem hMG nach Downregulation im langen Protokoll—Eine Analyse von 24.764 ART-Zyklen in Deutschland. J Reprod Med Endocrinol. 1994;4:284-8.
21. Hughes E, Collins J, Vandekerckhove P. Ovulation induction with urinary follicle stimulating hormone versus human menopausal gonadotropin for clomiphene-resistant polycystic ovary syndrome. Cochrane Database Syst Rev. 2000;(2):CD000087.

22. Coomarasamy A, Afnan M, Cheema D, van der Veen F, Bossuyt PMM, van Wely M. Urinary HMG versus recombinant FSH for controlled ovarian hyperstimulation following an agonist long down-regulation protocol in IVF or ICSI treatment: a systematic review and meta-analysis. Hum Reprod. 2008;23:310-5.
23. Al-Inany HG, Abou-Setta AM, Aboulghar MA, Mansour RT, Serour GI. Efficacy and safety of human menopausal gonadotrophins versus recombinant FSH: a meta-analysis. Reprod Biomed Online. 2008;16:81-8.
24. Lehert P, Schertz JC, Ezcurra D. Recombinant human follicle stimulating hormone produces more oocytes with low total dose per cycle in assisted reproductive technologies compared with highly purified HMG: a meta-analysis. Reprod Biol Endocrinol. 2010;8:112.
25. Filicori M, Cognigni GE, Taraborrelli S, Spettoli D, Ciampaglia W, De Fatis CT, et al. Luteinizing hormone activity in menotropins optimizes folliculogenesis and treatment in controlled ovarian stimulation. J Clin Endocrinol Metab. 2001;86(1):337-43.
26. Abd-Elaziz K, Duijkers I, Stockl L, Dietrich B, Klipping C, Eckert K, et al. A fully human recombinant FSH (Follitropin epsilon): two phase 1 randomized placebo and comparator controlled pharmacodynamic trials. Hum Reprod. 2017; 32(8):1639-47.
27. Andersen AN, Nelson SM, Fauser BCJM, Gracia-Velasco A, Klein BM, Arce JC. Individualized versus conventional ovarian stimulation for in vitro fertilization: a multicenter, randomized, controlled, assessor-blinded, phase 3 noninferiority trial. Fertil Steril. 2017;107(2):387-96.
28. Brinsden P, Akagbosu F, Gibbons LM, Lancaster S, Gourdon D, Engrand P, et al. A comparison of the efficacy and tolerability of two recombinant human follicle-stimulating hormone preparations in patients undergoing in vitro fertilization-embryo transfer. Fertil Steril. 2003;73:114-6.
29. Devroey P, Boostanfar R, Koper NP, Mannaerts BMJL, Ijzerman-Boon PC, Fauser BCJM, et al. A double blind non-inferiority RCT comparing corifollitropin alpha and rFSH during first seven days of ovarian stimulation using GnRH antagonist protocol. Hum Reprod. 2009;24(12):3063-72.
30. Balasch J, Fabergues F, Penarrubia J, Creus M, Manau D, Vidal E, et al. Outcome from consecutive assisted reproduction cycles in patients treated with recombinant follitropin alfa filled-by-bioassay and those treated with recombinant follitropin alfa filled-by-mass. Reprod Biomed Online. 2004;8:408-13.
31. Hugues JN, Barlow DH, Rosenwaks Z, Cédrin-Durnerin I, Robson S, Pidoux L, et al. Improvement in consistency of response to ovarian stimulation with recombinant human follicle stimulating hormone resulting from a new method for calibrating the therapeutic preparation. Reprod Biomed Online. 2003;6:185-90.
32. Ludwig M, Diedrich K. Evaluation of an optimal luteal phase support protocol in IVF. Obstet Gynecol Scand. 2001;80:452-66.
33. van Wely M, Kwan I, van der Veen F, Thomas J, Vail A, Van der Veen F, et al. Recombinant FSH versus urinary gonadotrophins for ovarian hyperstimulation in IVF and ICSI cycles. A systematic review and meta-analysis. Hum Reprod. 2009;24:S1-34.
34. Out HJ, Braat DD, Linsten BM, Gurgan T, Bukulmez O, Gökmen O, et al. Increasing the daily dose of recombinant follicle stimulating hormone (Puregon) does not compensate for the age-related decline in retrievable oocytes after ovarian stimulation. Hum Reprod. 2000;15:29-35.
35. Ludwig M, Katalinic A, Banz C, Schröder AK, Löning M, Weiss JM, et al. Tailoring the GnRH antagonist ceterorelix acetate to individual patients' needs in ovarian stimulation for IVF: results of a prospective, randomized study. Hum Reprod. 2002;17(11):2842-5.
36. Nelson SM, Yates RW, Lyall H, Jamieson M, Traynor I, Gaudoin M, et al. Anti-Müllerian hormone based approach to controlled ovarian stimulation for assisted conception. Hum Reprod. 2009;24:867-75.
37. Al-Inany HG, Youssef MA, Aboulghar M, Broekmans F, Sterrenburg M, Smit J, et al. Gonadotropin-releasing hormone antagonists for assisted reproductive

technology. Cochrane Database Syst Rev. 2011;5:CD001750.

38. Pu D, Wu J, Liu J. Comparison of GnRH antagonist versus GnRH agonist protocol in poor ovarian responders undergoing IVF. Hum Reprod. 2011;26(10):2742-9.
39. Humadian P, Ejdrup BH, Westergaard LG, Andersen CY. 1,500 IU human chorionic gonadotrophins administered at oocyte retrieval rescues the luteal phase when gonadotrophins-releasing hormone agonist is used for ovulation induction: a prospective randomised controlled study. Fertil Steril. 2010;93:847-54.
40. Howles CM. Predictive factors of ovarian reserve. Reprod Biomed Online. 2008; 16(S2):pS-5.
41. Pouwer AW, Farquhar C, Kremer JA. Long acting FSH versus daily FSH for women undergoing assisted reproduction. Cochrane Database Syst Rev. 2012;6:CD009577.
42. Cozzolino M, Vitagliano A, Cecchino GN, Ambrosini G, Gracia-Velasco A. Cori-follitropin alfa for ovarian stimulation in in-vitro fertilization: a systematic review and meta-analysis of review and meta-analysis of randomized controlled trials. Fertil Steril. 2019;111(4):722-33.
43. Kobayashi M, Nakano R, Ooshima A. Immunohistochemical localization of pituitary gonadotrophins and gonadal steroids confirms the 'two cell two gonadotrophins hypothesis of steroido-genesis in the human ovary. J Endocrinol. 1990;126(3):483-8.
44. Fanchin R, Righini C, Olivennes F, Taieb J, de Ziegler D, Frydman R. Computerized assessment of endometrial echogenicity: clues to the endometrial effects of premature progesterone elevation. Fertil Steril. 1999;71(1):173-81.
45. Bosch E. Recombinant human FSH and recombinant human LH in a 2:1 ratio combination: a new tool for ovulation induction. Exp Rev Obstet Gynecol. 2009;4(5):491-8.
46. Hillier SG. Current concepts of the roles of follicle stimulating hormone and luteinizing hormone in folliculogenesis. Hum Reprod. 1994;9:188-91.
47. Hughes JN, Soussis J, Calderon I, Balasch J, Anderson RA, Romeu A, et al. Recombinant LH study group 2005. Does the addition of recombinant LH in WHO group II anovulatory women over-responding to FSH treatment reduce the number of developing follicles? A dose-finding study. Hum Reprod. 2005;20:629-35.
48. Mochtar MH, Van der Veen F, Zeich M, van Wely M. Recombinant luteinizing hormone (rLH) for controlled ovarian hyperstimulation in assisted reproductive cycles. Cochrane Database Syst Rev. 2007;2:CD005070.
49. Howles CM. Luteinizing hormone supple-mentation in ART. In: Kovacs G (Ed). How to Improve Your ART Success Rates. Cambridge, UK: Cambridge University Press; 2011. pp. 99-104.
50. Lisi F, Rinaldi L, Fischel S, Lisi R, Pepe G, Picconeri MG, et al. Use of recombinant FSH and recombinant LH in multiple follicular stimulation for IVF: a preliminary study. Reprod Biomed Online. 2001;3(3):190-4.
51. Loumaye E, Engrand P, Howles CM, O'Dea L. Assessment of the role of serum luteinizing hormone an estradiol response to follicle stimulating hormone on in vitro fertilization treatment outcome. Fertil Steril. 1997;67: 889-99.
52. Tesarik J, Mendoza C. Effects of exogenous LH administration during ovarian stimulation of pituitary down regulated young oocyte donors on oocyte yield and develop-mental competence. Hum Reprod. 2002; 17:3129-37.
53. Loumaye E, Engrand P, Shoham Z, Hillier SG, Baird DT. Clinical evidence for an LH 'ceiling' effect induced by administration of recombinant human LH during the late follicular phase of stimulated cycles in World Health Organization type I and type II anovulation. Hum Reprod. 2003;18:314-22.

54. Marrs R, Meldrum D, Muasher S, Schoolcraft W, Werlin L, Kelly E. Randomized trial to compare the effect of recombinant human FSH (follitropin alfa) with or without recombinant human LH in women undergoing assisted reproduction treatment. Reprod Biomed Online. 2004;8:175-82.
55. Humadian P, Bungum M, Bungum L, Andersen CY. Effects of recombinant LH supplementation in women undergoing assisted reproduction with GnRh agonist down-regulation and stimulation with recombinant FSH: an opening study. Reprod Biomed Online. 2004;8:635-43.
56. De Placido G, Alviggi C, Mollo A, Strina I, Ranieri A, Alviggi E, et al. Effects of recombinant LH (rLH) supplementation during controlled ovarian stimulation(COH) in normogonadotrophic women with an initial inadequate response to recombinant FSH (rFSH) after pituitary downregulation. Clin Endocrinol. 2004;60:637-43.
57. Thuesen LL, Loft A, Egeberg AN, Smitz J, Petersen JH, Andersen AN. A randomized controlled dose-response pilot study of addition of hCG to recombinant FSH during COS for in vitro fertilization. Hum Reprod. 2012;27(10):3074-84.

8

Chapter

Gonadotropin-releasing Hormone Analogs

GONADOTROPIN-RELEASING HORMONE AGONISTS

INTRODUCTION

Premature luteinizing hormone (LH) surge was the common problem in assisted reproductive technology (ART) leading to cancellation of cycles and decreased pregnancy rate in the initial phase of ART era. Premature LH surge occurs because of positive feedback mechanism due to high estrogen level that is a result of multiple follicular developments. Hence, agonist was tried on the patient to resolve the problem.[1] Gonadotropin-releasing hormone agonist (GnRHa) decreases the follicle-stimulating hormone (FSH) and LH secretion from the pituitary and prevents the LH surge. It also abolishes FSH secretion, so the follicle develops only through exogenous FSH which allows the development of an optimum number of follicles by adjusting the dose of FSH.

MECHANISM OF ACTION (TABLE 1)

Gonadotropin-releasing hormone agonist causes flare-up effect initially followed by downregulation. This flare-up effect causes increased secretion of FSH and LH initially followed by decrease in their secretion if the analog is continued. Within 12 hours of administration, it liberates a high amount of FSH (5-fold increase) and LH (10-fold increase).[2] The flare-up effect can be used for short protocol and ovulation trigger.

The decrease in FSH and LH secretion is because of internalization of receptor–agonist complex and there is a reduction in the number of receptors causing reduction in FSH and LH content and release.[3]

Routes of administration: Gonadotropin-releasing hormone agonist, as mentioned in **Table 1**, can be given subcutaneously, intranasally, as depot preparation, as intramuscular (IM) injection, or as implants. Intranasal is better than daily subcutaneous (SC) injections but in rhinitis and allergy, absorption varies from patient to patient. The depot preparation as well as daily preparation achieved the same estradiol (E2) level, oocyte quality, fertilization, and pregnancy rates. But depot preparation causes prolonged desensitization, so the dose of gonadotropin and days needed are more for stimulation.[4] The effect of depot preparation may last for 8 weeks after the injection[5] and this is the reason for giving low implantation and pregnancy rate. The depot preparation might interfere with luteal phase and embryo development. In a recent meta-analysis, it has been found that pregnancy rates are same, but it required longer days of stimulation and more number of gonadotropins and therefore not advocated in terms of cost-effectiveness.[4]

Lahat et al. reported a high incidence of attention-deficit hyperactivity disorder in long-term follow-up of children exposed to GnRHa early in pregnancy especially as depot preparation.[6]

TABLE 1: Dose and route of administration of different GnRh agonists.

GnRHa	*Dose*	*Route*
Decapeptyl	100–500 mg/day	SC
Triptorelin	3.75 mg depot	IM
Naperelin	400 mg bd	Nasal
Goserelin	3.6 mg/month	SC/implant
Buserelin	300–400 mg	Intranasal
	200–500 mg	SC
Leuprolide	0.5–1 mg daily	SC
	3.75 ng/month	IM

(GnRHa: gonadotropin-releasing hormone agonist; IM: intramuscular; SC: subcutaneous)

GONADOTROPIN-RELEASING HORMONE AGONIST PROTOCOLS FOR ASSISTED REPRODUCTIVE TECHNOLOGY

- Long protocol
- Short protocol
- Ultrashort protocol
- Microdose protocol

Long Protocol

Gonadotropin-releasing hormone agonist is started from the midluteal phase, i.e., Day 21 of the cycle. Leuprolide acetate 1 mg daily can be given to the patient or a depot preparation of 3.75 mg can be given. This 1-mg dose is continued till the patient gets periods. Normally, the patient gets period after 7–10 days. The period comes when there is adequate downregulation. At this stage, the E2 level will be between 30 and 50 pg/mL. LH < 2.5 IU/L and endometrium will be single line (<4 mm). Gonadotropins are started from Day 2 of menstruation. The dose is decided based on ultrasound parameters in our practice, but other workers may decide the dose of gonadotropins based on anti-Müllerian hormone (AMH) levels or age and AMH together. As the pituitary is already downregulated, the dose of GnRHa can be reduced to half in the daily dose protocol (0.25–0.5 mg daily). This dose is given till the day of ovulation trigger. According to Nelson et al.,[7] a long protocol is best used for normal responding patients having AMH levels between 5 and 15 pmol/L.

The advantage of a long protocol is that it almost abolishes unwanted LH surge, prevents cancellation of cycles, and improves pregnancy rates that were about 20–30%.[8] With this long protocol, follicles develop depending on exogenous FSH dosage so there is complete elimination of endogenous control of sequences of follicular recruitment and selection. This leads to synchronization of the cohort of follicles, and the time for pickup can be adjusted. Majority of the studies have proved that a long protocol gives better results than short or ultrashort protocols.[9] The disadvantage of this protocol is that it requires more total doses of gonadotropins and longer duration of treatment. As there is initial flare-up for about 3 days because of an increase in FSH and LH, there may be cyst formation. High E2 and LH due to this may rescue corpus luteum giving high progesterone levels on the starting day of gonadotropin stimulation. In these cases, stimulation may have to be delayed till the cyst and corpus luteum resolve. Corpus luteum can lead to luteinization of small follicles and in some cases may also cause ovulation. Pretreatment with oral contraceptive (OC) pills for 14 days prior to starting GnRHa can reduce the cyst formation without negative effect on pregnancy rates.[10] But recent studies have shown that prior treatment with OC pills can reduce the pregnancy rates.

Downregulation can be confirmed by:

- Estradiol < 30 pg/mL
- LH < 2.5 IU/L
- Progesterone < 2 ng/mL
- Endometrial thickness < 4 mm

Short Protocol

In short protocol, 1 mg of leuprolide acetate is given daily from Day 1 or 2 of the menstrual cycle. Gonadotropins are started from Day 2 or Day 3, i.e., 1 day after the agonist is started. Agonist is continued till the day of trigger with gonadotropins. This protocol is used for poor responders and the advantage is that the initial flare-up effect can be used for development of the follicle. It is less expensive and has a lower incidence of ovarian hyperstimulation syndrome (OHSS), but does not give a big homogeneous cohort of follicles. The other disadvantage is that it can also rescue the corpus luteum of the previous cycle. It can cause luteinization of small follicles because of high levels of progesterone due to high FSH and LH and can also lead to ovulation from bigger mature follicles. Prolonged downregulation for >28 days may improve the endometrial receptivity and may increase the pregnancy rate. Quiet endometrium in postmenopausal patients also increases the pregnancy rate. Therefore, OC pills or progesterone should be given before starting the short protocol.[11]

Ultrashort Protocol

In ultrashort protocol, GnRHa is started from Day 1–2 of the menstruation in a dose of 0.5–1 mg/day. It is given for 3 days only. Gonadotropins are started from Day 2 or 3, i.e., 1 day after GnRHa is started. In this protocol, the advantage of the flare-up effect is taken for stimulation of the follicles. It decreases the dose of agonist as well as gonadotropins and thus decreases the cost and risk of OHSS. However, the disadvantage is the higher chance of a premature LH surge as the agonist is not continued. This also gives poor pregnancy rates.

Microdose Flare Protocol

Microdose flare protocol is the short protocol in which the dose of agonist is reduced to quarter of the short protocol. Instead of 200 µg of daily dose, only 50 µg is given daily.[12] Moreover, GnRHa can be stopped when gonadotropin is started. Suppression lasts up to gonadotropin introduction, but more studies are required for this protocol.[13,14]

CLINICAL APPLICATION OF GONADOTROPIN-RELEASING HORMONE AGONIST

The long protocol has a better pregnancy rate than short or ultrashort protocol.[15,16] Pregnancy rates are equivalent to antagonist protocols.[17] It has low cycle cancellation and high oocyte recovery rates. But it is associated with high gonadotropin consumption, increased cost due to increased days of stimulation, increased incidence of OHSS, and cyst formation. Ultrashort protocols are used for poor responders, but have poor pregnancy rates because of premature LH surge.

All GnRHa protocols cause luteal phase defect, and judicious luteal support should be given. This is discussed in the Chapter 23. GnRHa can be used as ovulation trigger. This is also discussed in detail in the Chapter 10.

When a long protocol is used, there is profound suppression of LH. When recombinant FSH (rFSH) is used for stimulation of follicles, in a subgroup of patients, supplementation of LH can improve the pregnancy rate. Comparison of short protocol or microdose protocol for poor responders versus antagonist protocol shows that there is no difference in pregnancy outcome.

There is no clear-cut advantage of GnRHa + gonadotropins than gonadotropins alone.[18] The advantages of agonist therapy are as follows:

- Multiple follicles, more embryos
- Prevents LH surge due to high E2
- No spontaneous ovulation
- Less cycle cancellation
- Flexibility of time to start stimulation and ovum pick up

There is no advantage of discontinuing GnRHa earlier. It may have a deleterious effect.[19,20] A continuous-long protocol in the luteal phase has given higher pregnancy rates.[21] But the short protocol increases the ovarian response. However, early release of androgen declines oocyte quality giving lower pregnancy rates.[22]

Delaying human chorionic gonadotropin (hCG) trigger for >2 days after more than three follicles of >17 mm diameter, are seen by ultrasound, is associated with poor pregnancy rates.[23]

Other uses of GnRHa are as follows:

- *Ovulation trigger*
- *Endometriosis*: For 3 months before in vitro fertilization (IVF)
- *Fibroid*: Not used as primary treatment
- *Precocious puberty*: Depot preparation are used
- Gonadal protection during chemotherapy[24]
- Metabolic prostatic cancer
- Breast cancer
- Hirsutism

CARRY HOME MESSAGE

- The long protocol abolishes the LH surge.
- Initial flare-up is utilized in short and ultrashort protocols.
- Pregnancy rates are highest in long protocol than short or ultrashort protocol.
- The long protocol can cause cyst formation, rescue corpus luteum with high progesterone, and requires more gonadotropins for stimulation.
- Daily doses are better than depot preparation in the long protocol.
- Ovarian hyperstimulation syndrome incidence is high in the long protocol.
- Judicious luteal support is required in agonist trigger.
- Because of low LH, the subgroup is benefitted by adding LH.

GONADOTROPIN-RELEASING HORMONE ANTAGONIST

INTRODUCTION

Premature LH surge was common in up to 20–50% of cases of IVF with gonadotropin stimulation. With the advent of GnRHa in the early 1980s,[25] it was the breakthrough in prevention of LH surge and allowed consultants for more flexible oocyte retrievals.[26] GnRHa was available at that time, but did not get much popularity due to allergic reaction due to its histamine-release property.[27] The use of GnRHa became universal in the 1980s, 1990s, and 2000s. But the development of third-generation antagonist has completely changed the line of treatment in ART.

MECHANISM OF ACTION

There are two different antagonists available commercially since 1999: (1) Cetrorelix (cetrotide from Merck) and (2) ganirelix (Orgalutran from Organon). It acts as a complete blocker for GnRH receptors and so blocks native GnRH that ultimately stops the release of FSH and LH from pituitary. It immediately blocks gonadotropin release and its action is reversible. LH falls by 70% and FSH by 30% within 6 hours of antagonist administration. Complete reversal of action occurs in 24–72 hours. The incidence of LH surge is extremely rare if the dose is not missed. Any imminent LH surge is blocked within 6–8 hours of administration.

ENDOCRINE CHANGES IN THE ANTAGONIST CYCLE

The progesterone level may be high (5% cases) on the day of stimulation in a spontaneous ovulatory cycle. Even if we postpone the stimulation for 1 or 2 days, the progesterone level will normalize but the pregnancy rates are low compared with normal levels.[28] The same is true if the E2 level is high because of the follicular cyst on Day 2. In both these situations, postponing of IVF cycle is advisable.

DOSAGE OF ANTAGONIST

- Daily dose scheme (Day 1-5-6-7)
- Single-dose scheme (depot)

In a daily dose scheme, 0.25 mg of cetrorelix or ganirelix is given daily. In a single-dose scheme, cetrorelix is given as 3-mg dose that inhibits LH surge for 4 days. Both daily dose and single-dose schemes give an equivalent pregnancy rate.[29] The fixed protocol is also known as French protocol. It is given on Day 7. It lasts for 4 days. If there are no mature follicles to give trigger, a single dose of 0.25 mg cetrorelix is given till the day of trigger.[30] In the fixed protocol, the antagonist is started from Day 6, 0.25 mg cetrorelix. The disadvantage of the fixed day is in polycystic ovary syndrome (PCOS) patients and poor responders. Here, if follicular development is unnecessarily late, more antagonists are used and may also increase the consumption of gonadotropins.

TIMING OF ANTAGONIST

Gonadotropin-releasing hormone antagonist can be given as a fixed protocol or flexible protocol. The argument for a fixed protocol is the knowledge that after certain days of stimulation with gonadotropins, LH starts rising in majority of the patients and so it should be started on fixed days routinely. Formerly, it was considered as the 6th day of stimulation.[31] But now recent studies have shown that it should be started from Day 5 of stimulation.[32] A fixed protocol is simpler and requires less monitoring (also known as Ludwig's protocol). The flexible antagonist protocol depends on endocrine and ultrasound criteria, which indicate the rise of LH. Antagonist is given when the size of the follicle is ≥14 mm.[33] The advantage of flexible criteria is that it can avoid unnecessary administration of GnRH antagonist and gonadotropin from Day 5 when LH surge is not going to occur as the follicle development was inadequate. There is no significant difference in the clinical pregnancy rate in flexible as well as the fixed protocol.[34,35] The flexible protocol should not start after Day 8. In patients with PCOS, the LH level is high even before antagonist is added in the fixed or flexible protocol. This early rise of LH may be detrimental and decrease the pregnancy rates so antagonist is started earlier, i.e., Day 2 has an advantage in these patients.

Breakthrough in LH surge can occur in spite of GnRH antagonist in patients with diminished ovarian reserve, but the dose of antagonist can be doubled in the subsequent cycle. When the LH level is <300 pg/mL or >1,100 pg/mL on the day of start of antagonist, it gives poor results.[36]

ADVANTAGES OF ANTAGONIST

- It is patient-friendly and has a high efficacy.
- There is no estrogen deprivation or cyst formation.
- The action of antagonist is immediate.
- The incidence of OHSS is decreased with the antagonist. It is decreased to >50%.[37] When the antagonist is used for downregulation, an agonist can be used as a trigger and this reduces the risk of OHSS to almost zero.[38] Here, all eggs are frozen or judicious luteal support is given.
- Coasting is very effective in the antagonist protocol with equivalent pregnancy rates.[39]
- It can avoid oocyte retrievals on weekends and avoid initiation of many cycles and the load for the center. Stimulation can be started on Day 3 instead of Day 2 and can give trigger also a day later.
- It has no teratogenic or other adverse effects on implantation or embryonic development.[40]
- The duration of treatment is short and the dose of gonadotropin is also reduced, thus reducing the cost of treatment.

DISADVANTAGES OF ANTAGONIST

- Delay of hCG for more than 2 days after three follicles of 17 mm on ultrasound is associated with a significantly decreased probability of pregnancy.[23]
- Pretreatment with OC pills is not to be used in antagonist cycles as there is a decreased probability of pregnancy when OC pills are used and it also increases the duration of stimulation required and cost to the patient.[41] Apart from pregnancy rate, it results in higher pregnancy loss and so OC pills' pretreatment is not recommended.[42] But the short course of 10–12 days does not affect the results.
- The lower pregnancy rate in the antagonist cycle reported earlier in some studies was because clinicians were less trained in using antagonist and a learning curve was required.[43]

EVIDENCE FOR GONADOTROPIN-RELEASING HORMONE AGONIST/ ANTAGONIST (TABLE 2)[44]

In the initial trials, the Cochrane library suggested that the use of antagonist was associated with a significantly lower chance of pregnancy compared to agonists.[45] But the explanation given by the German registry was that antagonists were used in poor responders as well as in patients having multiple failures and aged patients. So, the results of antagonists in terms of clinical pregnancy were poor.[46] In 2011, the Cochrane group published that there was no significant difference in the clinical pregnancy rate in the antagonist group and agonist group. The recent meta-analysis suggested that the use of antagonist is justified because of the equivalent pregnancy rate with agonist and increased safety in antagonist cycles.[47,48] Pregnancy rates were the same with flexible protocols as compared to long protocols. Similarly, even fixed protocols of antagonist had the same clinical pregnancy rates.[49] It is clear from this publication that the GnRHa era has come to an end.

TABLE 2: Comparison of agonists and antagonists.

GnRH agonist	*GnRH antagonist*
Molecular effects	
Downregulation of receptors	Inhibition of receptors without any activation
Desensitization of pituitary	Competitive antagonism
Flare-up response initially followed by downregulation	Immediate suppression
Slowly reversible response	Rapid reversible response
Clinical implications	
Longer IVF regimen	Shorter IVF regimen
Time-consuming and more expensive	Less time and less expensive
More injections, inconvenient to the patient	Fewer injections increase patient compliance
No endogenous LH surge	Induction of endogenous LH

(GnRH: gonadotropin-releasing hormone; IVF: in vitro fertilization; LH: luteinizing hormone)

Antagonists are administered in the later half of the follicular phase and hence profound suppression of pituitary does not occur. So, this is very useful in poor responders. Antagonist is the drug of choice in poor responders. This protocol is as effective as short, ultrashort, or microdose protocol.[12] GnRH antagonist versus long protocol was studied in a meta-analysis which analyzed that the antagonist protocol gives higher oocytes yield.[50] Addition of letrozole also decreases cancellation and total gonadotropin dosage.[51]

RECENT ADVANCES IN ANTAGONIST USAGE

- It can be used in a modified natural cycle or mild stimulation IVF.[52]
- Agonist trigger with a freeze-all policy can completely abolish OHSS.[37]
- Reinitiation of antagonist in case of severely established OHSS is possible.[53]
- Long-acting FSH can be used in antagonist cycles making stimulation more simplified. In 2018, the United States Food and Drug Administration (US FDA) has approved oral GnRHa. This is very useful in estrogen-dependent diseases, for oral contraception, and also for postcoital contraception. All noncontraceptive uses can be replaced by orally acting antagonists. Daily injections can be avoided and it abolishes the LH surge, so it will be a "game changer."

DOSAGE OF GONADOTROPINS

The starting dose of 150 IU is generally considered optimum for typical normal responding patients. Pregnancy rates are not increased by using higher doses.[54] Stimulation can be started from Day 2 or 3 while in mild stimulation, it is to be started from Day 5. There is no need to increase the dose of FSH from the day of antagonist initiation. There is no increase in pregnancy rate by increasing gonadotropin dosage.[55,56] The addition of LH at the time of initiation of antagonist has not given increased pregnancy rates in three meta-analyses.[57,58] LH is added only in the subgroup of patients as discussed in Chapter 13.

ADDITION OF LUTEINIZING HORMONE IN OVULATION INDUCTION

Low LH levels in antagonist cycles are not the indication of the addition of LH.[59] Clomiphene citrate with FSH or human menopausal gonadotropin (hMG) in the antagonist protocol had a lower pregnancy rate and were not cost-effective too.[60]

LUTEAL SUPPORT IN THE ANTAGONIST CYCLE

Formerly, it was believed that the antagonist cycle does not require luteal support, but because of gonadotropin stimulation irrespective of the analog used all patients required luteal support.[61] But E2 supplementation did not increase the pregnancy rate.[62]

Progesterone for prevention of LH surge: Medroxyprogesterone acetate (MPA) can be used to prevent ovulation without compromising oocyte quality. It is started from Day 7 or the lead follicle is 14 mm in dose of 5 mg twice a day.[63,64]

Luteal Phase Estrogen Pretreatment

Luteal phase pretreatment in antagonist cycle programming gives flexibility for starting day and weekends can be avoided for oocyte retrieval. Estradiol valerate is administered 2 mg bd from Day 25 of the previous cycle onwards during 6–10 days. Pregnancy rates arc comparable with control group. So stimulation can be started on Day 2-3-4-5.[65]

Antagonist in Gynecological Conditions

- 3 mg cetrorelix is administered weekly for 8 weeks. E2 is maintained between 50–60 pg/mL. It reduces the size of fibroids and surgery can be avoided or postponed.[66]
- Linzagolix reduces size and pain of adenomyosis. It can be used in patients resistant to ulipristal acetate. It reduces E2 and endometrial thickness and can be an alternative to surgery.[67]
- Elagolix, relugolix and linzagolix are used for reduction in size of fibroid which is dose dependent. It reduces E2 level and so add-back therapy id given to relieve symptoms of hypoestrinism.
- Elagolix is tried as 15 mg/day as low dose of 200 mg twice daily (high dose) in endometriosis.[68]
- Antagonists are useful in endometrial and ovarian cancer and in prostate cancer in male.

CARRY HOME MESSAGE

- Agonist can be used as a trigger in the antagonist cycle.
- The incidence of OHSS is extremely rare.
- The pregnancy rate is the same as the agonist cycle in spite of a low E2 level with antagonist.
- The treatment cost is reduced because of the lesser number of days of stimulation in the antagonist cycle.
- The antagonist is very useful in the mild stimulation protocol, poor responders, or modified natural cycles.
- Luteal support is a must in all antagonist cycles.

REFERENCES

1. Porter RN, Smith W, Craft IL, Abdulwahid NA, Jacobs HS. Induction of ovulation for in-vitro fertilization using buserelin and gonadotropins. Lancet. 1984;2:1284-5.
2. Lemey A, Maheror F. Development and application of LHRH agonist (Buserelin) as a new therapeutic approach for endometriosis. Fertil Steril. 1984;41:863-74.
3. Pelletier G, Dube D, Guy J, Séguin C, Lefebvre FA. Binding and internalization of a luteinizing hormone-releasing hormone agonist by rat gonadotrophic cells. A radioautographic study. Endocrinology. 1982;111:1068-76.
4. Albuquerque LE, Saconato H, Maciel MC. Depot versus daily administration of

gonadotrophin releasing hormone agonist protocols for pituitary desensitization in assisted reproduction cycles. Cochrane Database Syst Rev. 2005;25(1):CD002808.

5. Broekmans FJ, Bernardus RE, Berkhout G, Schoemaker J. Pituitary and ovarian suppression after early follicular and mid-luteal administration of a LHRH agonist in a depot formulation: Decapeptyl CR. Gynecol Endocrinol. 1992;6:153-61.
6. Lahat E, Raziel A, Friedler S, Schieber-Kazir M, Ron-El R. Long-term follow-up of children born after inadvertent exposure to long acting gonadotrophin releasing hormone agonist in early pregnancy. Hum Reprod. 1999;14:2656-60.
7. Nelson SM, Yates RW, Lyall H, Jamieson M, Traynor I, Gaudoin M, et al. Anti-Müllerian hormone based approach to controlled ovarian stimulation for assisted conception. Hum Reprod. 2009;24:867-75.
8. Akagbosu FT. The use of GnRH agonists in infertility. In: Brinsden R (Ed). A Textbook of In Vitro Fertilization and Assisted Reproduction, 2nd edition. USA: Parthenon Publishing; 1999. pp. 83-9.
9. Tan SL. Luteinizing hormone-releasing hormone agonist for ovarian stimulation in assisted reproduction. Curr Opin Obstet Gynecol. 1994;6:166-72.
10. Biljan MM, Mahutte NG, Dean N, Hemmings R, Bissonnette F, Tan SL. Effects of pretreatment with an oral contraceptive on the time required to achieve pituitary suppression with gonadotrophin-releasing hormone analogues and on subsequent implantation and pregnancy rates. Fertil Steril. 1998;70(6):1063-9.
11. Cedrin-Durnerin I, Bulwa S, Herve F, Martin-Pont B, Uzan M, Hugues JN. The hormonal flare up following gonadotrophin-releasing hormone agonist administration is influenced by a progesterone pretreatment. Hum Reprod. 1996;11:1859-63.
12. Kahraman K, Berkar B, Atabekoglu CS, Sonmezer M, Cetinkaya E, Aytac R, et al. Microdose gonadotropin-releasing hormone agonist flare up protocol versus multiple dose gonadotropin-releasing hormone antagonist protocol in poor responders undergoing intracytoplasmic sperm injection-embryo transfer cycle. Fertil Steril. 2009;91(6):2437-44.
13. Filicori M, Flamigini C, Cognigni GE, Falbo A, Arnone R, Capelli M, et al. Different gonadotropin and leuprorelin ovulation induction regimen markedly affect follicular fluid hormone levels and folliculogenesis. Fertil Steril. 1996;65:387-93.
14. Pantos K, Meimeth-Damianaki T, Vaxevanoglou T, Kapetanakis E. Prospective study of modified GnRH long protocol in an IVF program. Fertil Steril. 1994;64:709-13.
15. Frydman R, Belaisch-Allart J, Parneix I, Forman R, Hazout A, Testart J. Comparison between flare up and down regulation effect of luteinizing hormone-releasing hormone agonists in in vitro fertilization program. Fertil Steril. 1988;50:471-5.
16. Maheshwari A, Caserta D, Siristatidis CS, Bhattacharya S. Gonadotropin-releasing hormone agonist protocols for pituitary suppression in assisted reproduction. Cochrane Database Syst Rev. 2011;(8): CD006919.
17. Arslan M, Bocca S, Mirkin S, Barroso G, Stadtmauer L, Oehninger S. Controlled ovarian hyperstimulation protocols for in vitro fertilization: two decades of experience after the birth of Elizabeth Carr. Fertil Ateril. 2005;84(3):555-69.
18. School DC, Pijlman B, Stijnen T, Fauser BC. Effects of gonadotropin releasing hormone agonist addition to gonadotropin induction of ovulation in polycystic ovary syndrome patients. Eur J Obstet Gynecol Reprod Biol. 1992;45:53-8.
19. Cedrin-Durnerin I, Bidart JM, Robert P, Wolf JP, Uzan M, Hugues JN. Consequences on gonadotropin secretion of an early discontinuation of gonadotropin releasing hormone agonist administration in short-tern protocol for in vitro fertilization. Hum Reprod. 2000;15:1009-14.
20. Dirnfeld M, Fruchter O, Yshai D, Lissak A, Ahdut A, Abramovici H. Cessation of gonadotropin-releasing hormone analogue (GnRH-a) upon down-regulation versus conventional long GnRH-a protocol in poor

responders undergoing in vitro fertilization. Fertil Steril. 1999;72:406-11.

21. Fujii S, Sato S, Fukui A, Kimura H, Kasai G, Saito Y. Continuous administration of gonadotropin releasing hormone agonist during the luteal phase in IVF. Hum Reprod. 2011;16:1671-5.
22. Loumaye E, Coen G, Pampfer S, Vankrieken L, Thomas K. Use of gonadotropin releasing hormone agonist, during ovarian stimulation leads to significant concentration of peptide in follicular fluids. Fetil Steril. 1989;52:256-63.
23. Kolibianakis EM, Albano C, Camus M, Tournaye H, Van Steirteghem AC, Devroey P. Prolongation of follicular phase in in vitro fertilization results in a lower ongoing pregnancy rate in cycles stimulated with recombinant follicle-stimulating hormone and gonadotropin releasing hormone antagonists. Fertil Steril. 2004;82:102-7.
24. Chen H, Li J, Cui T. Adjuvant gonadotropin-releasing hormone analogues for chemotherapy induced premature ovarian failure in premenopausal women. Cochrane Database Syst Rev. 2011;(11):CD008018.
25. Janssens RM, Lambalk CB, Vermeiden JP, Schats R, Bernards JM, Rekers-Mombarg LT, et al. Dose-finding study of triptorelin acetate for prevention of a premature LH surge in IVF: a prospective, randomized, double-blind placebo-controlled study. Hum Reprod. 2000;15:2333-40.
26. Meldrum DR. Ovulation induction protocols. Arch Pathol Lab Med. 1992;116:406-9.
27. Rivier J. Novel antagonist of GnRH: a compendium of their physicochemical properties, activities, relative potencies and efficacy in humans. In: Insler V, Lunenfeld B (Eds). GnRH Analogues: The State of The Art 1993, 1st edition. New York, USA: Parthenon Publishing; 1993. pp. 13-26.
28. Kolibianakis EM, Venetis CA, Bontis J, Tarlatzis BC. Significantly lower pregnancy rates in the presence of progesterone elevation in patients treated with GnRH antagonists and gonadotrophins: a systematic review and meta-analysis. Curr Pharm Biotechnol. 2102;13:464-70.
29. Lee TH, Wu MY, Chen HF, Chen MJ, Ho HN, Yang YS. Ovarian response and follicular development for single dose and multiple dose protocols for gonadotropin releasing hormone antagonist administration. Fertil Steril. 2005;83:1700-7.
30. Olivennes F, Fanchin R, Bouchard P, Selva J, Frydman R. Scheduled administration of gonadotropin-releasing hormone antagonist (Cetrorelix) on day 8 of in vitro fertilization cycles: a pilot study. Hum Reprod. 1995;10(6):1382-6.
31. Borm G, Mannaerts B. Treatment with the gonadotropin releasing hormone antagonist ganirelix in women undergoing ovarian stimulation with recombinant follicle stimulating hormone is effective, safe and convenient: results of a controlled, randomized, multicenter trial. The European Orgalutran Study group. Hum Reprod. 2000;15:1490-8.
32. A double-blind, randomized, dose-finding study to assess the efficacy of the gonadotrophin-releasing hormone antagonist ganirelix (Org 37462) to prevent premature luteinizing hormone surges in women undergoing ovarian stimulation with recombine T follicle stimulating hormone (Puregon). Hum Reprod. 1998;13:3023-31.
33. Ludwig M, Katalinic A, Banz C, Schröder AK, Löning M, Weiss JM, et al. Tailoring the GnRH antagonist cetrorelix acetate to individual patient's needs in ovarian stimulation for IVF: results of a prospective, randomized study. Hum Reprod. 2002;17(11):2842-5.
34. Kolibianakis EM, Venetis CA, Kalogeropoulou L, Papanikolaou E, Tarlatzis BC. Fixed versus flexible gonadotropin releasing hormone antagonist administration in in vitro fertilization: a randomized controlled trial. Fertil Steril. 2011;95:558-62.
35. Escudero E, Bosch E, Crespo J, Simón C, Remohí J, Pellicer A. Comparison of two different starting multiple dose gonadotropin releasing hormone antagonist protocols in a selected group of in vitro fertilization-embryo transfer patients. Fertil Steril. 2004;81:562-6.
36. Brianna M, Schumaker L, Merseseau JE, Steiner AZ. Cycle day oestrogen level and lead

follicular size: analysis of 27790 IVF cycles to determine optimal start criteria for GnRh antagonist. Fertil Steril. 2018;109:633-7.
37. Kolibianakis EM, Collins J, Tarlatzis BC, Devroey P, Diedrich K, Griesinger G. Amongst patients treated for IVF with gonadotropins and GnRH analogues, is the probability of live birth dependent on the type of analogue used? A systematic review and meta-analysis. Hum Reprod Update. 2006;12:651-71.
38. Griensinger G, Diedrich K, Tarlatzis BC, Kolibianakis EM. GnRH antagonists in ovarian stimulation for IVF in patients with poor response to gonadotropins, polycystic ovary syndrome, and high risk of hyperstimulation: a meta-analysis. Reprod Biomed Online. 2006;13:628-38.
39. Aboulghar MA, Mansour RT, Amin YM, Al-Inany HG, Aboulghar MM, Serour GI. A prospective randomized study comparing coasting with GnRH antagonist administration in patients at risk for severe OHSS. Reprod Biomed Online. 2007;15:271-9.
40. Fluker M, Grifo J, Leader A, Levy M, Meldrum D, Muasher SJ, et al. Efficacy and safety of ganirelix acetate versus leuprolide acetate in women undergoing controlled ovarian hyperstimulation. Fertil Steril. 2001;75(1):38-45.
41. Griesinger G, Kolibianakis EM, Venetis C, Diedrich K, Tarlatzis B. Oral contraceptive pretreatment significantly reduces the ongoing pregnancy likelihood in gonadotropin-releasing hormone antagonist cycles: an updated meta-analysis. Fertil Steril. 2010;94:2382-4.
42. Kolibianakis EM, Papanikolaou EG, Camus M, Tournaye H, Van Steirteghem AC, Devroey P. Effect of oral contraceptive pill pretreatment on ongoing pregnancy rates in patients stimulated with GnRH antagonists and recombinant FSH for IVF: a randomized controlled trial. Hum Reprod. 2006;21:352-7.
43. Homburg R. Controlled ovarian stimulation for IVF and ICSI. Ovulation Induction and Controlled Ovarian Stimulation: A Practical Guide. Switzerland: Springer International Publishing; 2014. pp. 143-59.
44. Thakker SK, Allahbadia G, Allahbadia A. GnRH agonists versus GnRH antagonists for ovarian stimulation: pros and cons. In: Allahbadia G, Merchant R (Eds). Manual of Ovulation Induction and Ovarian Stimulation Protocols, 3rd edition. New Delhi: Jaypee Brothers Medical Publishers Ltd.; 2016. pp. 181-9.
45. Al-Inany H, Aboulghar M. Gonadotropin-releasing hormone antagonists for assisted conception. Cochrane Database Syst Rev. 2001;4:CD001750.
46. Griesinger G, Felberbaum R, Diedrich K. GnRH antagonists in ovarian stimulation: a treatment regimen of clinicians' second choice? Data from the German national IVF registry. Hum Reprod. 2005;20:2373-5.
47. Tarlatzis BC, Fauser BC, Kolibianakis EM, Diedrich K, Devroey P. GnRH antagonists in ovarian stimulation for IVF. Hum Reprod Update. 2006;12:333-40.
48. Al-Inany HG, Aboulghar M, Mansour R, Serour GI. Optimizing GnRH antagonist administration: meta-analysis of fixed vs flexible protocol. Reprod Biomed Online. 2005;10:567-70.
49. Al-Inany HG, Youssef MA, Aboulghar M, Broekmans F, Sterrenburg M, Smit J, et al. Gonadotropin-releasing hormone antagonists for assisted reproductive technology. Cochrane Database Syst Rev. 2011;(5):CD001750.
50. Franco JG Jr, Baruffi RL, Mauri AL, Petersen CG, Felipe V, Cornicelli J, et al. GnRH agonist versus GnRH antagonist in poor ovarian responders: a meta-analysis. Reprod Biomed Online. 2006;13:618-27.
51. Ozmen B, Sonmezer M, Atabekoglu CS, Olmus H. Use of aromatase inhibitors in poor responder patients receiving GnRH antagonist protocols. Reprod Biomed Online. 2009;19:478-85.
52. Pelinck MJ, Knol HM, Vogel NEA, Arts EGJM, Simons AHM, Heineman MJ, et al. Cumulative pregnancy rates after sequential treatment with modified natural cycle IVF followed by IVF with controlled ovarian stimulation. Hum Reprod. 2008;23:1808-14.

53. Lainas T, Sfontouris IA, Zorzocilis IZ, Petsas GK, Lainas GT, Alexopoulou E, et al. Live births after management of severe OHSS by GnRH antagonist administration in luteal phase. Reprod Biomed Online. 2009;19:789-95.
54. Wikland M, Bergh C, Borg K, Hillensjö T, Howles CM, Knutsson A, et al. A prospective randomized comparison of two starting doses of recombinant FSH in combination with cetrorelix in women undergoing ovarian stimulation for IVF/ICSI. Hum Reprod. 2001;16:1676-81.
55. Propst AM, Bates GW, Robinson RD, Arthur NJ, Martin JE, Neal GS. A randomized controlled trial of increasing recombinant follicle-stimulating hormone after initiating a gonadotropin releasing hormone antagonist for in vitro fertilization-embryo transfer. Fertil Steril. 2006;86:58-63.
56. Aboulghar MA, Mansour RT, Serour GI, Al-Inany HG, Amin YM, Aboulghar MM. Increasing the dose of human menopausal gonadotropins in the day of GnRH antagonist administration: randomized controlled trial. Reprod Biomed Online. 2004;8:524-7.
57. Baruffi RL, Mauri AL, Petersen CG, Martins AM, Cornicelli J, Cavagna M, et al. Recombinant LH supplementation to recombinant FSH during induced ovarian stimulation in the GnRH antagonist protocol: a meta-analysis. Reprod Biomed Online. 2007;14:14-25.
58. Mochtar MH, Van der V, Ziech M, van Wely M. Recombinant luteinizing hormone (rLH) for controlled ovarian hyperstimulation in assisted reproductive cycles. Cochrane Database Syst Rev. 2007;(2):CD005070.
59. Kolibianakis EM, Collins J, Tarlatzis B, Devroey P. Are endogenous LH levels during ovarian stimulation for IVF using GnRH analogues associated with the probability of ongoing pregnancy? A systematic review. Hum Reprod Update. 2006;12:3-12.
60. Engel JB, Ludwig M, Felberbaum R, Albano C, Devroey P, Diedrich K. Use of Cetrorelix in combination with clomiphene citrate and gonadotropins: a suitable approach to 'friendly' IVF? Hum Reprod. 2002;17:2011-26.
61. Beckers NG, Macklon NS, Eijkemans MJ, Ludwig M, Felberbaum RE, Klaus Diedrich K, et al. Nonsupplemented luteal phase characteristics after the administration of recombinant human chorionic gonadotropin, recombinant luteinizing hormone, or gonadotropin- releasing hormone (GnRH) agonist to induce final oocyte maturation in in vitro fertilization patients after ovarian stimulation with recombinant follicle stimulating hormone and GnRH antagonist co-treatment. J Clin Endocrinol Metab. 2003;88:4186-92.
62. Kolibianakis EM, Venetis CA, Papanilolaou E, Diedrich K, Tarlatzis BC, Griesinger G. Estrogen addition to progesterone for luteal phase support in cycles stimulated with GnRH analogues and gonadotropins for IVF: a systematic review and meta-analysis. Hum Reprod. 2008;23:1346-54.
63. Yildiz S, Turkgeldi E, Angun B, Eraslan A, Urman B. Comparison of a novel flexible progestin primed ovarian stimulation protocol and the flexible gonadotrophin releasing hormone antagonist protocol for assisted reproductive technology. Fertil Steril. 2019;112(4):677-83
64. Begueria R, Garcia D, Vassena R, Rodriguez A. Medroxyprogesterone acetate versus ganirelix in oocyte donation: a randomized controlled trial. Hum Reprod. 2019;34(5):872-80.
65. Blockeel C, Engels S, De Vos M et al. Oestradiol valerate pretreatment in GnRH antagonist cycles: a randomized controlled trial. Reprod Biomed Online. 2012;24(3):272-80.
66. Kupker W, Felberbaum RE, Krapp M, et al. Use of GnRh antagonists in the treatment of endometriosis. Reprod Biomed Online. 2002;5(1):12-6.
67. Donnez O, Donnez J. Gonadotrophin releasing hormone antagonist (linzagolix): a new therapy for uterine adenomyosis. Fertil Steril. 2020;114(3):640-4.
68. Taylor HS, Giudice LC, Lessey BA, et al. Treatment of endometriosis associated pain with elagolix m an oral GnRh antagonist. N Engl J Med. 2017;377:28-40.

9 Chapter

Monitoring of Ovulation Induction by Ultrasound

INTRODUCTION

Ultrasound is the modality of choice for monitoring of the patients undergoing assisted reproductive technology (ART). It gives a precise idea about the morphological changes and also about the hormonal changes occurring during the entire cycle when Doppler is also used for monitoring. The hormonal changes first reflect as vascular changes and then as morphological changes. Therefore, if vascular changes are observed with Doppler, the need of hormonal assessments for cycle monitoring can be omitted.

The purpose of follicular tracking is:

- To evaluate ovarian response to stimulation
- To decide the correct time of ovulation trigger and intrauterine insemination (IUI) or ovum pickup.

Follicles up to 2-mm diameter grow independent of gonadotropins, follicle stimulating hormone (FSH).[1] These are secondary antral follicles that recruit from the primordial follicles to preantral follicles and secondary antral follicles under the effect of androgen. Further development of the follicle is only possible in the presence of appropriate levels of gonadotropins. Before day 5 of the cycle, selection of the dominant follicle occurs.

Between Days 5 and 7, the dominance of the follicle becomes apparent. A follicle that is 10–12 mm in size is known as a dominant follicle, and it is this follicle that is most likely to grow to become a mature follicle and others become atretic **(Fig. 1)**. It is interesting to know that often the first largest follicle seen on a baseline scan is not the dominant follicle. This is possible when the follicle is a residual follicle of the previous cycle. The dominant follicle can be differentiated from the residual follicle of the previous cycle by Doppler. Blood flows close to the follicle can be seen by Doppler when the follicle becomes dominant (approximate size of 10 mm).

A scan is always done on the day gonadotropin is started. If there is a follicle of >10 mm, the patient is called back when the follicle is likely to reach 18 mm. This can be estimated because a follicle that is of >10 mm in diameter is a dominant follicle and it grows at a rate of 2–3 mm/day.[2]

It has no internal echogenicity and has thin (pencil line-like) walls and is not only

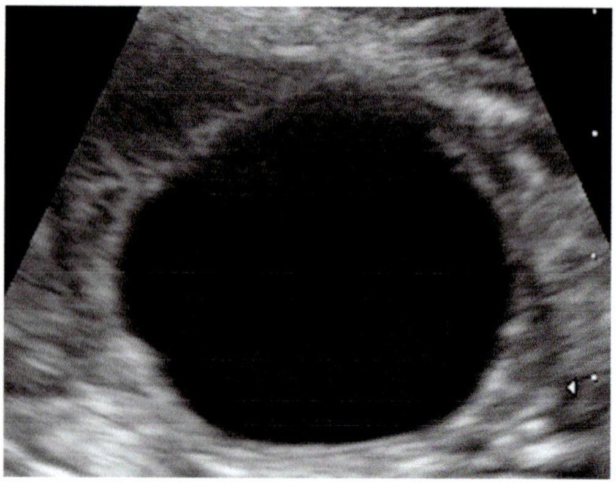

Fig. 1: B-mode ultrasound image of a mature follicle.

more likely to become the leading follicle but will also give a mature healthy ovum. If all the follicles are <10 mm on the day gonadotropin is started, the patient is called after 5 days. As the dominant follicle grows, it starts pulling vascularity toward itself.[3,4]

ULTRASOUND FEATURES OF PREOVULATORY FOLLICLE (TABLE 1)

B-Mode Features of a Mature Follicle

The follicular diameter is measured as a single diameter when the follicle is seen as a round structure, or three orthogonal diameters must be measured and their mean is used as follicular diameter, if it appears oval. Anatomical maturity of the follicle may be considered from the follicular diameter of 16–18 mm and consequently Doppler assessment is done to assess the functional maturity of the follicle. A follicular size of 17–18 mm is considered optimum for the gonadotropin-stimulated cycle whereas for clomiphene citrate (CC)-stimulated cycles, a minimum size of 18–20 mm is required.[5] It has been observed that the functional maturity in the follicle may be achieved later than the anatomical maturity. On B-mode ultrasound, a good-quality follicle is identified by thin isoechoic walls, regular round shape, and no echogenicity in the lumen. A thin hypoechoic rim surrounding the follicle and sometimes (about 35–40%) cumulus-like shadow may be seen in the follicle approximately 24–36 hours before ovulation.

Low-level linear echoes are seen inside the follicle parallel to the wall about 6–10 hours before rupture due to separation of the innermost cell layer of the follicle, as the initiation of the process of ovulation **(Fig. 2)**.[2]

Doppler Features of a Good Preovulatory Follicle

An increase in the perifollicular vascularity of the dominant follicle in the theca layer starts developing as early as the 8th day of the cycle in a normal length cycle. Fall in perifollicular resistance index (RI) starts 2 days before ovulation, reaches nadir at ovulation, remains low for 4 days, and then with gradual rise reaches 0.5 in the mid-luteal phase.[6]

When functionally mature, on color Doppler, the follicle shows blood vessels

TABLE 1: Ultrasound features of preovulatory follicle and endometrium.

	Follicle	*Endometrium*
Size/thickness	16–18 mm	8–10 mm
Morphology	Thin wall, no internal echoes, halo	Grade A/B
Vascualrity	Three fourth of the circumference	Zone 3–4
RI	0.4–0.48	<0.5
PSV	>10 cm/s	–
Uterine artery PI	–	<3.2
Volume	3–7 cc	3–7 cc
3D morphology	Cumulus	Intact endometrium–myometrium junction
3D PD	More symmetrical, the better	Higher, the better

(PD: pulse Doppler; PI: pulsatility index PSV: peak systolic velocity; RI: resistive index)

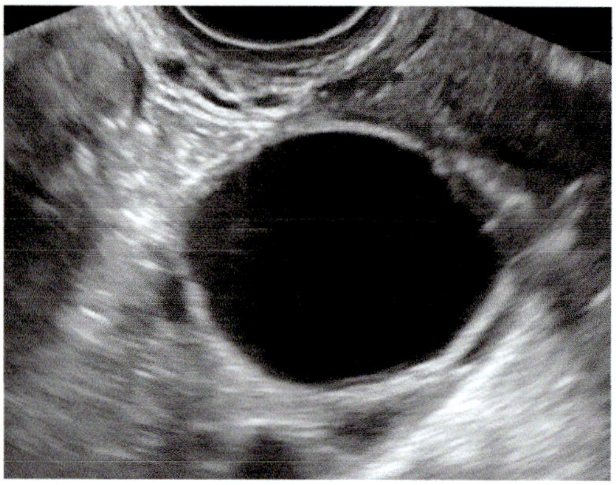

Fig. 2: B-mode ultrasound image of a follicle of which rupture is impending showing the mild separation of inner wall at 2 o' clock and 6 o' clock positions.

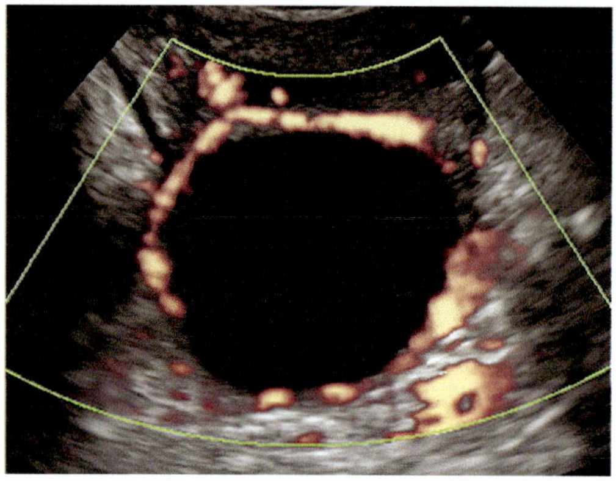

Fig. 3: Perifollicular vascularity seen on color Doppler.

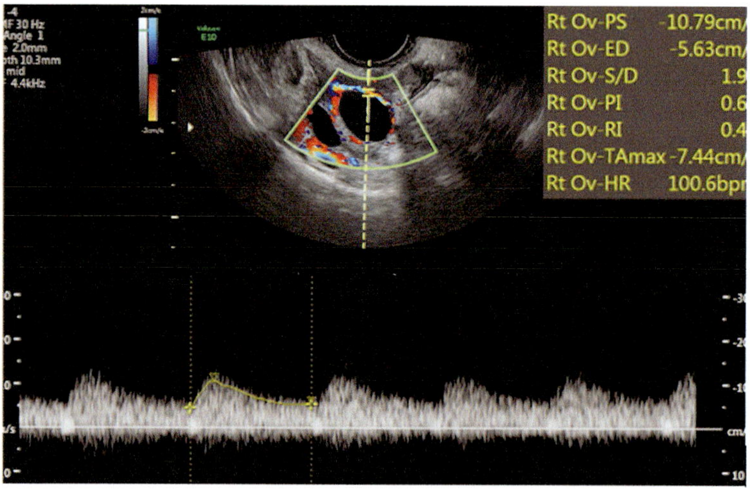

Fig. 4: Pulse Doppler image of the low-resistance perifollicular flow.

covering at least two-thirds to three-fourths of the follicular circumference **(Fig. 3)**. Chui et al. graded the follicular flow as grade 1–4, when in a single cross area slice the flow covered <25%, 25–50%, 50–75%, and >75% of the follicular circumference. The conception was related to grade 3–4 vascularity.[7]

On pulse Doppler, these blood vessels show RI of 0.4–0.48[7] and peak systolic velocity (PSV) of >10 cm/s **(Fig. 4)**.

The pulse repetition frequency (PRF) settings for color Doppler are set at 0.3 and wall filter at the lowest. The perifollicular vessels are only those that obliterate the follicular wall with color. If the follicular wall is seen and the vessel is seen just besides it, it is not a perifollicular vessel. Ovarian flow correlates well with oocyte recovery rates and hence may be useful in determining the most appropriate time to administer human chorionic gonadotropin (hCG). It has been quoted in a study by Nargund et al.[7,8] that embryos produced by fertilization of the ova obtained from the follicles that had a perifollicular PSV of < 10 cm/s are less likely to be grade 1 embryos and also have a higher chance of chromosomal malformations. In the same study, it has been shown that the probability of developing a grade 1 or 2 embryo is 75% if PSV was >10 cm/s, 40% if PSV was <10 cm/s, and 24% if there was no perifollicular flow. There is yet another study that supports this finding. Oocytes from severely hypoxic follicles are associated with a high frequency of abnormalities of organization of chromosomes on metaphase spindle and may lead to segregation disorders and catastrophic mosaics in embryo.[9] Our data of more than 1,000 IUI cycles has shown that when the perifollicular RI > 0.53 and PSV < 9 cm/s, 12 hours before ovulation trigger, the conception rates were only 8.3% and 10%, respectively, as compared to 32.8% and 28.2%, respectively, and individually when perifollicular RI < 0.50 and PSV > 11 cm/s.[10] Therefore, we have always preferred to wait with no extra medication when the patient is on CC stimulation or continue with the same dose of gonadotropin till we get desired perifollicular RI and PSV, though sometimes the follicular size may reach up to 22–24 mm. Almost 90% of the times, the desired RI and PSV are reached by the time the follicular size is 22–24 mm maximum.

In IVF cycles when there are multiple follicles, trigger is planned when there are at least three follicles between 18 and 16 mm and at least three follicles in either ovary show the Doppler parameters as stated above.

On 3D ultrasound, the follicular volume of 3–7.5 cc has been found to be optimum in our study.[11] This agrees with the study by Wittmack et al. which says: that in in vitro fertilization and embryo transfer (IVF-ET) cycles, follicles with a mean follicular diameter of 12–24 mm are associated with optimal rates of oocyte recovery, fertilization, and cleavage.[12] This corresponds to the follicular volumes between 3 and 7 mL. The accuracy of 3D US for measurement of follicular volume compared to the standard 2D techniques by comparing the volume of individual follicles estimated by both methods, 3D ultrasound with virtual organ computer-aided analysis (VOCAL) gave much more accurate measurements[13] **(Fig. 5)**.

The 3D ultrasound is especially useful to assess the follicular size in IVF cycles with multiple follicles. Since there are multiple follicles compressed by each other, these do not appear round in shape. Follicular diameter, therefore, cannot be a reliable parameter for follicular size. Follicular volume can be calculated on 3D ultrasound with Sono automated volume calculation (AVC) software. This software color-codes the follicles to calculate the number of follicles correctly. Moreover, it also calculates the three longest orthogonal diameters, mean diameter, and volume of the individual follicle. This information is not only useful to assess the time of trigger but is also useful to decide the type of trigger. When there are more than three follicles of between 11 and 14 mm in both the ovaries in the IUI cycle stimulated with gonadotropins apart from the mature follicles and when there are more than four follicles of between 11 and 14 mm in both the ovaries apart from mature follicles of 16 mm and larger, hCG is not considered as the trigger.

Cumulus is a reliable sign that indicates the presence of a fertilizable ovum in the follicle. The appearance of the intrafollicular cumulus-like structures by 3D ultrasound was correlated with the recovery rate of the mature oocytes.[14]

Feichtinger et al. in their study have shown the presence of cumulus in follicles >15 mm by 3D ultrasound.[15]

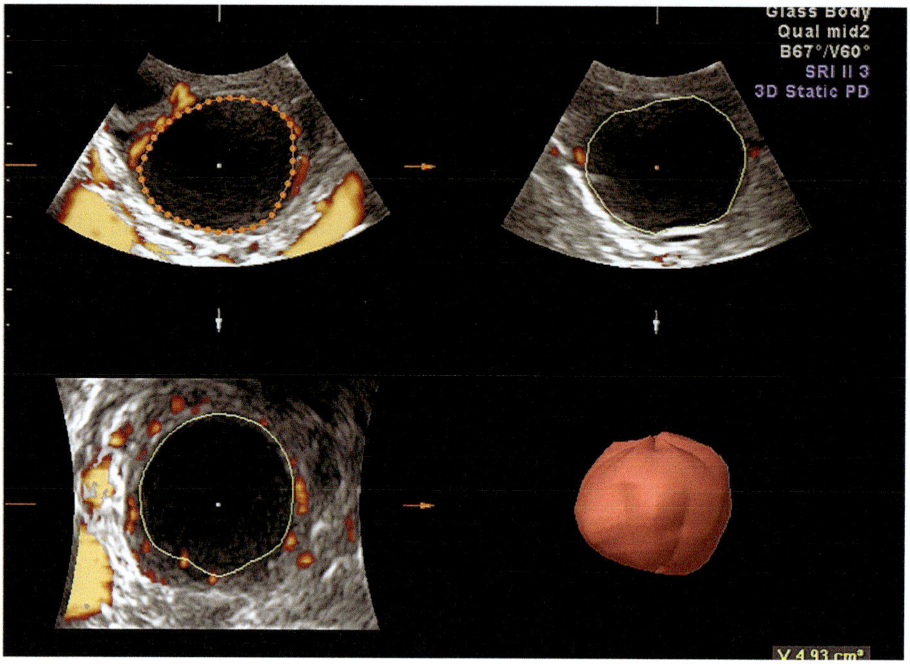

Fig. 5: 3D ultrasound acquired by the VOCAL calculated volume of the follicle.

It has been shown that follicular fluid concentrations of leptin and follicular angiogenesis-related factors are inversely related to the stromal blood flow index.[16] It has also been suggested that the follicles containing oocytes capable to produce a pregnancy have a perifollicular vascular network more uniform and distinctive.[17] Quantification of power Doppler information within a 3D model of an ovarian follicle can be performed using the "histogram facility". Three indices of vascularity can be generated: (1) the vascularization index (VI), which represents the ratio of power Doppler information within the total data relative to both color and gray information; (2) the flow index (FI), which is proportional to the power Doppler signal intensity; and (3) the vascularization flow index (VFI), which reflects a combination of the first two indices.

In our study,[11] we have found perifollicular VI between 6 and 20 and perifollicular FI > 35 as most optimum. 68.4% of patients conceived when the VI was between 6 and 18 and 50% when it was between 18 and 20. However, the pregnancy rates were <25% when VI was <6 and only 7.4% when VI was >20. It was only 7.4% of patients with FI < 27 who conceived whereas beyond 27, the conception rates rose consistently. It was 50% with FI between 27 and 35, 70% when FI was between 35 and 43, and almost all patients had conceived when FI was >43. Although it is possible to assess the follicular flow as expressed by the PSV and perifollicular color map,[18] it is the 3D power Doppler that gives the most precise information about the vascularization and follicular blood flow.[19] A study by Kupesic and Kurjak shows that when the ratio of FV to blood FI (FV/FI) is between 0.4 and 0.6, the pregnancy rates are 39%; if the ratio is >0.6, it is 52%; and when <0.4, it is only 21%.[20]

Human chorionic gonadotropin (hCG) plays a major role in inducing the influx of blood within follicles. At the luteinizing hormone (LH) surge, the perifollicular PSV is 10 cm/s. This means that if the follicle is said to be functionally mature when PSV is 10 cm/s, that is, the time when the LH surge starts and under the effect of that LH, the perifollicular PSV keeps on rising constantly.[21] This derives that a rising PSV with steady low RI suggests that the follicle is close to rupture. Vascular changes at the time of impending ovulation include increased vascularity of the inner wall of the follicle and a coincident surge in blood velocity just prior to eruption.[21] Our unpublished study of 350 IUI cycles has shown that when the perifollicular PSV was >20 cm/s, double IUI at 12–14 hours after trigger and 36–38 hours after trigger has given much higher pregnancy rates as compared to single IUI at 36–38 hours after trigger [presented at the International Society of Ultrasound in Obstetrics and Gynecology (ISUOG), 2006].

Implantation has been seen as the weakest link in the success of infertility treatment. The endometrium is a receptor organ for the majority of the hormones involved in the fertility and, therefore, the study of its morphology and vascularity is thought to explain the mysteries of implantation failure. Therefore, like follicle, the endometrium is also assessed by transvaginal 2D ultrasound and color Doppler before planning for hCG during any ARTs.

ULTRASOUND FEATURES OF PREOVULATORY ENDOMETRIUM (TABLE 1)

B-Mode Features of Endometrium with Good Receptivity

On transvaginal ultrasonography (TVS), an endometrial thickness of a minimum of 6 mm is required on the day of ovulation trigger, but 8–10 mm is optimum. Endometrial thickness has a more negative predictive value for implantation.[22]

In gonadotropin-stimulated cycles, the endometrial thickness is greater than in spontaneous cycles.[23] The growth rate of endometrial thickness in stimulated cycles is as follows:

- *Days 7–9 of stimulation*: 1.9 mm
- *Days 9–11*: 0.9 mm
- *Day 11 till hCG*: 0.6 mm
- *hCG till ET*: 0.5 mm

Even when pregnancy occurs with an endometrial thickness of 6–8 mm on the day of trigger, the rates of preclinical miscarriage (biochemical pregnancy) and clinical miscarriage were 21.9% and 15.6%, respectively, as compared to 0% and 12.9%, respectively, when the endometrial thickness was >8 mm.[24]

It is measured from the outer margin of anterior hyperechoic line of the endometrium to outer margin of posterior hyperechoic line of the endometrium, excluding the junctional zone and perpendicular to the long axis of endometrium and at the broadest part, which in normal endometrium is 1–2 cm inferior to the fundal end of endometrium. However, in a CC-stimulated cycle, the endometrial thickness may be less in the days immediately after CC is taken because of blocked estrogen receptors and its antiestrogenic effect. But during the late proliferative phase, endometrial thickness increases at a faster rate than in spontaneous cycles as the estrogen receptors are released because of the weaning effect of CC, and also because of increased estrogen due to multifollicular growth.

The morphology of the endometrium is as important as the thickness of the endometrium. In all the healthy endometria, the endometrial–myometrial interface is always seen as a clear hypoechoic halo surrounding the whole endometrium. Breach or irregularity of the endometrio–myometrial junction is an indication of unhealthy endometrium and therefore poor receptivity.

Popularly multilayered endometrium is considered as a desired endometrial pattern. Morphologically, the endometrium is graded as grade A **(Fig. 6A)**, when it is a triple-line endometrium with the intervening area as hypoechoic as the anterior myometrium. The echogenicity is attributed to the development of multiple vessels penetrating in the endometrium producing multiple tissue interfaces and therefore causing the echogenicity and also due to glycogen storage in the endometrial columnar epithelium. The endometrium is graded as grade B **(Fig. 6B)** when it is multilayered or triple line with a hypoechoic intervening area. Grade C endometrium would be a homogeneous isoechoic endometrium **(Fig. 6C)**.[25] Though some studies have shown no significant difference in pregnancy rates among different morphological patterns. According to literature evidence and our experience, different morphological patterns of the endometrium can be related to the estradiol levels. As the estradiol level increases, the endometrium becomes a triple line, increases in thickness, and progresses from grade B to grade A and then to grade C with supraphysiological levels of estradiol as occurs in multifollicular development.

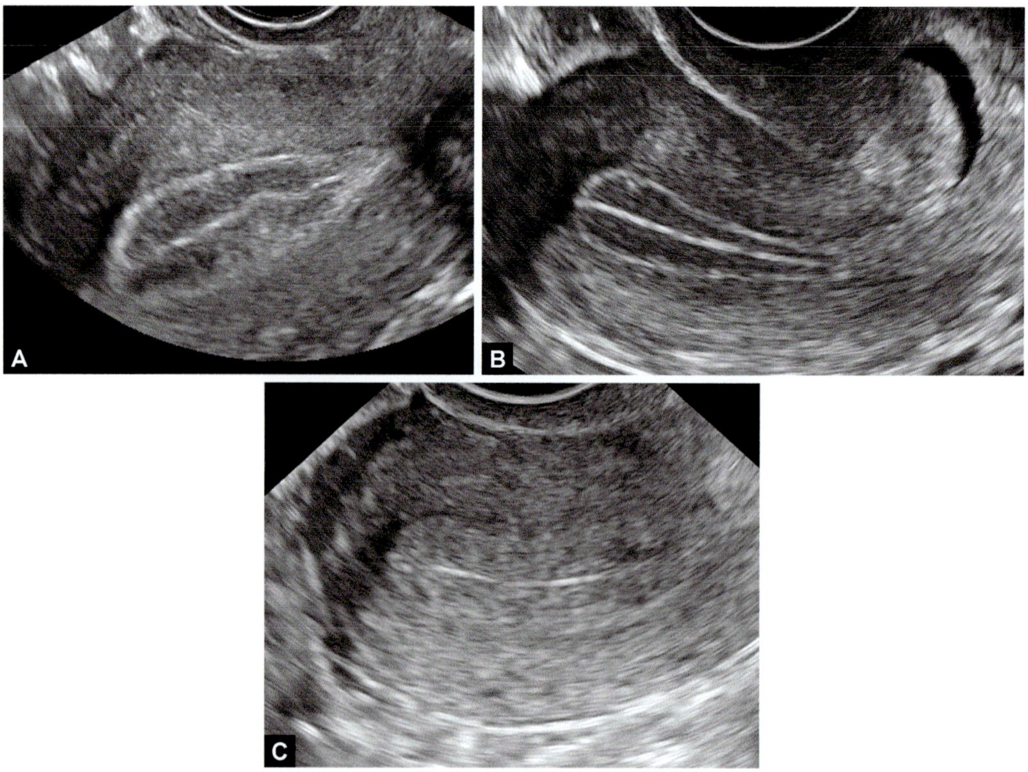

Figs. 6A to C: (A) B-mode ultrasound image of grade A endometrium; (B) B-mode ultrasound image of grade B endometrium; (C) B-mode ultrasound image of grade C endometrium.

Doppler Features of Endometrium with Good Receptivity

There are several reports by different groups[26] that agree on the fact that implantation rates can be more correlated with the vascularity of the endometrium rather than the thickness and morphology of the endometrium.

Segmental uterine artery perfusion demonstrates a significant correlation with hormonal and histological markers of uterine receptivity, reaching the highest sensitivity for subendometrial blood flow.[20]

On the color Doppler, the endometrium, which is mature, shows vascularity in Zones 3 and 4 or may be called subendometrial and endometrial layers **(Fig. 7)**.

The zones of vascularity are defined according to Applebaum[26] as: Zone 1 when the vascularity on power Doppler is seen only at endometrium–myometrium junction, Zone 2 when vessels penetrate through the hyperechogenic endometrial edge, Zone 3 when these reach the intervening hypoechogenic zone, and Zone 4 when these reach the endometrial cavity (central line). But a particular zone can be called vascularized only when at least 5 mm^2 area of that zone is vascularized. Below this cutoff for Zones 3 and 4, the pregnancy rates are extremely low.[27]

Another comparison of two studies have also shown similar results for pregnancy rates in relation to vascularity zones:[28]

- Zone 1 3.5—7.5% 5.2%
- Zone 2 15.8—29.7% 28.7%
- Zone 3 24.2—47.8% 52%
- Zone 4 67.3—74%

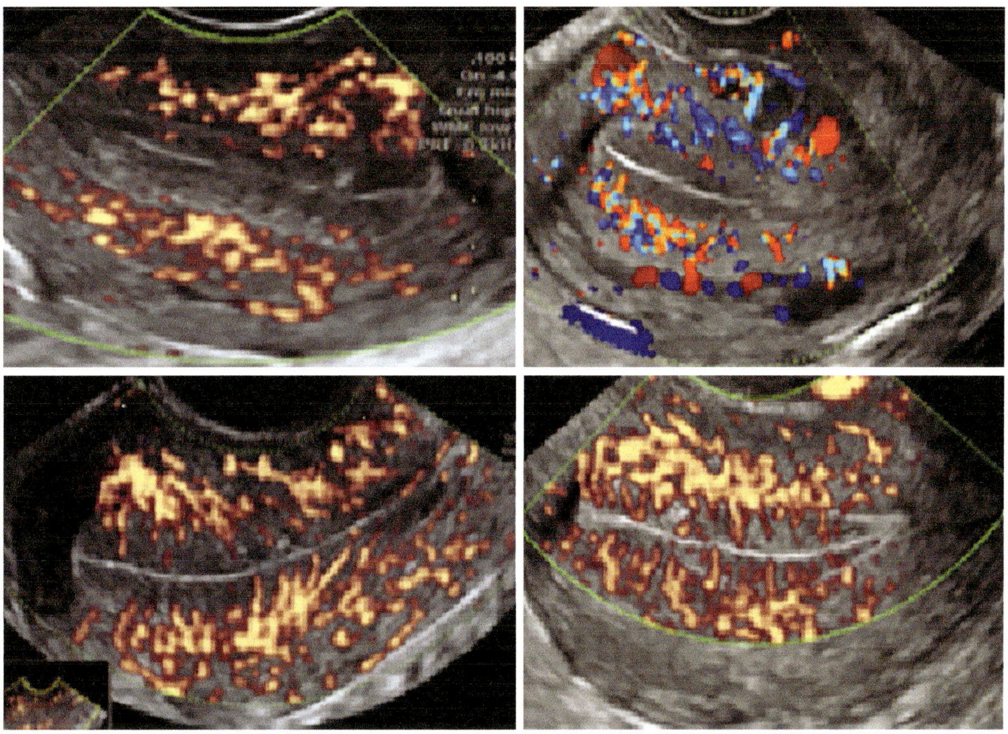

Fig. 7: Power Doppler images of the grade 1–4 endometrium.

Endometrial Vascularity: Its Relation to Implantation and Abortion Rates[29]

Vascularity in	Zone 1	Zone 2	Zone 3	Zone 4
% of patients	6.69%	20.73%	58%	14.47%
βhCG	19%	21.87%	39.77%	70.14%
Gestational sac	9.6%	14.58%	36.8%	68.65%
Abortions	50%	23.8%	5.6%	1.5%

Zaidi et al. found that the absence of flow in the endometrial and subendometrial zones on the day of trigger indicates the total failure of implantation.[30]

The vessels that reach the endometrium are the spiral arteries. The pulse Doppler of these arteries should have an RI < 0.6 for the endometrium to be called mature for implantation.

While the reported correlation between vascularity in the endometrium and subendometrium and pregnancy rates is controversial, it has been concluded in two studies that no difference was found in patients with good prognosis for cycle outcome, but in patients with poor embryo quality, better endometrial vascularity seemed to improve the cycle outcome.[31,32]

Though yet another study has shown that when pregnancy is achieved in the absence of endometrial and subendometrial flow more than half of these pregnancies will finish as spontaneous miscarriage.[28]

The pulse Doppler of these arteries indicating RI between 0.49 and 0.59 and pulsatility index (PI) between 1.1 and 2.3 has also been reported to be a good prognostic factor.[33]

The vessels that reach the endometrium should cover ≥5 mm^2 area of the endometrium, and this is considered a good prognostic factor.[27]

Moreover, the pulse Doppler analysis of the uterine artery waveform is done and its PI should be <3.2 **(Fig. 8)**.

Several authors have shown that the optimum uterine receptivity was obtained when the average PI of the uterine artery was between 2 and 3 on the day of transfer or on the day of trigger.[34,35]

Coulam et al. have also shown that no pregnancy was achieved after ET when uterine artery PI was >3.3 in an IVF program also.[36]

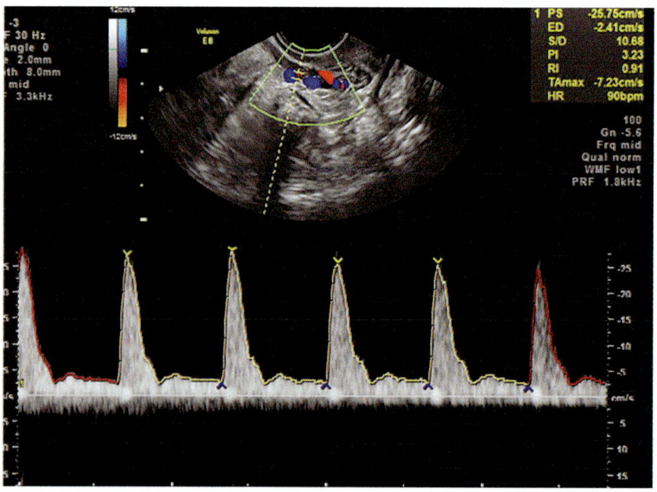

Fig. 8: Pulse Doppler image showing high-resistance uterine artery flow waveform.

Cacciatore et al. suggest that implantation is unlikely when PI is >3.3 and RI is >0.95 or when no velocities are seen at the end of the diastole.[37] In such cases, therefore in IUI cycles, trigger is withheld or postponed.

Endometrial volume by 3D ultrasound volume calculation of the endometrium may help to correlate the cycle outcome with quantitative parameters rather than endometrial thickness.[12] This is done by the software VOCAL.

A study by Raga et al.[38] shows that pregnancy and implantation rates were significantly lower when endometrial volume <2 mL, while no pregnancy was achieved when the endometrial volume was <1 mL. A study by Kupesic et al. also shows no pregnancy when the endometrial volume was <2 mL or when it exceeded 8 mL.[33]

If these parameters are not reached, the cycle is not canceled but only delayed. Stimulation is continued till these parameters are achieved. In case the PSV of the follicle starts rising with low RI, it means that the ovulation is impending. In such a situation, in spite of inadequate endometrial parameters, the trigger is given, but the patient is also explained that the results cannot be as good as they would be if every parameter was optimal. If the follicle grows beyond 23–24 mm and still perifollicular flow is not adequate, the trigger is planned and the patient may be given a choice of either timed intercourse or IUI, after proper explanation about the results.

SECRETORY PHASE ASSESSMENT

Rupture of the follicle leads to the formation of the corpus luteum. Corpus luteum is responsible for progesterone production. The functional efficacy of the corpus luteum can be assessed by Doppler by assessing the pericorpus luteal vascularity.

Segmental uterine and ovarian artery perfusion demonstrates a significant correlation with histological and hormonal markers of uterine receptivity and may aid assessment of the luteal phase defect.[39] A clear correlation between RI of corpus luteum and plasma progesterone levels has been seen in the natural cycle. RI of the corpus luteum can therefore be used as an adjunct to the plasma progesterone assay as an index of luteal function.[40]

A corpus luteum that is functionally normal and produces an adequate amount of progesterone shows corpus luteal flow: RI 0.35–0.50 and PSV 10–15 **(Fig. 9)**.

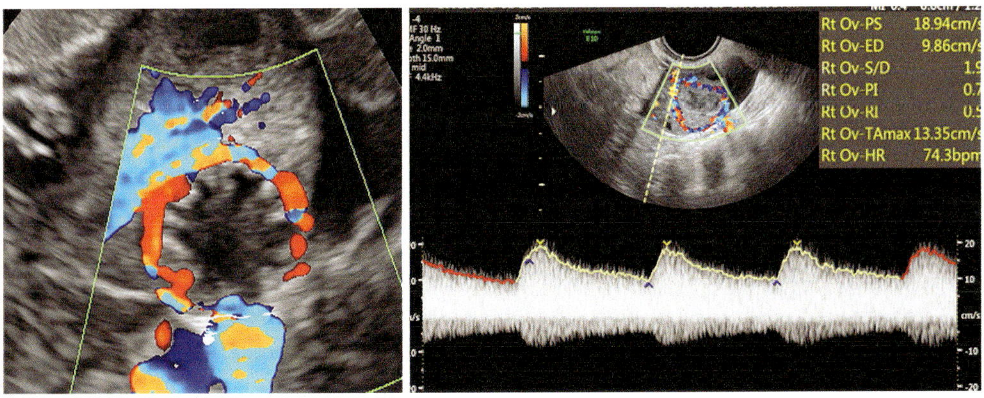

Fig. 9: Normal corpus luteal flow seen on color Doppler and pulse Doppler.

The receptor organ for progesterone is also endometrium as it is for estrogen and its vascular studies can be a reliable clue to adequate progesterone production. Endometrium becomes hyperechoic as a result of progesterone exposure. Soon after the rupture of the follicle, the outer margin of the endometrium starts becoming fluffy and blurred. With adequate progesterone levels, which are achieved in the mid-luteal phase, the spiral arteries show RI of 0.48–0.52 (low-resistance flow) and uterine artery shows PI of 2.0–2.5. This PI is lower than in the preovulatory phase because of smooth muscle relaxing effect of progesterone. Inadequate progesterone production and corpus luteal inadequacy are suggested by high-resistance flow in corpus luteal vessels.[40]

However, high spiral artery resistance would suggest an inadequate response of endometrium to progesterone. This is because of inadequate progesterone receptors in the endometrium or because of local endometrial causes, such as endometrial injury or chronic endometritis.

In the luteal phase defect because of low progesterone levels, the resistance in the pericorpus luteal vessels is high. Because of low progesterone levels, there is inadequate relaxation of the muscularis of the uterine artery and therefore the uterine artery resistance is high along with higher resistance in its branches—the spiral vessels.

The difference in corpus luteal flow and spiral artery flow in normal cycle and luteal phase defect has been mentioned in **Tables 2 and 3**.[39]

The secretory scan is especially helpful for pinpointing the cause of failure of treatment and change the protocol if required in the next cycle, e.g., hCG for luteal support in case of corpus luteal failure, more closer monitoring of the cycle and proper time of trigger for luteinized unruptured follicle, and modification in the stimulation protocol for inadequate progesterone receptors in endometrium.

TABLE 2: Corpus luteal Doppler parameters throughout the cycle in normal cases and in LPD.

	Normal	*LPD*
Perifollicular	0.56 ± 0.06	0.58 ± 0.04
LH peak day	0.44 ± 0.04	0.58 ± 0.04
Midluteal phase	0.42 ± 0.06	0.58 ± 0.04
Late luteal phase	0.50 ± 0.04	0.58 ± 0.04

(LH: luteinizing hormone; LPD: luteal phase defect)

TABLE 3: Endometrial Doppler parameters throughout the cycle in normal cases and LPD.

Phase	*Control RI*	*LPD RI*
Periovulatory	0.53 ± 0.04	0.70 ± 0.06
Midluteal	0.50 ± 0.02	0.72 ± 0.06
Late luteal	0.51 ± 0.04	0.72 ± 0.04

(LH: luteinizing hormone; LPD: luteal phase defect; RI: resistance index)

CORRELATION OF PROGESTERONE WITH ULTRASOUND FINDINGS

The blurring of the outer margin of multi-layered endometrium suggests initiation of progesterone secretion **(Fig. 10)**.

Low-resistance flow in corpus luteum with echogenic endometrium **(Figs. 11A and B)** and low-resistance endometrial vascularity in the midluteal phase suggest a normal luteal phase.

High-resistance corpus luteal flow suggests corpus luteal inadequacy. High-resistance endometrial flow in the mid-luteal phase suggests either inadequate progesterone levels or inadequate progesterone receptors in the endometrium.

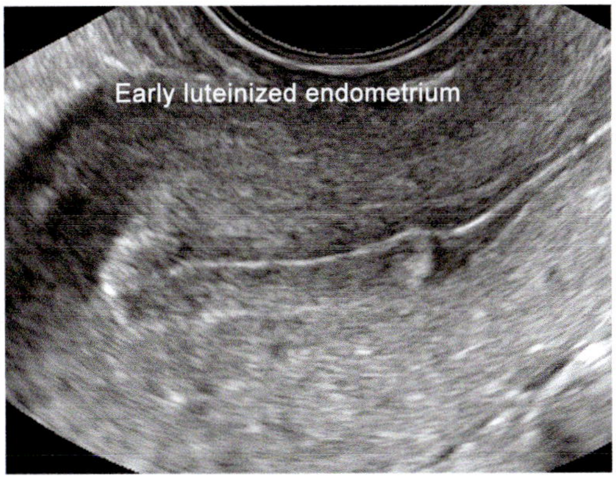

Fig. 10: Endometrium of early luteal phase seen on B-mode ultrasound. Blurring of the outer margins of multilayered endometrium can be seen.

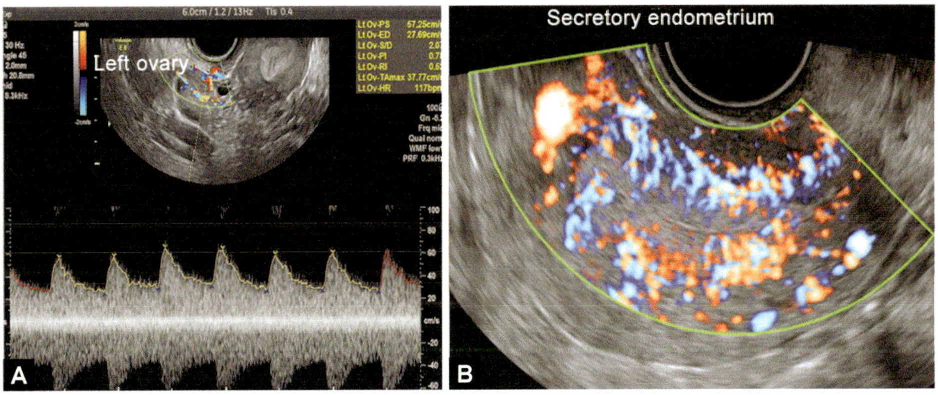

Figs. 11A and B : (A) Low-resistance blood flow of the corpus luteum demonstrated on pulse Doppler; (B) HD power Doppler showing blood flow in the secretory endometrium.

CONCLUSION

Ultrasound is an excellent tool for the assessment of the menstrual cycle. Hormonal changes occurring day-to-day during the menstrual cycle reflects as morphological and vascular changes in the ovary and the uterus. Assessing these changes by transvaginal ultrasound and Doppler and correctly interpreting can explain the hormonal basis of these changes. Ultrasound with Doppler can thus be used as the only modality for cycle assessment in patients undergoing ART and may be of help to reduce the cost of the cycle by avoiding certain hormonal assessments and still maintaining close and accurate watch on the hormonal changes occurring during the treatment cycle.

REFERENCES

1. Hackeloer BJ, Sallam HN. Ultrasound scanning of ovarian follicles. Clin Obstet Gynecol. 1983;10:603-20.
2. Hackeloer BJ, Fleming R, Robinson HP. Correlation of ultrasonic and endocrinological assessment of human follicular development. Am J Obstet Gynecol. 1979; 135:122.
3. Zaidi J, Barber J, Kyei-mensah A, Bekir J, Campbell S, Tan SL. Relationship of ovarian stromal blood flow at the baseline ultrasound scan to subsequent follicular response in an

in vitro fertilization program. Obstet Gynecol. 1996;88:779-84.

4. Engmann L, Sladkevicius P, Agrawal R, Bekir JS, Campbell S, Tan SL. Value of ovarian stromal blood flow velocity measurement after pituitary suppression in the prediction of ovarian responsiveness and outcome of in vitro fertilization treatment. Fertil Steril. 1999;71:22-9.
5. Luciano GN, Tarek AG. Ultrasonography and IVF. In: Rizk Botros RMB (Ed). Ultrasonography in Reproductive Medicine and Infertility. UK: Cambridge University Press; 2010. pp. 193-201.
6. Jokubkeine L, Sladkevicius P, Rovas L, Valentine L. Assessment of changes in volume and vascularity of ovaries during the normal menstrual cycle using three dimensional power Doppler ultrasound. Hum Reprod. 2006;21:2661-8.
7. Nargund G, Doyle PE, Bourne TH, Parsons JH, Cheng WC, Campbell S, et al. Ultrasound-deviced indices of follicular blood flow before HCG administration and prediction of oocyte recovery and preimplantation embryo quality. Hum Reprod. 1996;11:2512-17.
8. Nargund G, Bourne TH, Doyle PE, Parsons J, Cheng W, Campbell S, et al. Association between ultrasound indices of follicular blood flow, oocyte recovery and preimplantation embryo quality. Hum Reprod. 1996;11:109-13.
9. Van Blerkom, Antezak M, Schrader R. The developmental potential of human oocyte is related to the dissolved oxygen content of follicular fluid: association with vascular endothelial growth factor levels and perifollicular blood flow characteristics, Hum Reprod. 1997;12(5):1047-55.
10. Panchal SY, Nagori CB. Pre-hCG 3D and 3D power Doppler assessment of the follicle for improving pregnancy rates in intrauterine insemination cycles. J Hum Reprod Sci. 2009;2:62-7.
11. Panchal SY, Nagori CB. Can 3D PD be a better tool for assessing the pre HCG follicle and endometrium? A randomized study of 500 cases. Presented at 16th World Congress on Ultrasound in Obstetrics and Gynecology, 2006, London. J Ultrasound Obstet Gynecol. 2006;28(4):504.
12. Wittmack FM, Kreger DO, Blasco L, Tureck RW, Mastroianni L Jr Lessey BA. Effect of follicular size on oocyte retrieval, fertilization, cleavage and embryo quality in in vitro fertilization cycles: a 6 year data collection. Fertil Steril. 1994;62:1205-10.
13. Kyei-Mensah A, Zaidi J, Pittrof R, Shaker A, Campbell S, Tan SL. Transvaginal three dimensional ultrasound reproducibility of ovarian and endometrial volume measurements. Fertil Steril. 1996;66:718-22.
14. Poehl M, Hohlagschwandtner M, Doerner V, Dillinger B, Feichtinger W. Cumulus assessment by three dimensional ultrasound for in vitro fertilization. Ultrasound Obstet Gynecol. 2000;16:251-3.
15. Feichtinger W. Transvaginal three-dimensional imaging for evaluation and treatment of infertility. In: Merz E (Ed). 3D ultrasound in obstetrics and gynaecology. Philadelphia, PA: Lippincott Williams & Wilkins; 1998. pp. 37-43.
16. Wu MH, Tsai SJ, Pan HA, Hsiao KY, Chang FM. Three dimensional power doppler imaging of ovarian stromal blood flow in women with endometriosis undergoing in vitro fertilization. Ultrasound Obstet Gynecol. 2003;21:480-5.
17. Vlaisavljevic V, Reljic M, Gavric Lovrec V, Zazula D, Sergent N. Measurement of perifollicular blood flow of the dominant preovulatory follicle using three-dimensional power Doppler. Ultrasound Obstet Gynecol. 2003;22:520-6.
18. Merce LT. Ultrasound markers of implantation. Ultrasound Rev Obstet Gynecol. 2002;2:110-23.
19. Merce LT, Barco MJ, Kupesic S, Kurjak A. 2D and 3D power Doppler ultrasound from ovulation to implantation. In: Kurjak A, Chervenak F (Eds). Textbook of Perinatal Medicine. London: Parthenon Publishing; 2005.
20. Kupesic S, Kurjak A. Prediction of IVF outcome by three-dimensional ultrasound. Hum Reprod. 2002;17:950-5.
21. Bourne TH, Jurkovic D, Waterstone J, Campbell S, Collins WP. Intrafollicular blood flow during human ovulation. Ultrasound Obstet Gynecol. 1991;1:53-9.

22. Dickey RP, Olar TT, Taylor SN, Curole DN, Harrigill K. Relationship of biochemical pregnancy to preovulatory endometrial thickness and pattern in patients undergoing ovulation induction. Hum Reprod. 1993; 8:327-30.
23. Yagel S, Ben-Chetrit A, Anteby E, Zacut D, Hochner-Celnikier D, Ron M. The effect of ethinyl oestradiol on endometrial thickness and uterine volume during ovulation induction by clomiphene citrate. Fertil Steril. 1992;57:33-6.
24. Boue J, Boue A, Lazar P. Retrospective and prospective epidemiological studies of 1500 karyotyped spontaneous human abortions. Tetralogy. 1973;12:11-26.
25. Smith B, Porter R, Ahuja K, Craft I. Ultrasonic assessment of endometrial changes in stimulated cycles in an in vitro fertilization and embryo transfer program. J In Vitro Fert Embryo Transf. 1984;1:233-38.
26. Applebaum M. The 'steel' or 'teflon' endometrium - ultrasound visualization of endometrial vascularity in IVF patients and outcome. Presented at The third World Congress of Ultrasound in Obstetrics and Gyneacolgy. Ultrasound Obstet Gynecol. 1993;3(Suppl 2):10.
27. Yang JH, Wu MY, Chen CD, Jiang MC, Ho HN, Yang YS. Association of endometrial blood flow as determined by a modified color Doppler technique with subsequent outcome of in vitro fertilization. Hum Reprod. 1999;14:1606-10.
28. Chein LW, Au HK, Chen PL, Xiao J, Tzeng CR. Assessment of uterine receptivity by the endometrial-subendometrial blood flow distribution pattern in women undergoing IVF-ET. Fertil Steril. 2002;78:245-51.
29. Nagori C, Panchal S. Endometrial vascularity: its relation to implantation rates. Int J Infertil Fetal Med. 2012;3(2):48-50.
30. Zaidi J, Campbell S, Pittrof R, Tan SL. Endometrial thickness, morphology, vascular penetration and velocimetry in predicting implantation in an in vitro fertilization program. Ultrasound Obstet Gynecol. 1995;6:191-8.
31. Merce LT, Barco MJ, Bau S, Troyano JM. Prediction of ovarian response and IVF/ICSI outcome by three-dimensional ultrasonography and power Doppler angiography. Eur J Obstet Gynecol Reprod Biol. 2007;132:93-100.
32. Merce LT, Barco MJ, Bau S, Troyano JM. Are endometrial parameters by three-dimensional ultrasound and power Doppler angiography related to in vitro fertilization/embryo transfer outcome? Fertil Steril. 2008;89(1):111-7.
33. Kupesic S, Bekavac I, Bjelos D, Kurjak A. Assessment of endometrial receptivity by transvaginal color Doppler and three-dimensional power Doppler ultrasonography in patients undergoing in vitro fertilization procedures. J Ultrasound Med. 2001;20:125-34.
34. Steer CV, Campbell S, Tan SL, Crayford T, Mills C, Mason BA, et al. The use of transvaginal color flow imaging after in vitro fertilization to identify optimum uterine conditions before embryo transfer. Fertil Steril. 1992;57:372-6.
35. Zaidi J, Pittrof R, Shaker A, Kyei-Mensah A, Campbell S, Tan SL. Assessment of uterine artery blood flow on the day of human chorionic gonadotrophin administration by transvaginal color Doppler ultrasound in an in vitro fertilization program. Fertil Steril. 1996;65:(37):7-81.
36. Coulam CB, Stern JJ, Soenksen DM, Britten S, Bustillo M. Comparison of pulsatility indexes on the day of oocyte retrieval and embryo transfer. Hum Reprod. 1995;10:82-4.
37. Cacciatore B, Simberg N, Fusaro P, Tiitinen A. Transvaginal Doppler study of uterine artery blood flow in in vitro fertilization embryo transfer cycles. Fertil Steril. 1996;66:130-4.
38. Raga F, Bonilla-Musoles F, Casan EM, Klein O, Bonilla F. Assessment of endometrial volume by three-dimensional ultrasound prior to embryo transfer: clues to endometrial receptivity. Hum Reprod. 1999;14:2851-4.
39. Kupesić S, Kurjak A, Vujisić S, Petrović Z. Luteal phase defect: comparison between Doppler velocimetry, histological and hormonal markers. Ultrasound Obstet Gynecol. 1997;9(2):105-12.
40. Glock JL, Brumsted JR. Color flow pulsed Doppler ultrasound in diagnosing luteal phase defect. Fertil Steril. 1995;64:500-4.

10 Chapter

Ovulation Trigger

INTRODUCTION

Appropriate timing, adequate duration, and adequate amplitude of midcycle surge are the prerequisites for human female fertility. This midcycle follicle-stimulating hormone (FSH) and luteinizing hormone (LH) surge cause ovulation. In human beings, only LH surge can cause ovulation but in animals, both FSH and LH surge are mandatory to induce ovulation. The role of the FSH surge in humans has not been adequately understood till date.

FUNCTIONS OF LUTEINIZING HORMONE SURGE

Functions of LH surge are as follows:

- It induces mucinification of cumulus oophorus allowing oocyte release.
- It provokes the resumption of oocyte meiosis, which is arrested at the prophase of the first meiotic division and is converted to metaphase II. This is essential for fertilization.
- LH surge triggers follicular rupture. It induces a shift from estradiol secretion to progesterone secretion from granulosa cells.
- LH surge upregulates growth factors such as vascular endothelial growth factor (VEGF) and fibroblast growth factor. It stimulates cytokines involved in implantation.

Midcycle surge is governed by gonadotropin-releasing hormone (GnRH), estrogen, progesterone, and peptide hormones such as gonadotropin surge attenuating factor. Mural granulosa cells have LH receptors. LH stimulates epidermal growth factor in granulosa cells. These then act on cumulus cells that trigger oocyte maturation.

NATURAL LUTEINIZING HORMONE SURGE

Oocytes before LH surge are arrested at the prophase of the first meiotic division. LH surge reinitiates the arrested meiosis and triggers ovulation. A normal midcycle LH surge lasts for 48.7 ± 9.3 hours.[1]

Luteinizing hormone surge has three phases:

1. Rapid ascending phase—14 hours
2. Peak plateau—14 hours
3. Long descending phase—20 hours

Luteinizing hormone surge is greater than FSH surge. The LH level reaches 10–20 times higher than the basal LH level. The mean peak value is 46 ± 16 IU/L. LH pulse frequency remains the same as in the early proliferative phase, but the amplitude is high. Though the duration and amplitude of LH are different in different individuals. The sudden endogenous LH surge is due to positive feedback mechanism to a high estrogen level, i.e., 150 pg/mL/follicle. The increased amplitude of LH and FSH pulse is thought to be facilitated by positive feedback of estrogen on kisspeptin neurons in anteroventral periventricular nuclei of the hypothalamus and upregulation of GnRH receptors in the anterior pituitary. The serum progesterone starts rising after 12 hours of LH surge and plateaus up to ovulation and once again starts rising after ovulation. Ovulation occurs after 36 hours of the onset of LH surge. So, progesterone increases in two steps. Similarly, androstenedione and testosterone surge also occur two and four times, respectively, at the time of LH surge.[1]

Seibel et al. found that an oocyte starts maturing after 18 hours of the onset of LH surge and majority of oocytes retrieved after 25 hours reach meiosis after injection of human chorionic gonadotropin (hCG).[2] So, the threshold level of resumption of meiosis is 14–18 hours and to obtain the oocytes with metaphase II after aspiration, at least 28 hours are required after the onset of the surge.

The threshold amplitude of LH surge for oocyte maturation is quite low. Only 5% of LH peak concentration is required for meiosis and sufficient luteinization. The rest is required for triggering ovulation.[3] This means that actually in assisted reproductive technology (ART) because ovum pick-up is done, a very low dose of LH instead of 10,000 hCG may suffice. This will drastically reduce the incidence of ovarian hyperstimulation syndrome (OHSS), but no actual study data is available on ART with low-dose LH or hCG.

SEQUENCE OF HORMONAL EVENTS AT MIDCYCLE

- The onset of LH and FSH surge occurs abruptly.
- It is associated with estrogen peak.
- It occurs 12 hours after the estrogen peak.
- The duration of FSH and LH surge is 48 hours.
- LH surge has ascending limb lasting for 14 hours and is associated with the rise in progesterone and decline in estradiol.
- Then it has a plateau of 14 hours.
- Descending limb lasts for 20 hours associated with progesterone rise. This is after 36 hours of the onset of FSH and LH surge.
- The level of LH 100 IU and FSH 25–30 IU is considered normal.

INDICATIONS OF SURROGATE LUTEINIZING HORMONE SURGE

- Hypogonadotropic hypogonadism (WHO I)
- Hypothalamic-pituitary dysfunction (WHO II)

  Here, correct timing and amplitude of LH surge are absent after FSH-induced follicular growth.[4] Multiple follicular development prevents LH surge in stimulated cycles. It is said that gonadotropin surge-inhibiting factor, inhibin, and other nonsteroidal factors prevent FSH and LH surge which is otherwise induced by estrogen. GnRH analog can counter this surge.[5]
- Pretreatment with GnRH agonist (GnRHa) prevents LH surge and so surrogate LH surge is required.
- In patients undergoing intrauterine insemination (IUI), it is required to time IUI. Moreover, it lasts for 2 days giving a better pregnancy rate. Routine use of hCG, i.e., surrogate LH surge, is not found beneficial unless some intervention is to be done like IUI.[6,7]

FACTORS OF OVULATION TRIGGER

Ovulation trigger can be given by:

- hCG
- GnRHa
- Recombinant LH

Human Chorionic Gonadotropin Surge

Characteristics

- It has two to four times more binding affinity than LH.
- It has a biological half-life of >24 hours as compared to 60 minutes for endogenous LH. This is so because the beta-subunit of hCG is highly glycosylated and has a longer half-life.
- It stimulates the secretion of VEGF, which causes OHSS.
- Subcutaneous or intramuscular routes have the same serum levels and the same pregnancy rates.[8]
- hCG is used for ovulation triggers for about 30 years. It activates the same receptors as of LH on the corpus luteum.
- Bioavailability is less in obese women after giving hCG and so for obese women, 10,000 IU is the standard dose for trigger instead of 5,000 IU.
- No difference in oocyte yield is found with 5,000 IU or 10,000 IU of hCG.[9]
- Delayed hCG administration in the agonist or antagonist cycle gives a poor pregnancy rate according to some studies, but others have similar results.

Indications

- *Gonadotropin therapy*: Endogenous FSH and LH surge is attenuated in women treated with exogenous gonadotropins in spite of high estradiol levels. So, exogenous hCG is required for final maturation[10,11]
- To plan IUI at a particular time
- WHO group I where only hCG can be used
- Agonist cycle in ART.

Functions

- Resumes meiosis to metaphase II
- Follicular rupture and expulsion of ova
- Formation of corpus luteum for progesterone production.

Advantages

When hCG is used, it causes high levels of estradiol and progesterone and leads to normal luteal phase. The effect of hCG lasts for 5–8 days. So, it initiates and maintains progesterone production more efficiently than natural LH surge and there are less chances of luteal phase defects (LPDs).

Role of FSH Surge

- It induces LH receptor formation on granulosa cells that helps in oocyte maturation and corpus luteum formation.
- This may be a reason for a minimal increase in the metaphase II oocytes with agonist trigger.
- It enhances inhibin secretion that helps in the maturation of ova.
- FSH surge is not required for the formation of LH receptors in stimulated cycles because the increased level of FSH in the follicular phase in these patients leads to the formation of LH receptors and only hCG trigger suffices.

Side Effects

- Because of a longer half-life, hCG results in sustained luteotropic effect and development of multiple corpora lutea with very high estradiol and progesterone levels compared to spontaneous cycles. These high levels of estradiol and progesterone are detrimental to implantation. Because of multiple corpora lutea, there is a supraphysiological level of progesterone in the early luteal phase. The progesterone level reaches peak about 3 days after the oocyte collection. In a natural cycle, progesterone reaches to peak in the midluteal phase. So, the high progesterone on 3 days after ovum pick-up may be detrimental for implantation.

This explains why frozen embryo transfer gives better results.

- hCG trigger overstimulates corpora lutea and produces more estradiol that decreases endogenous LH and this can cause a luteal phase defect.[12,13]
- Multiple follicular rupture causes multiple pregnancies.
- Sustained effect of hCG causes OHSS in patients having an excessive response to gonadotropins. hCG stimulates VEGF which is the direct cause of OHSS.[14]
- However, it is very frustrating to withhold hCG to avoid OHSS and multiple pregnancy and will be waste of time and money as well as the number of canceled cycles will be in high proportion.
- hCG rise after subcutaneous injection is slower than intramuscular injection and slower than GnRHa trigger.

Therefore, in cases with high chance of OHSS, GnRHa is given as ovulation trigger, instead of hCG in the antagonist cycle.

Unphysiological effects of hCG:

- hCG bolus trigger induces a rapid increase in the progesterone level that reaches to peak after 12–24 hours. This level in the natural cycle is reached only in the midluteal phase.
- Natural peak is 40–60 IU with 25 IU/mL in 12 hours. hCG causes peak in 48 hours of up to 130–300 IU, i.e., about 10 times higher or even more depending on the dose and body mass index (BMI).
- Peak concentration of progesterone is advanced by 2 days that may lead to early endometrial advancement.

Majority of women experience a pronounced drop in progesterone concentration from the day it peaks until the day of implantation, i.e., fall from ovum pick-up + 4 days to ovum pick-up + 6 days.

- There is huge variability in progesterone concentration in the early luteal phase, and the sensitivity of hCG differs considerably.
- 5–6 days after ovum pick-up, the majority of women show hCG levels below the physiological concentration of LH during luteal phase causing low progesterone secretion.
- Progesterone measurement after 12–24 hours of trigger will guide for luteal support in the cycle.

Key points of progesterone secretion after hCG:

- Speed by which progesterone rises exceeds between 12 and 24 hours. In the natural cycle, it is only 5 nmol/L during the first 24 hours.
- Peak concentration of progesterone is reached after the trigger.
- Day of peak concentration varies from ovum pick-up day 3 and ovum pick-up day 4, i.e., early in 85% of cases. No pregnancy if endometrial advancement is >3 days.

Progesterone must appear at the right time and in the right amount to facilitate successful implantation, not too early, not too late, and not too low.

Recombinant hCG

- It has a structure similar to that of hCG.
- Absorption, distribution, and metabolism are the same as hCG.
- It is in a pure form and is theoretically safe.
- The maximum concentration is reached within 12–24 hours and the biological half-life is 38 hours.
- Efficacy and safety are the same according to the Cochrane review.[15]
- There is no difference in OHSS rate.
- The efficacy of recombinant hCG (rhCG) is similar to urinary hCG (uhCG) clinically.
- Adverse reactions are not documented.

- The accepted dose of uhCG is 5,000–10,000 IU. The rhCG dose is 250 μg that has the same activity as that of 6,500 IU of uhCG. rhCG has no allergic reaction and there is no failure of ovulation. It has ease of administration for patients and improved efficacy for ovulation and luteal phase support.

Gonadotropin-releasing Hormone Agonist

Characteristics

- It produces LH surge as efficiently as hCG for oocyte maturation and this was first suggested by Itskovitz in 1988.[16]
- It produces FSH surge also with LH surge, in contrast to hCG, but the role of FSH surge has not been established in humans. It has already been established in rats.[17] Both the surges are higher than with hCG surge.
- There is no difference in oocyte maturation and ovulation.
- LH surge due to GnRHa is 24–36 hours as compared to natural surge, which is 48 hours in length, and hCG surge is for 6 days.
- It has only two phases. It has a short ascending limb of >4 hours and long descending limb of >20 hours.[18] The initial rise is because of flare-up. It leads to LH surge with a high peak value and shorter duration than natural LH and hCG.
- Multiple doses do not prolong surge.
- The inhibition of surge is due to gonadotropin surge attenuating factor and inhibin that is induced by estradiol and this inhibition is replaced by GnRHa. It can induce LH surge in the antagonist cycle indicating that the pituitary response to GnRHa is preserved.[19]

Vascular endothelial growth factor and other substances such as angiopoietin 2 (destabilizing factor) are significantly decreased in the follicular fluid after GnRHa trigger. This plays a major role in decreasing OHSS.[20] GnRHa trigger increases antiestrogenic factors and helps in decreasing the risk of OHSS.

Advantages

Estradiol and progesterone levels are lower but can be managed by replacement. Instead, if the levels are supraphysiological, these are detrimental for implantation.[12,13]

- The short duration of surge of 24–36 hours is more physiological and only few follicles are converted into corpus luteum.[21]
- It reduces the risk of OHSS because of complete luteolysis[22] and decreased expression of VEGF.
- Pituitary response to GnRHa is preserved even in an antagonist cycle. OHSS-free clinics concept uses antagonist to prevent premature LH surge with agonist trigger.[23] Here GnRHa replaces antagonist and gives flare-up effect and releases FSH and LH from pituitary.
- For donors, it is the best-accepted protocol.
- It causes FSH surge and the FSH surge promotes the formation of LH receptors in luteinizing granulosa cells, nuclear maturation, and cumulus expansion.[24] It is useful in the luteinized unruptured follicle (LUF).
- More metaphase II (MII) oocytes are recovered with GnRHa than hCG trigger according to some studies.[25,26] But other studies do not find the difference.

Disadvantages

Gonadotropin-releasing hormone agonist trigger causes direct pituitary downregulation resulting in reduced levels of LH, insufficient to sustain adequate corpus luteal activity.

This will lead to a reduced luteal phase progesterone level that will not allow optimum implantation.[27] It causes a short luteal phase and LPD in all cases because of the short duration of LH surge. This shorter duration of LH cannot rescue luteal function because of the reduced amount of FSH and LH. The same amount can complete meiosis. Serum LH is <2 IU/mL after 4 days. So, it is not a direct effect on corpus luteum. Withdrawal of LH for ≥3 days causes luteolysis and so corpus luteal viability can be preserved only for 3 days without LH support.

- Even with luteal supplementation, 25% will still have luteal insufficiency.
- Minimum 600 mg progesterone/day is required which adds the cost in IUI cycles.
- It cannot be used in WHO group I patients.
- It cannot be used in downregulated patients.
- It has lower circulatory estradiol and progesterone in the luteal phase than hCG.
- There is a reduced live birth rate and ongoing pregnancy rate with GnRHa trigger than with hCG trigger in the antagonist protocol in spite of progesterone support.[28] In some studies, a lower implantation rate due to lower oocyte maturation and reduced oocyte and embryo competence is documented.
- Inadequate response:
  - There is a suboptimal response after trigger with GnRHa in patients having a basal level of LH < 1–2.2 IU/mL.[29]
  - When LH < 15 IU/mL after 10–12 hours of the trigger with GnRHa, this is a suboptimal response. The lower LH on the day of trigger also gives suboptimal response. This is common when progesterone is used to prevent LH surge. Adding 1,000–1,500 IU of hCG is very useful.[29] Dual trigger with trigger doses up to 5,000 IU does not improve the results.
  - Patients with a higher BMI give suboptimal response whereas lower BMI < 22 kg/m^2 also give poor response.
  - When the progesterone level is <3.5 ng/mL, the response of GnRHa is inadequate. The progesterone level should be between 5 and 10 ng/mL.
  - A high total dosage of gonadotropin can give an inadequate response (3,800 IU). This inadequate response is because of hypothalamic failure.

The benefit of LH surge is that it promotes LH receptor formation in luteinizing granulosa cells, resumption of meiosis, and cumulus expansion. The oocyte yield is always better with FSH and LH dual surge than only hCG.

It is observed that when LH surge is <15 mIU/mL, it results in lower oocyte retrieval rate and poor cycle outcome. A lower LH level on the day of trigger is also a risk factor for suboptimal response. Adding 1,000 IU of hCG with agonist, i.e., dual trigger in high responders with E2 < 4,000 pg/mL, improves live birth rate without OHSS. But if E2 > 4,000 IU, only estrogen with progesterone is given to support the luteal phase.[30] Along with age, false trigger, and poor ovarian reserve, suboptimal response to GnRHa may be the cause of empty follicle syndrome.

So, suboptimal responders are those in whom serum LH is <15 mIU/mL, approximately 10 hours after GnRHa trigger. Suboptimal responders have higher BMI and lower basal FSH and LH levels (<2.27 mIU/mL).[29] Dual trigger for final oocyte maturation improves the oocyte retrieval rate of suboptimal responders to GnRHa.[31] Suboptimal response is detected when there are no eggs retrieved after puncturing many follicles. This is due to hypothalamic cause, when the LH level is low. Here we can give hCG trigger and can get good results in terms of ova and pregnancy rate. This is common in patients having low BMI (22 kg/m^2) and baseline LH < 1 mIU/mL and higher dose of gonadotropins. Whenever there is a failed trigger, the LH level is <15 mIU/mL and progesterone <3.5 ng/mL, 8–12 hours after trigger. It is found that appropriate elevated post-trigger progesterone concentration with low LH can still result in successful oocyte retrieval, but low progesterone with normal LH concentration >15 mIU/mL might suggest an inadequate response. There is no effect of long-term oral contraceptive (OC) pills for this effect.[32]

Contraindications

- *Hypothalamic dysfunction*: In these patients in spite of GnRHa trigger, endogenous surge is absent or very low. So, oocyte maturation does not occur. So, these are not good candidates for GnRHa trigger.
- Women who have long-term suppression of hypothalamus and pituitary may have failed or may have suboptimal response because they may not be able to mount an optimal LH surge after GnRHa trigger.[33]
- Patients having low FSH and LH basal levels.
- Low LH on the day of trigger.
- Long-term oral contraceptions.[33]

How to Treat Luteal Phase Defect

- Progesterone and/or estradiol replacement can be done. Luteal phase support with vaginal progesterone 600 mg/day and oral estradiol 4 mg/day has given poor results. Only progesterone vaginal or intramuscular without estrogen has also given poor results. The pregnancy rate is 7.9% compared to 30% with hCG.[34] Serum progesterone level > 20 ng/mL and E2 > 200 pg/mL should be maintained.[35] Intramuscular progesterone 50 mg with estradiol 6 mg is given for 10 weeks.
- Humaidan's group administered 1,500 IU of hCG on the day of oocyte retrieval after agonist trigger.[26] It has given an equivalent pregnancy rate as hCG trigger and decreases pregnancy loss. In this study, no case of OHSS occurred when follicles sized 11 mm or larger, were <25. This idea came with the observation that if E2 > 4,000 IU, pregnancy rates are high with agonist trigger and here the LH is high on the day of the trigger. This high LH may rescue few corpus lutea and improve implantation. But if E2 is <4,000 IU, there may be a benefit with 1,000–1,500 IU of hCG without OHSS.
- Even in normal responders, the freeze-all policy and transfer in the next cycle are also acceptable[36] but pregnancy rates are the same.
- Freeze all is the policy for suspected OHSS cases but occasional patients including oocyte donors may get OHSS due to mutation in FSH, LH, or GnRH receptors.[26]
- Garcia-Velasco has reported a 50% pregnancy rate in patients of high-risk OHSS, when after freezing, embryos were transferred in the next cycle.[36,37]

Indications

- Polycystic ovarian syndrome (PCOS) patients, when multiple follicles develop
- In ART cycles where agonists are not used for downregulation
- Those who do not want a fresh embryo transfer
- Fertility preservation
- For those who want preimplantation genetic screening (PGS)/placental growth

factor (PGF) as this automatically means frozen transfer
- Prematurely elevated progesterone level
- Oocyte donors
- Risk of OHSS

Dosage

There are various regimens:
- Single subcutaneous injection 500–1,000 µg of leuprolide acetate
- Two injections of 500–1,000 µg of leuprolide acetate, 12 hours apart
- Intranasal buserelin 50–200 pg and triptorelin 0.2 mg.
- It is found that higher doses do not improve the number and quality of oocytes.[37] Unfortunately which compound, which dose, and when to give are not standardized.

Recombinant Luteinizing Hormone

- The biological half-life is 1 hour and the terminal half-life is 10–12 hours which is quite low than hCG which is 5 hours and 30 hours. Recombinant human LH (rhLH) of 2,500–5,000 IU can induce adequate follicular maturation, corpus luteal formation, and pregnancy without development of OHSS. It more closely mimics natural LH surge than hCG.[38]
- Implantation rate is significantly higher than hCG because of the better quality of embryos.
- It is extremely costly and ampoules of 75 IU only are available. The dose required for trigger is 15,000 IU (750 µg)–30,000 IU (1,500 µg).

RECENT ADVANCES

- *Orally active analog of LH*: Low molecular weight (LMW)—LH agonist has a similar mode of action but shorter half-life than hCG. It abolishes the possibility of OHSS as it has no action on vascular changes and does not induce the production of VEGF.[39]
- *Dual trigger* ***(Flowchart 1)***:
  - *FSH + hCG*: Adding 450 IU of FSH along with 10,000 hCG triggers

Flowchart 1: Treatment strategies in patients with a high risk of OHSS.

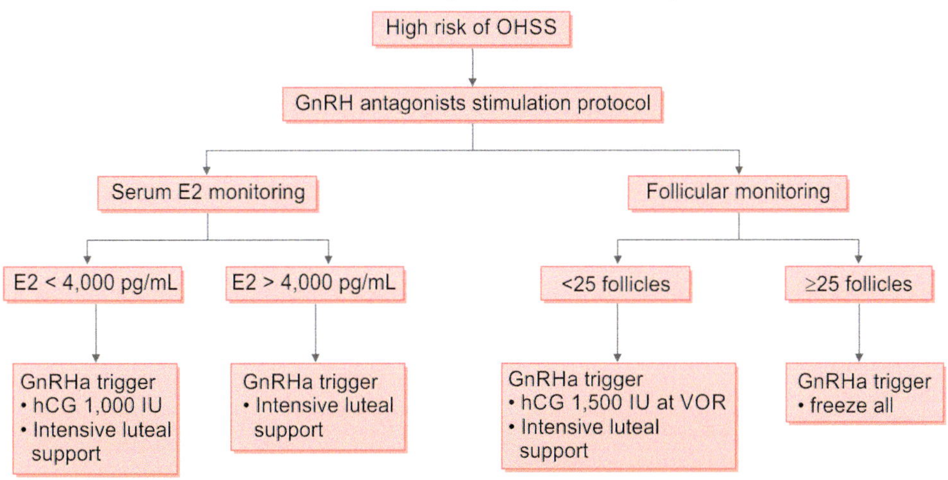

(GnRHa: gonadotropin-releasing hormone agonist; hCG: human chorionic gonadotropin; OHSS: ovarian hyperstimulation syndrome; VOR: vaginal oocyte retrieval)

improved fertilization rate. But there was no statistical difference in the critical pregnancy rate with controls.[40] The idea is to have FSH surge along with LH surge. This was also confirmed by the latest study of Qi Qui in 2020 that FSH addition with hCG does not increase the pregnancy rate.[41]

- *Agonist + hCG*: In the study of high risk of OHSS patients, 4 mg of leuprolide acetate and hCG (1,000–2,500 IU) gave the pregnancy rate of 53%.[42] hCG in dual trigger helps in meiosis of follicles but granulosa cells are refractory during this period and so it does not help in luteal support. It may cause OHSS.
  With routine use of 5,000 IU of hCG, 0.2 mg of decapeptyl was given. The pregnancy rate was 36% as compared to hCG alone which had only 22%.[29]

- Low-dose hCG 125 IU from Day 2 or 6 daily up to throughout the luteal phase has given good results.[43]

Role of Kisspeptin

- Kisspeptin stimulated hypothalamic-pituitary-ovarian (HPO) axis.
- It can cause LH surge for 12–14 hours.
- It is given 36 hours prior to ovum pick-up in a dose of 9.6 nmol/kg.
- Sometimes, the second dose of injection Kisspeptin is given 10 hours after the first dose to sustain the LH surge.
- It reduces the chance of OHSS as it does not produce overresponse.
- It allows fresh embryo transfer.
- It directly inhibits VEGF production.
- Kisspeptin is secreted because of positive feedback of E2 during the preovulatory period.
- Kisspeptin analog can be used for trigger.
- Kisspeptin antagonist can control tonic LH in PCOS.

CARRY HOME MESSAGE

- LH surge is mandatory for ovulation.
- FSH surge is useful, but its role is not understood.
- hCG surge is required in controlled ovarian hyperstimulation (COH) and IUI cycles.
- In IVF, because of the risk of OHSS, hCG is not favored.
- hCG surge does not require luteal support.
- GnRHa as ovulation trigger avoids OHSS.
- It causes luteal phase defect that requires judicious luteal support.
- 1,500 IU of hCG can rescue corpus luteum in agonist trigger when given at the time of pick-up or IUI.
- Recombinant LH for trigger is very costly.
- Dual trigger with agonist and hCG is beneficial.

REFERENCES

1. Hoff JD, Quigley ME, Yen SS. Hormonal dynamics at midcycle: a reevaluation. J Clin Endocrinol Metab. 1983;57:792-6.
2. Seibel MM, Smith DM, Levesque L, Borten M, Taymor ML. The temporal relationship between the luteinizing hormone surge and human oocyte maturation. Am J Obstet Gynecol. 1982;142:568-72.
3. Peluso JJ. Role of amplitude of gonadotropin surge in the rat. Fertil Steril. 1990;53:150-4.
4. Seibel MM, Kamrava MM, McArdle C, Taymor ML. Treatment of polycystic ovary disease with chronic low dose follicle stimulating hormone. Biochemical changes and ultrasound correlation. Int J Fertil. 1984;29:39-43.
5. Kol S, Lewit N, Itskovitz J. Ovarian hyperstimulation: effects of GnRH analogues. Ovarian hyperstimulation syndrome after using gonadotropin-releasing hormone analogue as a trigger of ovulation: causes and implications. Hum Reprod. 1996; 11(6):1143-4.
6. Clark L, Stranger J, Brinsmead M. Prolonged follicle stimulation decreases pregnancy rates after in vitro fertilization. Fertil Steril. 1991;55:1192-4.

7. Tan SL, Balen A, el Hussein E, Mills C, Campbell S, Yovich J. A prospective randomized study of the optimum timing of human chorionic gonadotropin administration after pituitary desensitization in in vitro fertilization. Fertil Steril. 1992;57: 1259-64.
8. Elkind-Hirsch KE, Bello S, Esparcia L, Phillips K, Sheiko A, McNichol M. Serum human gonadotropin levels are correlated with body mass index rather than route of administration in women undergoing in vitro fertilization-embryo transfer using human menopausal gonadotropin and intracytoplasmic sperm injection. Fertil Steril. 2001;75:700-4.
9. Shaltout AM, Eid MS, Shohayeb AA. Does triggering ovulation by 5000 IU of hCG affect ICSI outcome? Middle East Fertil Soc J. 2006;11:99-103.
10. Ferrareti AP, Garcia JE, Acosta AA, Jones GS. Serum luteinizing hormone during ovulation induction with human menopausal gonadotropin for in vitro fertilization in normally menstruating women. Fertil Steril. 1983;40:743-7.
11. Schenken RS, Hodgen GD. Follicle-stimulating hormone induced ovarian hyperstimulation in monkeys: blockage of luteinizing hormone surge. J Clin Endocrinol Metab. 1983;57:50-5.
12. Gidley-Baird AA, O'Neill C, Sinosich MJ, Porter RN, Pike IL, Saunders DM. Failure of implantation in human in vitro fertilization and embryo transfer patients: the effects of altered progesterone/estrogen ratios in human and mice. Fertil Steril. 1986;45:69-74.
13. Forman R, Fries N, Testart J, Belaisch-Allart J, Hazout A, Frydman R. Evidence for an adverse effect of elevated serum estradiol concentrations on embryo implantation. Fertil Steril. 1988;49:118-22.
14. Christenson LK, Stouffer RL. Follicle-stimulating hormone and luteinizing hormone/chorionic gonadotropin stimulation of vascular endothelial growth factor production by macaque granulosa cells from pre- and periovulatory follicles. J Clin Endocrinol Metab. 1997;82:2135-42.
15. Youssef MA, Al-Inany HG, Aboulghar M, Lam WS. Recombinant versus urinary human chorionic gonadotrophin for final oocyte maturation triggering in IVF and ICSI cycles. Cochrane Database Syst Rev. 2011;(4):CD003719.
16. Itskovitz J, Boldes R, Barlev A, Erlik Y, Kahana L, Brandes JM. The induction of LH surge and oocyte maturation by GnRH analogue (buserelin) in women undergoing ovarian stimulation for in vitro fertilization. Gynecol Endocrinol. 1988;2(Suppl 1):165.
17. Moor RM, Osborn JC, Cran OG, Walters DE. Selective effect of gonadotropins on cell coupling, nuclear maturation oocytes. Embryol Exp Morphol. 1981;61:347-65.
18. Scheele F, van der Meer M, Lambalk CB, Schoute E, Schoemaker J, Hompes PG. Exploring the recovery phase after treatment with gonadotropin-releasing hormone agonist. Gynecol Reprod Biol. 1995;62(2):221-4.
19. Olivennes F, Fanchin R, Bouchard P, Taieb J, Frydman R. Triggering of ovulation by gonadotropin- releasing hormone agonist in patients pretreated with GnRH antagonist. Fertil Steril. 1996;66(1):151-3.
20. Cerrillo M, Rodriguez S, Mayoral M, Pacheco A, Martínez-Salazar J, Garcia-Velasco JA. Differential regulation of VEGF after final oocyte maturation with GnRH agonist versus hCG. A rationale for OHSS reduction. Fertil Steril. 2009;91(4 Suppl):1526-8.
21. Emperaire J, Ruffie A. triggering ovulation with endogenous luteinizing hormone may prevent the ovarian hyperstimulation syndrome. Hum Reprod. 1991;6:506-10.
22. Monroe SE, Henzl MR, Martin MC, Schriock E, Lewis V, Nerenberg C, et al. Ablation of folliculogenesis in women by a single dose of gonadotropin-releasing hormone agonist: significance of time in cycle. Fertil Steril. 1985;43:361-8.
23. Albano C, Smitz J, Camus M. Comparison of different doses of gonadotropin-releasing hormone antagonist Cetrorelix during controlled ovarian hyperstimulation. Fertil Steril. 1997;67:917-22.

24. Zelinski-Wooten MB, Hutchison JS, Hess DL, Wolf DP, Stouffer RL. Follicle-stimulating hormone alone supports follicle growth and oocyte development in gonadotropin-releasing hormone antagonist-treated monkeys. Hum Reprod. 1995;10(7):1658-66.
25. Humaidan P, Bungum L, Bungum M, Hald F, Agerholm I, Blaabjerg J, et al. Reproductive outcome using a GnRH antagonist (cetrorelix) for luteolysis and follicular synchronization in poor responder IVF/ICSI patients treated with a flexible GnRH antagonist protocol. Reprod Biomed Online. 2005;11(6):679-84.
26. Humaidan P, Ejdrup Bredkjaer H, Westergaard LG, Andersen CY. 1,500 IU human chorionic gonadotropin administered at oocyte retrieval rescues the luteal phase when gonadotropin-releasing hormone agonist is used for ovulation induction: a prospective, randomized, controlled study. Fertil Steril. 2010;93:847-54.
27. Yding Anderson C, Vilbour Anderson K. Improving luteal phase after ovarian stimulation reviewing new options. Reprod Biomed Online. 2014;28:552-9.
28. Humaidan P, Papanikolaou EG, Kyrou D, Alsbjerg B, Polyzos NP, Devroey P, et al. The luteal phase after GnRH-agonist triggering of ovulation: present and future perspectives. Reprod Biomed Online. 2012;24:134-41.
29. Lu X, Hong Q, Sun L, Chen Q, Fu Y, Ai A, et al. Dual trigger for final oocyte maturation improves the oocyte retrieval rate of suboptimal responders to gonadotropin-releasing hormone agonist. Fertil Steril. 2016;106:1356-62.
30. Shapiro BS, Daneshmand ST, Garner FC, et al. Gonadotropin-releasing hormone agonist combined with a reduced dose of human chorionic gonadotropin for final oocyte maturation in fresh autologous cycles of in- vitro fertilization. Fertil Steril. 2008;90(1):231-3.
31. Elbaek HO, Alsbjerg B, Laursen R, Povlsen BB, Mikkelsen AT, Andersen CY, et al. The exogenous progesterone-free luteal phase in IVF—exploring a new concept. Hum Reprod. 2014;29(i326):502.
32. Chen SL, Ye DS, Chen X, Yang XH, Zheng HY, Tang Y, et al. Circulating luteinizing hormone level after triggering oocyte maturation with GnRH agonist may predict oocyte yield in flexible GnRH antagonist protocol. Hum Reprod. 2012;27:1351-6.
33. Meyer L, Murphy LA, Gumer A, Reichman DE, Rosenwaks Z, Cholst IN. Risk factors for a suboptimal response to gonadotropin-releasing hormone agonist trigger during in-vitro fertilization cycles. Fertil Steril. 2015;104(3):637-42.
34. Griesinger G, Diedrich K, Devroey P, Kolibianakis EM. GnRH agonist for triggering final oocyte maturation in the GnRH antagonist ovarian hyperstimulation protocol: a systematic review and meta-analysis. Hum Reprod Update. 2006;12(2): 159-68.
35. Engmann L, DiLuigi A, Schmidt D, Nulsen J, Maier D, Benadiva C. The use of gonadotropin releasing hormone (GnRH) agonist to induce oocyte maturation after cotreatment with GnRH antagonist in high-risk patients undergoing in-vitro fertilization prevents the risk of ovarian hyperstimulation syndrome: a prospective randomized controlled study. Fertil Steril. 2008;89(1):84-91.
36. Aflatoonian A, Oskouian H, Ahmadi S, Oskouian L. Can fresh embryo transfers be replaced by cryopreserved-thawed embryo transfers in assisted reproductive cycles? A randomized controlled trial. J Assist Reprod Genet. 2010;27:357-63.
37. Garcia-Velasco JA. Agonist trigger: what is the best approach? Agonist trigger with vitrification of oocytes or embryos. Fertil Steril. 2012;97(3):527-8.
38. Vuong TN, Ho MT, Ha TD, Phung HT, Huynh GB, Humaidan P. Gonadotropin-releasing hormone agonist trigger in oocyte donors co-related with a gonadotropin-releasing hormone antagonist: a dose finding study. Fertil Steril. 2016;105(2):356-63.
39. Manau D, Fabergues F, Arroyo V, Jiménez W, Vanrell JA, Balasch J. Hemodynamic changes induced by urinary human chorionic gonadotropin and recombinant luteinizing hormone used for inducing final follicular

maturation and luteinization. Fertil Steril. 2002;78:1261-7.
40. Van de Lagemaat R, Raafs BC, van Koppen C, Timmers CM, Mulders SM, Hanssen RGJM. Prevention of the onset of ovarian hyperstimulation syndrome (OHSS) in the rat after ovulation induction with a low molecular weight agonist of the LH receptor compared with hCG and rec-LH. Endocrinology. 2011; 152:4350-7.
41. Qui Q, Huang J, Li Y, Chen X, Lin H, Li L, et al. Does an FSH surge at the time of hCG trigger improve IVF/ICSI outcomes? A randomized, double-blinded, placebo controlled study. Hum Reprod. 2020; 35(6):1411-20.
42. Lamb JD, Shen S, McCulloch C, Jalalian L, Cedars MI, Rosen MP. Follicle-stimulating hormone administered at the time of human chorionic gonadotropin trigger improves oocyte developmental competence in in vitro fertilization cycles: a randomized, double-blind, placebo-controlled trial. Fertil Steril. 2011;95(5):1655-60.
43. Chang FE, Beall SA, Cox JM, Ritcher KS, DeCherney AH, Levy MJ. Assessing the adequacy of gonadotropin-releasing hormone agonist leuprolide to trigger oocyte maturation and management of inadequate response. Fertil Steril. 2016;106: 1093-100.

11

Chapter

Ovulation Induction in Hypogonadotropic Hypogonadism

INTRODUCTION

Hypogonadotropic hypogonadism (HH) is hypothalamo-pituitary failure, ovulatory dysfunction [classified by the World Health Organization (WHO) as group I type of anovulation]. It is the condition in which secretions of gonadotropins from the pituitary are so low that there is no growth of follicles in the ovary and so no estrogen production. The classical finding is a very low estrogen level along with anovulation and amenorrhea and no withdrawal bleed with progesterone.

The recent studies have shown that kisspeptin regulates gonadotropin-releasing hormone (GnRH) secretion.[1] It has been documented that central and peripheral administration of kisspeptin increases follicle-stimulating hormone (FSH) and luteinizing hormone (LH) secretion by activating GnRH neurons.

CAUSES

- *Hypothalamic causes*:
  - Extremely low body weight—anorexia nervosa or sudden severe crash dieting
  - Strenuous exercises such as dancing and running
  - Kallmann syndrome (isolated GnRH deficiency)
  - Psychiatric disorders—anxiety
  - Stress
- *Pituitary causes*:
  - Surgery—hypophysectomy or trauma
  - Radiation to brain
  - Sheehan's syndrome
  - Pituitary tumors
  - Empty sella syndrome
  - Extrapituitary lesions—tumors such as craniopharyngioma, glioma, and meningioma
  - Isolated FSH or LH deficiency
- *Systemic diseases (chronic illnesses)*:
  - Renal failure
  - Cirrhosis
  - Beta thalassemia
  - Sarcoidosis and tuberculosis
  - Meningoencephalitis
  - Syphilis
  - Agonist, antagonist, and steroids
- Idiopathic

DIAGNOSIS

- *On history and examination*: Small uterus and ovaries and other signs of hypoestrinism
- *Blood investigations*: Low estradiol (E2), low LH, low or normal FSH, and thyroid function tests
- *According to the cause*:
  - GnRH stimulation test
  - MRI
  - Renal ultrasound

DIFFERENTIAL DIAGNOSIS

- Polycystic ovarian syndrome (PCOS)
- Hyperprolactinemia (HPRL)
- Isolated hypothyroidism
- Premature ovarian failure (POF)

MANAGEMENT

Hormone Replacement Therapy

Hormone replacement therapy is given to all the patients of HH after menarche, even when fertility is not a concern. Estrogen and progesterone are given cyclically. It is protective against osteoporosis and cardiovascular diseases. It helps in the development of genital organs. Moreover with this priming, treating her for fertility becomes easier. Vitamin D and calcium are also given simultaneously.

Management for Desiring Pregnancy

- Pulsatile GnRH therapy
- Gonadotropins therapy

Pulsatile Gonadotropin-releasing Hormone Therapy

Gonadotropin-releasing hormone is the neurohormone synthesized by nerve endings in the anterior hypothalamus. It goes to the pituitary and releases FSH and LH. It has a very short half-life and is released in a pulsatile fashion. The frequency and amplitude of the pulse are changed by various factors that affect the hypothalamus. This is usually assessed by LH pulse that reflects the GnRH release. GnRH is released once in 60 minutes in the follicular phase and once in 4 hours in the luteal phase. The amount, timing, and pulsatile release of GnRH determine the pattern of ovulatory cycle by the release of hormones (FSH and LH) from the anterior pituitary.

When pituitary is intact, GnRH can be given in a pulsatile manner for FSH and LH release in patients with idiopathic hypothalamic failure. This can be done through an infusion pump by the subcutaneous or intravenous route. The dose is 15–20 µg subcutaneously or 5–10 µg intravenously every 60–90 minutes. This is an effective therapy for ovulation induction in hypothalamic amenorrhea and may give pregnancy rates of up to 80%. In these patients, the ovulation trigger with human chorionic gonadotropin (hCG) is not required.[2] The infusion pump can be withdrawn in the luteal phase and luteal support can be given till the menstruation or till pregnancy occurs.

This treatment has an advantage over gonadotropin therapy, that it leads to monofollicular development, and therefore the incidence of multiple pregnancy is <5% and the risk of ovarian hyperstimulation syndrome (OHSS) is rare **(Box 1)**. Multiple pregnancies may occur only when hCG is given as an ovulation trigger.[3] It does not even require a fancy expensive monitoring system. But the difficulty of this treatment is fixing and using the infusion pump, which is inconvenient and expensive and may also lead to thrombophlebitis if used for the intravenous route **(Box 2)**. But if acceptable to the patient, it is a better treatment option in terms of low multiple pregnancies and low OHSS rate. Though this treatment option is not commonly used. It has been replaced by gonadotropin therapy.

Box 1: Advantages of GnRH therapy.

- High ovulation rate
- Pregnancy rate 80–90%
- Low OHSS
- Low multiple pregnancy rate
- No monitoring required
- Low abortion rate

(GnRH: gonadotropin-releasing hormone; OHSS: ovarian hyperstimulation syndrome)

Box 2: Disadvantages of GnRH therapy.

- Use of infusion pump
- Thrombophlebitis
- Skin reaction, hematoma
- Development of antibodies

(GnRH: gonadotropin-releasing hormone)

Gonadotropin Therapy

Gonadotropin therapy is useful in HH patients of either hypothalamic or pituitary origin. FSH and LH/hCG is a more effective combination in these cases rather than FSH alone.[4]

When only FSH is given, there will be good follicular development but the estrogen level will be low and ovulation may not occur. The endometrial development is also inadequate. For both these reasons, oocyte fertilization and conception rates are low.[5]

According to the two-cell-two-gonadotropin hypothesis, LH is required to produce androgen from theca cells and these androgens under the influence of FSH will be converted into estrogen. In HH patients, LH is absent or very low and thus no androgen is available for estrogen production **(Box 3)**.[6,7]

The dose of gonadotropins is very high and the response to the ovary is very slow because ovaries are not exposed to endogenous gonadotropins and FSH receptors on the ovary are also less.

So, the stimulation is done by either human menopausal gonadotropin (HMG) or FSH and recombinant LH (rLH) or FSH combined with low dose hCG **(Box 4)**.

A woman with a basal serum level of LH of <1.2 IU/L suggests more severe deficiency of LH and would benefit from LH supplementation.[8,9]

In a standard protocol, HMG is usually started in the dose of 150 IU daily or 150 IU recombinant FSH (rFSH) with 75 IU rLH for 5 days. If the E2 level is increased, the same dose is continued, otherwise a 33% increase in the dose is done every 5 days.[10] The response is considered optimum when one follicle of 17–18 mm develops or an E2 level of >400 IU/L is achieved and the midluteal progesterone level reaches 25 nmol/L. Ovulation trigger is given with hCG 10,000.[10]

Box 3: Role of adding LH with FSH in HH patients.

- Dose-related increase in androgen and E2 from rFSH-induced follicles
- Increases sensitivity to FSH
- Enhances luteinization when exposed to hCG

(FSH: follicle-stimulating hormone; HH: hypogonadotropic hypogonadism; LH: luteinizing hormone; rFSH: recombinant FSH; hCG: human chorionic gonadotropin)

Box 4: Most accepted regime for hypogonadotropic hypogonadism patients.

- Confirm diagnosis by FSH, LH, and E2
- Start HMG 150 IU or rFSH 150 IU + rLH 75 IU
- If LH < 1.2 IU/mL, use higher doses of LH
- After 7 days of E2, if increases continue the same dose
- If no E2 rise, increase 33% of the existing dose
- Ovulation trigger by 10,000 IU of hCG or 250 rhCG
- Luteal support by progesterone or hCG

(FSH: follicle-stimulating hormone; HMG: human menopausal gonadotropin; LH: luteinizing hormone; rhCG: recombinant human chorionic gonadotropin; rFSH: recombinant FSH)

For ovulation trigger, hCG is a must because endogenous LH is absent and in this case, GnRH antagonist is of no use. Luteal support with progesterone or hCG 2,000 IU every 3–4 days is a must as endogenous LH is absent.

The dose of LH is as follows:

- The daily dose of 75 IU of rLH is sufficient. A high dose > 225 IU of LH causes atresia of follicles indicating ceiling effect of LH.[4]
- The majority of the patients require only 75 IU of LH, but few patients may require 225 IU LH. Shoham et al. in a randomized double-blind, placebo-controlled trial confirmed the validity of 1.2 IU/L as a cutoff and efficacy of 75 IU as the effective dose for LH supplementation for patients having severe LH deficiency.[11] The rise of E2 due to LH helps in endometrial development, implantation, and pregnancy. Individual FSH and LH injections are better than HMG

for monofollicular development. The fixed ratio of FSH and LH in HMG gives multifollicular development. High doses of rLH in the final stage of maturation after 11–12 mm allow one follicle to mature and others to undergo atresia, resulting in monofollicular development when FSH and LH are used separately.

- Priming with rLH, 300 IU for 7 days, before FSH stimulation has shown no beneficial effect in terms of follicular development and pregnancy.[12] But pretreatment with LH may require a lower dose of FSH and the level of LH may remain high during stimulation. This may be due to its effect on pituitary LH secretion in idiopathic HH due to the secretion of kisspeptin that is a potent stimulator for gonadotropin secretion. The results reported in HH are 89% and 72% after 6 and 7 ovulatory cycles, respectively.[13,14] The ovarian response in HH patients may not be affected so much with age like in other infertile patients. Hence, the dose schedule options are:
    - 7 days HMG 150–225 according to body weight and then increase after 7 days if no response
    - *Step-up + step-down protocol*: Day 1–2 (150 mg) and Day 3–7 (75 mg). From Day 8 and onwards, according to the response, the dose is individualized. Normally, the FSH/LH ratio should be 2:1 in the first half and then should be reversed in the second half.[15]

ADDITIONAL STRATEGIES (BOX 5)

Several patients with HH may not respond to the conventional HMG protocol and may require additional drugs. Those documented are:

Box 5: Additional strategies.

- Additional growth hormone or IGF-1
- Pretreatment with estrogen
- Pretreatment with estrogen and progesterone

(IGF-1: insulin-like growth factor 1)

- *Growth hormone (GH) or insulin-like growth factor 1 (IGF-1)*: GH deficiency is one of the causes for poor response to HMG in HH patients. GH has a direct effect on follicle maturation and amplifies the action of FSH and LH.[16] Adding GH to the patients not responding to HMG results in the development of more follicles and ovulation. It also reduces the daily dose and treatment duration with HMG.[16] GH deficiency may also be the causative factor in patients with unexplained infertility or poor responders.
- *Pretreatment with estrogen*: Patients with HH, who do not conceive with a conventional protocol with HMG, may respond well and give good pregnancy rates by adding estrogen and progesterone cyclically. In one study, 22 out of 30 patients conceived with this protocol.[17]

In the hypoestrogenic environment, HMG seems to be less effective and so prior treatment with estrogen and progesterone combination results in high estrogen environment and gives better pregnancy rates. It promotes cervical mucus and endometrium for better response to gonadotropins.[16] Adding conjugated estrogen with HMG also gives better pregnancy rates.

RECENT ADVANCES (BOX 6)

- *Long-acting compounds*: Daily injection of gonadotropins is not accepted by the patients and it increases stress and treatment burden. Long-acting drugs may be preferred to the same. Follitropin alpha, long-acting FSH, can replace daily FSH injections for the first 7 days of ovulation induction.[18]
- *Kisspeptin/GPR54 complex*: Exogenous kisspeptin GPR54 stimulates the hypothalamo-pituitary-gonadal axis in

Box 6: Recent advances in treatment.

- Long-acting FSH
- Exogenous kisspeptin
- *ERK* and *ERK2* gene mutation

(FSH: follicle-stimulating hormone)

normal females.[19] If it is particularly given during the preovulatory period, a rise in LH is pronounced.[16] Kisspeptin may be a promising drug in the future for ovulation induction in HH patients. It causes a lower incidence of OHSS. An oral GPR54 agonist has been developed and it will have an advantage over gonadotropin injections.

- *ERK1* and *ERK2* signal-regulated kinases have been found out between LH surge and ovulation.[20] It leads to a decrease in cyclic adenosine monophosphate (AMP) between cumulus and oocytes. Cyclic AMP represses the resumption of meiosis and maturation of oocyte. So, the reduction of cyclic AMP results in the resumption of meiosis and ovulation. These *ERK1* and *ERK2* gene mutation may cause infertility. This gene research will help in in vitro maturation and in vitro fertilization (IVF).

CARRY HOME MESSAGE

- Classical features of HH are low estrogen with amenorrhea and anovulation with low FSH and LH levels.
- Hormone replacement therapy is given when fertility is not an issue.
- Pulsatile GnRH therapy and gonadotropin replacement are the options.
- HMG or rFSH and rLH individually can be used, but individual doses are more useful.
- rLH in high doses can help in monofollicular development in the latter half of stimulation.
- Pretreatment with estrogen is not much useful.
- Pretreatment with LH reduces FSH dose during stimulation.
- Growth hormone can be used in poor responders.
- Follitropin alpha and long-acting compounds have future hope.
- Kisspeptin regulated GnRH secretion and is the newer research for management.

REFERENCES

1. Dungan HM, Clifton DK, Steiner RA. Minireview: Kisspeptin neurons as central processors in the regulation of gonadotropin-releasing hormone secretion. Endocrinology. 2006;147:1154-8.
2. Homburg R, Eschel A, Armar NA, Tucker M, Mason PW, Adams J, et al. One hundred pregnancies after treatment with pulsatile luteinizing hormone releasing hormone to induce ovulation. Br Med J. 1989;298:809-12.
3. Braat DD, Schoemaker R, Schoemaker J. Life table analysis of fecundity of intravenously gonadotropin-releasing hormone treated patients with normogonadotropic and hypogonadotropic amenorrhea. Fertil Steril. 1991;55:266-71.
4. The European Recombinant Human LH Study Group. Recombinant human luteinizing hormone (LH) to support human follicle-stimulating hormone (FSH)-induced follicular development in LH and FSH deficient an ovulatory women: a dose-finding study. J Clin Endocrinol Metab. 1998;83:1507-14.
5. Balasch J, Miro F, Burzaco I, Casamitjana R, Civicon S, Ballescá JL, et al. The role of luteinizing hormone in human follicle development and oocyte fertility: evidence from in vitro fertilization in a woman with long standing hypogonadotropic hypogonadism and using recombinant human follicle stimulating hormone. Hum Reprod. 1995;10:1678-83.
6. Thompson EL, Patterson M, Murphy KG, Smith KL, Dhillo WS, Todd JF, et al. Central and peripheral administration of kisspeptin-10 stimulates the hypothalamo-pituitary-gonadal axis. J Neuroendocrinol. 2004;16:850-8.
7. Fevold HL. Synergism of follicle stimulating hormone and luteinizing hormones in producing estrogen secretion. Endocrinology. 1941;28:33-6.
8. Shoham Z, Balen A, Patel A, Jacobs HS. Results of ovulation induction using human menopausal gonadotropin or purified follicle stimulating hormone in hypogonadotropic hypogonadism patients. Fertil Steril. 1991;56:1048-53.

9. O'dea L, the US Recombinant Human LH Study Group. Recombinant LH in support of recombinant FSH in female hypogonadotropic hypogonadism-evidence of threshold effect. Fertil Steril. 2000; 74(Suppl 1):836.
10. Messinis IE. Ovulation induction: a mini review. Hum Reprod. 2005;20:2688-97.
11. Shoham Z, Smith H, Yeko T, O'Brien F, Hemsey G, O'Dea L. Recombinant LH (lutropin alfa) for the treatment of hypogonadotropic women with profound LH deficiency: a randomized double-blind, placebo-controlled, proof-of-efficacy study. Clin Endocrinol (Oxf). 2008;69:471-8.
12. Balasch J, Fabregues F, Carmona F, Casamitjana R, Tena-Sempere M. Ovarian luteinizing hormone promising preceding follicle stimulating hormone stimulation: clinical and endocrine effects in women with long term hypogonadotropic hypogonadism. J Clin Endocrinol Metab. 2009;94:2367-73.
13. Flukar MR, Urman B, Mackinnon M, Barrow SR, Pride SM, Yuen BH. Exogenous gonadotropin therapy in World Health Organization groups I and II ovulatory disorders. Obstet Gynecol. 1994;83:189-96.
14. Tadokoro N, Vollenhoven B, Clark S, Baker G, Kovacs G, Burger H, et al. Cumulative pregnancy rates in couples with an ovulatory infertility compared with unexplained infertility in an ovulation induction programme. Hum Reprod. 1997;12:1939-44.
15. Krause BT, Ohlinger R, Haase A. Lutropin alpha, recombinant human luteinizing hormone for the stimulation of follicular development in profoundly LH-deficient hypogonadotropic hypogonadal women: a review. Biologics. 2009;3:337-47.
16. Hull KL, Harvey S. Growth hormone: roles in female reproduction. J Endocrinol. 2001;168:1-23.
17. Yildrim M, Noyan V, Tiras MB. Estrogen-Progestogen pre-treatment before HMG induction in hypogonadotropic patients. Int J Gynecol Obstet. 2000;71:249-50.
18. Fauser BC, Mannaerts BM, Devroey P, Leader A, Boime I, Baird DT. Advances in recombinant DNA technology: corifollitropin alfa, a hybrid molecule with sustained follicle-stimulating activity and reduced injection frequency. Hum Reprod Update. 2009;15:309-21.
19. Dhillo WS, Chaudhri OB, Thompson EL, Murphy KG, Patterson M, Ramachandran R, et al. Kisspeptin-54 stimulated gonadotropin release most potently during the preovulatory phase of the menstrual cycle in women. J Clin Endocrinol Metab. 2007;92:3958-66.
20. Fan HY, Liu Z, Shimada M, Sterneck E, Johnson PF, Hedrick SM, et al. *MAPK3/1 (ERK1/2)* in ovarian granulosa cells are essential for female fertility. Science. 2009;324:938-41.

Chapter 12

Ovulation Induction in Polycystic Ovarian Syndrome

INTRODUCTION

Patients with polycystic ovarian syndrome (PCOS) have a high antral follicle count (AFC) and also have high stromal vascularity, both of which make them more prone to ovarian hyperstimulation syndrome (OHSS). This is one of the most dreaded complications of ovulation induction. Therefore, ovulation induction in PCOS requires careful assessment of the patient and careful consideration before deciding on the ovulation induction protocols. Moreover, insulin resistance, high androgen, and high luteinizing hormone (LH)—the major components of the PCOS—are also challenges for ovulation induction in these patients.

Approximately 20–30% of women in the reproductive age group have polycystic ovaries (PCO) and about half of these have signs and symptoms of PCOS. The earliest description of PCO appears to date from 1845 as "sclerocystic ovaries."[1] According to the European Society for Human Reproduction and Embryology/American Society for Reproductive Medicine (ESHRE/ASRM) consensus 2003[2] (Rotterdam criteria), the diagnosis of PCOS consists of at least two of the following three criteria:

1. Oligo- and/or anovulation
2. *Hyperandrogenism*: Biochemical and/or clinical
3. *PCO on ultrasound [excluding other causes such as congenital adrenal hyperplasia (CAH)]*: This means an ovary that is 10 cc in volume and/or has more than 12 antral follicles.

Polycystic ovarian syndrome, apart from its endocrinal component, as mentioned in the Rotterdam criteria, also has a metabolic component. The chief components of clinical criteria are irregular menstrual cycles due to oligo-ovulation or anovulation, acne, hirsutism and in severe cases acanthosis nigricans due to hyperandrogenemia. Some of these patients may be very obese or absolutely thin lean. Most important among the hormonal criteria are high androgen, high LH, and high anti-Müllerian hormone (AMH). The serum prolactin level is high in 30–40% of PCOS due to high estrogen, the source of which is peripheral conversion of estrone from high androgen **(Flowcharts 1 and 2)**.

POLYCYSTIC OVARIES ON ULTRASOUND

Polycystic ovaries on ultrasound mean an ovary that is 10 cc in volume and/or has more than 12 antral follicles according to the Rotterdam criteria. But the recent literature evidences mention that the number of antral follicles may be changed to 26 per ovary in

Flowchart 1: Androgen metabolism.

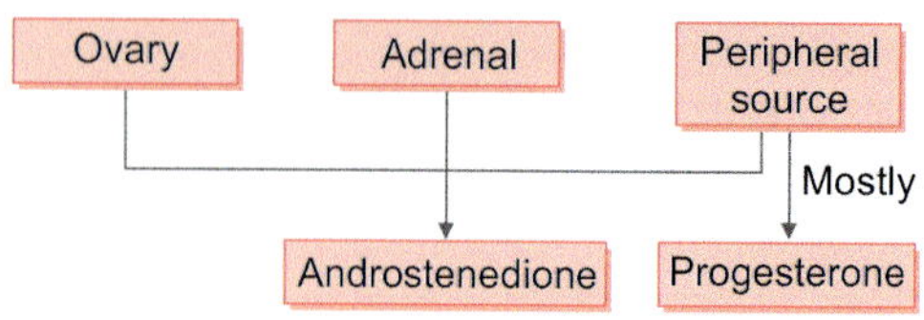

Flowchart 2: Adrenal androgen.

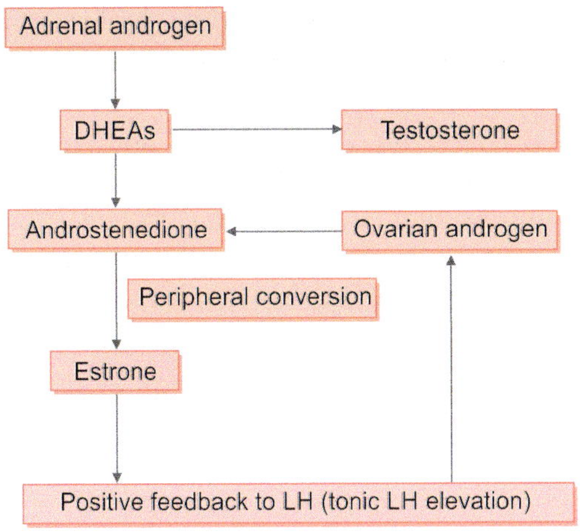

(DHEAs: dehydroepiandrosterones; LH: luteinizing hormone)

Flowchart 3: Serine phosphorylation.

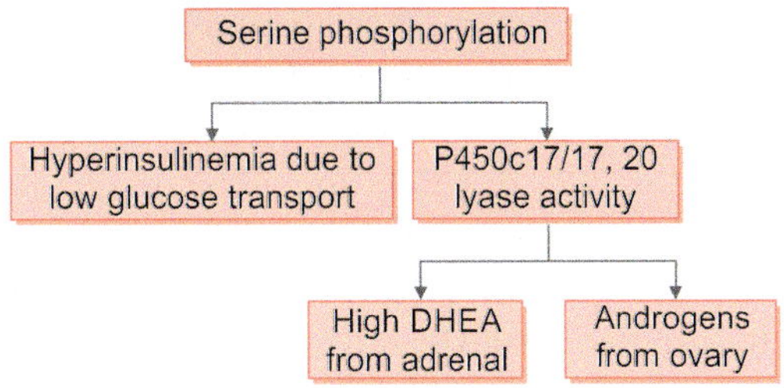

(DHEA: dehydroepiandrosterone)

a frank manifestation of PCOS.[3] There are several studies that have mentioned that the volume of 10 cc may be needed to be reconsidered as patients with smaller ovaries have also been found to have PCOS in a considerable percentage of cases.[4] Moreover, a recent study has also mentioned variation in the cutoffs for follicle number and ovarian volume for different age groups.[5]

AFC is an important marker for PCO, but the same number cannot be applicable to age groups. Superior diagnostic performance with improved balance of sensitivity and specificity compared to single threshold.[6]

The metabolic derangements that are commonly seen in patients with PCOS are hyperinsulinemia and hyperlipidemia.

Insulin resistance is because of:

- Serine phosphorylation of beta-chain of insulin receptor **(Flowchart 3)**.
- Serine phosphorylation of ovarian and adrenal cytochrome P450c17 enzyme **(Flowchart 3)**
- This activates 17-hydroxylase and 17,20-lyase activities, which help in androgen synthesis. This leads to high androgen. About 15% of women with PCO also have adrenal hyperandrogenism.
- Increase in insulin-like growth factor-1 (IGF-1) IGF-1 augments androgen production due to high LH.

CLINICAL PATHOLOGY

- Insulin resistance leads to hyperinsulinemia.
- This increases the androgen level directly from ovary and adrenals.
- Indirect rise of androgen is also a result of high LH.
- Hyperinsulinemia inhibits sex hormone-binding globulin (SHBG) synthesis from the liver giving a high-free androgen level.
- Hyperinsulinemia and hyperandrogenemia cause anovulation and late sequelae of PCOS.

OPTIONS FOR OVULATION INDUCTION IN POLYCYSTIC OVARIAN SYNDROME PATIENTS

The comprehensive treatment of PCOS may include correction of both metabolic and endocrinal components. In this chapter, the ovulation induction options are discussed for PCOS patients. Ovulation induction in PCOS women is different than ovulation induction in non-PCOS women. In PCOS women, fertility is compromised not only because of oligo anovulation, but also due to poor ovum quality owing to high LH and in turn high insulin levels. These patients also have a risk of ovarian hyperstimulation due to high androgen levels and they also have higher abortion rates due to both bad ovum quality and poor endometrial vascularity. This means improving fertility and ovulation induction in these cases should have a holistic approach to decrease insulin, androgen, and LH and also to decrease the risk of OHSS and abortion rates. The options for ovulation induction in PCOS patients are as follows:

- Weight loss
- Clomiphene citrate (CC)
- Letrozole
- Insulin-lowering drugs
- Glucocorticoids
- Gonadotropins
- Gonadotropin-releasing hormone (GnRH) antagonist
- GnRH agonist (GnRHa)
- Ovarian drilling
- In vitro fertilization/in vitro maturation (IVF/IVM)

Weight Loss

It is the first line of treatment in obese PCOS patients. Central obesity is more common to cause metabolic changes. These patients typically have a waist-to-hip ratio of 0.7–0.8 which is an android type of obesity. Obesity, as is known, cannot be judged by just the weight. The best parameter to assess obesity is body mass index (BMI). The normal BMI range is 20-24.9 kg/m^2, whereas when it is between 25 and 29 kg/m^2, the individual is called overweight.

When BMI is >30 kg/m^2, it indicates obesity[7] and BMI of <20 kg/m^2 is also considered low and abnormal.

It is the weight loss and decrease in the fat that cause improvement of insulin resistance, decrease in androgen levels, and resumption of ovulation. During the initial period of calorie restriction, preferential loss of intra-abdominal fat occurs due to increased lipolysis and its high metabolic activity.[8,9] Only 5% of the total body weight loss is important to induce ovulation.[10] It reduces 30% of visceral fat. This regains reproductive functions in 60–100% of cases. Weight loss reduces hyperinsulinemia and hyperandrogenemia and increases SHBG. It improves the sensitivity for ovulation induction drugs. It also reduces clomiphene resistance. Weight loss decreases the rate of abortions. A retrospective study of 5,019 cycles of IVF revealed that obesity was associated with longer durations and increased amounts of gonadotropin stimulation, increased frequency of cycle cancellation for inadequate response, and lower oocyte yields.[11]

Kulkarni et al, have mentioned that change in diet composition with urbanization has great influence on the phenotype of PCOS in western Indian population. It has resulted into more severe phenotype of PCOS and is likely to have implications on fertility outcome. Lifestyle changes can revert this effect.[12]

Weight loss is an effective way of treating fertility-related complications of PCOS and therefore must be emphasized. It can be achieved by diet control, exercise, group therapy, behavioral counseling, pharmacological treatment, and bariatric surgery. Antiobesity drugs are considered an experimental therapy for the purpose of improving fertility. Bariatric surgery is also still experimental in this context, and pregnancy should not be allowed for 12 months after the surgery though it may help to improve gestational diabetes. So, it is a teamwork that is required to help the patient to lose weight. But a normal weight PCOS patient may not benefit from weight loss. The role of preconceptional counseling of overweight women was emphasized by the second international workshop group and was endorsed by ESHRE and ASRM held in Thessaloniki in Greece in 2007.

ESHRE/ASRM recommendations:
- 5–10% of weight loss by energy deficit of 30% or 500–700 kcal/day to prevent weight gain
- 150 min/wk of moderate exercise or 75 min/wk of vigorous exercise
- For weight loss, double the time of moderate and vigorous exercise.
- Antiobesity drugs are considered experimental.
- Bariatric surgery is also still experimental and pregnancy should not be allowed for 12 months after the surgery.
- Weight loss and metformin prior to IVF increases pregnancy rate.

Clomiphene Citrate

Clomiphene citrate induces ovulation in 70–80% of cases with a 30–40% pregnancy rate and gives a 30% cumulative live birth rate.[13-15] CC acts on the hypothalamus to secrete GnRH, which in turn gives follicle-stimulating hormone (FSH) and LH. In PCOS patients, LH is otherwise also high and is a cause of bad oocyte quality. Therefore, if on Day 8–9 of the cycle, LH > 10 IU in the first CC-treated cycle, it is not used in the subsequent cycle.[16] Patients who do not respond to 150 mg of CC are CC-resistant cases. This occurs in 15–40% of PCOS patients.[17]

Clomiphene is used for obese PCOS for ovulation induction when BMI > 30 kg/m^2. Metformin in these cases is added when there is clomiphene resistance.

ESHRE-ASRM guidelines:
- Clomiphene has a lower pregnancy rate than letrozole and gonadotropins.
- Clomiphene plus gonadotropins does not have a higher pregnancy rate.
- CC can be used in obese patients with BMI > 30 kg/m^2 with anovulatory infertility.
- Metformin can be added to CC-resistant cases.
- Risk of multiple pregnancy is increased.

Letrozole

Letrozole is considered as the first line of treatment for ovulation induction in women with PCOS.

This is a very good alternative to CC. It causes borderline hypoestrinism and hyperandrogenism. The mechanism has already been discussed in Chapter 6 in this book. A fall in estrogen levels leads to a rise in FSH and LH levels that stimulates follicular development. The resultant rise in estrogen has a negative feedback mechanism and it reduces FSH and LH, thus allowing monofollicular development. Hyperandrogenism caused by letrozole increases the sensitivity of the follicle to FSH. Letrozole with gonadotropins is a synergistic combination without decreasing the pregnancy rate.[18]

There are several reports that indicate that letrozole is better than CC for ovulation induction in PCOS[19,20] and some reports have shown that letrozole is at least as effective as CC for ovulation induction.[21,22] The advantages of letrozole in PCOS patients are monofollicular development, lesser incidence of multiple pregnancy, lesser risk of OHSS, and lower abortion rates due to fall in LH levels and no effect on cervical mucus and endometrium.

Letrozole or CC + metformin are equally effective for ovulation induction and achieving pregnancy in CC-resistant cases. But letrozole is better tolerated and therefore preferred.[23]

ESHRE-ASRM guidelines:
- Letrozole should be considered as first-line therapy for ovulation induction in PCOS.
- Live birth rate increases by 40–60%.
- Letrozole resistance is less than CC.
- Risk of multiple pregnancy is less with letrozole.

Insulin-lowering Drugs (Insulin Sensitizers)

Insulin resistance in PCOS patients causes hyperinsulinemia, which in turn stimulates theca cells of the ovary to secrete more androgen, through LH. Androgen further recruits more follicles and leads to more LH again establishing a vicious cycle. Hyperinsulinemia in women with obesity contributes to anovulation by increased ovarian androgen secretion.[24] More than half of PCOS patients have insulin resistance. Insulin sensitizers such as metformin will reduce the insulin levels and thus will break the cycle and hence help in correcting the hormonal balance.

Earlier metformin was thought to be a useful drug for ovulation induction in PCOS patients. But recent reports indicate that when metformin is used as the only drug for ovulation induction in PCOS patients, the live birth rate is only 7.2% as compared to that with CC which is 22.5%.[25] Findings of two randomized controlled trials (RCTs) indicated that metformin does not increase live birth rates above those observed with CC alone.[26]

It has also been proved that metformin does not lower the dose of CC required when it is used in combination with CC.[26] CC, therefore, is the most appropriate first line of treatment for ovulation induction in PCOS patients. It is interesting to know that anthropometrical data and metabolic characteristics do not give grounds for adjustment of the dose of metformin as its efficacy is not dose-dependent, but side effects are. Therefore, metformin should be preferred in the lowest possible doses.[27] ESHRE/ASRM 2007 consensus on the use of metformin as an agent for ovulation induction shows that there is no clear evidence that the addition of metformin to CC as a primary therapy for induction of ovulation has a beneficial effect.[28]

Therefore, the use of metformin in PCOS should be restricted to women with glucose intolerance and frank type II diabetes.[29] Addition of metformin to gonadotropins has no advantage in improving ovulation rates, pregnancy rates, live birth rates, multiple pregnancy rates, or incidence of OHSS **(Box 1)**.[30,31]

Box 1: Metformin and infertility.

- CC is better than metformin for ovulation induction
- Combination of CC and metformin does not increase pregnancy rate[26]
- Combination does not lower the dose requirement of CC
- Metformin combined with gonadotropin does not have a better outcome than gonadotropin alone
- If given in resistant PCOS patients, it decreases the sensitivity to ovulation induction drugs
- Incidence and severity of OHSS are reduced by 6–12 weeks of pretherapy with metformin
- It does not reduce the abortion rate[26]

(CC: clomiphene citrate; OHSS: ovarian hyperstimulation syndrome; PCOS: polycystic ovarian syndrome)

Metformin in Patients for IVF

There are several papers that indicate no difference in pregnancy rates in metformin and nonmetformin groups in IVF patients.[31,32] Though it is a common practice for gynecologists and endocrinologists to administer or sustain metformin treatment in infertile patients with PCOS scheduled for IVF, irrespective of their basal metabolic status or clinical efficacy of treatment. In patients with PCOS and poor ovarian reserve, metformin worsened the response to gonadotropins and it should be stopped before starting controlled ovarian hyperstimulation for IVF.[33]

In a meta-analysis that evaluated the effectiveness of metformin as a cotreatment during IVF cycles in women with PCOS, metformin reduced the risk of OHSS by approximately 75%.[34] Another study also confirms that in patients with PCOS, who are at a high risk for OHSS and who have been stimulated with gonadotropins for IVF cycles, metformin reduces the risk of OHSS by modulating the ovarian response to stimulation.[35] It reduces the number of small follicles and reduces IGF-1 in follicular fluids.[36] It reduces days of coasting and lowers estradiol (E2) level giving a positive impact on fertilization and pregnancy rate.[37] A study by Kjøtrød et al. concludes that metformin (1,000–1,500 mg) treatment for 12 weeks before and during IVF or intracytoplasmic sperm injection (ICSI) in nonobese women with PCOS significantly increases pregnancy and live birth rates compared with placebo.[38]

Metformin after Conception

The safety of metformin in pregnancy has not been established. A large prospective RCT has shown that when metformin is continued in early pregnancy, it does not decrease the miscarriage rate.[22] Indirect data from a recent meta-analysis has shown no significant benefit of pregestational metformin administration on abortion risk in patients with PCOS, when either used as monotherapy or in combination with other fertility drugs.[39] Metformin crosses the placenta, and a significant level is found in fetal serum. Therefore, metformin should be stopped after the pregnancy test until more consistent data are available.

Vega et al. have documented in their study that insulin has direct toxicity on human placenta, particularly on early trophoblast and it is protected by metformin. Continuition of metformin during pregnancy may be beneficial and may help prevent pregnancy loss. Though larger studies may be required to prove the same.[40]

Metformin in Clomiphene Citrate-Resistant Cases

In a meta-analysis, metformin + CC showed a higher ovulation rate and pregnancy rate than CC alone in CC-resistant obese PCOS patients.[41] CC with metformin and laparoscopic ovarian diathermy have similar pregnancy rates in CC-resistant cases.[42] This combination results in modest ovulation and should be tried before gonadotropins in developing countries.[23]

Metformin for young patients with PCOS has a long timeline to achieve pregnancy. It is a drug of choice in PCOS patients who do not want to conceive immediately. Its action is gradual and within 6 months, it establishes ovulatory cycles by decreasing insulin and androgen levels. Another advantage of metformin is that it decreases the incidence of multiple pregnancy with ovulation induction drugs. If the patient does not conceive when on metformin, the option of CC remains open for her. A recent meta-analysis revealed that metformin does not result in weight loss among overweight and obese PCOS patients.[19,43] Addition of metformin to lifestyle had no significant benefit on ovulation and circulating androgen levels.[44] Role of metformin has been summarized in **Box 2**.

Box 2: Role of metformin in PCOS.

- Metformin has a systemic and local effect
- It is used in type II diabetes and decreases hyperinsulinemia
- It decreases lipolysis, hepatic gluconeogenesis, and glucose absorption and so decreases the requirement of insulin
- It increases the sensitivity of target cells to insulin
- It acts on theca cells and decreases androgen, which in turn decreases the luteinizing hormone level
- Metformin does not cause weight loss[43]
- Lifestyle management is superior over metformin in prophylaxis of diabetes[47]
- Oral contraceptive (OC) pill is superior for menstrual irregularities, endometrial hyperplasia, and malignancy[48]

Other Insulin Sensitizers

Insulin sensitizers, pioglitazone and rosiglitazone, and other drugs such as acarbose or D-chiro-inositol have not been found superior over metformin and so their routine use for infertile patient has not been established. The safety of all these drugs during pregnancy is still not established.

- Pioglitazone in a dose of 30–50 mg/day and rosiglitazone in a dose of 4–8 mg/day may be used in combination with metformin in patients who are resistant to metformin.[45] Acarbose is also as effective as metformin in a dose of 100 mg in clomiphene-resistant PCOS.[46]
- D-chiro-inositol in a dose of 1,200 mg/day for 6–8 weeks corrects ovulatory dysfunction. The safety of all these drugs during pregnancy is still not established. The addition of metformin to lifestyle had no significant benefit on ovulation and circulating androgen levels.[44]

According to ASRM guidelines 2018, inositol in any form should be considered currently as an experimental therapy for PCOS, with emerging evidence on efficacy highlighting the need for further research.

ESHRE/ASRM guidelines:

- Metformin does not give a good pregnancy rate.
- It is added in CC resistant cases particularly with BMI > 30 kg/m^2
- It reduces OHSS in a dose of 1500 mg from the previous cycle.
- Other insulin sensitizers are considered experimental.

Glucocorticoids

Half of PCOS patients have an adrenal component in hyperandrogenism and is evidenced by increased dehydroepiandrosterone sulfate (DHEA-S).[49] This is secreted from zona reticularis of the adrenal cortex. These patients are resistant to 150 mg of CC and may also require higher doses of gonadotropins. To improve intraovarian androgen milieu, reduction of circulating and intraovarian androgen is required. It is only then that ovulation may occur. Only adrenal androgen can be reduced effectively with glucocorticoids and so it is extensively tried in the resistant PCOS. Dexamethasone 0.5 mg is given continuously for 3 months as the ovarian follicle takes 100 days for complete development. The dose can be titrated with testosterone or DHEA levels.

Dexamethasone 0.5 mg daily can be added for 3–6 months in these patients along with CC. Dexamethasone leads to water retention in patients. Waterlogging can be reduced by adding diuretics once a week or decreasing the dose of dexamethasone to 0.25 mg or drug may also be discontinued after ovulation. Serious complications are extremely rare and so this drug must be tried in obese CC-resistant PCOS.

Gonadotropins

Gonadotropins are used as second-line pharmacological agents in women with

PCOS who have failed first-line oral ovulation induction therapy. But it can be used as the first line of therapy after proper counseling. It is always used in preference to Clomiphene + Metformin therapy and in clomiphene-resistant cases to improve ovulation and live birth rates. According to ASRM 2018 guidelines, gonadotropins should be combined with metformin for better results.

Gonadotropins are indicated in patients with CC failure with high LH and having antiestrogenic effect of CC. It has a higher pregnancy rate than CC + metformin.[23,50] As LH is already high in PCOS patients, in nondownregulated cycles, it is advisable to use FSH as the ovulation-inducing gonadotropin in PCOS patients. Bioactivity of highly purified urinary FSH (uFSH-HP) and recombinant FSH (rFSH) is also higher than other preparations and dose required will be also less of these preparations.

Specific bioactivity of gonadotropins has been shown in **Table 1**.

Recombinant FSH does not have inhibiting substances like FSH. It has more basic isoforms, higher consistency, and has less batch-to-batch variations. Because of high bioactivity, the dose requirement is less. Though no significant difference is seen in the live birth rate comparing the uFSH and rFSH.[51]

Recombinant Follicle-stimulating Hormone versus Human Menopausal Gonadotropin

The meta-analysis of eight RCTs conforming rFSH to human menopausal gonadotropin (hMG) has shown that rFSH has 50% higher pregnancy rates.[52] The FINVAT report 1999 also showed that the pregnancy rates were higher with rFSH than with hMG. The prospective study of 24,000 assisted reproductive technology (ART) cycles from Germany also showed a higher birth rate and lower dosage with rFSH than hMG.[53] But a Cochrane review in 2009 shows a nonsignificant higher live birth rate with hMG as compared to rFSH.[51]

Chronic Low-dose Protocol

In PCOS patients, gonadotropins are used as a chronic low-dose protocol. The incidence of OHSS is reduced from 4.6% to 1% and the multiple pregnancy rate is reduced to 5.7% as compared to 22–34% using this protocol. A uniovulatory cycle rate of 70% is achieved with rFSH with the chronic low-dose protocol.[54] The basic concept of a chronic low-dose protocol is the threshold theory which demands the attainment and maintenance of follicular development with exogenous FSH without exceeding the threshold requirement of the ovary.

TABLE 1: Specific bioactivity of gonadotropins.

hMG (1950)	8 IU/mg of protein
uFSH (1980)	100–150 IU/mg of protein
uHMG-HP	2,000 IU/mg of protein
uFSH-HP (1982)	9,000 IU/mg of protein
rFSH (1995)	10,000 IU/mg of protein

(hMG: human menopausal gonadotropin; uHMG-HP: highly purified urinary hMG; uFSH-HP: highly purified urinary follicle-stimulating hormone; rFSH: recombinant FSH)

In a chronic low-dose protocol, 37.5 IU of rFSH is started from Day 5 of the cycle. The same dose is continued for 14 days. Increasing the dose before 14 days loses the advantages of a chronic low-dose protocol. Though ovulation monitoring is done during this period and in most of the cases, a mature follicle develops within these 14 days. If it does not, then the dose of gonadotropin is increased by 37.5 IU for another 7 days. If the follicle does not develop even at 37.5 IU, rFSH is increased after another 7 days till the mature follicle is achieved.[55] This protocol gives monofollicular development and therefore higher pregnancy rates. Multifollicular development leads to high E2 and progesterone levels, their altered ratios, and therefore low implantation rates.

Professors Roy Homburg and Collin Howles published a study in 2005 stating that if low-dose rFSH is used as the first line of treatment for ovulation induction, the pregnancy rates can be doubled to that of CC. This study showed a clear superiority of low-dose FSH over CC for treating anovulatory patients with PCOS. In the first cycle, pregnancy rates are 30% with rFSH as compared to 14% with CC, and in the second cycle, it is 50% with rFSH as compared to 32% with CC.[55] This explains that the time to achieve pregnancy is significantly reduced. If cost is not a prohibiting factor, rFSH in a chronic low-dose protocol is to be preferred over CC.

The chronic low-dose protocol is also described as a chronic low-dose step-up protocol. In those patients who have a high FSH threshold, the chronic low-dose step-down protocol is used. This protocol has a higher cancellation and complication rate.[56]

Even an ultra-low-dose step-up protocol with only 10 IU of rFSH is useful.[57] In patients who have a high FSH threshold, the chronic low-dose step-down protocol is used. But this regimen has a higher cancellation and complication rate.[56] Multifollicular development in PCOS is not because of differential FSH threshold but is because of the availability of more FSH sensitive antral follicles in the cohort as compared to normal ovaries.[58] The chronic ultra-low-dose protocol gave very good results when as small as 8.3 IU of FSH was given in incremental doses. It reduces the cost and gives monofollicular development with low cycle cancellation rates.[57]

Chronic Low-dose Step-down Protocol

It activates preovulatory follicles by surpassing the FSH threshold. Once the follicles develop, the dose of FSH is reduced because the number of days of FSH in FSH windows decides the number of recruited follicles. So because of the shorter half-life of FSH, dose reduction will limit the number of growing follicles. As the follicle grows, the sensitivity for FSH increases and so requires a lower dose of FSH. This will allow monofollicular development and leads to atresia of other follicles.[59]

How is It Given?

About 75–150 IU of FSH is given for 4–5 days initially and minimum of 5–7 days are required to have a steady level of FSH. The dose is decreased as soon as the ovarian reaction is seen on ultrasound, e.g., 10 mm of follicle, monofollicular development and avoids OHSS. The dose is reduced by 37.5 IU for 2 days and then again reduced by 37.5 IU. Initiation of follicular growth is expected when serum levels of FSH are from 6.5 to 10.4 U/L. This assay is useful in poor responders.[50] It is concluded that monofollicular development and ovulation are achieved more effectively in the chronic step-up protocol than the step-down protocol.[60] So the step-down protocol is the second-line backup protocol for PCOS. Estrogen and progesterone injection in the luteal phase maintains the pregnancy rate.[61]

Multifollicular development in PCOS is common not because of the difference of FSH threshold but these contain twice the number of available FSH-sensitive antral follicles in the cohort as compared to normal ovary.[58]

We have found a combination of letrozole with rFSH very useful. It is cost-effective as it reduced the consumption of rFSH and also gives monofollicular development. Letrozole is given from Day 3 to 7 and rFSH is started from Day 8. This regimen decreases the incidence of OHSS and multiple pregnancies with comparable results as those of rFSH alone.

ESHRE-ASRM recommendations:

- Gonadotropins are the second line of treatment in PCOS after letrozole.
- Gonadotropins can be considered as first line of treatment after counseling as they have very high pregnancy rates.
- These are better than CC + metformin for improving ovulation rate, pregnancy rate, and live birth rate.
- Metformin can be added to gonadotropins to improve ovulation.
- Ovarian drilling should be offered as an alternative before starting gonadotropins after proper counseling of benefits and risks.
- Low-dose gonadotropins give monofollicular development.

Gonadotropin-releasing Hormone Antagonist

In PCOS patients, there is a tonic rise of LH, particularly in thin lean PCOS patients. There is also a possibility of premature LH surge because of high estrogen levels. The advantage of the GnRH antagonist protocol is the growth of fewer follicles, leading to lower peak E2 levels and lower risk of OHSS.[62,63] Moreover, the risk of OHSS is also reduced as there is an option of using the GnRH agonist as a trigger. It has also been proved that the dose of gonadotropins required is also less in GnRH antagonist protocols.[64] Antagonist is started when at least one follicle has grown to 14 mm, to prevent LH surge, and is continued till the follicle matures, i.e., the day of hCG. If antagonist is started early and the LH level is not high at that time, the follicle will regress, as a certain amount of LH is required for the final stages of maturation of the follicle. Gonadotropin dose does not require increment when antagonist is started. Antagonist also helps in the correct timing of intrauterine insemination (IUI). But antagonist is not to be added if premature LH surge is not documented in the previous cycle or there is no proof of raised LH on ultrasound. In IVF cycles, GnRH antagonist can be used as a fixed or flexible protocol. In the fixed protocol, GnRH antagonist is started on Day 6 of the stimulation whereas in flexible protocol, it is started when the lead follicle is >13 mm or the serum E2 levels are >600 pg/mL. Antagonist used is Ganirelix or Cetrotide 0.25 mg daily. Similar conception rates can be achieved in long agonist and flexible GnRH antagonist protocols.[65] But with the antagonist protocol, the incidence of severe OHSS is reduced to 50%.[62,63]

- Oral contraceptive (OC) pills pretreatment for 2–3 months was used to decrease LH in PCOS patients, but it may be detrimental to cycle outcome in the antagonist cycle.[66]
- Micronized E2 2 mg BD for 10 days before the expected menstruation or from the midluteal phase may decrease FSH and LH and a good cohort of the follicles can be achieved.

Box 3: Advantages of antagonist protocol.

- Lower risk of OHSS has 50% compared to agonist protocol
- Gonadotropin-releasing hormone agonist can be used for ovulation trigger
- It gives equivalent pregnancy rates
- It decreases the amount of gonadotropin used
- Estradiol concentration is lower on the day of hCG

- Norethisterone 10 mg/day can be used to schedule the cycle as it decreases the LH level.
- In IVF patients early administration of GnRh antagonist may possibly lead to benefit due to decreased incidence if moderate-to-severe OHSS with better pregnancy rate. It may be due to reduced LH and E2 in early follicular phase. It also causes synchronization of follicles.[67]

Stimulation can also be started after 4–5 days of OC pills, 3–5 days of progesterone, and 1–2 days after estrogen.[68]

The advantages of the antagonist protocol are given in **Box 3**.

Gonadotropin-releasing Hormone Agonist

Gonadotropin-releasing hormone agonist is used for ovulation trigger in PCOS patients. It induces a sustained release of LH from the pituitary gland that lasts for 24 hours.[69] (This is effective to induce preovulatory oocyte maturation.)[70] The advantage is that the duration of action of GnRH agonist is shorter (24–36 hours) than hCG and is similar to natural surge.[71] It leads to a lesser rise in E2 and progesterone levels and therefore gives better implantation rates and the chance of OHSS is also reduced. But when agonist is used as a trigger, the chance of luteal phase defect is very high due to lower circulating luteal E2 and progesterone.[72] Some may also have early luteolysis and a short luteal phase.[73] Luteal support is, therefore, mandatory in these cases. GnRHa for downregulation is an established treatment in IVF cycles, but should not be used in IUI cycles for the same purpose. This is so because downregulation in IUI cycles increases gonadotropin consumption, multiple pregnancy rate, and incidence of OHSS, without any benefit. For IVF cycles also, the recent studies have shown that downregulation with antagonist is a better option in PCOS patients. It significantly reduces the risk of OHSS and also prevents supraphysiological levels of estrogen which may be an important cause for implantation failure.

Antagonist + Agonist Protocol

In PCOS patients, GnRH antagonist is used for downregulation and agonist is then used for oocyte trigger. Agonist when used as a trigger has 24–36 hours' duration of action. It leads to lower FSH and LH resulting in luteal phase deficiency. Therefore, luteal support with 1,500 IU hCG, every third day, can be used[74] along with progesterone. This protocol decreases the risk of OHSS significantly. According to recent studies, even dual trigger may be given. As per this protocol, agonist trigger is backed by 1,500 IU of hCG on the day of oocyte retrieval.[74] This decreases the chance of luteal phase defect but should not be used when the follicles are plenty. When follicles are plenty, "freeze-all" policy is most successful.[75]

Skorupskaite et al. demonstrated interactive regulation of GnRH/LH secretion by neurokinin B, kisspeptin in PCOS and NKB system mediates aspects of estrogenic feedback. So kisspeptin infusion can increase LH secretion and pulsatility in direct relation to E2 exposure. But if NK3R antagonist is added, though LH response to kisspeptin is preserved, its relationship to E2 is not.[76]

Triggering final oocyte maturation with kisspeptin is a novel therapeutic option to enable the use of fresh embryo transfer in women at a high risk of OHSS. This is because kisspeptin results in a shorter duration of LH exposure (12–14 hours) without the risk of increasing possibility of OHSS. Second dose of kisspeptin after 10 hours improves the yield of oocytes.[77]

Ovarian Drilling

Laparoscopic ovarian drilling (LOD) is considered second-line treatment in clomiphene-resistant cases and first-line treatment when laparoscopy is done for some other reason in a patient with PCOS and anovulation. Counseling must be done to discuss the pros and cons of the treatment. Ovarian drilling is an effective tool for ovulation induction for PCOS patients. The advantage of ovarian drilling is that it induces unifollicular development without the risk of OHSS or high-order multiple pregnancies[78] and its beneficial effects can last for up to 9 years.[79] Cochrane review says that both 12 months' pregnancy rate after drilling and 6 months' gonadotropin stimulation have similar pregnancy rates.

It has also been quoted by Professor Roy Homburg that spontaneous pregnancy can occur after several years of drilling. Ovarian drilling gives 70–80% of ovulation rate and 60% of pregnancy rates.[80]

A Cochrane database analysis of four RCTs comparing LOD with gonadotropin therapy showed similar cumulative pregnancy rates 6–12 months after LOD and after 3–6 months of gonadotropin therapy.[81]

How Ovarian Drilling Works?

Various explanations have been described in the literature as to why drilling works. But the most accepted theory is that drilling decreases the androgen level by destroying ovarian stroma. This decrease in androgen will decrease LH and change the FSH/LH ratio. Stein-Leventhal had long back suggested that the larger the ovary, a larger portion of its stroma needs to be removed to decrease androgen and insulin levels. So, what I have found in my practice is that only four punctures do not work in majority of cases. The larger the stromal volume, the larger amount of stroma needs to be destroyed, and therefore more punctures need to be done to decrease the androgen levels to effective limits. Ovarian drilling leads to the destruction of the stromal cells which in turn reduces androgen production and decreases stromal blood flow, leading to fall in serum levels of vascular endothelial growth factor (VEGF) and IGF-1. On drilling along with the stroma, small follicles are also destroyed, which leads to a fall in AMH levels and therefore increases the sensitivity of follicles to FSH.[79,78] Failure of ovarian drilling in women with relatively high-power Doppler indices along with high levels of AMH may be due to the severity of PCOS in these women. It is possible that the extent of follicle destruction by LOD in these women was not enough to reduce intraovarian AMH to a level consistent with resumption of ovulation.[83] Another study has also shown that adjusted diathermy dose based on ovarian volume for LOD of PCOS has better reproductive outcome compared with fixed thermal dosage.[84] This means that measuring AMH and ovarian stromal three-dimensional (3D) power Doppler blood flow for women with anovulatory PCOS undergoing ovarian drilling may provide a useful tool in evaluating the outcome of ovarian drilling.[85]

The mechanism of action of ovarian drilling is given in **Box 4**.

Box 4: Mechanism of action in ovarian drilling.

- Decreases androgen levels because of the destruction of stroma
- Decreases LH level directly proportional to pregnancy rate after LOD
- Increases FSH level
- Decreases estrogen level and gives feedback to FSH
- Reverses LH/FSH ratio
- Temporary decrease in inhibin level
- Local and systemic effects promote ovulation
- Subcapsular cyst has high androgen-rich fluid that is released and decreases androgen levels

(FSH: follicle-stimulating hormone; LH: luteinizing hormone; LOD: laparoscopic ovarian drilling)

Box 5: Guidelines of experts in Thessaloniki in Greece in 2007 for laparoscopic ovarian drilling.

- Laparoscopic ovarian drilling achieves unifollicular development with no risk of ovarian hyperstimulation syndrome and high-order multiple pregnancies
- It is a one-time treatment
- Intensive monitoring is not required
- It is as effective as gonadotropin therapy
- Adhesions formation, destruction of ovarian tissue, and surgery-related complications are minimal
- Surgery should be performed by expert personnel

Method

It may be done with unipolar cautery, dipping 4 mm into the ovarian stroma, and has excellent results similar to laser therapy.[86] Various other methods have been described in the literature without added advantage. Newer methods for ovarian drilling that are being tried now are transvaginal hydrolaparoscopic drilling, ultrasound-guided transvaginal ovarian needle drilling (UTND), and laparoscopic ovarian multineedle intervention (LOMNI). The purpose for trials on these procedures is to ease out the ovarian drilling into a less invasive and a simple procedure.

The guidelines of experts in Thessaloniki in Greece in 2007 for LOD are given in **Box 5**.

Advantages

- Ovarian drilling is especially indicated in PCOS patients who are resistant to CC. If ovarian drilling is done before starting gonadotropin therapy, the dose of gonadotropin required can be decreased and the risk of OHSS and multiple pregnancy is reduced. As it destroys stroma and decreases the androgen and in turn the LH levels, it improves the ovum quality and decreases the risk of abortions, the incidence of which is higher in PCOS patients as compared to non-PCOS patients. Ovarian drilling is a one-time procedure and therefore is a suitable method to facilitate ovulation induction in PCOS patients who cannot repeatedly come for monitoring or follow-up.
- The mean treatment costs per live birth within 8–12 months after initial treatment are significantly lower per live birth when treatment is started with laparoscopic electrocautery compared with when started with ovulation induction with rFSH, and electrocautery is a rational treatment for clomiphene-resistant PCOS.[79] Laparoscopic electrocautery of the ovaries is as effective as ovulation induction with FSH treatment in terms of live births, but reduces the need for ovulation induction or ART in a significantly higher proportion of women and increases the chance for the second child.[87]

Disadvantages

- In spite of being significantly advantageous, ovarian drilling has been widely blamed for postprocedure ovarian failure. Though the risk is probably exaggerated.

Ovarian failure after ovarian drilling is possible only when it is done in an ovary that does not have stromal excess or is not a polycystic ovary. Therefore, it is important and essential to do baseline ultrasound scan prior to laparoscopy, and diagnosis of PCO is confirmed and preferable stromal volume is also calculated. Api et al. have concluded in their study that there was no concrete evidence of a decreased ovarian reserve nor premature ovarian failure associated with LOD in women with PCOS.[88]

- *Adhesions*: Pelvic or ovarian adhesions are seen in 40–60% of cases and they do not depend on the number of punctures. But they do not change the pregnancy rate and adhesiolysis does not improve pregnancy rates.[89]

Variations in the Method of Ovarian Drilling

Newer methods for ovarian drilling—under trials:

- *Transvaginal hydrolaparoscopic drilling*: Ovarian drilling by hydrolaparoscopy is an effective treatment in CC-resistant PCOS and it has given 76% pregnancy rates within a period of 7.2 months.[90]
- *Ultrasound-guided transvaginal ovarian needle drilling*: It gives equivalent results. But safety and efficacy require further studies.
- *Laparoscopic ovarian multineedle intervention*: This was devised by Kaya and associates.[91]
- Transvaginal ultrasound-guided follicular aspiration of subcapsular cysts without causing significant stromal damage has yielded a 50–85% ovulation rate, thus proving that removal of androgen from follicular fluid helps to decrease LH and revert LH/FSH ratio.[92]

But LOD gives better results than all other alternative techniques.

Unilateral drilling has been suggested by some workers with an argument that it has an advantage of a short procedure time, minimized adhesions, and ovarian tissue damage, but still induces activity in both ovaries.[92] Though according to other authors, this requires further evaluation.[93] In a latest study, Sunj et al. have shown that unilateral ovarian drilling using thermal doses adjusted to the ovarian volume (60 J/cc) was more effective than bilateral drilling done with constant thermal doses for both ovaries.[94] We have not even seen significant adhesions after drilling during cesarean section of the patients in whom we have done ovarian drilling. Ovarian malignancy after drilling has not been proved.

The major concern though is that how many punctures should be done per ovary. According to Adam Balen and Armar's technique, four punctures for 4 seconds at 40 W should be done in each ovary.[95] According to Naether et al.,[96] 5–20 punctures for 1 second at 400 W and according to Gjonnaess,[97] 5–8 punctures for 5–6 seconds at 300–400 W should be done. If the above data is closely observed and analyzed, puncture duration is decreased when the power of current (Watts) is increased and a number of punctures are less if each puncture is continued for a longer time.

In our unpublished study that was conducted from 2002 to 2009, the total number of patients with PCOS enrolled was 2,733. Out of these, 134 patients did not turn up after the initial investigations and 2,699 patients were taken for study. Out of these 2,699 patients, 1,566 patients had come after taking treatment for subfertility for more than a year. In all the patients, a baseline ultrasound scan was done on Day 2–3 of the cycle to assess the ovarian volume, stromal volume, and the number of antral follicles and in these patients insulin resistance was also confirmed prior to the procedure. Depending on the stromal volume value, 20–40 punctures with 400 W unipolar cautery were done in each ovary and the results are displayed in **Table 2**.

It is seen in **Figure 1** that the number of cycles for conception is fewer when ovarian drilling is done. I would like to emphasize that there was not a single case of ovarian failure in this series.

High intensity focused ultrasound was tried by Shehata et al. for PCOS patients as noninvasive option of ovarian drilling. But larger studies are required to prove its efficacy.[98]

TABLE 2: Results of 20–40 punctures with 400 W unipolar cautery—in each ovary.

	No drilling	*With drilling*
Conceived	882 (55.68%)	828 (74.26%)
Not conceived	702	287
Total	1,584	1,115

ESHRE-ASRM recommendations 2018:

- It is the second line of therapy like gonadotropins in letrozole-resistant cases.
- If laparoscopy is indicated for some other reason, then it can be considered as the first treatment option.
- The risks, costs, and benefits should be discussed with the patient.

In Vitro Fertilization and In Vitro Maturation

According to 2018 ASRM guidelines, IVF is offered as a third-line treatment for PCOS and anovulatory infertility. The main advantage is achieved with SET and multiple pregnancies can be avoided. The patient must be counseled for the cost and the risk of OHSS. Antagonist cycles are always preferred instead of agonist protocols that required lower dose of gonadotropins and lower incidence

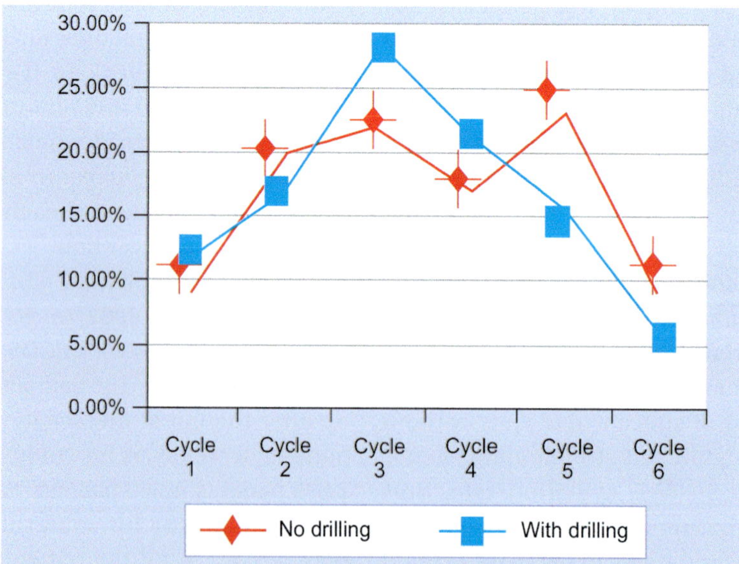

Fig. 1: Conception rate against the number of treatment cycles.

of OHSS. Apart from this, there is always a chance to give agonist trigger and "freeze all" can be adopted. For prevention of OHSS in agonist or antagonist cycle, metformin is recommended from the previous cycle in a dose of 1,000–2,550 mg daily. The period for IVM is 24–48 hours in culture media with FSH and hCG. Thereafter, ICSI is done on these mature oocytes. The initial study has documented 8.9 oocytes/retrieval, 64% of maturation rate, 45% of fertilization rate after IVF/ICSI, 15.3% pregnancy rate per transfer, and 7.3% live birth rate.[66] The challenges may be adequate laboratory conditions and learning skills for the clinician doing the ovum pick-up and also the embryologist.

Polycystic Ovarian Syndrome and Assisted Reproductive Technology

Role of ART in polycystic ovarian syndrome has been shown in **Box 6**.

ESHRE/ASRM guidelines:

- IVF is the third line of therapy after the first and the second line fail.
- IVF is effective and single embryo transfer (SET) can minimize multiple pregnancy rate.
- Risks, costs, and benefits should be discussed with the patient.

Box 6: Polycystic ovarian syndrome and assisted reproductive technology.

- Polycystic ovarian syndrome is not an indication for assisted reproductive technique
- Treat anovulation as a cause of infertility
- Assisted reproductive technique is indicated for associated pathology
- Assisted reproductive technique is preferred for single embryo transfer and to avoid multiple pregnancies
- Fresh cycle transfer has poor results due to high E2 and progesterone
- Freeze-all is the preferred approach

- Antagonist protocol and agonist trigger with freeze all can avoid OHSS completely.
- Exogenous LH is not required in PCOS.
- All FSH preparations have given good results.
- Antagonist protocol is preferred over agonist for duration of treatment, cost and risk of OHSS.
- hCG is to be used in lower doses.
- Metformin 1,000–2,500-g can be used to decrease the risk off OHSS in agonist cycle.

In Vitro Maturation (Box 7)

IVM refers to retrieval of oocytes as GV or metaphase I stage from follicle after follicle priming. IVM is the future for PCOS patients, as it is a 100% OHSS-free treatment. The treatment cost is low as the consumption of gonadotropins is very low.

Indications

- Risk of OHSS
- Estrogen sensitive cancers

Box 7: In vitro maturation.

- IVM should be done in properly indicated patients only as results are not as good as conventional ART.
- It is an alternative method for women who need shorter stimulation , fewer injections and lesser monitoring and drug cost.
- It has a learning curve for operator and embryologist.
- It is good for patients with high AFC.
- Vitrification of immature oocyte is not done due to poor results.
- ICSI is preferred.
- There is suboptimal nuclear and cytoplasmic maturation and so more research is required.
- Sufficicient data is lacking for developmental outcome and malformations.
- ASRM-2021 guidelines.

For Fertility Preservation

Repeated assisted reproduction failure due to resistant ovary syndrome.

Follicular priming for IVM can be done by three methods:

1. Low dose FSH is given for 3–6 days followed by retrieval on Day 7–10 without hCG.
2. Use only hCG (single injection 10,000 IU) to prime intermediate sized follicles 36 hours before oocyte retrieval.
3. Minimal FSH stimulation before hCG priming.

The initial study has documented 8.9 oocytes/retrieval, 64% of maturation rate, 45% of fertilization rate after IVF/ICSI, 15.3% pregnancy rate per transfer, and 7.3% live birth rate.[60] The challenges may be adequate laboratory conditions and learning skills for the clinical doing the ovum pick-up and also the embryologist. Recent studies have shown pregnancy rates of 33–39%.[99] Clinical pregnancy rates are highest when FSH and hCG are both used for priming. Freeze all have higher pregnancy rates than fresh transfer.[100] Follicles are picked up to 10 mm size because the larger size causes atresia of other follicles. Needle size is 16–18 guage and pressure to be maintained between 80 and 120 µg.

The recent development in IVM is inclusion of pre-IVM step. Before moving the egg to IVM media, 2 hours of incubation is required. It helps oocyte to remain in GV stage for 24 hours and blocks the resumption of meiosis. This helps in cytoplasmic maturation and improves oocyte competence. This improves the chances of getting good quality blastocysts.[101] But in birth groups, live birth rates and neonatal outcomes are nearly the same.[102]

CARRY HOME MESSAGE

- Weight loss is the first line of treatment.
- Clomiphene is the time-tested drug.
- Letrozole is the first line therapy for infertility in patients with PCOS.
- Adding metformin has no advantage on ovulation induction, though corrects the metabolic component and thus supports the pregnancy better in CC-resistant cases.
- Glucocorticoids may be useful in CC-resistant PCOS patients.
- Chronic low-dose FSH protocol is a very effective ovulation induction method for PCOS patients. It is second-line therapy.
- Agonist may be used as an ovulation trigger.
- Antagonists to prevent premature LH surge are very useful in thin, lean PCOS both in IUI and in IVF cycles.
- Ovarian drilling has excellent results in the best hands. IVF is the third line of treatment.
- IVM is the future.

REFERENCES

1. Dr Thatcher. Defining PCOS—a perspective. The American Infertility Association Newsletter, February 2001.
2. Rotterdam ESHRE/ASRM-Sponsored PCOS Consensus Work Group. Revised 2003 consensus on diagnostic criteria and long-term health risks related to polycystic ovarian syndrome. Hum Reprod. 2004;19(1):41-7.
3. Lujan ME, Jarrett BY, Brooks ED, Reines JK, Peppin AK, Muhn N, et al. Updated ultrasound criteria for polycystic ovary syndrome: reliable thresholds for elevated follicle population and ovarian volume. Hum Reprod. 2013;28(5):1361-8.
4. Lam PM, Raine-Fenning N. Role of three-dimensional ultrasonography in polycystic ovary syndrome. Hum Reprod. 2006;21(9):2209-15.
5. Kim HJ, Adams JM, Gudmundsson JA, Arason G, Pau CT, Welt CK. Polycystic ovary morphology: age-based ultrasound criteria. Fertil Steril. 2017;108(3):548-53.
6. Ahmed AK, Quinn M, Kao CN, Greenwood E, Cedars MI, Hudleston HG. Improved diagnostic performance for the diagnosis of polycystic ovary syndrome using age stratified criteria. 2019;111(4):787-93.

7. Erel CT, Senturk LM. The impact of body mass index on assisted reproduction. Curr Opin Obstet Gynecol. 2009;21:228-35.
8. Park HS, Lee K. Greater beneficial effects of visceral fat reduction compared with subcutaneous fat reduction on parameters of the metabolic syndrome: A study of weight reduction programmes in subjects with visceral and subcutaneous obesity. Diabet Med. 2005;22:266-72.
9. Smith SR, Zachwieja JJ. Visceral adipose tissue: a critical review of intervention strategies. Int J Obes Relat Metab Disord. 1999;23:329-35.
10. Homburg R. Understanding the problems of treating PCOS. In: Homburg R (Ed). Ovulation Induction and Controlled Ovarian Stimulation: A Practical Guide, 2nd edition. Switzerland: Springer International Publishing; 2014. pp. 65-72.
11. Fedorscak P, Dale PO, Stroreng R, Ertzeid G, Bjercke S, Oldereid N, et al. Impact of overweight and underweight on assisted reproduction treatment. Hum Reprod. 2004;19:2523-8.
12. Kulkarni SD, Patil AN, Gudi A, Homburg R, Conway GS. Changes in diet composition with urbanization and its effect on the polycystic ovarian syndrome phenotype in a western Indian population. Fertil Steril. 2019;112(4):758-62.
13. Hammond MG. Monitoring techniques for improved pregnancy rates during clomiphene ovulation induction. Fertil Steril. 1984;42: 499-508.
14. Dickey RP, Taylor SN, Curole DN, Rye PH, Pyrzak R. Incidence of spontaneous abortion in clomiphene pregnancies. Hum Reprod. 1996;11:2623-8.
15. Glyser M, March CM, Mishell DR Jr, Bailey EJ. A decade's experience with an individualized clomiphene treatment regimen including its effect on the postcoital test. Fertil Steril. 1982;37:161-7.
16. Panda B, Mohapatra L, Sahu MC, Padhy RN. Success in pregnancy through intrauterine insemination at first cycle in 300 infertile couples: An analysis. J Obstet Gynecol India. 2014;64(2):134-42.
17. National Collaborating Center for Women's and Children's Health/National Institute for Clinical Excellence. Fertility: assessment and treatment for people with fertility problems. London (UK): RCOG Press; 2004.
18. Ozdemir U, Ozaksit G, Cakir Gungor AN, Aydogan M. Letrozole usage adjuvant to gonadotropins for ovulation induction for patients with clomiphene citrate failure. Arch Gynecol Obstet. 2013;288(2):445-8.
19. Begum MR, Ferdous J, Begum A, Quadir E. Comparison of efficacy of aromatase inhibitor and clomiphene citrate in induction of ovulation in polycystic ovarian syndrome. Fertil Steril. 2009;92:853-7.
20. Badawy A, Elnashar A, El-Ashry M, Shahat M. Gonadotropin-releasing hormone agonists for prevention of chemotherapy-induced damage: a prospective randomized study. Fertil Steril. 2009;91:694-7.
21. Badawy A, Abdel Aal I, Abulatta M. Clomiphene citrate or letrozole for ovulation induction in women with polycystic ovarian syndrome: a prospective randomized trial. Fertil Steril. 2009;92:849-52.
22. Casper RF. Letrozole versus clomiphene citrate: which is better for ovulation induction? Fertil Steril. 2009;92(3):858-9.
23. Abu Hashim H, Wafa A, El Rakhawy M. Combined metformin and clomiphene citrate versus highly purified FSH for ovulation induction in clomiphene-resistant PCOS women: a randomized controlled trial. Gynecol Endocrinol. 2011;27(3):190-6.
24. Bohler H Jr, Mokshagundam S, Winters SJ. Adipose tissue and reproduction in women. Fertil Steril. 2010;94:795-825.
25. Creanga AA, Bradley HM, McCormick C, Witkop CT. Use of metformin in polycystic ovary syndrome: a meta-analysis. Obstet Gynecol. 2008;111(4):959-68.
26. Legro RS, Barnhart HX, Schlaff WD, Carr BR, Diamond MP, Carson SA, et al. Clomiphene, metformin or both for infertility in the polycystic ovary syndrome. N Engl J Med. 2007;356:551-66.
27. Falghesu AM, romualdi C, Di Florio C, Sanna S, Tagliaferri V, Gambineri A, et al. Is there a dose-response relationship of metformin

treatment in patients with polycystic ovary syndrome? Results from a multicentric study. Hum Reprod. 2012;27(10):3057-66.
28. Moll E, Bossuyt Patrick MM, Korevaar JC, Lambalk CB, van der Veen F. Effect of clomiphene citrate plus metformin and clomiphene citrate plus placebo on induction of ovulation in women with newly diagnosed polycystic ovary syndrome: randomized double-blind clinical trial. BMJ. 2006;332(7556):1485.
29. Nestler JE. Metformin in the treatment of infertility in polycystic ovarian syndrome: an alternative perspective. Fertil Steril. 2008;90(1):14-6.
30. Palomba S, Orio F Jr, Falbo A, Manguso F, Russo T, Cascella T, et al. Prospective parallel randomized double-blind, double-dummy controlled clinical trial comparing clomiphene citrate to metformin as the first-line treatment for ovulation induction in nonobese anovulatory women with polycystic ovary syndrome. J Clin Endocrinol Metab. 2005;90:4068-74.
31. Costello MF, Chapman M, Conway U. A systematic review and meta-analysis of randomized controlled trials on metformin co-administration during gonadotropin ovulation induction or IVF in women with polycystic ovary syndrome. Hum Reprod. 2006;21:1387-99.
32. Kjotrod SB, von During V, Carlsen SM. Metformin treatment before IVF/ICSI in women with polycystic ovary syndrome; a prospective, randomized, double-blind study. Hum Reprod. 2004;19:1315-22.
33. Palomba S, Falbo A, Di Cello AD, Cappiello F, Tolino A, Zullo F. Does metformin affect the ovarian response to gonadotropins for in vitro fertilization treatment in patients with polycystic ovary syndrome and reduced ovarian reserve? A randomized controlled trial. Fertil Steril. 2011;96(5):1128-33.
34. Tso LO, Costello MF, Albuquerque LE, Andriolo RB, Freitas V. Metformin treatment before and during IVF or ICSI in women with polycystic ovary syndrome. Cochrane Database Syst Rev. 2009;2:CD006105.
35. Palomba S, Falbo A, Carrillo L, Villani MT, Orio F, Russo T, et al. Metformin reduces the risk of ovarian hyperstimulation syndrome in patients with polycystic ovary syndrome during gonadotropins-stimulated in vitro fertilization cycles: a randomized controlled trial. Fertil Steril. 2011;96(6):1384-90.
36. Stadtmauer LA, Toma SK, Riehl RM, Talbert M. Metformin treatment of patients with polycystic ovary syndrome undergoing in vitro fertilization improves outcomes and is associated with modulation of insulin-like growth factors. Fertil Steril. 2001;75:505-9.
37. Stadtmauer LA, Toma SK, Riehl RM, Talbert M. The impact of metformin therapy on ovarian stimulation and outcome in 'coasted' patients with polycystic ovary syndrome undergoing in-vitro fertilization. Reprod Biomed Online. 2002;5:112-6.
38. Kjøtrød SB, Carlsen SM, Rasmussen PE, Holst-Larsen T, Mellembakken J, Thurin-Kjellberg A, et al. Use of metformin before and during assisted reproductive technology in non-obese young infertile women with polycystic ovary syndrome: a prospective, randomized, double-blind multi-centre study. Hum Reprod. 2011;26(8):2045-53.
39. Palomba S, Falbo A, Orio F, Zullo F. Effect of preconceptional metformin on abortion risk in polycystic ovary syndrome: a systematic review and meta-analysis of randomized controlled trials. Fertil Steril. 2009;92:1646-58.
40. Vega M, Mauro M, Williams Z. Direct toxicity of insulin on the human placenta and protection by metformin. Fertil Steril. 2019;111(3):489-95.
41. Wang LL, Ren W, Cheng QF, Fan XD. Therapeutic effect of metformin for clomiphene-resistant infertility patients with polycystic ovary syndrome: a systematic analysis. Zhonghua Fu Chan Ke Za Zhi. 2012;47(9):659-63.
42. Abu Hashim H, El Lakany N, Sherief L. Combined metformin and clomiphene citrate versus laparoscopic ovarian diathermy for ovulation induction in clomiphene-resistant women with polycystic ovary syndrome: a randomized controlled trial. J Obstet Gynecol Res. 2011;37(3):169-77.

43. Lord JM, Flight IH, Norman RJ. Metformin in polycystic ovary syndrome: systematic review and meta-analysis. BMJ. 2003;327:951-3.
44. Ladson G, Dodson WC, Sweet SD, Archibong AE, Kunselman AR, Demers LM, et al. The effects of metformin with lifestyle therapy in polycystic ovary syndrome: a randomized double-blind study. Fertil Steril. 2011;95(3):1059-66.
45. Glueck CJ, Moreira A, Goldeberg N, Sieve L, Wang P. Pioglitazone and metformin in obese women with polycystic ovary syndrome not optimally responsive to metformin. Hum Reprod. 2003;18:1618-22.
46. Sonmez AS, Yasar L, Savan K, Koç S, Özcan J, Toklar A, et al. Comparison of the effects of acarbose and metformin use on ovulation rates in clomiphene citrate-resistant polycystic ovary syndrome. Hum Reprod. 2005;20(1):175-9.
47. Knowler WC, Barrett-Connor E, Fowler SE, Hamman RF, Lachin JM, Walker EA, et al. Reduction in the incidence of type 2 diabetes with lifestyle intervention or metformin. N Engl J Med. 2001;346:393-403..
48. Costello MF, Shrstha B, Eden J, Johnson NP, Sjoblom P. Metformin versus oral contraceptive pill in polycystic ovary syndrome: a Cochrane review. Hum Reprod. 2007;22:1200-9
49. Lobo RA, Granger LR, Davajan V, Mishell Jr DR. An extended regimen of clomiphene citrate in women unresponsive to standard therapy. Fertil Steril. 1982;37:762-6.
50. Van Weissenbruch MM, Schoemaker HC, Drexhage HA, Schoemaker J. Pharmacodynamics of human menopausal gonadotropin (hMG) and follicle stimulating hormone (FSH). The importance of the FSH concentration in initiating follicular growth in polycystic ovary-like disease. Hum Reprod. 1993;8(6):813-21.
51. Van Wely M, Kwan I, Van der Veen F, Thomas J, Vail A, van der Veen F, et al. Recombinant FSH versus urinary gonadotrophins for ovarian hyperstimulation in IVF and ICSI cycles. A systematic review and meta-analysis. Hum Reprod. 2009;Suppl 1:i134.
52. Daya S, Gunby J, Hughes EG, Collins JA, Sagle MA. Follicle-stimulating hormone versus human menopausal gonadotropin for in vitro fertilization cycles: a meta-analysis. Fertil Steril. 1995;64:347-54.
53. Ludwig M, Rabe T, Buhler K, et al. Wirksamkeit von recombinantem humane FSH in Vergleigh zu urinarem hMG nach Downregulation im langen Protokoll—eine Analyse von 24,764 ART-Zyklen in Deutschland. J Reproduction Med Endocrinol. 1994;4:284-8.
54. Homburg R, Howles CM. Low-dose FSH therapy for anovulatory infertility associated with polycystic ovarian syndrome: rationale, results, reflections and refinements. Hum Reprod Update. 1999;5(5):493-9.
55. Homburg R, Hendriks ML, Konig TE, Anderson RA, Balen AH, Brincat M, et al. Clomifene citrate or low-dose FSH for the first-line treatment of infertile women with anovulation associated with polycystic ovary syndrome: a prospective randomized multinational study. Hum Reprod. 2012; 27(2):468-73.
56. Van Santbrink EJ, Fauser BC. Urinary follicle-stimulating hormone for normogonadotropic clomiphene-resistant anovulatory infertility: prospective, randomized comparison between low dose step-up and step-down dose regimens. J Clin Endocrinol Metab. 1997;82(11):3597-602.
57. Van der Meer M, Hompes P, de Boer J, Schats R, Schoemaker J. Cohort size rather than follicle-stimulating hormone threshold levels determines ovarian sensitivity in polycystic ovary syndrome. J Clin Endocrinol Metab. 1988;83:423-6.
58. Orvieto R, Homburg R. Chronic ultra-low-dose follicle-stimulating hormone regimen for patients with polycystic ovary syndrome: one click, one follicle, one pregnancy. Fertil Steril. 2009;91(Suppl 4):1533-5.
59. diZerega GS, Hodgen GD. The primate ovarian cycle: suppression of human menopausal gonadotropin-induced follicular growth in the presence of the dominant follicle. J Clin Endocrinol Metab. 1980;50(5):819-25.

60. Christin-Maitre S, Hugues JN; Recombinant FSH Study Group. A comparative randomized multicentric study comparing the step-up versus step-down protocol in polycystic ovary syndrome. Hum Reprod. 2003;18:1626-31.
61. Engmann L, DiLuigi A, Schmidt D, Nulsen J, Maier D, Benadiva C. The use of gonadotropin-releasing hormone (GnRH) agonist to induce oocyte maturation after cotreatment with GnRH antagonist in high-risk patients undergoing in vitro fertilization prevents the risk of ovarian hyperstimulation syndrome: a prospective randomized controlled study. Fertil Steril. 2008;89:84-91.
62. Al-Inany HG, Youssef MA, Aboulghar M, Broekmans F, Sterrenburg M, Smit J, et al. Gonadotrophin-releasing hormone antagonists for assisted reproductive technology. Cochrane Database Syst Rev. 2011;(5):CD001750.
63. Kolibianakis EM, Collins J, Tarlatzis BC, Devroey P, Diedrich K, Griesinger G. Among patients treated for IVF with gonadotropins and GnRH analogues, is the probability of live birth dependent on the type of analogue used? A systematic review and meta-analysis. Hum Reprod Update. 2006;12:651-71.
64. Navot D, Bergh PA, Laufer N. Ovarian hyperstimulation syndrome in novel reproductive technologies: prevention and treatment. Fertil Steril. 1992;58:249-61.
65. Lainas RG, Sfontouris IA, Zorzovilis IZ, Petsas GK, Lainas GT, Alexopoulou E, et al. Flexible GnRH antagonist protocol versus GnRH long agonist protocol in patients with polycystic ovarian syndrome treated for IVF: a prospective randomized controlled trial (RCT). Hum Reprod. 2010;25(3):683-9.
66. Kolibianakis EM, Papanikolaou EG, Camus M, Tournaye H, Van Steirteghem AC, Devroey P. Effect of oral contraceptive pill pretreatment on ongoing pregnancy rates in patients stimulated with GnRH antagonists and recombinant FSH for IVF. A randomized controlled trial. Hum Reprod. 2006;21:352-7.
67. Shin JJ, Parl KE, Choi YM, Kim HO, Choi CH, Lee WS, Cho JH. Early gonadotropin-releasing hormone antagonist protocol in women with polycystic ovary syndrome: a preliminary randomized trial. Clin Exp Reprod Med. 2018;45(3):135-42.
68. Cedrin-Durnerin I, Bstandig B, Parneix I, Bied-Damon V, Avril C, Decanter C, et al. Effects of oral contraceptive, synthetic progesterone or natural estrogen pretreatments on the hormonal profile and the antral follicle cohort before GnRH antagonist protocol. Hum Reprod. 2007;22(1):109-16.
69. Casper RF, Sheehan KL, Yen SS. Gonadotropin-estradiol responses to a superactive luteinizing hormonereleasing hormone agonist in women. J Clin Endocrinol Metab. 1980;50:179-81.
70. Itskovitz J, Boldes R, Levron J, Erlik Y, Kahana L, Brandes JM. Induction of preovulatory luteinizing hormone surge and prevention of ovarian hyperstimulation syndrome by gonadotrophin-releasing hormone agonist. Fertil Steril. 1991;56:213-20.
71. Scheele F, van der Meer M, Lambalk CB, Schoute E, Schoemaker J, Hompes PG. Exploring the recovery phase after treatment with gonadotropin-releasing hormone agonist for ovulation induction in polycystic ovarian syndrome: three pilot trials. Eur J Obstet Gynecol Reprod Biol. 1995;62(2):221-4.
72. Itskovitz J, Boldes R, Barlev A, Erlik Y, Kahana L, Brandes JM. The induction of LH surge and oocyte maturation by GnRH analogue (buserelin) in women undergoing ovarian stimulation for in vitro fertilization. Gynecol Endocrinol. 1988;2(Suppl 2):165.
73. Gonen Y, Balkier H, Powell W, Casper CF. Use of gonadotropin-releasing hormone agonist to trigger follicular maturation for in vitro fertilization. J Clin Endocrinol Metab. 1990;71:918-22.
74. Humadian P, Ejdrup Bredkjaer H, Westergard LG, Andersen CY. 1,500 IU human chorionic gonadotropin administered at oocyte retrieval rescues the luteal phase when gonadotropin-releasing hormone agonist is used for ovulation induction: a prospective, randomized, controlled study. Fertil Steril. 2010;93:847-54.

75. Griesinger G, Schultz L, Bauer T, Broessner A, Frambach T, Kissler S. Ovarian hyperstimulation syndrome prevention by gonadotropin-releasing hormone agonist triggering of final oocyte maturation in a gonadotropin-releasing hormone antagonist protocol in combination with a 'freeze-all' strategy: a prospective multicentric study. Fertil Steril. 2011;95:2029-33.
76. Skorupskaite K, George JT, Veldhuis JD, Millar RP, Anderson RA. Kisspeptin and neurokinin B interactions in modulating gondotrophin secretion in women with polycystic ovary syndrome. Hum Reprod. 2020;35(6):1421-31.
77. Balen A. Surgical treatment of polycystic ovarian syndrome. Best Pract Res Clin Endocrinol Metab. 2006;20:271-80.
78. Abbara A, Clarke S, Islam R, Prague JK, Comninos AN, Narayanaswamy S, et al. A second dose of kisspeptin-54 improves oocyte maturation in women at high risk of ovarian hyperstimuation syndrome: a Phase 2 randomized controlled trial. Hum Reprod. 2017;32(9):1915-24.
79. Amer SA, Banu Z, Li TC, Cooke ID. Long-term follow-up of patients with polycystic ovary syndrome after laparoscopic ovarian drilling: endocrine and ultrasonographic outcomes. Hum Reprod. 2002;17:2851-7.
80. Homburg R. Ovulation Induction and Controlled Ovarian Stimulation: A Practical Guide, 2nd edition. Switzerland: Springer International Publishing; 2014. pp. 109-13.
81. Farquhar C, Vandekerkhove P, Lilford R. Laparoscopic "drilling" by diathermy or laser for ovulation induction in anovulatory polycystic ovarian syndrome. Cochrane Database Syst Rev. 2001;(4):CD001122.
82. Amer SA, Li TC, Leder WL. The value of measuring anti-Mullerian hormone in women with anovulatory polycystic ovary syndrome undergoing laparoscopic ovarian diathermy. Hum Reprod. 2009;92:1586-93.
83. Nardo LG, Gelbaya TA, Wilkinson H, Roberts SA, Yates A, Pemberton P. Circulating basal anti-Mullerian hormone levels as predictor of ovarian response in women undergoing ovarian stimulation for in vitro fertilization. Fertil Steril. 2009;92:1586-93.
84. Mahmoud S, Kamal MM, Hamed MD. Laparoscopic ovarian drilling in polycystic ovary syndrome: efficacy of adjusted thermal dose based on ovarian volume. Fertil Steril. 2011;95:1115-8.
85. Elmashad AI. Impact of laparoscopic ovarian drilling on anti-Mullerian hormone levels and ovarian stromal blood flow using three-dimensional power Doppler in women with anovulatory polycystic ovarian syndrome. Fertil Steril. 2011;95(7):2342-6.
86. Donesky B, Adashi E. Surgically induced ovulation in the PCO syndrome: ovarian wedge resection revisited. Fertil Steril. 1995;63:439-63.
87. Nahuis MJ, Lohuis EO, Bayram N, Bayram N, Hompes P, Oosterhuis GJE, et al. Long-term follow-up of laparoscopic electrocautery of the ovaries versus ovulation induction with recombinant FSH in clomiphene citrate-resistant women with polycystic ovary syndrome: an economic evaluation. Hum Reprod. 2012;27(12):3577-82.
88. Api M. Is ovarian reserve diminished after laparoscopic ovarian drilling? Gynecol Endocrinol. 2009;25:159-65.
89. Mercorio E, Mercorio A, Di Spiezio Sardo A, Barba GV, Pellicano M, Nappi C. Evaluation of ovarian adhesion formation after laparoscopic ovarian drilling by second-look minilaparoscopy. Fertil Steril. 2008; 89:1229-33.
90. Gordts S, Gordts S, Puttemans P, Valkenburg M, Campo R, Brosens I. Transvaginal hydrolaparoscopy in the treatment of polycystic ovary syndrome. Fertil Steril. 2009;91(6):2520-6.
91. Kaya H, Sezik M, Ozkaya O. Evaluation of a new surgical approach for the treatment of clomiphene citrate-resistant infertility in polycystic ovary syndrome: laparoscopic ovarian multi-needle intervention. J Minim Invasive Gynecol. 2005;12(4):355-8.
92. Balen AH, Jacobs HS. A prospective study comparing unilateral and bilateral laparoscopic ovarian diathermy in women

with polycystic ovary syndrome. Fertil Steril. 1994;62(5):921-5.

93. Fernandez H, Morin-Surruca M, Torre A, Faivre E, Deffieux X, Gervaise A. Ovarian drilling for surgical treatment of polycystic ovary syndrome: a comprehensive review. Reprod Biomed Online. 2011;22:556-68.
94. Sunj M, Canic T, Baldani DP, Tandara M, Jeroncic A, Palada I. Does unilateral laparoscopic diathermy adjusted to ovarian volume increase the chances of ovulation in women with polycystic ovary syndrome? Hum Reprod. 2011;28(9):2417-24.
95. Armar NA, McGarrigle HH, Honour J, Holownia P, Jacobs HS, Lachelin GC. Laparoscopic ovarian diathermy in the management of anovulatory infertility in women with polycystic ovaries: endocrine changes and clinical outcome. Fertil Steril. 1990;53:45-9.
96. Naether OG, Fischer R, Weise HC, Geiger-Kötzler L, Delfs T, Rudolf K. Laparoscopic electrocoagulation of ovarian surface in infertile patients with polycystic ovarian disease. Fertil Steril. 1993;60:88-94.
97. Gjonnaess H. The course and outcome of pregnancy after ovarian electrocautery with PCOS: the influence of body weight. Br J Obstet Gynecol. 1989;96:714-9.
98. Shehata IA, Ballard JR, Casper AJ, Hennings LJ, Cressman E, Ebbinni ES. High intensity focused ultrasound for potential treatment of polycystic ovary syndrome: toward a noninvasive surgery. Fertil Steril. 2014;101(2):545-51.
99. Ho VNA, Pham TD, Le AH, Ho TM, Vuong LN. Live birth rate after human chorionic gonadotropin priming in vitro maturation in women with polycystic ovary syndrome. J Ovarian Res. 2018;11:70.
100. Orgtga-Hrepich C, Stoop D, Guzman L, van Landuyt L, Tournaye H, Smitz J, et al. A "freeze all" embryo strategy after in vitro maturation: a novel approach in women with polycystic ovary syndrome. Fertil Steril. 2013;100:1002-7.
101. Sánchez F, Lolicato F, Romero S, De Vos M, Van Ranst H, Verheyen G, et al. An improved IVM method for cumulus-oocyte complexes from small follicles in polycystic ovary syndrome patients enhances oocyte competence and embryo yield. Hum Reprod. 2017;32:2056-68.
102. Vuong LN, Le AH, Ho VNA, Pham TD, Sanchez F, Romero S, et al. Live births after oocyte in vitro maturation with a prematuration step in women with polycystic ovary syndrome. J Assist Reprod Genet. 2020; 37:347-57.

13

Chapter

Ovulation Induction in Poor Responders

INTRODUCTION

Management of a poor responder is one of the greatest challenges in assisted reproductive technology (ART) management. This is so primarily because there is no clear-cut standard definition of poor responders. Different definitions and consensus include age, ovarian reserve tests, and previous response to gonadotropins as measures to diagnose poor responders. Moreover, the success of an ART cycle is directly related to the number of embryos transferred.[1]

CAUSES OF POOR RESPONSE

There are different causes of poor response, which are as follows:

- Age
- Ovarian surgery
- Advanced endometriosis
- Endometrioma
- Obesity
- Previous pelvic infection
- Smoking
- Postchemotherapy and postradiotherapy
- Family history of early menopause
- Genetic conditions (Turner syndrome)
- Follicle-stimulating hormone (FSH) receptor polymorphism

Bologna Criteria Consensus

The European Society of Human Reproduction and Embryology (ESHRE) consensus definition (2011) states that the presence of any two of the following three features is deemed necessary to define poor response:[2]

1. Advanced maternal age (>40 years) or any other risk factor for poor ovarian reserve.
2. A previous poor response to stimulation (<3 oocytes) or expected poor response when no previous stimulation is done.
3. Abnormal ovarian reserve tests [antral follicle count (AFC) 5–7 follicles, anti-Müllerian hormone (AMH) 0.5–1.0 ng/mL].

Age

Age > 37 years is the most important predictor of low response. The cohort of follicles decreases giving a poor pregnancy rate. All other causes of poor ovarian response are to be considered in young patients.

Bologna criteria have been criticized because of the following:

- Definition of the poor ovarian responder (POR) has also the same threshold of three or fewer oocytes.
- Selection of age is an arbitrary selection of 40 years.
- Ignorance of oocyte quality and other factors, such as smoking and medical disorders, is not included. So, it is not widely accepted.

The markers for poor ovarian reserve are as follows:

- Anti-Müllerian hormone < 3 pmol/mL
- Total AFC > 5

- Less than three developing follicles or three oocytes retrieved after ovarian stimulation are defined as poor responders.[3,4]

All other markers are supportive and are not used routinely.

TREATMENT OPTIONS (BOX 1)

Increasing Gonadotropin Dosage

The dose is increased with an idea that it will overcome the effect of aging (decline in AFC). Earlier studies suggested that increasing the dose of urinary gonadotropins from 300 to 450 IU can improve the results in terms of pregnancy rate and less chances of cycle cancellation. But this was not confirmed in other studies.[5,6] Klinkert et al. increased the dose of recombinant FSH (rFSH) to double in women having AFC < 5, but did not document any benefit. So, increasing the dose of gonadotropin to >300 IU does not help in poor responders. Proper diagnosis of poor responders can avoid cancellation and decide the correct line of treatment.[7] In a prospective study, it was concluded that there was no difference in the clinical pregnancy rate per transfer, irrespective of the stimulating dose of 300, 450, 600 IU FSH/day in gonadotropin-releasing hormone (GnRH) agonist microdose flare-up protocol.[7] The ovarian response is determined by the number of follicles available for recruitment than by circulating gonadotropin levels. On the contrary, higher doses give poor-quality oocytes in the normal responding ovary.[8] The type of gonadotropin, i.e., rFSH, human menopausal gonadotropin (HMG), or urinary FSH (uFSH), has not shown any statistical difference in the pregnancy rate.[9] Step-down regime means decreasing the dose of gonadotropin from 450 to 300–150 IU as follicles develop. This regime gives the same results without compromising cycle outcome and also has an economic benefit.[10] A higher dose of FSH also affects endometrial receptivity. A modified natural cycle or with a low dose of gonadotropin[11] with oral agents has given the same results as high-dose gonadotropins used for ovulation induction. This means that higher doses of gonadotropins do not increase the number of oocytes retrieved. In frozen embryo transfer (FET) cycles, results are better than high gonadotropin cycles. This indicates that a high dose affects the endometrial receptivity.

Box 1: Treatment options in poor responders.

- Increase gonadotrophic dose
- GnRH agonist flare protocol
- LH supplementation
- GnRH agonist stop protocol
- Microdose GnRH agonist in the luteal phase
- Luteal phase FSH + agonist
- GnRH agonist microdose flare
- GnRH antagonist
- Estrogen priming
- Clomiphene citrate
- Letrozole
- L-arginine
- Growth hormone
- Glucocorticoids
- Pre-IVF androgen
- Natural cycle IVF
- Aspirin
- Pyridostigmine
- Other therapies
- Donor oocytes
- Pretreatment OC pills
- IVM

(FSH: follicle-stimulating hormone; GnRH: gonadotropin-releasing hormone; IVF: in vitro fertilization; IVM: in vitro maturation; LH: luteinizing hormone; OC: oral contraceptive)

Gonadotropin-releasing Hormone Agonist: Flare-up Protocol or Short Protocol

The initial stimulating effect on endogenous gonadotropin release is observed when an agonist is given at the beginning of the menstrual cycle. Later on, the GnRH agonist suppresses the premature luteinizing hormone (LH) surge. So considering this physiological effect, some workers started giving GnRH agonist and gonadotropin from the beginning of the cycle in the early follicular phase. Earlier trials did report a higher pregnancy rate;[12] others failed to demonstrate an improved ovarian response or cycle outcome.[13] GnRH agonist flare-up does not improve results even with prior oral contraceptive (OC) pills. The results of the flare-up protocol are similar to the antagonist protocol.[14] So, the flare-up protocol in poor responders does not improve the result. One of the theories put forward is atresia of the follicles induced by increase in LH and progesterone. FSH that is produced by agonist flare-up is not much bioactive. But in some studies, the flare-up protocol has given better results than long protocols.[15] Here, GnRH agonist (1 mg leuprolide acetate) is given from the first day and stopped after 3 days and gonadotropins are started from Day 3 or 4.

Gonadotropin-releasing Hormone Agonists: Luteinizing Hormone Supplementation

Profound suppression of gonadotropins occurs after the midluteal GnRH agonist protocol. Several groups have evaluated the outcome by adding 75–150 IU of LH daily from day 6 of stimulation in long protocol as well as flare-up protocol. Unfortunately, this protocol is not beneficial in improving the ovarian response and pregnancy rate.[16,17] So the addition of LH in poor responders does not improve the outcome.[18] There is a subset of patients in whom LH supplementation can improve the results. They are with profound LH suppression and poor responders.[19] In a study by Humaidan et al., rFSH + rLH gives a similar number of eggs to rFSH alone, though pregnancy failure is less with rFSH + rLH combination.[20] In poor ovarian reserve patients, this group has been classified as "low prognosis" patients who may (1) have suboptimal response (4–9 oocytes instead of 10–15 oocytes) or (2) be hyporesponsive requiring higher doses of gonadotropins.

Gonadotropin-releasing Hormone Agonists: Stop Protocols and Reduced Dose

A long luteal GnRH agonist protocol suppresses gonadotropin secretion. If it is continued after menstruation, it profoundly suppresses gonadotropin secretion and may inhibit subsequent response with controlled ovarian hyperstimulation (COH). It has been tried to assess the response after stopping the GnRH agonist before starting gonadotropins. A prospective study by Faber et al. showed the pregnancy rate of 24% per transfer and 12.5% cancellation rate with LH surge in only one patient.[21] However, Gracia-Valesco et al. reported that cancellation, pregnancy, and implantation rates are the same as the long protocol and stop protocol. But higher numbers of mature oocytes are obtained as well as a reduced dose of gonadotropins is required with the stop protocol.[22] Similar results can be obtained by a long protocol of 0.5 mg leuprolide acetate that is reduced to 0.25 mg after downregulation.[23]

Minidose Luteal Phase Gonadotropin-releasing Hormone Agonist

A decreasing dose of the GnRH agonist in the luteal phase prior to gonadotropin stimulation theoretically will improve the response after stimulation, as suppression will be less. Feldberg et al. tried with triptorelin 0.5 mg before menstruation and then 0.1 mg daily and in another group 0.1 mg before menstruation and 0.05 mg after menstruation. Improved results were observed with decreasing dose.[24] Leuprolide acetate is given as 1 mg in the midluteal phase and 0.5 mg after menstruation. Instead if 0.5 mg is given in the midluteal phase and 0.25 mg after menstruation in a long protocol improves ovarian response with a lesser dose of gonadotropins.[23]

Luteal Phase FSH + GnRH Agonist

Selection of the follicle is done in the luteal phase of the preceding cycle. So, if FSH is given during the luteal phase, it may give a better response in poor responders. In one study, more mature oocytes were obtained when FSH and GnRH agonist were started together in the midluteal phase.[25] Further studies are required to assess the efficacy of this protocol.

Dual Stimulation (DuoStim)

It is also very useful in poor responders. Ovulation induction is done in follicular phase and after pickup also. Stimulation in the luteal phase significantly increases the number of final transferable blastocysts in the natural cycle. This strategy may be applied in other situations where obtaining competent oocytes is an urgent need.[26]

Gonadotropin-releasing Hormone Agonist: Microdose Flare

When using microdose flare protocol, the lowest dose of agonist is given, which can stimulate endogenous FSH secretion and inhibits LH surge. As low as 0.25 mg leuprolide acetate can be used to achieve adequate levels of gonadotropins.[27] Pretreatment with oral pills or progesterone can reduce progesterone and raise androgen. In one study, Surrey et al. introduced 40 µg leuprolide acetate twice daily. This reduced cycle cancellation from 73 to 31.6%. According to this study, when the age was >40 years, a pregnancy rate of 18.2% was achieved.[27,28] So, a microdose flare-up protocol is very useful in poor responders. But with natural cycle in vitro fertilization (IVF) and stop protocol, the results were similar to the microdose flare-up protocol.[29,30] Comparing microdose flare-up protocol and antagonist protocol, the microdose flare-up protocol has a higher pregnancy rate.[31,32] But two randomized cohort trials failed to demonstrate any beneficial effect of microdose flare-up protocol when compared with the antagonist protocol with regard to the number of cycles and pregnancy rates.[6,14]

Gonadotropin-releasing Hormone Antagonist

Gonadotropin-releasing hormone antagonist will inhibit untoward LH surge and progesterone rise. It can be used as a fixed protocol from Day 6 of stimulation or when the lead follicle is 14 mm in diameter. It does not cause suppression in the early follicular phase. Several prospective randomized trials have evaluated antagonist in comparison with alternative regimes in poor responders. Cheung et al. did not get statistical significant difference in pregnancy rates.[31]

No significant difference was seen between antagonist and microdose protocols while some of the studies got better results with microdose flare protocol.[14,30] The main advantage of antagonist is that it does not cause prolonged suppression in the early follicular phase, which is the crucial time for poor responders. It also suppresses LH and progesterone rise and so decreases the cancellation of cycles. It is the protocol of choice as it decreases the time for stimulation as well as the total amount of gonadotropins required. As the results are equivalent to other protocols, the antagonist protocol is preferred due to other advantages. In the luteal phase antagonist protocol, an antagonist is added for 3–5 days before the expected day of menstruation and continued for 4–7 days. Stimulation is started with 300–450 IU and when the lead follicle reaches 14 mm, the antagonist is restarted till the day of trigger. The advantage in this case is that it causes luteolysis before the period. Here, FSH is not sufficiently reduced and a cohort of recruitable follicles remains. This has improved the results.[33]

Gonadotropin-releasing Hormone Antagonist with Agonist

In this protocol, an agonist is given for 3 days after period and then gonadotropins are given with a flexible antagonist protocol or an agonist can be given in the midluteal phase and stopped after menstruation. Then gonadotropin with a flexible antagonist protocol is used. None of these regimes has any advantage over the antagonist protocol.

Estrogen Priming and Antagonist Treatment

Estradiol administration in the luteal phase may induce FSH receptor formation in poor responders and follicles become responsive to gonadotropins in coordination. Estradiol is administered as a 0.1-mg transdermal patch or 4-mg daily estradiol valerate in the luteal phase. The GnRH antagonist is introduced 2 days later and continued for 3 days. Then gonadotropins are given for ovulation induction. An antagonist is reintroduced at a lead follicle size of 14 mm. An ongoing pregnancy rate of 26% was achieved by this protocol.[34] Compared with the microdose flare-up protocol, there is no statistically significant difference in the clinical pregnancy rate.[35] Estradiol valerate 4 mg/day can be given from Day 21 of the luteal phase and continued till Day 3 of menstruation or up to the day of trigger. This may increase the pregnancy rate in poor responders,[36] but other studies have not shown similar results.[37]

Clomiphene Citrate

Adding clomiphene citrate (CC) induces endogenous gonadotropin secretion that helps in poor responders. This is used in the antagonist protocol. In a study comparing the long protocol with clomiphene and antagonist protocol, a better pregnancy rate was observed with a lower cancellation rate in the antagonist protocol.[38] The theoretical disadvantage of the effect of CC on endometrial development must be considered and in other studies, the results are disappointing.[30]

Letrozole

Letrozole is added with an idea that it increases androgen by preventing aromatization to estrogen. This androgen sensitizes the follicle to FSH and this may help to reduce the dose of FSH. Letrozole can be given from Day 3 to 7 in a dose of 2.5 mg. Gonadotropins are given simultaneously. The antagonist protocol is used, but in comparison with microflare protocols, this protocol is inferior considering all aspects[39] though some studies have shown better results with letrozole.[40] Implantation rates may be higher as compared to CC, but lower numbers of matured oocytes are obtained in letrozole with the antagonist protocol.[40]

L-arginine

L-arginine is based on the function of nitric oxide. It enhances periovulatory vasodilatation. The dose is 16 g daily. It has been claimed to improve pregnancy rates.[41]

Growth Hormone

Growth hormone is produced centrally by pituitary and locally by ovary. It increases the local production of insulin-like growth factor 1 (IGF-1) and oocyte competence **(Box 2)**. IGF-1 improves the response of granulosa cells to FSH and helps in oocyte maturation and steroidogenesis. In a meta-analysis by Kolibiankis, it has been shown that adding growth hormone decreases the cycle cancellation and improves the pregnancy rates. But the studies included were heterogeneous.[42] Further, well-controlled randomized studies have failed to demonstrate beneficial effect. It is useful in IGF-1 deficiency, i.e., hypogonadotropic hypogonadism. The growth hormone is given in a dose of 4–12 IU subcutaneous from the day of stimulation with gonadotropins. This adds to the cost of the treatment without improving results. Similarly, the growth hormone stimulating factor is also not beneficial in the treatment of poor responders. Even the recent study in July 2020 has shown that growth hormone supplementation may improve some reproductive outcomes in poor responders but not live birth rate.[43]

Box 2: Actions of growth hormone.

- It promotes steroidogenesis (recruits follicles)
- It promotes gametogenesis
- This acts directly or through IGF-1 and by increasing the sensitivity to IGF-2
- It indirectly upregulates LH receptors
- It increases progesterone production
- The DNA repair capacity in oocyte is increased

(DNA: deoxyribonucleic acid; IGF-1: insulin-like growth factor 1; LH: luteinizing hormone)

Glucocorticoids

Glucocorticoids stimulate the secretion of growth hormone and IGF-1. Giving dexamethasone 1 mg daily in the long protocol causes a lower cycle cancellation rate, but no difference in implantation or pregnancy rates has been found.[44]

Pre-IVF Androgens

Androgen sensitizes the follicle to gonadotropin stimulation. In women, upregulation of FSH receptors before stimulation may enhance follicular responsiveness to exogenous gonadotropins and this allows majority of the antral follicles to develop into dominant or mature follicles rather than undergoing atresia. This increase in FSH receptors increases LH receptors also in the later phase, giving good oocyte maturation.[45] Dehydroepiandrosterone (DHEA) is secreted from the zona reticularis of adrenal cortex and ovarian theca cells. It is a prohormone in ovarian steroidogenesis. It may reduce the aneuploidy rate and so may decrease the miscarriage rate.[46] In two randomized controlled trials, transdermal testosterone application was done. 12.5-mg transdermal testosterone gel is applied for 21 days in the cycle preceding controlled ovarian stimulation (COS) with an antagonist. The dose can be 20 mg/kg/day given 5 days prior to stimulation.[47] It did not show improvement in oocytes, embryo quality, implantation rate, or pregnancy rates.[48,49] DHEA supplementation, especially above the age of 35 years, is associated with a decreased miscarriage rate in women with diminished ovarian reserve (DOR). DHEA may improve pregnancy rates, but the effect of DHEA on the oocyte quality has not been adequately studied **(Box 3)**. There is no statistical improvement in ovarian response markers, ovarian response to low-dose gonadotropins, or IVF outcome in pretreatment DHEA in poor responders.

Box 3: Possible mechanism of DHEA.

- Improves the pool of primordial follicles
- Increases IGF-1 during stimulation
- Increases steroid production, testosterone, and estrogen
- Sensitizes FSH receptors
- Effect is cumulative and more antral follicles are exposed to treatment
- Modulates the level of AMH expression
- Delays the effect of ovarian aging
- May augment endometrial function[50]

(AMH: anti-Müllerian hormone; DHEA: dehydroepiandrosterone; FSH: follicle-stimulating hormone; IGF-1: insulin-like growth factor 1)

Natural Cycle In Vitro Fertilization

In this protocol, no gonadotropins are given. Only hCG is given when the follicle matures and pickup is done after 34–35 hours. A pregnancy rate of 17% per transfer can be achieved.[50] This has a very low pregnancy rate with only one embryo available for transfer and many a times, no ovum is retrieved. Early LH surge is very common in a natural cycle. The number of cycles tried for the pregnancy is too many and has a psychological impact on the patient. Ovum donation may be preferred to this in most cases.

Mild Ovarian Stimulation

In poor responder groups, mild ovarian stimulation is more cost-effective and patient friendly than conventional IVF and should be considered for poor responders over 37 years of age.[51] Modified natural cycle is also a good option for young poor responders or older patients.

Aspirin

Aspirin is to improve the blood supply and the results are disappointing.[52] Aspirin has three modes of actions: (1) Increases capillary blood flow to endometrium, (2) produces anti-inflammatory effect, and (3) reduces uterine contractions. But results are not improved as the uterine artery resistance remains unaffected.[53]

Pyridostigmine (Growth Hormone-releasing Factor)

Pyridostigmine is given in a dose of 120 mg/day. It is an acetylcholinesterase inhibitor. It leads to increase in acetylcholine, which increases the growth hormone. It is given from Day 21 of the previous cycle till the day of trigger. Compared with placebo, it showed better pregnancy rates.[54] But other studies showed limited success.

Acupuncture

Current literature does not provide sufficient evidence that adjuvant acupuncture improves IVF clinical pregnancy rates.[54]

Ovum Donation

Ovum donation can be offered in poor responders as an alternative or in case of the failure of retrieving eggs.

Pretreatment with Oral Contraceptive Pills

It has several advantages, which are as follows:

- It produces estrogen environment.
- It increases sex hormone-binding globulin (SHBG) and decreases the androgen level helping in preventing apoptosis.
- It decreases LH and so there is follicular synchronization.
- It decreases progesterone rise during the preovulatory period.
- It decreases FSH and LH and thus downregulates pituitary.

Add-on treatments are introduced into routine practice before these have been shown to improve live birth rates. They may cause more expense and still worsen the results. Strong evidence is required before add-ons are introduced to regular treatment. Associated risks and uncertainties must be explained to the prospective patients.[55]

CARRY HOME MESSAGE

- Poor responders should be correctly identified by Bologna criteria.
- Increasing gonadotropin dosage is not useful.
- Long protocol and flare-up protocol are not useful in poor responders.
- Microdose protocol gives better results.
- Gonadotropin-releasing hormone antagonist with estrogen priming is good alternative.
- Addition of letrozole rather than CC can improve pregnancy rates.
- Growth hormone simply increases the cost of treatment.
- Aspirin, pyridostigmine, glucocorticoids, and acupuncture may have a supportive effect but have to still prove their role in improving pregnancy rates.
- OC pills may help some patients by reducing LH in the patients.
- Pre-IVF androgen does not give better results in oocytes and fertilization rate, but decreases abortion rate.

REFERENCES

1. Zhang M, Bu T, Tian H, Li X, Wang D, Wan X, Wang Q, et al. Use of cumulative live birth rate per total number of embryos to calculate the success of IVF in consecutive IVF cycles in women aged ≥ 35 years. BioMed Research International; 2019. https://doi.org/10.1155/2019/6159793.
2. Land J, Yarmilinskaya MI, Dumoulin JC, Evers JL. High dose hMG stimulation in poor responder does not improve in vitro fertilization outcome. Fertil Steril. 1996;65(5):951-65.
3. Pandian Z, McTavish AR, Aucott L, Hamilton MP, Bhattacharya S. Interventions for 'poor responders' to controlled ovarian hyperstimulation (COH) in in-vitro fertilization (IVF). Cochrane Database Syst Rev. 2010;(1):CD004379.
4. Karande VC, Jones GS, Veeeck LL, Muasher SJ. High dose follicle stimulating hormone stimulation at the onset of the menstrual cycle does not improve the in vitro fertilization outcome in low responder patients. Fetil Steril. 1990;53:486-9.
5. Klinkert ER, Broekmans FJ, Looman CW, J D F Habbema JDF, Velde ER. Expected poor responders on the basis of an antral follicle count do not benefit from higher starting dose of gonadotrophins in IVF treatment: a randomized controlled trial. Hum Reprod. 2005;20:611-5.
6. Schmidt DW, Bremmer T, Orris JJ, Maier DB, Benadiva CA, Nulsen JC. A randomized prospective study of microdose leuprolide versus ganirelix in in vitro fertilization cycles for poor responders. Fertil Steril. 2005;83:1568-71.
7. Berkkanoglu M, Ozgur K. What is the optimum maximal gonadotropin dosage used in micro-dose flare up cycles in poor responders? Fertil Steril. 2010;94(2):662-5.
8. Ben-Rafael Z, Benadiva CA, Ausmanas M, Barber B, Blasco L, Flickinger GL, et al. Dose of human menopausal gonadotropin influences the outcome of an in vitro fertilization program. Fertil steril. 1987;48: 964-8.
9. Eskandar M, Jaroudi K, Jambi A, Archibong EI, Coskun S, Sobande AA. Is recombinant follicle-stimulating hormone more effective in IVF poor responders than human menopausal gonadotropins? Med Sci Monit. 2004;10(1):16-9.
10. Cedrin-Durnerin I, Bstandig B, Herve F, Wolf J, Uzan M, Hugues J. A comparative study of high fixed-dose and decremental-dose regimes of gonadotropins in a minidose gonadotropin-releasing hormone agonist flare protocol for poor responders. Fertil Steril. 2000;73:1055-6.
11. Youssef MA, van Wely M, Al Inany H, Madani T, Jahangiri N, S Khodabakhshi S, et al. A mild ovarian stimulation strategy in women with poor ovarian reserve undergoing IVF: A multicenter randomized non-inferiority trial. Hum Reprod. 2017;32(1):112-8.

12. Katayama KP, Roesler M, Gunnarson C, Stehlik E, Jagusch S. Short-term use of gonadotropin releasing hormone agonist (leuprolide) for in vitro fertilization. J In Vitro Fert Embryo Trans. 1988;5:332-4.
13. Gindoff PR, Hall JL, Stillman RJ. Ovarian suppression with leuprolide acetate: comparison of luteal, follicular, and flare up administration in controlled ovarian hyperstimulation for oocyte retrieval. J In Vitro Fert Embryo Trans. 1990;7:94-7.
14. Akman MA, Erden HF, Tosun HB, Bayazit N, Aksoy E, Bahceci M. Comparison of agonistic flare up protocol and antagonistic multiple-dose protocol in ovarian stimulation of poor responders: result of prospective randomized trial. Hum Reprod. 2001;16:868-70.
15. Padilla SL, Dugan K, Maruschak V, et al. Use of flare up protocol with high dose human follicle stimulating hormone and human menopausal gonadotropins for in vitro fertilization in poor responders. Fertil Steril. 1996;65:796-9.
16. Barrenetxea G, Agirregoikoa JA, Jimenez MR, de Larruzea AL, Ganzabal T, Carbonero K. Ovarian response and pregnancy outcome in poor responder women: a randomized controlled trial on the effect of luteinizing hormone supplementation in in vitro fertilization cycles. Fertil Steril. 2008;89:546-53.
17. Fabregues F, Creus M, Penarrubia J, Manau D, Vanrell JA, Balasch J. Effects of recombinant human luteinizing hormone supplementation on ovarian stimulation and the implantation rate in down-regulated women of advanced reproductive age. Fertil Steril. 2006;85:925-31.
18. Hill MJ, Levy G, Levens ED. Does exogenous LH in ovarian stimulation improve assisted reproduction success? An appraisal of the literature. Reprod Biomed Online. 2012;24(3):261-71.
19. Levi DP, Navarro JM, Schattman GL, Davis OK, Rosenwaks Z. The role of LH in ovarian stimulation. Exogenous LH: let's design the future. Hum Reprod. 2000;15(11):2258-65.
20. Humaidan P, Chin W, Rogoff D, D'Hooghe T, Longobardi S, Hubbard J, et al. Efficacy and safety of follitropin alfa/lutropin alfa in ART: a randomized controlled trial in poor ovarian responders. Hum Reprod. 2017;32:544-55.
21. Faber BM, Mayer J, Cox B, JonesD, Toner JP, Oehninger S, et al. Cessation of gonadotropin-releasing hormone agonist therapy combined with high dose gonadotropin stimulation yields favorable pregnancy results in low responders. Fertil Steril. 1998;69:826-30.
22. Gracia-Valesco JA, Isaza V, Requena A, Martínez-Salazar FJ, Landazábal A, Remohí J, et al. High dose of gonadotropins combined with stop versus non-stop protocol if GnRH analogue administration in low responder IVF patients: a prospective, randomized, controlled trial. Hum Reprod. 2000;15:2292-6.
23. Olivennes F, Righini C, Fanchin R, Torrisi C, Hazout A, Glissant M, et al. A protocol using a low dose of GnRH agonist might be the best protocol for patient a with high FSH concentrations on day 3. Hum Reprod. 1996;11(6):1169-72.
24. Feldberg D, Farhi J, Ashkenazi J, Dicker D, Shalev J, Ben-Rafael Z. Minidose gonadotrophic-releasing hormone agonist is the treatment of choice in poor responders with high follicle-stimulating hormone levels. Fertil Steril. 1994;62:343-6.
25. Ubaldi FM, Capalbo A, Vaiarelli A, Cimadomo D, Colamaria S, Alviggi C, et al. Follicular versus luteal phase ovarian stimulation during the same menstrual cycle (DuoStim) in a reduced ovarian reserve population results in a similar euploid blastocyst formation rate: new insight in ovarian reserve exploitation. Fertil Steril. 2016;105(6):1488-95.
26. Deaton JL, Bauguess P, Huffman CS, Miller KA. Pituitary response to early follicular-phase minidose gonadotrophic-releasing hormone agonist (GnRHa) therapy: evidence for a second flare. J Assist Reprod Genet. 1996;13:390-4.
27. Surrey ES, Bower J, Hill DM, Ramsey J, Surrey MW. Clinical and endocrine effects of a microdose GnRH agonist flare regimen administered to poor responders who are undergoing in vitro fertilization. Fertil Steril. 1998;69:419-24.

28. Detti L, Williams DB, Robins JC, Maxwell RA, Thomas MA. A comparison of three downregulation approaches for poor responders undergoing in vitro fertilization. Fertil Steril. 2005;84:1401-5.
29. Demirol A, Gurgan T. Comparison of microdose flare-up and antagonist multiple-dose protocol for poor responder patients: a randomized study. Fertil Steril. 2009;92(2):481-5.
30. Schoolcraft WB, Surrey ES, Minjarez DA, Stevens JM, Gardner DK. Management of poor responders: can outcomes be improved with novel gonadotropin-releasing hormone antagonist/letrozole protocol? Fertil Steril. 2008;89(1):151-6.
31. Cheung LP, Lam PM, Lok IH, Tak-Yu Chiu T, Yeung SY, Tjer CC, et al. GnRH antagonist versus ling GnRH agonist protocol in poor responders undergoing IVF: a randomized controlled trial. Hum Reprod. 2005;20:616-21.
32. Nilsson L, Andersen AN, Lindenberg S, Hausken J, Andersen CY, Kahn JA. Ganirelix for leuteolysis in poor responder patients undergoing IVF treatment: a Scandinavian multicenter 'extended pilot study'. Acta Obstet Gynecol Scand. 2010;89(6):828-31.
33. Dragisic KG, Davis OK, Fasouliotis SJ, Rosenwaks Z. Use of a luteal estradiol patch and a gonadotrophic-releasing hormone antagonist suppression protocol before gonadotrophic stimulation for in vitro fertilization in poor responders. Fertil Steril. 2005;84:1023-6.
34. Shastri SM, Schoyer KD, Barbieri EA, Kligman I, Davis O, Rosenwaks Z. Stimulation of the young poor responder: our experience with luteal estradiol/GnRH antagonist suppression versus a standard protocol (LP microdose Lupron). Fertil Steril. 2008;90(Suppl.1):S32.
35. Chang EM, Han JE, Won HJ, Kim YS, Yoon TK, Lee WS. Effect of estrogen priming through luteal phase and stimulation phase in poor responders in in vitro fertilization. J Assist Reprod Genet. 2012;29(3):225-30.
36. Aghahosseini M, Aleyassin A, Khodaverdi A, Esfahani F, Mohammadbeigi R, Movahedi S, et al. Estradiol supplementation during the luteal phase in poor responder patients undergoing in vitro fertilization: a randomized clinical trial. J Assist Reprod Genet. 2011;28(9):785-90.
37. D'Amato G, Caroppo E, Pasquadibisceglie A, Carone D, Vitti A, Vizziello GM. A novel protocol of ovulation induction with delayed gonadotrophic-releasing hormone antagonist administration combined with high-dose recombinant follicle-stimulating hormone and clomiphene citrate for poor responders and women over 35 years. Fertil Steril. 2004;81:1572-7.
38. Homburg R. Management of poor responders. Ovulation Induction and Controlled Ovarian Stimulation: A Practical Guide, 2nd edition. Switzerland: Springer International Publishing; 2014. pp. 159-68.
39. Yaralli H, Esinler I, Polat M, Bozdag G, Tiras B. Antagonist/letrozole protocol in poor ovarian responders for intracytoplasmic sperm injection: a comparative study with the microdose flare up protocol. Fertil Steril. 2009;92(1):231-5.
40. Battalgia C, Salvatori M, Maxia N, Petraglia F, Facchinetti F, Volpe A. Adjuvant L-arginine treatment for in vitro fertilization in poor responder patients. Hum Reprod. 1999;14:1690-7.
41. Kolibianakis E, Venetis C, Diedrich K, Tarlatzis BC, Griesinger G. Addition of growth hormone to gonadotropins in ovarian stimulation of poor responders treated by in vitro fertilization: a systematic review and meta-analysis. Hum Reprod Update. 2009;15:613-22.
42. Keay SD, Lenton EA, Cooke ID, Hull MG, Jenkins JM. Low dose dexamethasone augments the ovarian response to exogenous gonadotropins leading to a reduction in cycle cancellation rate in a standard IVF program. Hum Reprod. 2001;16:1861-5.
43. Barad D, Gleicher N. Effect of dehydroepiandrosterone on oocyte and embryo yields, embryo grade and cell number in IVF. Hum Reprod. 2006;21:2845-9.

44. Cozzolino M, Cecchino GN, Troiano G, Romanelli C. Growth hormone cotreatment for poor responders undergoing in vitro fertilization cycles: a systematic review and meta-analysis. Fertil Steril. 2020;114(1): 97-109.
45. Gliecher N, Weghofer A, Barad DH. Dehydroepiandrosterone (DHEA) reduces embryo aneuploidy: direct evidence from preimplantation genetic screening (PGS). Reprod Biol Endocrinol. 2010;10(8):140.
46. Kim CH, Howles CM, Lee HA. The effect of transdermal testosterone gel pre-treatment on controlled ovarian stimulation and IVF outcome in low responders. Fertil Steril. 2011;95(2):679-83.
47. Massim N, Cedrin-Durnerin S, Coussieu C, Galey-Fontaine J, Wolf JP, Hugues J-N. Effects of transdermal testosterone application on ovarian response to FSH in poor responders undergoing assisted reproduction technique-a prospective randomized double-blind study. Hum Reprod. 2006;21:1204-11.
48. Fabregues F, Penarrubia J, Creus M, Manau D, Casals G, Carmona F, et al. Transdermal testosterone may improve ovarian response to gonadotropins in low-responder IVF patients: a randomized clinical trial. Hum Reprod. 2009;24:349-59.
49. Gibson DA, Simitsidellis I, Kelepouri O, Critchley HOD, Saunders PTK. Dehydroepiandrosterone enhances decidualization in women of advanced reproductive age. Fertil Steril. 2018;109(4):728-34.
50. Mohsen IA, El Din RE. Minimal stimulation protocol using letrozole versus microdose flare-up GnRH agonist protocol in women with poor ovarian response undergoing ICSI. Gynecol Endocrinol. 2013;29(2):105-8.
51. Fraterelli JL, McWilliams GD, Hill MJ, Miller KA, Scott RT. Low dose aspirin use does not improve in vitro fertilization outcomes in poor responders. Fertil Steril. 2008;89(5):1113-7.
52. Lambers MJ, Hoozzemans Da, Schats R, Homburg R, Lambalk CB, Hompes PGA. Low dose aspirin in non-tubal IVF patients with previous failed conception: a prospective randomized double blind placebo-controlled trial. Fertil Steril. 2009;92:923-9.
53. Chung-hoon K, Hee-Dong C, Yoon-Seok C. Pyridostigmine cotreatment for controlled ovarian hyperstimulation in low responders undergoing in vitro fertilization-embryo transfer. Fertil Steril. 1999;71:652-7.
54. El-Toukhy T, Sunkara SK, Khairy M, Dyer R, Khalaf Y, Coomarasamy A. A systematic review and meta-analysis of acupuncture in in vitro fertilisation. BJOG. 2008;115(10): 1203-13.
55. Wilkinson J, Malpas P, Hammarberg K, Tsigdinos PM, Lensen S, Jackson E, et al. Do à la carte menus serve infertility patients? The ethics and regulation of in vitro fertility add-ons. Fertil Steril. 2019;112(6): 973-85.

14

Chapter

Mild Ovarian Stimulation in Assisted Reproductive Technology

INTRODUCTION

It was the belief of assisted reproductive technology (ART) consultants that the greater the number of eggs retrieved, the more the pregnancy rate. So, larger doses of gonadotropins were used for several years after ART practice started and most commonly, the long protocol was used. But this protocol is expensive and takes a longer duration for stimulation leading to more chances of ovarian hyperstimulation syndrome (OHSS) and multiple pregnancy.

Robert Edwards was the first person to advocate lower doses of gonadotropins, i.e., milder stimulation, patient-friendly, and safe approach in 1996. The balance between patient comfort, cost, and live birth rate is very important, and therefore this concept gradually became popular. The concept of the natural cycle in vitro fertilization (IVF) or minimal stimulation is very common in Japan and USA and some parts of Europe.

There are three groups of patients who can be benefitted from mild IVF:

1. Patients with limited income, particularly in developing countries
2. Patients with low ovarian reserve
3. Patients who do not want hormonal stimulation or cannot be given hormonal stimulation due to medical disorders.

In group 1, tubal infections are common in the lower socioeconomic class in developing countries and the only option left to them for fertility is ART. Natural cycle IVF is affordable to them. In group 2, eggs can be retrieved and collected over several cycles with mild stimulation and are cryopreserved. In these patients with advanced age, preimplantation genetic screening (PGS) can be done or single embryo transfer can be done later on.

The International Society of Mild Approaches in Assisted Reproduction (ISMAAR) defines mild IVF cycle, either as:

- Gonadotropins are administered at a lower dose and/or shorter duration throughout the cycle in which a gonadotropin-releasing hormone (GnRH) antagonist is given as cotreatment, or
- Stimulation with oral compounds, either alone or in combination with gonadotropins and GnRH antagonist.[1]

Ovulation induction and luteal support are the part of this protocol where the aim is to collect between two and seven eggs.[2]

VARIOUS PROTOCOLS

Natural Cycle IVF

In natural cycle IVF, the results are very poor, especially in older patients.[3] A pregnancy rate of approximately 7% is quoted in several papers.[4] About 4–11 natural cycles produce the same live birth rate as one conventional cycle. It is frustrating for the patient to accept negative results for several cycles. Therefore, it is not a preferred protocol.

Natural cycles are patient-friendly, cheap and safe, and no drugs are used but premature luteinizing hormone (LH) surge is very common. This may lead to cancellation of cycles in up to 20%. In many oocyte retrievals, one may not get a single ovum.

However, some authors have quoted that natural cycle IVF in poor responders is as effective as controlled ovarian hyperstimulation (COH) in terms of pregnancy rate and implantation rate with lower expense and better compliance.[5] The pregnancy rate per cycle and per transfer was 10% and 16–18%, respectively, according to these studies. This has been proved also in a meta-analysis by Daya et al.[6] This natural cycle IVF can be used for patients with breast cancer, kidney transplant, liver transplant, and thrombophilia.

Modified Natural Cycle

The initial reports of the modified natural cycle using mild stimulation and GnRH antagonist have also given disappointing results. In this protocol, a GnRH antagonist is started when the size of the lead follicle is 14 mm and at the same time gonadotropin (75–300 IU) is also started. It reduces the cycle cancellation as it prevents LH surge. Here, endogenous follicle stimulating hormone (FSH) rise is taken as an advantage. Ovulation trigger is done by 10,000 IU human chorionic gonadotropin (hCG) or recombinant hCG (rhCG) 250 µg. The pregnancy rate was 8.3%.[7] So, the results are disappointing in spite of a safe and patient-friendly protocol, and results are not significantly different from those of the natural cycle. The modified natural cycle is used in poor responders and advanced age patients.

Low-dose hCG instead of FSH can complete follicle maturity in a natural cycle. So, it can be applied in the modified natural cycle.[8]

Delayed Low-dose FSH with Antagonist (Mild IVF Cycle)

According to this protocol, FSH stimulation is started on Day 5–7 in a dose of 150 IU. An antagonist is given for prevention of LH surge, along with endogenous FSH in this protocol, but the multiple pregnancy rate is not reduced;[5] therefore, single embryo transfer is preferred. The cumulative pregnancy rate for 12 months and standard protocols are the same.[5] The quality of the egg is superior and the implantation rate is better as compared to the long protocol. Because the E2 level is low, the detrimental effect on endometrium, oocyte, and embryo is not observed. It is less expensive and gives a similar pregnancy rate.

Clomiphene Combined with Gonadotropins

In this protocol, clomiphene citrate (CC) is given in early phase of the cycle and then combined with gonadotropins. This decreases the requirement of gonadotropins and also the risk of OHSS. The results are similar to the conventional antagonist protocol.[9] If CC is given before Day 6 of the cycle, it helps in ovulation induction, but has a negative effect on the endometrium.[10] Instead if it is given after 6 days of the menstrual cycle, it has an inhibitory effect on LH surge and ovulation and probably no effect on endometrium. Therefore in premature LH surge, if CC is given around the time of ovulation, it can improve the quality of oocytes and maturation. In these cases, CC is given from Day 7. Agonist trigger is preferred in these cycles to prevent functional ovarian cysts. It does not cause luteal phase defect in natural cycles and corpus luteum is adequately functional to support the luteal phase. CC being antiestrogenic does not allow positive feedback of estrogen to release LH and so there is no progesterone surge.[11]

Aromatase Inhibitors with Gonadotropins

Aromatase inhibitors have a dual property. These chemicals prevent androgen to estrogen conversion by aromatization, leading to low estrogen that is beneficial for endogenous FSH production. An increased androgen level sensitizes the preantral and antral follicles to FSH. Letrozole 2.5–5 mg with gonadotropins gives promising results. It keeps estrogen close to the physiological range and that improves the implantation rate. Letrozole increases integrin expression and improves endometrial receptivity.

Low-dose Gonadotropins

In poor responder women, there is a fair evidence that the clinical pregnancy rate after IVF in conventional gonadotropin protocol is not different when compared to the mild stimulation protocol, i.e., when using low-dose gonadotropin protocol (≤150 IU/day).[12]

MILD VERSUS CONVENTIONAL PROTOCOL

- Dose requirement in the mild protocol is less and so the cost is low and less monitoring is required.
- In mild stimulation, a lesser number of follicles are produced (<8) and this gives a better implantation rate.[13]
- Endometrial receptivity is high because of lower estradiol (E2) in mild protocol. Otherwise, high E2 alters the uterine relaxing property of progesterone and prevents implantation.
- Abnormal and mosaic embryos are more common with the conventional protocol. This is because of increased meiotic segregation errors in early embryonic cleavage division.[14] Therefore, the aneuploidy rate is higher with the conventional protocol.
- The twin pregnancy rate is very low with mild stimulation.
- The incidence of OHSS is low with mild stimulation.
- Mild stimulation is more patient-friendly.
- In poor responders, natural cycle IVF or mild stimulation has an advantage.

American Society for Reproductive Medicine (ASRM) recommendations, 2018: In patients who are classified as poor responders and pursuing IVF, strong considerations should be given to a mild ovarian stimulation protocol (low-dose gonadotropin with or without oral agents) due to lower costs and comparable low pregnancy rates compared with traditional IVF stimulation.[15]

DISADVANTAGES OF MILD STIMULATION

- It may give mono- or bifollicular development in 15–20% of patients that may lead to cycle cancellation and give a lower pregnancy rate.
- Less embryos are available for cryopreservation.
- In some cases as LH is suppressed, the pregnancy rates are low. In these cases, hCG or human menopausal gonadotropin (hMG) or recombinant LH (rLH) is to be added.[16]
- A lower pregnancy rate can cause psychological problems.
- For ovum donors, mild stimulation should be mandatory. The risk/benefit ratio is lower with mild stimulation than

the risk mild stimulation as a cause of negative consequences for the donor are taken into account. The present practice of hyperstimulating donors, indicates the recipients' interest is put first. It is difficult to ignore the profit generated. It should not come as a surprise that many people feel increasingly uneasy about how oocyte donation is managed in this era of increasing commercialization of oocytes.[17]

CARRY HOME MESSAGE

- Conventional protocol is expensive and can cause OHSS and multiple pregnancy.
- Mild stimulation helps in low-income groups and patients having estrogen-dependent tumors.
- The aim is to collect 2–7 ova.
- Natural cycle IVF has a 7% pregnancy rate and results are poor.
- Modified natural cycle has the same results.
- Mild stimulation, i.e., 150 IU FSH, has sane results as the conventional protocol.
- CC + gonadotropins has the same results.
- Letrozole has the additional benefit of improving endometrial receptivity.

REFERENCES

1. Schipper I, Hop WC, Fauser BC. The follicle stimulating hormone (FSH) threshold/ window concept examined by different inventions with exogenous FSH during the follicular phase of the normal menstrual cycle: duration, rather than magnitude, of FSH increase affects follicle development. J Clin Endocrinol Metab. 1998;83:1292-98.
2. Nargund G, Fauser BC, Macklon NS, Ombelet W, Nygren K, Frydman R, et al. Rotterdam ISMAAR Consensus group on terminology for ovarian stimulation for IVF. Hum Reprod. 2007;22:2801-4.
3. Verberg MFG, Macklon NS, Nargund G, Frydman R, Devroey P, Broekmans FJ, et al. Mild ovarian stimulation for IVF. Hum Reprod Update. 2009;15:13-29.
4. Pelinck MJ, Hoek A, Simons AH, Heineman MJ. Efficacy of natural cycle IVF: a review of the literature. Hum Reprod Update. 2002;8:129-39.
5. Heijen EM, Eijkemans MJ, De Klerk C, Polinder S, Beckers NG, Klinkert ER, et al. A mild treatment strategy for in vitro fertilization: a randomized no-inferiority trial. Lancet. 2007;369:743-9.
6. Daya S, Gunby J, Hughes EG, Sagle MA, YoungLai EV. Natural cycles for in vitro fertilization: cost-effectiveness analysis and factors influencing outcome. Hum Reprod. 1995;10:1719-24.
7. Pelinck MJ, Vogel NE, Hoek A, Simons AHM, Arts EGJM, Mochtar MH, et al. Cumulative pregnancy rates after three cycles of minimal stimulation IVF and results according to subfertility diagnosis: a multicenter cohort study. Hum Reprod. 2006;21:2375-83.
8. Paulson RJ, Chung K, Quaas AM, Mucowski SJ, Jabara SI, Bendikson KA. Low dose human chorionic gonadotrophin alone can complete follicle maturity: successful application to modified natural cycle in vitro fertilization. Fertil Steril. 2016;105(5):1228-31.
9. Gibreel A, Maheshwari A, Bhattacharya S. Clomiphene citrate in combination with gonadotropins for controlled ovarian stimulation in women undergoing in vitro fertilization. Cochrane Database Syst Rev. 2012;(11):CD008528.
10. Wallace KL, Johnson V, Sopelak V, Hines R. Clomiphene citrate versus letrozole: molecular analysis of the endometrium in women with polycystic ovarian syndrome. Fertil Steril. 2011;96(4):1051-6.
11. Teramoto S, Kato O. Minimal ovarian stimulation with clomiphene citrate: a large scale retrospective study. Reprod Biomed Online. 2007;15(2):134-48.
12. Youssef MA, van Wely M, Al-Inany H, Madani T, Jahangiri N, Khodabakhshi S, et al. A mild ovarian stimulation strategy in women with poor ovarian reserve undergoing IVF: a multicenter randomized controlled trial. Hum Reprod. 2005;20:611-5.
13. Verberg MFG, Eijkemans MJC, Maklon NS, Heijnen EMEW, Baart EB, Hohmann FP, et al. The clinical significance of the retrieval

of a low number of oocytes following mild ovarian stimulation for IVF: a meta-analysis. Hum Reprod Update. 2009;15:5-12.
14. Baart EB, Martini E, Eijkemans MJ, Opstal DV, Beckers NGM, Verhoeff A, et al. Milder ovarian stimulation for in-vitro fertilization reduces aneuploidy in human pre-implantation embryo: a randomized controlled trial. Hum Reprod. 2007;22(4):980-8.
15. Practice Committee of the American Society of Reproductive Medicine. Comparison of pregnancy rates for poor responders using IVF with mild stimulation versus conventional IVF: a guideline. Fertil Steril. 2018;109(6):993-9.
16. Takahashi K, Mukaida T, Tomiyama T, Goto T, Oka C. GnRH antagonist improved blastocyst quality and pregnancy outcome after multiple failures of IVF/ICSI-ET with a GnRH agonist protocol. J Assist Reprod Genet. 2004;21(9):317-22.
17. Pennings G. Mild stimulation should be mandatory for oocyte donation. Hum Reprod. 2020;35(11):2403-7.

15

Chapter

Role of Luteinizing Hormone in Ovulation Induction

INTRODUCTION

Recent knowledge on luteinizing hormone (LH) has raised a lot of controversies regarding its usage in assisted reproductive technology (ART). With the use of gonadotropin-releasing hormone (GnRH) agonist as well as antagonist, LH levels are very low when LH is required for the final stages of development of an ovum. So, the use of analogs may be detrimental to the ova. The contradictory thing is that a growing follicle is more sensitive to LH and dependent on LH on the final stages of maturation, which is low due to analogs.[1] Some people advocate add-back LH from the midfollicular phase in the ovarian cycle and others have found no benefit of the addition of LH. However, the addition of recombinant LH (rLH) has shown better oocyte quality.[2]

ROLE OF LUTEINIZING HORMONE (FIG. 1)

- LH is required for follicular steroidogenesis. It helps theca cells to form androgen from the progesterone and pregnanolone.
- It helps in follicular maturation. In the final maturation stage of the follicle, only LH is enough for further growth of the follicle.
- It helps in ovulation. LH helps in rupture of the follicle and luteinization of the follicle. The corpus luteum starts secreting progesterone instead of estrogen after ovulation. LH peak prevents growth of the rest of the nondominant follicles.
- LH stimulates the corpus luteum and maintains luteal phase functions by adequate secretion of progesterone.

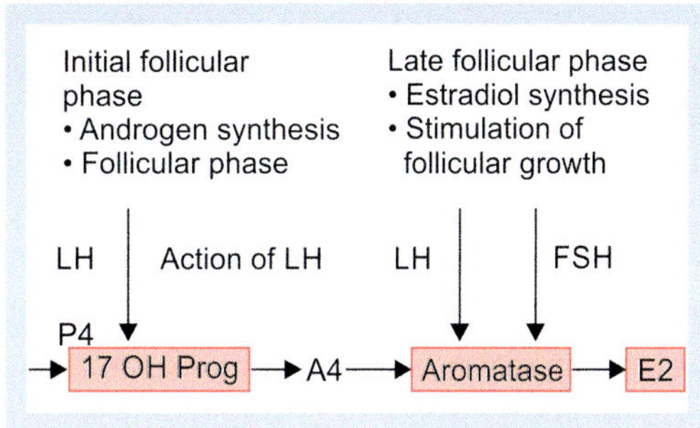

Fig. 1: Action of LH. (E2: estradiol; FSH: follicle-stimulating hormone; LH: luteinizing hormone)

PHYSIOLOGY OF LUTEINIZING HORMONE IN OVULATION

Two Cell–Two Hormone Theory[3]

Follicle-stimulating hormone (FSH) draws the cholesterol for its conversion into progesterone. Under the effect of LH, this progesterone is converted into androgen by theca cells. This androgen traverses to granulosa cells in the developing follicle, where due to aromatase activity androgen is converted into estrogen. For the final stage of development of follicle, both FSH and LH are required.[4,5]

Basic science, experiment, and clinical data have shown that LH is absolutely necessary for normal follicular development and oocyte maturation.[6] Therefore, in hypogonadotropic hypogonadism (HH), stimulation with only recombinant FSH (rFSH) gives a very poor fertilization rate and exogenous LH is required to optimize ovulation.[6]

At the intermediate follicular phase, LH receptors are detected in the granulosa compartment[3] and have an additive effect afterward. So, LH regulates both theca cells and granulosa cells. FSH and LH also control local production of growth hormones for folliculogenesis. The fluctuation of LH is responsible for the change in the estrogen level because of the change in androgen production. When the LH level is low, there will be low estradiol (E2) which will disturb endometrial preparation.

The rise of LH is beneficial as it converts progesterone to androgen that will aromatize to estrogen. So, more FSH leads to more production of progesterone from cholesterol and this is detrimental to implantation. So once LH receptors develop, i.e., after 10-mm size of the follicle, the dose of FSH can be decreased and further growth of the follicle is taken care of by LH. This is because there is no rise in progesterone; instead, it is decreased as it is converted to androgen and later on to estrogen. This high LH also takes care of the luteal phase.[7,8]

THERAPEUTIC WINDOW OF LUTEINIZING HORMONE[6]

Balasch and Fabregues[6] hypothesized that there is a LH ceiling, which may be associated with reproductive failure, e.g., polycystic ovary syndrome (PCOS) **(Fig. 2)**. During the second half of the follicular phase, when the FSH level decreases, the LH-dependent phase of the follicular development proceeds normally provided LH is above the threshold level and below the ceiling level. But the meta-analysis conducted by Mochtar et al. showed no significant difference in pregnancy rates in rLH and rFSH group and only rFSH group.[9] Studies have shown that the level of LH should be between 1.2 and 5.0 IU/L for optimal follicular development where endogenous LH is suppressed.[4]

The therapeutic aspects of LH can be discussed under the following heads:

- Age and LH
- Long protocol and LH
- Antagonist and LH

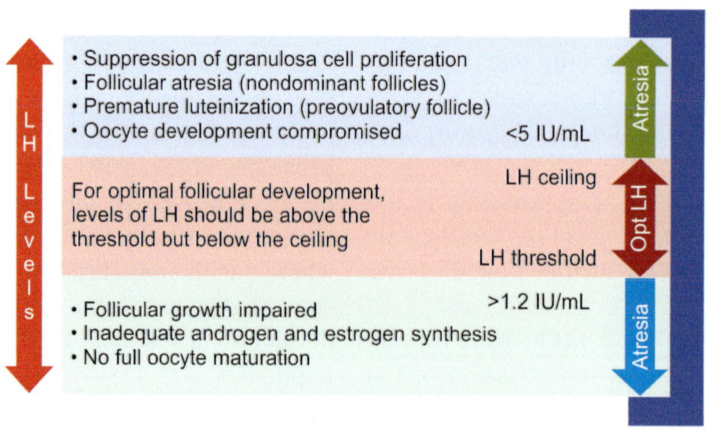

Fig. 2: Luteinizing hormone (LH) levels.

- Poor responders and LH
- Polycystic ovary syndrome and LH (high LH)
- FSH and LH polymorphism

Age and Luteinizing Hormone

There is a decline in the pregnancy rate after 35 years of age due to less number of ova available and increase in the incidence of aneuploidy. The deoxyribonucleic acid (DNA) content of the oocyte is lower after the age of 35 years. In these patients due to advanced age even with a high dose of FSH, there is a poor response. Moreover, a high FSH dose increases the conversion of cholesterol to progesterone, increasing the progesterone level. As there is LH deficiency or less bioactive LH available, progesterone is not converted to androgen. This progesterone excess leads to a low implantation rate. Here, LH supplementation will convert progesterone to androgen which will be aromatized to estrogen. Both low progesterone and high E2 will favor good endometrial development for implantation. Hill et al. suggest rLH supplementation after the age of 35 years.[10] At the Bourn Hall Clinic, London, they add rLH supplementation in stimulation protocol for women over 35 years of age. The Cochrane review reiterated the usefulness of rLH in poor responders and advance-aged women who are at risk of spontaneous abortion.[11] A recent meta-analysis by Hill et al. favors the addition of LH in ART in the advanced age group.[12]

Criteria to add LH on Day 6 of stimulation:[4]

- LH < 1.25 ng/mL on Day 6 of stimulation
- No follicle > 10 mm on Day 6 of stimulation
- Estradiol < 200 pg/mL
- Endometrial thickness < 6 mm

The disadvantage of LH in elderly people is that ovary has more stromal content, and excess LH may have adverse effects because of more sensitivity to stromal tissue. This excessive LH level further damages already aged oocytes. The LH level is high in elderly patients, but its bioactivity may be different in different patients. LH may have a ceiling effect on larger follicles. With menopause and advanced age, FSH and LH levels increase and these are biologically less active. The number of functioning LH receptors decreases with age. This biologically less active LH causes low estrogen because of low androgen production. Exogenous LH can correct this defect. There is always a discrepancy between immunoactive LH and bioactive LH levels. Bioactivity of LH decreases as age advances. Therefore, the serum levels of LH cannot decide which patients will require exogenous LH supplementation.

A meta-analysis by Kolibianakis et al. does not support the use of GnRH analog and also confirms no influence of rFSH + rLH or rFSH treatment.[13] Vuong et al. also did not find any difference when LH was added in women >35 years of age. So, LH is useful in only a subset of patients and that still needs definition.[14]

Alviggi et al. have stated in a systematic review that rLH supplementation is required in:

- Women between the age of 35 and 39 years
- Unexpected hyporesponse to rFSH monotherapy in patients having normal ovarian reserve parameters
- Poor responders with suppressed LH levels due to GnRH analogs, but the role of LH supplementation is controversial[15]
- In Poseidon group I, i.e., hyporesponse, and group II when age is 35–39 years with hyporesponse with normal antral follicle count (AFC) and anti-Müllerian hormone (AMH) (i.e., AFC > 5, AMH > 1.1) **(Fig. 3)**.[15]

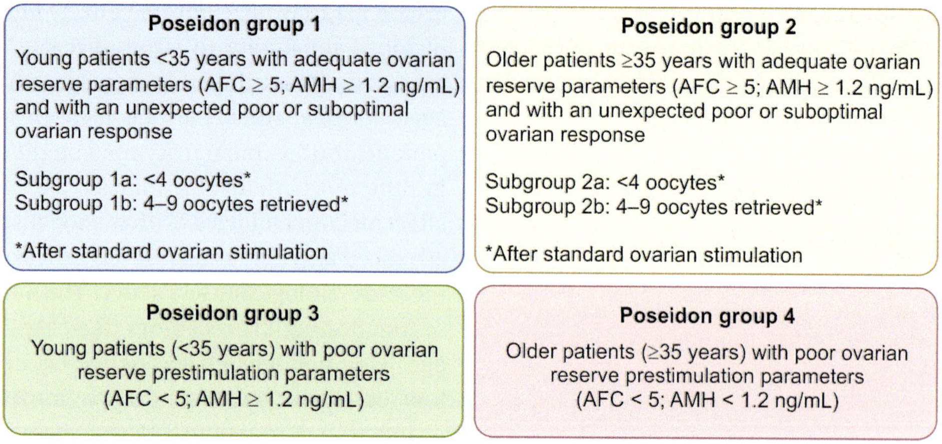

Fig. 3: Poseidon groups indicating in which patients would LH supplementation be required.[15]
(AFC: antral follicle count; AMH: anti-Müllerian hormone; LH: luteinizing hormone)

Long Protocol and Luteinizing Hormone

Long protocol in ART suppresses LH level, though not to zero level. It usually remains between 0.5 and 2.5 IU/L. Even with this low level of LH, rFSH can produce multiple follicular growth. Even when LH goes to <0.5 IU/L, there is no difference in pregnancy rates. Only <1% of LH receptors are required for normal response. In the presence of minimal stimulation by LH, FSH can activate signals modified by insulin-like growth factors (IGFs), which sustain androgen synthesis and can have ovarian androgen. Adding LH from day 6 routinely to all patients does not improve the pregnancy rate.[16] This low LH has no adverse effect on the ongoing pregnancy rate beyond 12 weeks. There is no cutoff value to identify the women requiring LH supplementation, so LH estimation is of no use. <1% of LH receptors should be occupied to achieve optimum ovarian response.[17] The optimum response is achieved when LH levels are between 0.5 and 1.5 IU/L.[18] Continuous administration of GnRH agonist helps to maintain a small amount of tonic LH secretion because each agonist injection may cause the release of a small amount of LH, but its bioactivity is less as compared to normal LH secreted. The reason of differential response to LH between the HH females and normogonadotropic (NG) women could be that the HH stage in NG women is much shorter (2–3 weeks) than that in HH women. The normal level of LH before pituitary suppression will prime the small follicles. So, follicles are less sensitive to a drop in LH level and respond to FSH irrespective of LH levels.

Antagonist Cycle and Luteinizing Hormone

There is a diversified opinion regarding the addition of LH in the antagonist cycle. The GnRH antagonist is started from Day 6 and addition of rLH does not improve the IVF outcome, but few reports suggest that adding LH or human menopausal gonadotropin (hMG) in antagonist cycle improves the results. A meta-analysis by Hill MJ et al. proved that adding LH will improve the results,[10] but fall of LH to >50% from early to midfollicular phase results in a lower birth rate. Low early and midfollicular phase LH had low E2, low oocyte yield, and low embryo development. So, LH is to be added if the level is <1.2 IU/L in the midfollicular phase.

Luteinizing Hormone in Poor Responders

Luteinizing hormone has an important role in poor responders. There is a subset of patients who are benefited from adding LH. The Asia Pacific Fertility Advisory Group[19] in 2011 strongly recommended rLH in cotreatment with rFSH in patients with a history of poor response in:

- Suboptimal response to stimulation on Day 6:
  - No follicle of >10 mm in size
  - Endometrial thickness of <6 mm
  - Estradiol level <200 pg/mL
- It may be beneficial in females of >35 years of age with a long agonist or antagonist protocol.[18]

An LH dose of 75 IU is sufficient in most cases, but a small percentage of women may require doses of LH up to 150–225 IU. Many studies including one by Musters et al. demonstrated that adding rLH to the ovulation induction protocol does not show any difference in top quality embryos or ongoing pregnancy rates.[20] Adding LH is more effective when there is an inadequate response to rFSH. Rather than increasing the dose of FSH, rLH is added and that results in more oocyte yield.[21] The ESPART (Efficacy and Safety of Pergoveris in ART) study showed that the live birth rate was higher in the recombinant human FSH (rhFSH)/rLH group compared to the rFSH group, in spite of the same number of eggs retrieved. The pregnancy outcome failure was significantly lower in the rhFSH/rhLH group and is helpful in improving the live birth rate.[22] The reason for the better outcome may be because of LH, which may reduce the rate of granulosa cell apoptosis. LH receptors are present in the endometrium during the window of implantation and play an important role in embryo-endometrium crosstalk during implantation. The positive effect of LH on embryo and endometrium helps in implantation in women above 35 years of age.

Luteinizing Hormone in Polycystic Ovary Syndrome

It has already been discussed that high LH can have a ceiling effect on ova, and this is observed in PCOS patients. This high LH is associated with reproductive failure. PCOS is a classical example of high LH with a poor pregnancy rate and a higher abortion rate due to the effect of LH on ovum quality and endometrial receptivity. High LH causes follicular atresia, premature luteinization, and poor oocyte quality due to high androgen levels. Preovulatory development of ova is dependent on the optimum level of LH, which is above the threshold and below the ceiling level. LH should be avoided as it can cause ovarian hyperstimulation syndrome (OHSS). Clomiphene citrate (CC) is the classical example for a lower pregnancy rate due to high LH. CC acts on the hypothalamus to secrete FSH and LH. This high LH is detrimental to ova. When endogenous LH is elevated, FSH alone is conceptually better.[23]

Follicle-stimulating Hormone and Luteinizing Hormone Polymorphism

The ovarian response to FSH differs from patient to patient due to FSH receptor polymorphism. FSH receptor gene is a marker for ovarian response. FSH receptor gene consists of two single nucleotide polymorphism (SNP) in axon-10 and changes two amino acids at positions 307 and 680. Women with 307 Ala and 680 Ser single-nucleotide polymorphisms (SNPs) show a reduced response to controlled ovarian hyperstimulation (COH). These patients require higher doses of FSH and are called poor responders.[24] In these cases after the development of a follicle of 10–11 mm, LH can be added instead of increasing the dose of FSH for better outcome and lower FSH delivery.

Luteinizing hormone polymorphism: The LH receptor gene carries as many as 282 SNPs.[25] In 1991, Petterson and Soderholm identified a common genetic LHβ variant or v-β-LH due to alterations in beta subunit gene leading to changes in amino acid sequence. There is more potency of LH activity of v-β-LH at the receptor site, but its duration of activity is shorter.[26] Presence of v-β-LH increases the requirement of FSH. These are the patients in whom exogenous LH is required for stimulation.[26] It is very common in Japanese patients. An endogenous LH level is not accurate to decide which patients will require LH supplementation.[27] Instead, v-β-LH can be used as a marker for ovarian response to rFSH. It helps the clinician to identify the patients who will require LH supplementation.[26] In genuine empty follicle syndrome, *LHCGR* gene mutations are responsible for no ova being retrieved on oocyte retrieval. It is inherited in the family. So, screening of mutation is useful.[28]

Human menopausal gonadotropin or luteinizing hormone: Studies have shown that rLH is better than hMG to be combined with FSH during ovarian stimulation. In hMG, the human chorionic gonadotropin (hCG), i.e., the LH activity, may be inconsistent and may affect oocyte maturation and affect pregnancy rates.[29]

Human menopausal gonadotropin: There are controversial results with hMG + rFSH for live birth rates. The only advantage is lesser number of ampoules of rFSH required resulting in lower cost of treatment, but if rLH is added instead of hMG it gives higher birth rates.[30] The hCG content is six times greater than that of LH. hCG, when given after a follicle size of 10 mm, has no effect on large follicles, but causes demise of smaller follicles.[31]

The disadvantages of hMG are as follows:
- Protein contamination
- Local allergic reaction
- Batch-to-batch inconsistencies
- Supply limitations
- Variable LH quality and bioavailability in different hMG preparations
- Much more hCG than LH activity (at least 10 times).

The characteristics of hCG are as follows:
- Serum half-life is two-fold
- More stable
- Slow degradation and high binding affinity to LH receptors
- 1 IU of hCG is six to eight times greater in bioactivity than 1 IU of LH
- Accumulates on daily injections.

Comparing Human Chorionic Gonadotropin and Luteinizing Hormone at the Molecular Level

- Different source
- Different molecular weight
- Different number of amino acids (AA) in beta chain
- Different number of glycosylation sites
- Different half-life.

Comparing Human Chorionic Gonadotropin and Luteinizing Hormone Functionally and Clinically

- Different effect on cyclic adenosine monophosphate (cAMP)
- Different gene expressions
- LH gives more oocytes/embryo

- Better quality of oocytes/embryo
- Difference in cumulative pregnancy rate with LH.

Administration of low-dose hCG 200 IU/day (100–400) replacing rFSH in the final days of ovarian stimulation reduces the consumption of gonadotropins without differences in oocyte yields and pregnancy outcome.[31] The reason is that a developing follicle becomes less dependent on FSH as it acquires LH responsiveness.[32] In a large series,[33] rFSH was discontinued when six follicles were >12 mm or E2 was >600 ng/L. rFSH was substituted by 200 IU of hCG. There was significant reduction in the total dose of FSH, but oocytes retrieved and pregnancy rates were the same.

CARRY HOME MESSAGE

- LH is strictly necessary for meiosis, rupture of the follicle, and luteal phase.
- LH promotes theca cells to produce androgen which is aromatized to estrogen by granulosa cells under the influence of FSH—two cell–two hormone theory.
- A small amount of LH is enough for follicular maturation in agonist downregulated cycles.
- The results are good when LH is >1.2 IU/L (threshold) and <5 IU/L (ceiling level).
- Adding LH improves the results when the LH level is low.
- LH receptors develop when the follicle is >10 mm in diameter and then LH can take over the function of FSH.
- With advanced age, LH supplementation gives better results because of less bioactive LH or LH polymorphism.
- High LH gives a poor pregnancy rate, and classical examples are PCOS and CC-induced cycles.
- Recombinant LH is more specific than hCG.

REFERENCES

1. Shoham Z. The clinical therapeutic window for luteinizing hormone in controlled ovarian stimulation. Dertil Steril. 2002;77(6):1170-7.
2. Ruvolo G, Bosco L, Pane A, Morici G, Cittadini E, Roccheri MC. Lower apoptosis rate in human cumulus cells after administration of recombinant luteinizing hormone to women undergoing ovarian stimulation for in vitro fertilization procedures. Fertil Steril. 2007;87(3):542-6.
3. Hillier SG, Whitelaw PF, Smyth CD. Follicular oestrogen synthesis: the 'two-cell, two-gonadotrophin' model revisited. Mol Cell Endocrinol. 1994;100:51-4.
4. O'Dea L, O'Brien F, Currie K, Hemsey G. Follicular development induced by recombinant luteinizing hormone (LH) and follicle stimulating hormone (FSH) in anovulatory women with LH and FSH deficiency: evidence of a threshold effect. Curr Med Res Opin. 2008;24(10):2785-93.
5. Vaskivuo T. Regulation of apoptosis in the female reproductive system (2002). [online] Available from: http://jultika.oulu.fi/files/isbn9514266676.pdf [Last accessed March, 2021].
6. Balasch J, Fabregues F. Is luteinizing hormone needed for optimal ovulation induction? Curr Opin Obstet Gynecol. 2002;14(3):265-74.
7. Voutilainen R, Tapanainen J, Chung BC, Matteson KJ, Miller WL. Hormonal regulation of P450scc (20,22-desmolase) and P450c17 (17 alpha-hydroxylase/17,20-lyase) in cultured human granulosa cells. J Clin Endocrinol Metab. 1986;63(1):202-7.
8. Palermo R. Differential actions of FSH and LH during folliculogenesis. Reprod Biomed Online. 2007;15(3):326-37.
9. Jayaprakasan K. Sono AVC. A novel method of automatic volume calculation. Ultrasound Obstet Gynecol. 2008;31:691-6.
10. Hill MJ, Levens ED, Levy G, Ryan ME, John M Csokmay, Alan H DeCherney, et al. The use of recombinant luteinizing hormone in patients undergoing assisted reproductive techniques with advanced reproductive age: a systematic review and meta-analysis. Fertil Steril. 2012;97(5):1108-14.
11. Mochtar MH, Van der Veen, Zeich M, van Wely M. Recombinant luteinizing hormone (rLH) for controlled ovarian hyperstimulation in assisted reproductive cycles. Cochrane Database Syst Rev. 2007;(2):CD005070.

12. Hill MJ, Levy G, Levens ED. Does exogenous LH in ovarian stimulation improve assisted reproduction success? An appraisal of the literature. Reprod Biomed Online. 2012;24(3):261-71.
13. Kolibianakis EM, Kalogeropoulou L, Griesinger G, Papanikolaou EG, Papadimas J, Bontis J, et al. Among patients treated with FSH and GnRH analogues for in vitro fertilization, is the addition of recombinant LH associated with the probability of live birth? A systematic review and meta-analysis. Hum Reprod Update. 2007;13:445-52.
14. Vuong TNL, Phung HT, Ho MT. Recombinant follicle-stimulating hormone and recombinant luteinizing hormone versus recombinant follicle-stimulating hormone alone during GnRH antagonist ovarian stimulation in patients aged ≥35 years: a randomized controlled trial. Hum Reprod. 2015;30(5):1188-95.
15. Alviggi C, Conforti A, Esteves SC, Andersen CY, Ernesto Bosch E, Bühler K, et al. Recombinant luteinizing hormone supplementation in assisted reproductive technology: a systematic review. Fertil Steril. 2018;109(4):644-64.
16. Kollibianakis EM, Collins J, Tarlatzis B, Papanikolaou E, Devroey P. Are endogenous LH levels during ovarian stimulation for IVF using GnRH analogues associated with probability of ongoing pregnancy? A systematic review. Hum Reprod Update. 2006;12:3-12.
17. Chappel SC, Howles C. Re-evaluation of the roles of luteinizing hormone and follicle-stimulating hormone in the ovulatory process. Hum Reprod. 1991;6:1206-12.
18. Wong PC, Qiao J, Ho C, Wiweko B, Takehara Y, Nadkarni PV, et al. Current opinion on use of luteinizing hormone supplementation in assisted reproduction therapy: an Asian perspective. Reprod Biomed Online. 2011;23(2):81-90.
19. Lahoud R, Al-Jefout M, Tyler J, Ryan J, Driscoll G. A relative reduction in mid-follicular LH concentrations during GnRH agonist IVF/ICSI cycles leads to lower live birth rates. Hum Reprod. 2006;21(10):2645-9.
20. Musters AM, van Wely M, Mastenbroek S, Kaaijk EM, Repping S, van der Veen F, et al. The effect of recombinant LH on embryo quality: a randomized controlled trial in women with poor ovarian reserve. Hum Reprod. 2012;27:244-50.
21. De Placido G, Alviggi C, Perino A, Strina I, Lisi F, Fasolino A, et al. Italian collaborative group on recombinant human luteinizing hormone. Recombinant human LH supplementation versus recombinant human follicle-stimulating hormone step up protocol during controlled ovarian stimulation in normogonadotropic women with initial inadequate response to rFSH. A multicenter, prospective, randomized controlled trial. Hum Reprod. 2005;20: 390-6.
22. Humaidan P, Chin W, Rogoff D, D'Hooghe T, Longobardi S, Hubbard J, et al. Efficacy and safety of follicular alfa/lutropin alfa in ART: a randomized controlled trial in poor ovarian responder. Hum Reprod. 2017;32:544-55.
23. Regan L, Owen EJ, Jacobs HS. Hypersecretion of luteinizing hormone, infertility and miscarriage. Lancet. 1990;336:1141-4.
24. Simoni M, Tempfer CB, Destenaves B, Fauser BCJM. Functional genetic polymorphisms and female reproductive disorders: Part I: Polycystic ovarian syndrome and ovarian response. Hum Reprod Update. 2008;14(5):459-84.
25. Themmen APN. An update of pathophysiology of human gonadotrophin subunit and receptor gene mutations and polymorphisms. Reproduction. 2005;130(30): 263-74.
26. Alviggi C, Clarizia R, Pettersson K, Mollo A, Humaidan P, Strina I, et al. Suboptimal response to GnRHa long protocol is associated with a common LH polymorphism. Reprod Biomed Online. 2009;18(1):9-14.
27. Loumaye E, Engrand P, Howles CM, O'Dea L. Assessment of the role of serum luteinizing hormone and estradiol response to follicle-stimulating hormone on in vitro fertilization treatment outcome. Fertil Steril. 1997;67:889-99.
28. Yuan P, He Z, Zheng L, Wang W, Li Y, Zhao H, et al. Genetic evidenc of 'genuine' empty

follicle syndrome: a novel effective mutation in the *LHCGR* gene and review of literature. Hum Reprod. 2017;32(4):944-53.

29. Carone D, Vizzillo G, Vitti A. Clinical outcomes of ovulation induction in WHO group I anovulatory women using r-hFSH/r-hLH in a 2:1 ratio compared to hMG. Hum Reprod. 2010;25:285-321.
30. Ferraretti AP, Ginarolli L, Magli MC, D'angelo A, Farfalli V, Montanaro N. Exogenous luteinizing hormone in controlled ovarian hyperstimulation for assisted reproduction techniques. Fertil Steril. 2004; 82(6):1521-6.
31. Filicori M, Cognigni GE, Tabarelli C, Pocognoli P, Taraborrelli S, Spettoli S, et al. Stimulation and growth of antral ovarian follicles by selective LH activity administration in women. J Clinical Endocrinol Metab. 2001;87:1156-61.
32. Sullivan MW, Stewart-Akers A, Krasnow JS, Berga SL, Zeleznik AJ. Ovarian responses in women to recombinant follicle-stimulating hormone and luteinizing hormone (LH): a role of LH in the final stages of follicular maturation. J Clin Endocrinol Metab. 1999;84:228-32.
33. Van Horne AK, Bates GW Jr, Robinson RD, Artgus NJ, Propst AM. Recombinant follicle-stimulating hormone (r-FSH) supplemented with low-dose human chorionic gonadotropin compared with r-FSH alone for ovarian stimulation for in vitro fertilization. Fertil Steril. 2007;88:1010-3.

16 Chapter

Preovulatory Progesterone in Ovulation Induction

INTRODUCTION

Controlled ovarian stimulation is done for in vitro fertilization-embryo transfer (IVF-ET). There is a marked increase in the estradiol (E2) level due to multifollicular development. Normally, the progesterone level sharply rises after the trigger that is given for final oocyte maturation. But, in some of the patients, there is premature luteinizing hormone (LH) surge and may lead to cycle cancellation in IVF. These premature LH surges can be prevented by routine use of gonadotropin-releasing hormone agonist (GnRHa) or antagonist in IVF cycles.

There is a subtle increase in serum progesterone at the time of human chorionic gonadotropin (hCG) in some of the patients, in spite of using agonist or antagonist in IVF cycles. The incidence of progesterone rise is as high as 35% in the agonist cycle[1] and up to 38% in the antagonist cycle.[2] So, this rise of progesterone is not premature luteinization and the follicle is not converted into corpus luteum. This is preovulatory progesterone rise, irrespective of the LH level.

PHYSIOLOGY

The growing follicle secretes a small amount of progesterone, which can be detected 2–3 days prior to the mid-cycle surge. It facilitates the follicle-stimulating hormone (FSH) and LH surge.[3] So, progesterone helps in a positive feedback mechanism along with E2 for LH and FSH surge.

In controlled ovarian stimulation, there are multiple follicles that collectively produce more progesterone than the natural cycle, irrespective of the agonist or antagonist used. As a response to the rise in progesterone from multiple follicles, in the latter half of the follicular phase, there is endogenous LH rise which is termed premature luteinization. But in these cases, LH surge occurs before progesterone rise. Progesterone rise occurs in spite of the use of agonist or antagonist, which indicates that the cause is different. Therefore, it is called premature elevation of progesterone and not premature luteinization.

PATHOGENESIS

The pathogenesis of this is poorly understood and there are various hypotheses given for expalantion:

- *Follicular LH level*: Some authors believe that the rise in the progesterone level is because of the rise in LH in the follicular phase.[4] In this case, pituitary desensitization is not complete and some amount of LH is always present. This LH stimulates granulosa cells to secrete progesterone in the late follicular phase, but it cannot trigger the ovulation.[5]
- *Accumulation of hCG from exogenous human menopausal gonadotropin (hMG)*: hMG that is given for ovulation induction has LH activity due to hCG added to it. This hCG accumulates in serum because of its long half-life, and this LH activity

stimulates granulosa cells to secrete progesterone.[6] These women had higher serum hCG levels and high progesterone in the same studies. If this hypothesis is true, recombinant FSH (rFSH) is a better drug than hMG for stimulation as rFSH has no LH-like activity and progesterone rise should not occur during stimulation.[7] Pure FSH with no LH activity gives higher rise of progesterone or the same as hMG.

- *Increased sensitivity of LH receptors of granulosa cells to FSH*: It is found that the higher the FSH exposure, the more the progesterone rise. This progesterone rise is because of increased LH sensitivity of granulosa cells in FSH-treated cycles.[2] The highest sensitivity of granulosa cells to FSH is due to increased E2 levels. This E2 stimulates the granulosa cells continuously in presence of FSH to secrete progesterone. So, a higher dose of FSH will cause more follicles to develop, which in turn gives more estrogen level that sensitizes granulosa cells to secrete progesterone level which is high in the preovulatory phase. Because of FSH and E2, the follicle develops LH receptors and so more follicles have more LH receptors and more progesterone. So, exogenous gonadotropins may lead to high progesterone levels.
- *Poor ovarian response and increased LH activity*: Premature progesterone rise is common in poor responder patients with increased LH sensitivity. But it was found that neither recombinant hCG (rhCG) nor recombinant LH (rLH) was responsible for this. It was due to the adverse reaction of the oocyte-cumulus complex.

CERTAIN FACTS ABOUT PROGESTERONE RISE

- The rise of progesterone is not related to the LH level as it may occur in agonist or antagonist cycles also when LH levels are very low.
- A positive correlation is found with the dose of FSH required for stimulation. Patients who required higher doses had a progesterone level of >1.5 ng/mL and these patients were more prone to ovarian hyperstimulation syndrome (OHSS) and vice versa.[8] A high FSH dose gives a high progesterone level irrespective of the agonist or antagonist cycle.
- High E2 levels and more number of oocytes collected are directly related to serum progesterone level elevation. This may be due to more FSH as the daily dose may give a good response. So, the initial high FSH dose induces strong steroidogenic activity in granulosa cells that cause a rise in the progesterone level.
- The LH-driven conversion to E2 by theca cells is prevented by agonist and antagonist. There are more numbers of follicles due to FSH stimulation. During this stage, progesterone is the intermediate product and is not converted to androgen and then E2. So, lack of LH activity also increases the progesterone level in the follicular phase that causes advancement of endometrium without any effect on the embryo. This advancement of endometrium gives reduced implantation.[9,10] So, this is contradictory to the hMG-induced progesterone rise hypothesis. In this case, when hMG is used, more LH activity will convert progesterone to androgen and then to estrogen giving a lower progesterone level. So, according to this explanation, the progesterone level will be lower in hMG cycles rather than rFSH.[11]
- Serum levels >1.5 ng/mL have a poor pregnancy rate due to endometrial advancement rather than its effect on

embryo and irrespective of stimulation or trigger has a low birth rate. So, transfer in a subsequent cycle of frozen-thawed embryo gives better results.[12] These findings have been confirmed by microarrays.

- If the threshold value is considered low as reported in certain studies, then there will be no low pregnancy rate with higher values of progesterone and results will be the same.
- If pre-hCG progesterone levels are high, alternative treatment is to give hCG earlier before progesterone rises. This treatment may be beneficial.[13]
- There is a contribution from the adrenal cortex also for the progesterone rise and there is some role of dexamethasone to suppress it. However, the study by Fanchin et al. proved that increase in progesterone seen during controlled ovarian stimulation was unaltered by dexamethasone treatment, thereby confirming that premature progesterone elevation results solely from the effect of exogenous gonadotropin to ovary and the number of mature follicles. Therefore, E2 and progesterone correlate on the day of the trigger.[14]
- Since premature progesterone elevation is commonly associated with a strong ovarian response to controlled ovarian stimulation, this subgroup often produces competent embryos, may override endometrial alterations, and maintain good pregnancy rates. These patients are good responders. But if progesterone is high with a weak ovarian response to controlled ovarian stimulation, a poor-quality embryo cannot compensate for endometrial changes by progesterone and these embryos should be frozen.
- Data obtained by direct immunoassay may often show high progesterone levels, but mass spectrometry may show lower levels. So measuring progesterone by different assays may have different results. In direct immunoassay, 17-OH hydroxyprogesterone is also measured along with progesterone and therefore shows high progesterone levels, leading to unrequired canceled ET in many cycles.

IMPACT OF THE PROGESTERONE LEVEL ON PREGNANCY

A progesterone level of 1.5 ng/mL is chosen as an arbitrary level. Pregnancy rates are low when the progesterone level is >1.5 ng/mL irrespective of the agonist or antagonist cycle and irrespective of the E2 level and total dose of gonadotropin. The patients who had progesterone level <1.5 ng/mL had higher pregnancy rates.[15] A meta-analysis by Venetis et al. has concluded that the progesterone level does not correlate with the cycle outcome.[16] But in this meta-analysis, the threshold value for high progesterone was kept as 0.9 ng/mL. So, the results are conflicting regarding the pregnancy outcome. A recent meta-analysis including several thousand IVF-ET cycles observed a detrimental effect on the pregnancy rate when the progesterone level exceeded 0.8 ng/mL.[17]

Since premature progesterone elevation is associated with strong controlled ovarian stimulation, this group often produces competent embryos. These good-quality embryos may override putative endometrial alterations. But in presence of a weak response, the poor-quality embryo cannot compensate for the alterations in endometrial receptivity induced by progesterone.

Flowchart 1: Two-cell–two-gonadotropin theory.

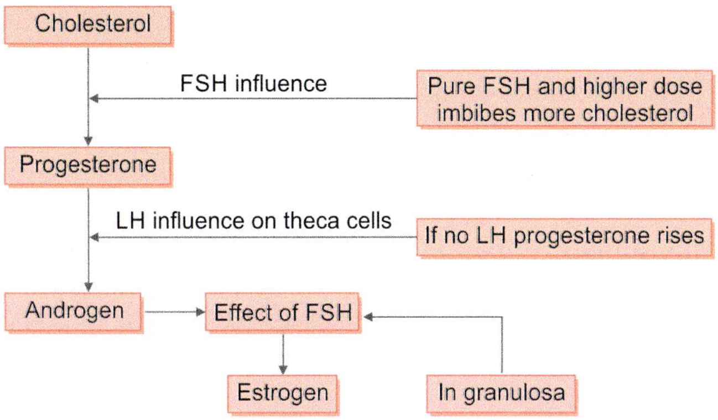

(FSH: follicle-stimulating hormone; LH: luteinizing hormone)

BIOCHEMISTRY ON BASIS OF TWO-CELL–TWO-GONADOTROPIN THEORY (FLOWCHART 1)

This theory explains that:

- The higher the FSH, the higher the progesterone level.
- If LH is absent, then progesterone is not converted to androgen and the progesterone level rises.
- Therefore, hMG-highly purified (HP) will give lesser progesterone rise.
- Progesterone and 17-OHP are terminal products and are not converted into androgen and E2.
- Their level is very high in follicular fluid, rather than in the serum (>1,000 times).
- Both the cells, granulosa cells and theca cells can produce progesterone and 17-OHP. Theca cells alone can produce androgen from CYP 17. But granulosa cells also have limited amount of CYP 19, i.e., aromatase, which converts it into estrogen.

So FSH has got the direct effect on increasing the progesterone level by upgrading 3β-hydroxysteroid dehydrogenase (3βHSD), in granulosa cells along with increase in E2

Flowchart 2: Progesterone.

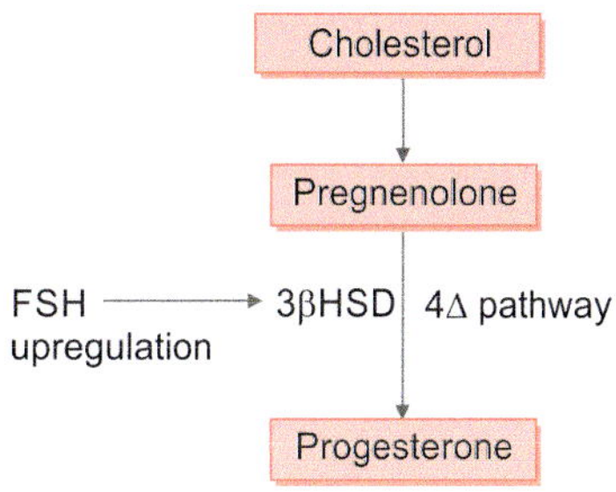

(3βHSD: 3β-hydroxysteroid dehydrogenase; FSH: follicle-stimulating hormone)

(Flowchart 2).[18] This progesterone goes to theca cells and is converted into androgen. This androgen goes to granulosa cells, where it is converted into estrogen but in limited amount.

EFFECT OF PROGESTERONE ON OOCYTE AND ENDOMETRIUM

The elevated progesterone level may impair the endometrial receptivity. It causes advancement of the endometrium, endometrial asynchrony, and change in endometrial gene expression.[19] The Bosch et al. group did not find any detrimental effect of high progesterone on oocyte in terms of fertilization, cleavage, or embryo quality.

The pregnancy rates were the same when the embryos of patients with high progesterone levels from donors were transferred to recipients or in the same patient in the subsequent cycle after cryopreservation.

So, it is concluded that low pregnancy rates due to elevated progesterone levels are due to their detrimental effect on the endometrium rather than oocyte or embryo irrespective of trigger or stimulation protocol. But recent two large retrospective analyses have reported different findings.[20,21]

In these studies, the top-quality embryos were less when the progesterone level was high either in the agonist or in the antagonist cycle.

RESCUE STRATEGIES FOR PROGESTERONE RISE

- Agonist and antagonist protocols do not make difference in the pregnancy rate in patients with progesterone rise.
- High doses of FSH increase progesterone rise. But the step-down regime decreases progesterone rise.
- If the dose of FSH is continued even after three follicles of >17 mm with delay of hCG, it causes more progesterone rise.
- Freeze all is the most accepted policy.
- If the baseline progesterone is high, dexamethasone can reduce the progesterone level.
- In high responders, the critical level of 1.5 ng/mL is higher.

Wang et al. hypothesized that follicles with and increased luteinizing hormone receptor (LHR) expression due to high FSH exposure during stimulation become hypersensitive to ovulation trigger resulting in high circulating early luteal phase progesterone levels and subsequently endometrial advancement and reduced reproductive outcome. So reducing the dose of FSH and agonist trigger instead of hCG may be useful because in case of few follicles.[22]

PATHWAY OF STEROID PRODUCTION IN OVARY

Pathway of steroid production in ovary is discussed in **Figure 1**.

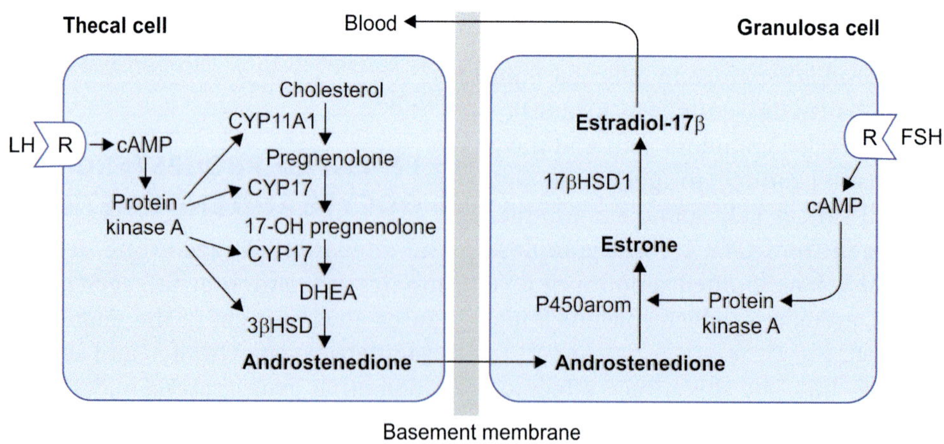

Fig. 1: Pathway of steroid production in ovary. (cAMP: cyclic adenosine monophosphate; DHEA: dehydroepiandrosterone: FSH: follicle-stimulating hormone; LH: luteinizing hormone)

Flowchart 3: Progesterone level is high during the preovulatory period.

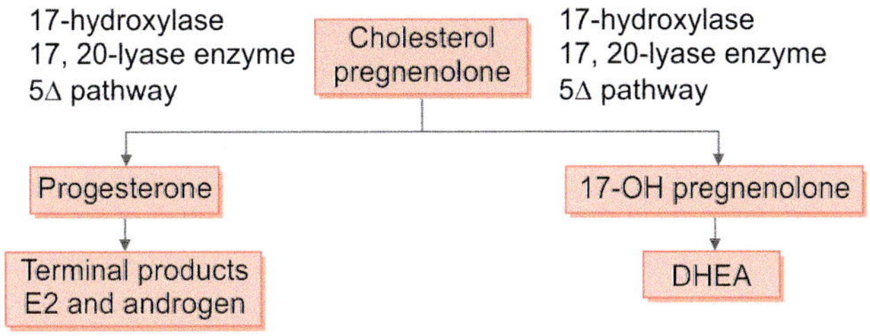

(DHEA: dehydroepiandrosterone)

CARRY HOME MESSAGE

- A serum level of 1.5 ng/mL of progesterone is considered as the most appropriate threshold irrespective of the agonist or antagonist cycle and the number of follicles received.
- Progesterone level >1.5 ng/mL gives a poor pregnancy rate as it affects endometrial receptivity rather than the embryo. In the process of elevation of the progesterone level, it may pass through the normal level which may lead to endometrial asynchrony and advancement of the endometrium.
- A higher progesterone level is seen with rFSH stimulation rather than hMG-HP. This is aggravated by more number of follicles[23] (Here the absence of LH in rFSH prevents conversion to androgen).
- If the progesterone level is >1.5 ng/mL, the "freeze-all" policy should be adopted. The embryos should then be transferred in the subsequent cycle.
- When the progesterone level is high during the preovulatory period, early hCG may be beneficial to the patient **(Flowchart 3)**.

REFERENCES

1. Edelstein MC, Seltman HJ, Cox BJ, Robinson SM, Shaw RA, Muasher SJ. Progesterone levels on the day of human chorionic gonadotropin administration in cycles with gonadotropin-releasing hormone agonist suppression are not predictive of pregnancy outcome. Fertil Steril. 1990;54:853-7.
2. Ubaldi F, Camus M, Smitz J, Bennink HC, Van Steirteghem A, Devroey P. Premature luteinization in in vitro fertilization cycles using gonadotropin-releasing hormone agonist (GnRHa) and recombinant follicle-stimulating hormone (FSH) and GnRH-a and urinary-FSH. Fertil Steril. 1996;66:275-80.
3. Chang RJ, Jaffe RB. Progesterone effect on gonadotropin release in women pretreated with estradiol. J Clin Endocrinol Metab. 1978;47:119-25.
4. Younis JS, Simon A, Laufer N. Endometrial preparation: lessons from oocyte donation. Fertil Steril. 1996;66:873-84.
5. Ubaldi F, Smitz J, Wisanto A, Joris H, Schiettecatte J, Derde MP, et al. Oocyte and embryo quality as well as pregnancy rate in intracytoplasmic sperm injection are not affected by high follicular phase serum progesterone. Hum Reprod. 1995;10:3091-6.
6. Copperman AB, Horowitz GM, Kaplan P, Scott RT, Navot D, Hofmann GE. Relationship between circulating human chorionic gonadotropin levels and premature luteinization in cycles of controlled ovarian hyperstimulation. Fertil Steril. 1995;63: 1267-71.
7. Shaw RW, Ndukew G, Imoedemhe DA, Bernard AG, Burford G. Twin pregnancy after pituitary desensitization with LHRH agonist and pure FSH. Lancet. 1985;326:506-7.
8. Bosch E, Labrata E, Crespo J, Simón C, Remohí J, Jenkins J, et al. Circulating progesterone levels and ongoing pregnancy rates in controlled ovarian stimulation cycles for in vitro fertilization: analysis of over 4000 cycles. Hum Reprod. 2010;25:2092-100.
9. Bosch E, Valencia I, Escudero E, Crespo, Simón C, Remohí J, et al. Premature luteinization during gonadotropin-releasing hormone antagonist cycles and its relationship with in vitro fertilization outcome. Fertil Steril. 2003;80:1444-9.
10. Bourgain C, Devroey P. The endometrium in stimulated cycles for IVF. Hum Reprod. 2003;9:515-22.

11. Anderson AN, Devrory P, Arce JC. Clinical outcome following stimulation with highly purified hMG or recombinant FSH in patients undergoing IVF: a randomized assessor-blind controlled trial. Hum Reprod. 2006;21:3217-27.
12. Fanchin R, Raghini C, Olivennes F, de Ziegler D, Selva J, Frydman R. Premature progesterone elevation does not alter oocyte quality in in vitro fertilization. Fertil Steril. 1996;65:1178-83.
13. Harada T, Yoshida S, Katagiri C, Takao N, Ikenari T, Toda T, et al. Reduced implantation rate associated with a subtle rise in serum progesterone concentration during the follicular phase of the cycles stimulated with a combination of a gonadotropin-releasing hormone agonist and gonadotrophin. Hum Reprod. 1995;10:1060-4.
14. Fanchin R, Raghini C, Olivennes F, Taieb J, de Ziegler D, Frydman R. Premature progesterone elevation and androgen elevations are not prevented by adrenal suppression in IVF. Fertil Steril. 1997;67: 115-9.
15. Bosch E, Labarta E, Crespo J, Simón C, Remohí J, Jenkins J, et al. Circulating progesterone levels and ongoing pregnancy rates in controlled ovarian stimulation cycles for In vitro fertilization-analysis of over 4000 cycles. Hum Reprod. 2010;25:2092-100.
16. Venetis CA, Kolibianakis EM, Papanikolaou E, Bontis J, Devroey P, Tarlatzis BC. Is progesterone elevation on the day of human chorionic gonadotropin administration associated with the probability of pregnancy in in vitro fertilization? A systematic review and meta-analysis. Hum Reprod Update. 2007;13:343-55.
17. Venetis CA, Kolibianakis EM, Bosdou JK, Tarlatzis BC. Progesterone elevation and probability of pregnancy after IVF: a systematic review and meta-analysis of over 60,000 cycles. Hum Reprod. 2013;19:433-57.
18. Oktem O, Akin N, Bildik G, Yakin K, Alper E, Balaban B, et al. FSH stimulation promotes progesterone synthesis and output from human granulosa cells without luteinization. Hum Reprod. 2017;32(3):643-52.
19. Smitz J, Anderson AN, Devroey P, Arce J-C, Merit Group. Endocrine profile in serum and follicular fluid differs after ovarian stimulation with HP-HMG or recombinant FSH in IVF patients. Hum Reprod. 2007; 22:676-87.
20. Huang B, Ren X, Wu L, Zhu L, Xu B, Li Y, et al. Elevated progesterone levels on the day of oocyte maturation may affect top quality embryo IVF cycles. PLoS One. 2016;11:e0145895.
21. Vanni VS, Somigliana E, Reschini M, Pagliardini L, Marotta E, Faulisi S, et al. Top quality blastocyst formation rates in relation to progesterone levels on the day of oocyte maturation in GnRH antagonist IVF/ICSI cycles. PLoS One. 2017;12:e0176482.
22. Wang NF, Skouby SO, Humadian P, Andersen CY. Response to ovulation trigger is correlated to late follicular phase progesterone levels: a hypothesis explaining reduced reproductive outcomes caused by increased late follicular progesterone rise. Hum Reprod. 2019;34(5):942-8.
23. Al-Inany HG, Abou-Setta AM, Aboulghar MA, Mansour RT, Serour GI. Highly purified hMG achieves better pregnancy rates in IVF cycles but not ICSI cycles compared with recombinant FSH: a meta-analysis. Gynecol Endocrinol. 2009;25:1-7.

17

Chapter

Hyperprolactinemia

INTRODUCTION

Prolactin is secreted from lactotrophs of the anterior pituitary. It is regulated by prolactin inhibitory factor (dopamine) secreted from the hypothalamus. Hyperprolactinemia is one of the common causes of oligoanovulation. Prolactin secretion inhibits gonadotropin-releasing hormone (GnRH) secretion leading to a decrease in follicle-stimulating hormone (FSH) and luteinizing hormone (LH) and so causes anovulation and amenorrhea.

EFFECT OF PROLACTIN ON REPRODUCTION

Prolactin acts directly on the ovary by its action on the aromatase enzyme causing menstrual irregularities. In the follicular phase, higher levels affect follicular growth and anovulation. In the luteal phase, it affects the corpus luteum function. An increased level causes poor endometrial development.

Estrogen increases prolactin secretion and is commonly seen in polycystic ovary syndrome (PCOS) as the estrogen level is high. A high prolactin level inhibits GnRH secretion, which in turn inhibits FSH and LH release leading to anovulation. A high prolactin level abolishes midcycle LH surge which is due to the positive effect of the rise in estrogen. This leads to luteal phase defect (LPD) and recurrent pregnancy loss.[1]

CAUSES OF HYPERPROLACTINEMIA

Physiological

Rapid eye movement (REM) sleep, pregnancy, coitus, nipple stimulation, stress, etc., cause high prolactin levels in the blood. The practical consideration is that if the breast is examined for galactorrhea, the blood test for prolactin should not be planned simultaneously with that. Similarly, serum prolactin levels should not be asked for very early in the morning, immediately after waking up. The prolactin level is at peak after 5–8 hours of sleep. In both these conditions, the prolactin level is raised. The collection of the blood sample for prolactin is therefore planned after 2 hours of waking up and before the breast is examined for secretions.

Drug Induced

The drugs that are known to cause a rise in prolactin levels are estrogen, methyldopa, phenothiazines, opiates, cimetidine, and oral contraceptive pills. It is due to the inhibition of dopamine release.

Pathological

The common causes are as follows:
- Idiopathic
- Prolactinoma
- Hypothalamo-pituitary tumors

- Polycystic ovary syndrome
- Hypothyroidism
- Renal failure

About 30% of the patients with PCOS have hyperprolactinemia.[2] Hyperprolactinemia in PCOS patients do not require specific treatment for high prolactin levels; treating PCOS will correct it. Similarly in hypothyroid patients, correction of the thyroid problem automatically corrects related hyperprolactinemia.

PRESENTATION AND DIAGNOSIS

- The most common presentation is galactorrhea.
- Oligoanovulation and infertility may be the cause for seeking medical advice.
- History of related drugs and illnesses should be ruled out.
- Hypothyroidism is to be excluded.
- Headache and visual disturbances are common in pituitary macroadenoma.
- Hyperprolactinemia without galactorrhea is because there is inadequate priming of the breast due to estrogen.[3]

INVESTIGATIONS

Prolactin Level

The normal prolactin level is <30 ng/mL. There are three different types of prolactin: (1) little (80%), (2) big, and (3) big-big. The bioactivity of prolactin is mostly due to little prolactin. At times, blood prolactin levels may be high without galactorrhea or amenorrhea and no other symptoms. This is due to high levels of big and big-big prolactin that have the least bioactivity. It does not require any treatment.

A blood prolactin level of 100–200 ng/mL may be due to pituitary microadenoma. A level >200 ng/mL is due to pituitary macroadenoma and this is symptomatic. If ovulation is present, then a high level of prolactin should be ignored.

Computed Tomography and Magnetic Resonance Imaging

To diagnose microadenoma that is <10 mm and macroadenoma that is >10 mm, computed tomography and magnetic resonance imaging are the investigations of choice.

Serum Thyroid-stimulating Hormone

Rule out hypothyroidism as increased thyroid hormone (TH) is associated with increased prolactin levels due to increased thyroid-stimulating hormone (TSH).

TREATMENT

Dopamine receptor agonists are very effective in normalizing prolactin levels. Commonly used drugs are bromocriptine and cabergoline.

Bromocriptine

Bromocriptine is started as a 1.25-mg daily dose and is increased by 1.25 mg to a maximum dose of 40 mg daily in divided doses till spontaneous menstruation occurs. Dopamine agonists can restore ovulatory cycles in 50–75% of cases. The same dose is continued till the patient conceives in cases of hyperprolactinemia. Once the normal level of prolactin is achieved, the test is repeated every 6 months.

Bromocriptine also reduces the tumor size in 3–6 months. So it is useful in symptomatic patients in pregnancy with prolactinoma. It is useful in nonoperable cases.

Cabergoline

Cabergoline is more patient-friendly than bromocriptine. It is administered in a twice-a-week dose and the results are comparable with bromocriptine. The initial dose is 0.25 mg twice a week and can be increased to 2 mg twice a week. It is effective in 70–80% of patients resistant or nontolerant to bromocriptine.[4] Gastrointestinal tract (GIT) and central nervous system (CNS) side effects are common and so the increase in dose is always gradual. Common contraindications are hypertension, valvular heart diseases, and fibrotic diseases. Vaginal preparations, slow-release oral tablets, and once-a-month preparations are under clinical trials. When used in infertile patients, pregnancy is achieved in almost 85% of cases. Quinagolide also gives equivalent results.

Cabergolin inhibits VEGF receptor-2 specifically and prevents increase in permeability. So it decreases vascular permeability. It is therefore useful in prevention of OHSS. The recommended dose is 0.5 mg for 8 days from the day of trigger. It has no effect on E2 level and also does not help in severe OHSS. It does not have a luteolytic effect and does not affect luteal angiogenesis also. It has no effect on fertilization, cleavage, implantation or clinical pregnancy rate.

In cases of macroadenomas, surgery or radiation is required in persistent and resistant cases or recurrent prolactinomas. For patients who do not require pregnancy, microadenomas may be left untreated.

EFFECT OF HYPER-PROLACTINEMIA IN FEMALE

- Oligoanovulation
- A decrease in FSH and LH secretion
- Increase in intraovarian androgens as it prevents aromatization
- LPD

TRANSIENT HYPERPROLACTINEMIA

Reduction in dopamine inhibitory effect raises prolactin and LH. Transient hyperprolactinemia is observed in normal prolactinemic patients with luteal insufficiency in 73% and galactorrhea in 80% of patients.[5]

This is commonly seen when clomiphene citrate is used for the stimulation protocol. In these cases, bromocriptine is given from Day 5 of the cycle till ovulation. This improves the endometrial thickness and vascularity. In normoprolactinemic patients, bromocriptine is not continued in the luteal phase otherwise it may lead to LPD due to its effect on corpus luteum. The dose of bromocriptine is 1.25 mg twice a day from Day 5 of the cycle till ovulation. Here cabergoline cannot be used as its effect lasts in the luteal phase and causes LPD. Decreasing the prolactin level improved the secretion of FSH and also the quality of the follicle.[6,7] Rise of prolactin in these cases is because of a high estrogen level and if bromocriptine is given to these patients, pregnancy rates up to 40% can be achieved as compared to 1% in controls.[8]

Infertile women with galactorrhea and normal prolactin level respond well to bromocriptine.[9]

The explanation for normal prolactin with galactorrhea is that the biologically active form of prolactin is not detected in immunoassay. The second explanation is exaggerated nocturnal spikes of prolactin secretion that are not recognized in random daytime samples.[9]

CARRY HOME MESSAGE

- Hyperprolactinemia without symptoms may be because of "big prolactin."
- Hyperprolactinemia in PCOS requires treatment of PCOS only.
- TSH must be evaluated before treating hyperprolactinemia.
- Microadenoma does not require surgery.
- Galactorrhea without hyperprolactinemia requires treatment.
- Spikers should be treated with bromocriptine.

REFERENCES

1. Cunha-Filho JS, Gross JL, Lemos NA, Lemos NA, Giugliani C, Freitas F, et al. Hyperprolactinemia and luteal insufficiency in infertile patients with mild and minimal endometriosis. Horm Metab Res. 2001;33(4):216-20.
2. Isik AZ, Gülekli B, Zorlu CG, Ergin T, Gökmen O. Endocrinological and clinical analysis of hyperprolactinemic patients with and without ultrasonically diagnosed polycystic ovarian changes. Gynecol Obstet Invest. 1997;43:183-5.
3. Balen A, Jacobs H. Anovulatory Infertility and Ovulation Induction, 2nd edition. Amsterdam: Elsevier; 2003. pp. 144-55.
4. Verhelst J, Abs R, Maiter D, van den Bruel A, Mark Vandeweghe M, Velkeniers B, et al. Cabergoline in the treatment of hyperprolactinemia: a study in 455 patients. J Clin Endocrinol Metab. 1999;84:2518.
5. Asukai K, Uemura T, Minaguchi H. Occult hyperprolactinemia in infertile women. Fertil Steril. 1993;60(3):423-7.
6. Yoshida K, Kayama F, Kimura Y, Kimura Y, Tamechika S, Satoh K, et al. The effect of occult hyperprolactinemia (OHP) on gonadotropin secretion system. Nihon Naibunpi Gakkai Zasshi. 1994;70(10):1101-14.
7. DeVane GW, Guzick DS. Bromocriptine therapy in normoprolactinemic women with unexplained infertility and galactorrhea. Fertil Steril. 1986;46:1026-31.
8. Ben-David M, Schenker JG. Transient hyperprolactinemia. A correctable cause of female idiopathic infertility. J Clin Endocrinol Metab. 1983;57:442-4.
9. Padilla SL, Person G, McDonough PG, Reindollar RH. The efficacy of bromocriptine in patients with ovulatory dysfunction and normoprolactinemic galactorrhea. Fertil Steril. 1985;44(5):695-8.

18 Chapter

Thyroid Disorders

INTRODUCTION

Thyroid disorders in women are associated with menstrual disorders and impaired fertility. The restoration of the euthyroid state after treatment shows a definite improvement in menstrual disorders and fertility.[1] Formerly, thyroid function tests were recommended for symptomatic women or with a family history of dysfunction. This approach may miss 30–35% of women with hypothyroidism. To screen all the patients, especially infertile and aged patients, and pregnancy patients for thyroid dysfunction is cost-effective and recommended by the American Association of Clinical Endocrinology (AACE).

HYPOTHYROIDISM AND REPRODUCTION

The normal thyroid-stimulating hormone (TSH) level is 0.45–4.5 mIU/L. Hypothyroidism is seen more often in females and increases with age.[2] Menstrual irregularities, spontaneous abortions, preterm deliveries, unexplained stillbirth, and infertility are the common manifestations in a woman. Menorrhagia is due to anovulation, poor muscle tone, and platelet dysfunction.

Infertility

- Almost 70% of infertility in a hypothyroid woman is due to anovulation.[3]
- Oligomenorrhea is the most common clinical presentation.
- It is found in women with unexplained infertility.
- Empirical treatment with thyroid hormones in euthyroid patients does not help in infertility management.
- Every woman after the age of 35 years should be screened for thyroid functions even though she is asymptomatic.

There is insufficient evidence that subclinical hypothyroidism (SCH) with normal TSH, i.e., TSH > 2.5 mIU/L, is associated with infertility.

TSH level > 4 mIU/L is associated with miscarriage, but there is insufficient evidence for a level between 2.5 and 4 mIU/L.

Mechanism of Action (Flowchart 1)

The exact mechanism of the effect of thyroid disorder on ovarian function is not known, but it has been postulated that thyroid hormone might have a direct action on ovarian physiology through receptors in granulosa cells. Thyroid has got synergistic action with follicle-stimulating hormone (FSH) causing a stimulatory effect on granulosa cells. Therefore, hypothyroid patients may have anovulation and may require higher doses for ovarian stimulation.

A normal level of thyroid has an optimum effect on FSH-modulated morphological differentiation of granulosa cells. So alteration in the thyroid level will deteriorate ovarian function.[4] According to John Lowe, hypothyroidism can cause a picture similar

Flowchart 1: Mechanism of action of thyroid-stimulating hormone (TSH).

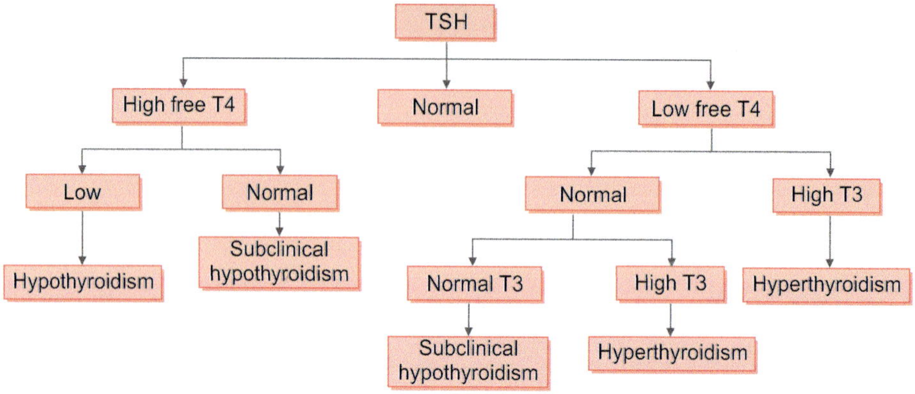

to polycystic ovarian syndrome (PCOS) causing anovulation. Replacement of thyroid hormone can resolve the functional small cysts and anovulation. A study by Muderis et al. confirmed the above findings.[5]

Whenever the TSH level is increased in hypothyroidism, there is an increase in the prolactin level that also causes anovulation. But here the treatment is thyroxine (T4) and not prolactin-lowering drugs.[6]

So, high TSH and low T4 confirm the diagnosis of hypothyroidism and low TSH and high T4 or triiodothyronine (T3) confirm the diagnosis of hypothyroidism. Once the diagnosis is established, the autoimmune disorder must be looked for. Antimicrobial antibody and antithyroid antibody and antithyroglobulin antibody are useful indicators of risk of progression.[7] But they rarely help as far as management is concerned. In patients with a recent onset of hypothyroidism and hypothalamo-pituitary disorders, T4 should be assessed along with TSH. Transient changes in TSH can be caused by glucocorticoids, dopamine, systemic illnesses, and psychiatric disturbances also. To decrease the miscarriage rate, levothyroxine is given in patients with thyroid antibodies if TSH is >2.5 mIU/L.

The upper limit of normal in most laboratories is 4 mIU/L for nonpregnant and 2.5 mIU/L for first trimester patients.

Treatment

Once the diagnosis of hypothyroidism has been established, replacement therapy with 25–50 μg of T4 is recommended, i.e., T4 to be given daily. The dose is increased by 25 μg daily after reassessment with a biochemical and clinical examination after 4 weeks. With proper dosage, the pregnancy rate can reach 64%, i.e., improved pregnancy rate and lower miscarriage rate.[8]

Subclinical Hypothyroidism

Subclinical hypothyroidism is defined as TSH higher than the upper limit of the normal range (4.5–5.0 mIU/L) with normal free T4 levels. During pregnancy, the upper limit is considered as 4 mIU/L but 2.5 mIU/L in the first trimester. There is a fair evidence that treatment of subclinical hypothyroidism when TSH is >4 mIU/L is associated with an improved pregnancy rate and a decreased miscarriage rate.[9] Though there are some studies which also suggest that the TSH values between 2.5 and 5 mIU/L are not associated with adverse IUI outcomes. It has no signs or symptoms with normal T3 and T4 with TSH between 7.5 and 10 mIU/L. The treatment of subclinical hypothyroidism is still controversial for infertility. Thyroxine is given to this group of patients as it has no negative effect and may improve fertility. The role of thyroid replacement on euthyroid patients in infertility has no proved value. But gonadotropin therapy and pregnancy may lead to subclinical hypothyroidism and may require T4.[10]

However, unless abnormal thyroid function can be documented by specific laboratory assessment, empiric treatment has no place. It does not help infertile patients in a euthyroid state.[11] The FASTER (First- and Second-Trimester Evaluation of Risk) trial did not show an adverse effect on the baby in subclinical hypothyroidism. Several studies recommend to maintain TSH between 0.5 and 2.0 mIU/mL.

American Society for Reproductive Medicine (ASRM) Practice committee consensus (2015):

- If the TSH concentration is more than the nonpregnant laboratory reference level (>4 mIU/L), the patient should be treated with levothyroxine to maintain a level < 2.5 mIU/L.
- If the TSH level is between 2.5 and 4 mIU/L, the management option is to monitor it or bring it <2.5 mIU/L.
- During the first trimester, it is advisable to treat when TSH is >2.5 mIU/L.
- Anti-thyroid peroxidase (TPO) is recommended when the repeated TSH value is 2.5 mIU/L.
- If anti-TPO antibodies are detected, the TSH level should be checked and treatment is considered if the TSH level is >2.5 mIU/L.

Evaluation of Therapy

The goal is to maintain the TSH in the lower half of the normal range. The full response of TSH to changes in T4 is relatively slow. A minimum of 8 weeks is necessary between changes in dosage and assessment of TSH. Then further evaluation is done in 4 weeks.

HYPERTHYROIDISM

Mechanism of Action

An elevated T4 level leads to an increased level of sex hormone-binding globulin (SHBG). Thus, an increased level of serum concentration of estradiol and testosterone is observed. The baseline levels of FSH and luteinizing hormone (LH) are also increased. There is attenuated midcycle LH surge, which causes oligoanovulation. It causes a wide range of menstrual disorders from menorrhagia to amenorrhea.

Subclinical hyperthyroidism is as common as subclinical hypothyroidism.

The most common cause of subclinical hyperthyroidism is excessive doses of T4.

Diagnosis

- *Clinical manifestations*: Tachycardia, exophthalmos, tremors, and enlarged thyroid gland
- After the diagnosis of thyroid disorder, a possible cause of the same may be diagnosed by ultrasound, radioactive iodine uptake, and antithyroid antibody.
- Screening is done by TSH assay.

Treatment

The goal is to establish a euthyroid state.

Medical Therapy

In infertile patients, medical therapy is recommended. The drugs used are carbimazole, propylthiouracil, or methimazole.

Dose schedule:

- *Carbimazole*: 10–20 mg 8 hourly
- *Propylthiouracil*: 100–200 mg 8 hourly
- *Methimazole*: 10–15 mg 8 hourly

Common side-effects are gastrointestinal (GI) symptoms, rashes, and agranulocytosis. These inhibit the organification of iodide and decrease the production of T4 and T3. The action is established in 2–4 weeks. The half-life of T4 is about 1 week and the gland has large stores of T4. The maximum effect occurs at 4–8 weeks. Once the patient becomes euthyroid, the dose is to be titrated and gradually reduced to a minimum of 5 mg daily, and then once the patient is euthyroid at that dose also, then the drug is discontinued. Symptomatic relief may be achieved by adding beta-blockers, i.e., propranolol 40–60 mg 6 hourly or nadolol 40–240 mg daily.

Carbimazole is better avoided in patients with asthma and cardiac failure. Relapse of hyperthyroidism can occur in 2 years. It can also be treated by surgery or irradiation, but pregnancy should be postponed for several months. Screening with a highly sensitive TSH assay is a must in all cases of infertility.

CARRY HOME MESSAGE

- Hypo- or hyperthyroidism causes ovulatory dysfunction.
- Hypothyroidism can cause hyperprolactinemia.
- Treatment of subclinical hypothyroidism is controversial.
- Drugs for thyroid are of no value in euthyroid patients.

REFERENCES

1. Longcope C. The male and female reproductive system in thyrotoxicosis. In: Bravermann LD, Utiger RD (Eds). Werner & Ingbar's The thyroid, 6th edition. Philadelphia: Lippincott; 1991. pp. 828-35.
2. Danese MD, Powe NR, Sawin CT, Ladenson, PW. Screening for mild thyroid failure at the periodic health examination. A decision and cost-effectiveness analysis. JAMA. 1996;276(4):285-92.
3. Goldsmith RE, Sturgis SH, Lerman J, Stanbury JB. The menstrual pattern of thyroid disease. J Clin Endocrinol Metab. 1962;12:846-55.
4. Marou T, Hayashi M, Matsuo H, Yamamoto T, Okada H, Mochizuki M. The role of thyroid hormone as a biological amplifier of the actions of follicle-stimulating hormone in the functional differentiation of cultures porcine granulosa cells. Endocrinology. 1987;121(4):1233-41.
5. Muderris II, Boztosun A, Oner G, Bayram F. Effect of thyroid hormone replacement therapy on ovarian volume and androgen hormones in patients with untreated primary hypothyroidism. Ann Saudi Med. 2011;31(2):145-51.
6. Madkar C, Balkawade NU, Dahiya PA. Thyroid pituitary and ovulation. In: Deshpande H (Ed). Practical Management of Ovulation Induction. New Delhi: Jaypee Brothers Medical Publishers; 2016. pp. 46-7.
7. Rao AR. Hyperprolactinemia and thyroid disorders. Principles and Practice of Assisted Reproductive Technology, 1st edition. New Delhi: Jaypee Brothers Medical Publishers; 2014. pp. 8127-37.
8. Oravec S, Hlavacka S. Disorders of thyroid function and fertility disorders. Ceska Gynekol. 2000;65(1):53-7.
9. ASRM practice committee 2015, Subclinical hypothyroidism in the infertile female population: a guideline. Fertil Steril. 2015;104(3): 545-53.
10. Mandel SJ. Thyroid function during gonadotropin therapy (Abstract). Presented at the 10th International Congress of Endocrinology. San Francisco: The Endocrine Society; 1996.
11. Speroff F, Fritz MA. Reproduction and the thyroid. Clinical Gynecologic Endocrinology and Infertility, 7th edition. New Delhi: Jaypee Brothers Medical Publishers; 2005. pp. 803-23.

19 Chapter

Adenomyosis

INTRODUCTION

Adenomyosis is a benign condition in which endometrial glands and stroma are detected in the myometrium. It is common in infertile patients and is often associated with endometriosis. It also often causes myometrial hyperplasia in the surrounding tissues.

BIRD'S DEFINITION[1]

Adenomyosis may be defined as the benign invasion of the endometrium into the myometrium, producing a diffusely enlarged uterus which microscopically exhibits ectopic non neoplastic, endometrial glands and stroma surrounded by the hypertrophic and hyperplastic myometrium.

There are no standard criteria for diagnosis and there is lack of evidence for the standard treatment.

SIGNS AND SYMPTOMS

- The patient may not have any signs and symptoms. These are often incidentally diagnosed.
- The signs and symptoms may be associated with congestive dysmenorrhea and menorrhagia.
- When associated with endometriosis, they cause pelvic pain.
- Adenomyosis is a common cause of infertility mostly due to implantation failure.
- On examination, the uterus is enlarged and globular and is tender on examination. It may be local or diffuse.

PATHOGENESIS

Adenomyosis is an estrogen-dependent gynecological disorder. There is invagination of endometrial basalis in the myometrium. This is due to:

- Altered immunoactivity
- Breaking of endometrium due to trauma
- Disturbance of the junctional zone (JZ)
- Metaplasia of embryonic pluripotent Mullerian remnants
- Metaplasia of adult stem cells.

There may be a combination of different processes.[2]

PRESENTATION

Adenomyosis may present as:

- Diffuse adenomyosis
- Focal adenomyosis
- Polypoid adenomyosis.

It ranges from a slightly thickened functional zone to full-thickness uterine adenomyosis.

CLASSIFICATION[3]

Classification of adenomyosis is given in **Table 1** and shown in **Figures 1A to K**.

TABLE 1: Classification of adenomyosis.

Adenomyosis subtype	*Definition*	*Figure*
Internal adenomyosis (Ai):		
Focal adenomyosis (Ai0)	Localized intramyometrial tiny cystic component with or without JZ bulging (unique or multiple)	**1A**
Superficial adenomyosis (Ai1)	Disseminated subendometrial tiny cystic component without JZ hypertrophy (symmetric or asymmetric)	**1B and C**
Diffuse adenomyosis (Ai2)	Disseminated intramyometrial tiny cystic component with JZ hypertrophy (symmetric or asymmetric)	**1D and E**
Adenomyomas (Ad):		
Intramural solid adenomyoma (Ad1)	Ill-defined myometrial lesion with tiny cystic component (hemorrhagic or not)	**1F**
Intramural cystic adenomyoma (Ad2)	Ill-defined myometrial lesion with hemorrhagic cystic cavity	**1G**
Submucosal adenomyoma (Ad3)	Ill-defined myometrial lesion with tiny cystic component and intracavitary protrusion	**1H**
Subserosal adenomyoma (Ad4)	Ill-defined subserosal myometrial lesion with tiny cystic component	**1I**
External adenomyosis (Ae):		
Posterior external adenomyosis (Ae1)	Ill-defined subserosal posterior myometrial mass associated with posterior deep endometriosis	**1J**
Anterior external adenomyosis (Ae2)	Ill-defined subserosal anterior myometrial mass associated with anterior deep endometriosis	**1K**

Note: asymmetric = predominant disseminated involvement by adenomyosis in one uterine wall; JZ = junctional zone; symmetric = disseminated involvement by adenomyosis in anterior and posterior uterine wall.

Source: Bazot M, Darai E. Role of transvaginal sonography and magnetic resonance imaging in the diagnosis of uterine adenomyosis. Fertil Steril. 2018;109(3):389-97.

INVESTIGATIONS

Ultrasound

Adenomyosis may be diffuse and focal.[4] When focal, it has ill-defined margins. It may cause symmetrical or asymmetrical thickening of myometrium. Depending on the severity of the adenomyosis, the uterus may or may not appear bulky. The affected myometrium shows a coarse heterogenous echogenicity with a "salt and pepper" appearance (hyperechoic areas, hypoechoic areas)[5] **(Fig. 2A)** and also shows cystic lesions. Myometrial cysts have 98% specificity and 78% accuracy for the diagnosis of adenomyosis **(Fig. 2B)**. Heterogenous echogenicity has a sensitivity of 88% for the diagnosis of adenomyosis.[4] Islands of endometrial tissue in the myometrium appear as endometrial buds **(Fig. 2C)**. Alternate vertical hyper- and hypoechoic zones appear, typically described as "rain in forest" or a "Venetian blind" appearance or fan shadows of the myometrium **(Fig. 2B)**. Echogenic flecks can be seen at the endometrial-myometrial junction. These are collapsed myometrial cysts.

The JZ is irregular or interrupted and in severe cases, inaccessible also. High-resolution ultrasound can now show the

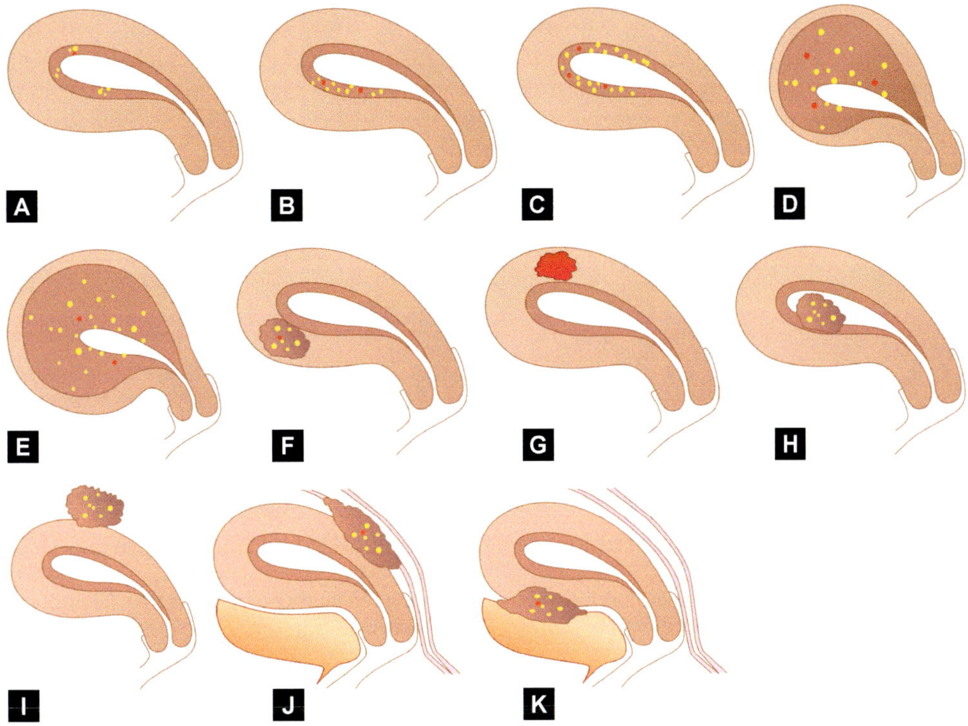

Figs. 1A to K: Magnetic resonance imaging classification of adenomyosis: different morphologic and locations of adenomyosis subtypes including internal adenomyosis, adenomyomas, and external adenomyosis. (A) Internal adenomyosis comprised focal or multifocal adenomyosis, (B) superficial asymmetric or (C) symmetric adenomyosis, and (D) diffuse asymmetric or (E) symmetric adenomyosis. Adenomyomas are related to intramural adenomyoma, (F) solid or (G) cystic and (H) submucosal or (I) Subserosal adenomyomas. External adenomyosis are represented by (J) posterior adenomyosis and (K) anterior associated respective with posterior and anterior deep endometriosis.
Source: Bazot M, Darai E. Role of transvaginal sonography and magnetic resonance imaging in the diagnosis of uterine adenomyosis. Fertil Steril. 2018;109(3):389-97.

endometrial strands extending into the myometrium, interrupting the JZ **(Fig. 2E)**. Adenomyotic uteri may commonly show an abnormal curvature of the fundal endometrial cavity, in a direction opposite to the normal direction of the fundus **(Fig. 2D)**. This is described as a question mark sign of the uterus.[6]

On color Doppler, the affected myometrium shows markedly increased vascularity with vascular dilatation **(Fig. 2F)**. The diameter of these vessels is larger than that of normal myometrium.[7]

Vascularity in adenomyosis is penetrating type translesional in distribution. Decreased uterine artery resistance and increased velocity are also noted.

Endometrial strands extending into the myometrium are also seen on 3D ultrasound (3D US). Adenomyosis shows radial or penetrating vascularity **(Figs. 3A and B)**. It is the JZ assessment that is assessed by the 3D US. Therefore, magnetic resonance imaging (MRI) was considered as an imaging modality for adenomyosis. The difference in the JZ thickness at two different places around the

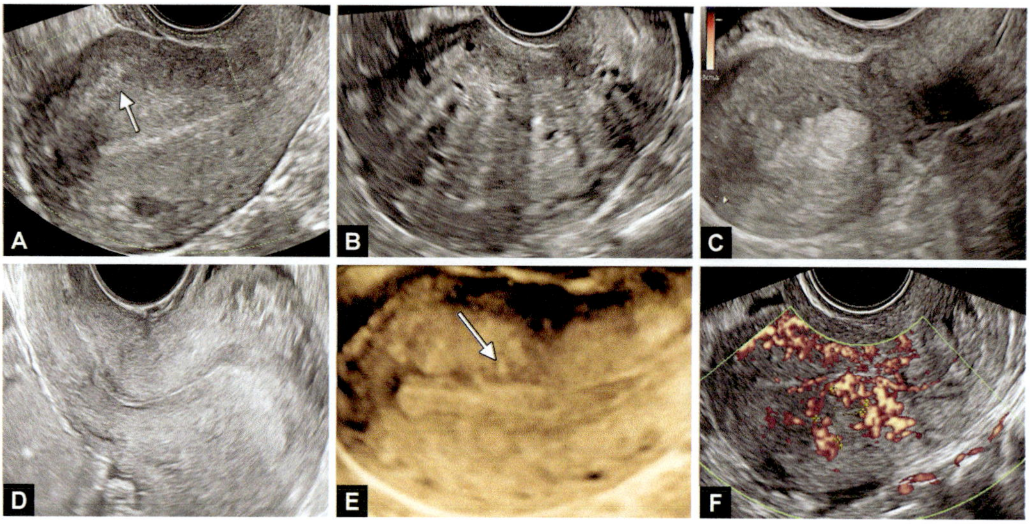

Figs. 2A to F: (A) Salt and pepper appearance in anterior myometrium (arrow); (B) Myometrial cysts (anechoic lesions) and fan shadows seen on a 2D ultrasound image of adenomyosis; (C) Endometrial bud seen on a B-mode ultrasound image; (D) Question mark sign in a retroverted retroflexed adenomyotic uterus; (E) Endometrial strands extending into the myometrium (arrow); (F) Power Doppler image of adenomyosis showing a deranged vascular pattern.

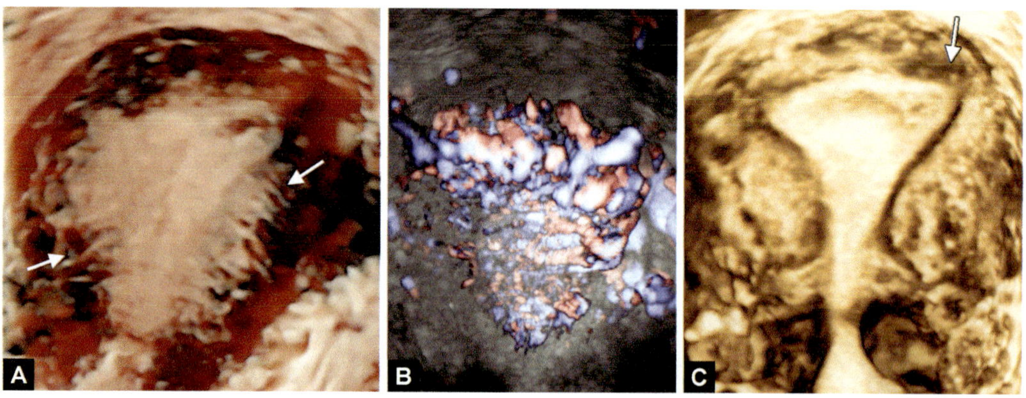

Figs. 3A to C: (A) 3D ultrasound rendered image showing endometrial strands extending into the myometrium; (B) Penetrating vascularity seen on 3D power Doppler in the adenomyotic uterus; (C) 3D ultrasound image showing irregularity of the JZ.

endometrium of >4 mm or a JZ thickness of 12 mm has 88% sensitivity and 85% accuracy for the diagnosis of adenomyosis.[8] Three-dimensional transvaginal ultrasonography (TVS) markers:[8,9] JZ difference >4 mm and JZ infiltration and distortion have been proven as highly sensitive markers for the diagnosis of adenomyosis **(Fig. 3C)**.

Magnetic Resonance Imaging

Magnetic resonance imaging was considered accurate because of the assessment of JZ thickening and myometrial involvement. But now 3D US gives an accurate idea about JZ and is considered at par with MRI.[10] Maximal JZ thickness (JZ_{max}) (12 mm)[11] was associated with a sensitivity and a specificity of 93% and 91%, respectively. However, other studies showed lower sensitivities (63–70%) and specificities (88–96%).[12,13]

To diagnose internal adenomyosis, it may be more useful to compare 3D T2-weighted MRI sequences with 2D T2-weighted MRI sequences to determine the JZmax. The JZmax thickness could also be evaluated by fat-sat suppressed T1-weighted MRI to determine its potential additional diagnostic value.

The main direct criterion for adenomyosis on MRI is the detection of tiny myometrial cysts related to islets of dilated ectopic endometrium. These high-intensity myometrial foci are embedded within the myometrium, most commonly in the inner myometrium, and display a high signal on T2 and a low signal on T1-weighted MRI.[11-14] However, myometrial cysts, although almost pathognomonic of adenomyosis, are detected in only about half of the cases on T2.[11,12] This low sensitivity (<50%) is mainly due to the limited spatial resolution of 2D fast spin echo (2D FSE) T2-weighted MRI. Breath-hold T2-weighted sequences in addition to conventional 2D turbo spin echo (2D TSE)-T2-weighted MR sequences optimize the accuracy of MRI and reduce inter-observer variability **(Figs. 4A and B)**.[15,16]

On MRI, external adenomyosis is diagnosed as an ill-defined subserosal posterior or anterior myometrial mass giving a hypointense signal on T2-weighted MRI. This lesion often contains high-intensity central cystic areas visible on T2- and sometimes on T1-weighted MRI.

An adenomyoma is diagnosed as an ill-defined myometrial mass that is hypointense on T2-weighted MRI. This lesion always contains high-intensity central cystic areas visible on T2- and sometimes on T1-weighted MRI.[17-19] Neither the JZ nor the uterine serosa is affected in the presence of an isolated adenomyoma.

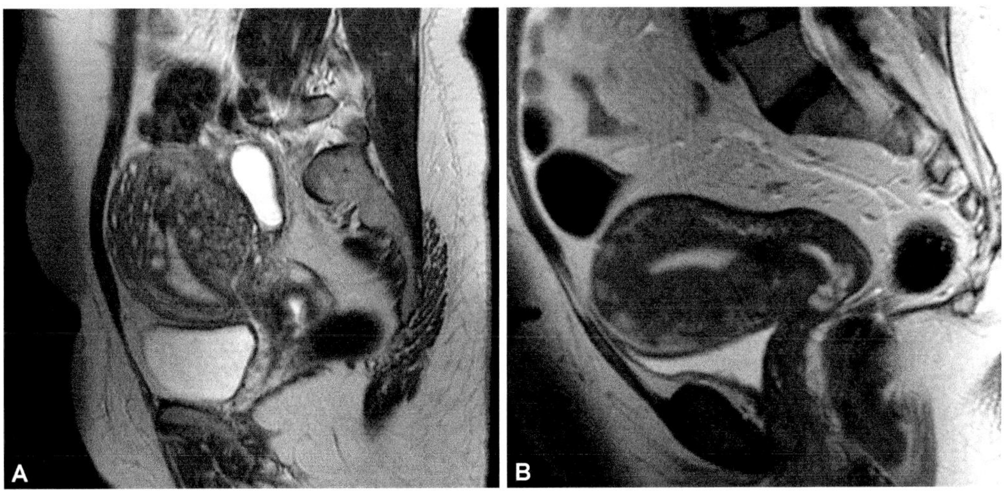

Figs. 4A and B: (A) Diffuse adenomyosis: Sagittal T2WI showing bulky uterus with poorly-defined endometrial-myometrial junctional zone with multiple hyperintense foci and linear strands in the anterior and posterior myometrium (Swiss cheese appearance); (B) Adenomyosis: Sagittal T2WI showing diffuse asymmetrical thickening of the endometrial-myometrial junctional zone, predominantly involving posterior wall myometrium of uterus (more than 12 mm in thickness) with hyperintense foci in myometrum (cystic changes/heterotopic endometrial glands).

Cystic adenomyoma is characterized by its predominant hemorrhage content. On MRI, cystic adenomyomas display homogeneously high-signal intensity on T1-weighted MRI.[20] The appearance on T2-weighted MRI is variable reflecting hemorrhage in different stages of organization.[20] In addition, fluid–fluid level and low signal rim on T2 are sometimes present.[20]

Histopathologically: Endometrial glands and stroma are seen in the myometrium, deeper than 2.5 mm. It is surrounded by hyperplastic and hypertrophic smooth muscle. Cysts are seen with hemolyzed red blood cells and siderophages.

Effect on Fertility[21]

The incidence of adenomyosis in infertile females is 20–25% as mentioned in different literature evidence. But in our practice, we have found it to be as common as 30% in the infertile population.

It interferes with implantation and reduces the likelihood ratio for clinical pregnancy by 28% within vitro fertilization/ intracytoplasmic sperm injection (IVF/ ICSI).[22] The endometrial glands that ectopically grow in myometrium have more estrogen and cause an inflammatory reaction and decrease the chance of implantation. Though some workers have reported no difference in pregnancy rates or implantation rate in women with or without adenomyosis.[23,24]

There are two distinct phenotypes of adenomyosis. Both have different etiopathologies and pathogenesis. Focal adenomyosis of the outer myometrium (FAOM) and diffuse adenomyosis. FAOM is significantly associated with primary infertility, where as diffuse adenomyosis has not found to be associated with fertility status.[25]

It causes early pregnancy loss and thus reduces the live birth rate.[26]

Management options for adenomyotic patients with infertility are given in the following text.

Surgical Treatment

- In cases with focal adenomyoma, surgical resection of the lesion is recommended and it is claimed to improve conception rates.[27] Surgery can be done laparoscopically or by laparotomy or by robotic surgery. If the lesion is nearer to the endometrium and smaller in size, it can be removed by resectoscope through hysteroscopy.
- *Myometrial reduction*: To reduce the bulk of the adenomyotic uterus, abnormal tissues are removed and then metroplasty is done laparoscopically or by laparotomy:
  - Classical reduction of anterior and posterior portions after midline incision (V-shaped resection).
  - Modified transverse H incision. It has a 50% pregnancy rate.[28]
  - Most popular is the triple-flap method developed by Osada et al.[28] It has reduced the risk of rupture during pregnancy.
- *Laparotomic surgery*:
  - Partial reduction surgery:
    - Wedge resection of the uterine wall: Recurrence rate is high with this surgery.
    - Modified reduction surgery: Adenomyomatous tissues are cut into small slices and the pregnancy rate after this surgery is good.
    - Transverse H incision of uterine wall: Pregnancy rates are good after this surgery.

- Complete adenomyosis excision:
  - Triple-flap method: Complete extraction of adenomyosis is done with this technique followed by reconstruction of the uterine cavity and uterine wall. It decreases the risk of uterine rupture.
  - Asymmetric dissection method: The risk of uterine rupture is higher with this method.
- *Laparoscopic surgery*:
  - For focal/nodular lesions, surgical excision of the lesion similar to fibroids.
  - Diffuse adenomyosis requires an advanced technique. Because of difficult surgery, it is preferably tackled by laparotomy.

Most of the uteri rupture due to electrically powered instruments used and are common after laparoscopic adenomyomectomy rather than laparotomy.

Factors causing uterine rupture: Rupture of the uterus is a very common complication after surgery for adenomyosis. Factors that affect the risk of rupture of the uterus are as follows:[29]

- Surgical technique used
- Extent and volume of the defect
- Method of repair of uterine wall and cavity
- Postoperative wound infection and hematoma
- Skill and experience of the surgeon.[30]

Medical Treatment

- Either GnRH agonist therapy alone or preoperative GnRH agonist therapy has given a poor pregnancy rate. But the GnRH agonist therapy is given in diffuse adenomyosis. Long-term GnRH agonist prior to IVF increases the clinical pregnancy rate.[31]
- It is best used after ovum pickup. A GnRH agonist is given for few months and then frozen embryo-transfer is done. This is the current strategy today.
- Medical management with Ulipristal (UPA) for one or two courses for 3 months each can be tried before assisted reproductive technology (ART) cycles. But the results are still not appreciable.
- *High-intensity focused ultrasound (HIFU)*: Magnetic resonance-guided, HIFU therapy, a modality established as a treatment option for fibroid, is currently under trial for adenomyosis also.[32]
- Surrogacy
- Letrozole, oral contraceptive pills, Danazol, Tamoxifen, and RU 486 are useful for pain relief and are under trial.

CARRY HOME MESSAGE

- Adenomyosis is estrogen-dependent and occurs due to invagination of the endometrium into myometrium due to injury or due to metaplasia or adult stem cells.
- The cause of infertility is implantation failure.
- Ultrasound is used as a modality of choice for diagnosis but MRI may be required in difficult-to-diagnose cases.
- Surgery is advisable in cases with a large globular uterus. The triple-flap method is the most accepted one and has the lowest incidence of uterine rupture.
- Long-term GnRH agonist therapy improves the pregnancy rate in the transfer of frozen embryos.
- Medical management with all other drugs can be used for relief of symptoms but does not help much to improve fertility.

REFERENCES

1. Bird CC, McElin T, Manalo-Estrella P. The elusive adenomyosis of the uterus. Am J Obstet Gynecol. 1972;112:583-93.
2. Gracia-Solares J, Donnez J, Donnez O, Dolmans MM. Pathogenesis of uterine adenomyosis: invagination or metaplasia. Fertil Steril. 2018;109:371-9.

3. Bazot M, Darai E. Role of transvaginal sonography and magnetic resonance imaging in the diagnosis of uterine adenomyosis. Fertil Steril. 2018;109(3):389-97.
4. Raine-Fenning N, Jayaprakasan K, Deb S. Three-dimensional ultrasonographic characteristics of endometriomata. Ultrasound Obstet Gynecol. 2008;31:718-24.
5. Aleem F, Pennisi J, Zeitoum K, Predanic M. The role of color Doppler in diagnosis of endometriomas. Ultrasound Obstet Gynecol. 1995;5:51-4.
6. Di Donato N, Bertoldo V, Montanari G, Zannoni L, Caprara G, Seracchioli R. Question mark form of uterus: a simple sonographic sign associated with presence of adenomyosis. Ultrasound Obstet Gynecol. 2015;46(1):126-7.
7. Perrot N, Mergui JL, Frey I, Bazot M, Uzan M. Adenomyosis: power Doppler findings.. Ultrasound Obstet Gynecol. 2001; 17(2):177-8.
8. Exacoustos C, Brienza L, Di Giovanni A, Szabolcs B, Romanini ME, Zupi E, et al. Adenomyosis: three-dimensional sonographic findings of the junctional zone and correlation with histology. Ultrasound Obstet Gynecol. 2011;37:471-9.
9. Kupesic S, Kurjak A, Pasalic L, Benic S, Ilijas M. The value of transvaginal colour Doppler in the assessment of pelvic inflammatory disease. Ultrasound Med Biol. 1995;21960:733-8.
10. Champaneria R, Abedin P, Daniels J, Balogun M, Khan KS. Ultrasound scan and magnetic resonance imaging for diagnosis of adenomyosis: systematic review comparing test accuracy. Acta Obstet Gynecol Scand. 2010;89(11):1374-84.
11. Reinhold C, McCarthy S, Bret PM, Mehio A, Atri M, Zakarian R, et al. Diffuse adenomyosis: comparison of endovaginal US and MR imaging with histopathologic correlation. Radiology. 1996;199:151-8.
12. Bazot M, Cortez A, Darai E, Rouger J, Chopier J, Antoine JM, et al. Ultrasonography compared with magnetic resonance imaging for the diagnosis of adenomyosis: correlation with histopathology. Hum Reprod. 2001; 16:2427-33.
13. Dueholm M, Lundorf E, Hansen ES, Sorensen JS, Ledertoug S, Olesen F. Magnetic resonance imaging and transvaginal ultrasonography for the diagnosis of adenomyosis. Fertil Steril. 2001;76:588-94.
14. Togashi K, Nishimura K, Itoh K, Fujisawa I, Noma S, Kanaoka M, et al. Adenomyosis: diagnosis with MR imaging. Radiology. 1988;166:111-4.
15. Bazot M, Darai E, Clement de Givry S, Boudghene F, Uzan S, Le Blanche AF. Fast breathhold T2-weighted MR imaging reduces interobserver variability in the diagnosis of adenomyosis. Am J Roentgenol. 2003;180:1291-6.
16. Krinsky G, DeCorato DR, Rofsky NM, Flyer M, Earls JP, Ambrosino M, et al. Rapid T2-weighted MR imaging of uterine leiomyoma and adenomyosis. Abdom Imaging. 1997;22:531-4.
17. Yamashita Y, Torashima M, Hatanaka Y, Takahashi M, Fukumatsu K, Tanaka N, et al. MR imaging of atypical polypoid adenomyoma. Comput Med Imaging Graph. 1995;19:351-5.
18. Byun JY, Kim SE, Choi BG, Ko GY, Jung SE, Choi KH. Diffuse and focal adenomyosis: MR imaging findings. Radiographics. 1999;19:S161-70.
19. Song SE, Sung DJ, Park BJ, Kim MJ, Cho SB, Kim KA. MR imaging features of uterine adenomyomas. Abdom Imaging. 2011; 36:483-8.
20. Troiano RN, Flynn SD, McCarthy S. Cystic adenomyosis of the uterus: MRI. J Magn Reson Imaging. 1998;8:1198-202.
21. Naftalin J, Hoo WL, Pateman K, Mavrelos D, Holland T, Jurkovic D. How common is adenomyosis? A prospective study of prevalence using transvaginal ultrasound in gynecology clinic. Hum Reprod. 2012; 27(12):3432-9.
22. Galliano D, Bellver J, Diaz-Gracia C, Simon C, Pellicer A. ART and uterine pathology: how relevant is the maternal side for implantation? Hum Reprod Update. 2015;21:13-38.

23. Vercellini P, Consonni D, Dridi D, Bracco B, Frattaruolo MP, Somigliana E. Uterine adenomyosis and in vitro fertilization outcome: a systematic review and meta-analysis. Hum Reprod. 2014;29(5):964-77.
24. Martinez-Conejero JA, Morgan M, Montesinos M, Fortuño S, Meseguer M, Simón C, et al. Adenomyosis does not affect implantation, but is associated with miscarriage in patients undergoing oocyte donation. Fertil Steril. 2011;96:943-50.
25. Bourdon M, Santulli P, Oliveira J, Marcellin L, Maignien C, Melka L, Bordonne C, et al. Focal adenomyosis is associated with primary infertility. Fertil Steril. 2020;114(6):1271-7.
26. Fernandez H, Higgins C, Vollenhoven BJ, Da Silva Costa F. The association between sonographically diagnosed adenomyosis and invitro fertilization embryo transfers. Fertil Steril. 2017;108(3):e260.
27. Kishi Y, Yabuta M, Taniguchi F. Who will benefit from uterus sparing surgery in adenomyosis associated subfertility? Fertil Steril. 2014;102(3):802-7.
28. Fujushita A, Masuzaki H, Khan KN, Kitajima M, Ishimaru T. Modified reduction surgery for adenomyosis. A preliminary report of the transverse H incision technique. Gynecol Obstet Invest. 2004;57:132-8.
29. Osada H, Siber S, Kakinuma T, Nagaishi M, Kato K, Kato O. Surgical procedure to conserve the uterus for future pregnancy in patients suffering from massive adenomyosis. Reprod Biomed Online. 2011;22:94-9.
30. Osada H. Uterine adenomyosis and adenomyoma, the surgical approach. Fertil Steril. 2018;109:466-7.
31. Vernuccini S, Luci S, Tosti C, Sorbi F, Petraglia F. Role of medical therapy in the management of uterus adenomyosis. Fertil Steril. 2018;109:398-405.
32. Chin W, Wallbridge J, Quinn S. MR guided focused ultrasound for the treatment of adenomyosis: current insights. Res Rep Focused Ultrasound. 2015;4:1-8.

20

Chapter

Endometriosis

INTRODUCTION

Endometriosis is an inflammatory disease associated with pelvic pain and is characterized by ectopic endometrial tissue outside the endometrial cavity. It is a very common disease of reproductive age group and its incidence in infertile patients may vary from 20 to 50%.[1]

PATHOGENESIS OF INFERTILITY IN PATIENTS WITH ENDOMETRIOSIS

In patients with endometriosis, monthly fecundability is reduced due to several different suggested mechanisms:

- Mechanical distortion of the tube and tubo-ovarian relationship.
- Abnormal folliculogenesis gives poor-quality oocytes which in turn decreases fertilization and decreases the possibility of a good-quality embryo.
- Luteinized unruptured follicle
- Decreased chances of implantation because of change in hormonal milieu and change in cytokines at the endometrial level.
- Luteal phase defect causes infertility and recurrent pregnancy loss also.
- Production of reactive oxygen species (ROS) in the peritoneum can cause deoxyribonucleic acid (DNA) fragmentation in sperms and motility of sperms is affected.[2] Changes in cytokines in the peritoneal fluid may change Th1/Th2 activity. There is increased angiogenesis.
- There is increased DNA damage to oocyte, sperm, and embryo, which affects fertilization, implantation, and increases miscarriage.[3]

CLINICAL FEATURES

The most common is infertility and chronic pain. Apart from infertility, the patient can have congestive dysmenorrhea, dyspareunia, dysmenorrhea, chronic pelvic pain, and painful bowel movements. It is the deep penetrating endometriosis (DIE) that leads to dysmenorrhea, dyspareunia, chronic pelvic pain, and often dysuria or pain on defecation if it involves bladder or bowel. When in the bladder, it may also involve:

- Ureteric insertion and may lead to obstruction and hydronephrosis.
- Symptoms will be related to the location of endometriosis, e.g., a patient with bladder endometriosis may have cyclical urinary symptoms.

Signs

On examination, there is pain, thickening, or nodule of uterosacral ligaments or restricted movements of the uterus according to the severity of the disease. On pervaginal examination, an ovarian cyst may be felt and rectovaginal endometriosis can also be palpated.

DIAGNOSIS

Ultrasound

Endometrioma: It has shaggy walls, internal echogenicities, ground-glass appearance, and linear echogenic flecks in its walls **(Fig. 1A)**. The echogenic flecks are believed to be cholesterol or hemosiderin deposits in the cyst walls. The fluid–fluid level is an apparent vertical fluid level **(Fig. 1B)**. Adhesions and pain on pressure with the probe are very common in patients with endometriosis. This leads to usually posteriorly placed ovaries. Sometimes when both ovaries are adherent posterior to the uterus, these are typically known as kissing ovaries **(Fig. 1C)**. One-third to one-half of the ovarian endometriotic cysts are bilateral. Solid areas may be sometimes seen, which may be blood clots. The streaming sign is often seen in endometriomas.

On Doppler

Scattered vascularity at ovarian hilus with moderate vascular impedance has been described in the literature. The ovarian hilar resistance index (RI) varies between 0.40 and 0.56. Vascularity is higher during menstruation and in symptomatic patients.[4] Avascular lesions indicate scarification and are less convenient for delivery of medication

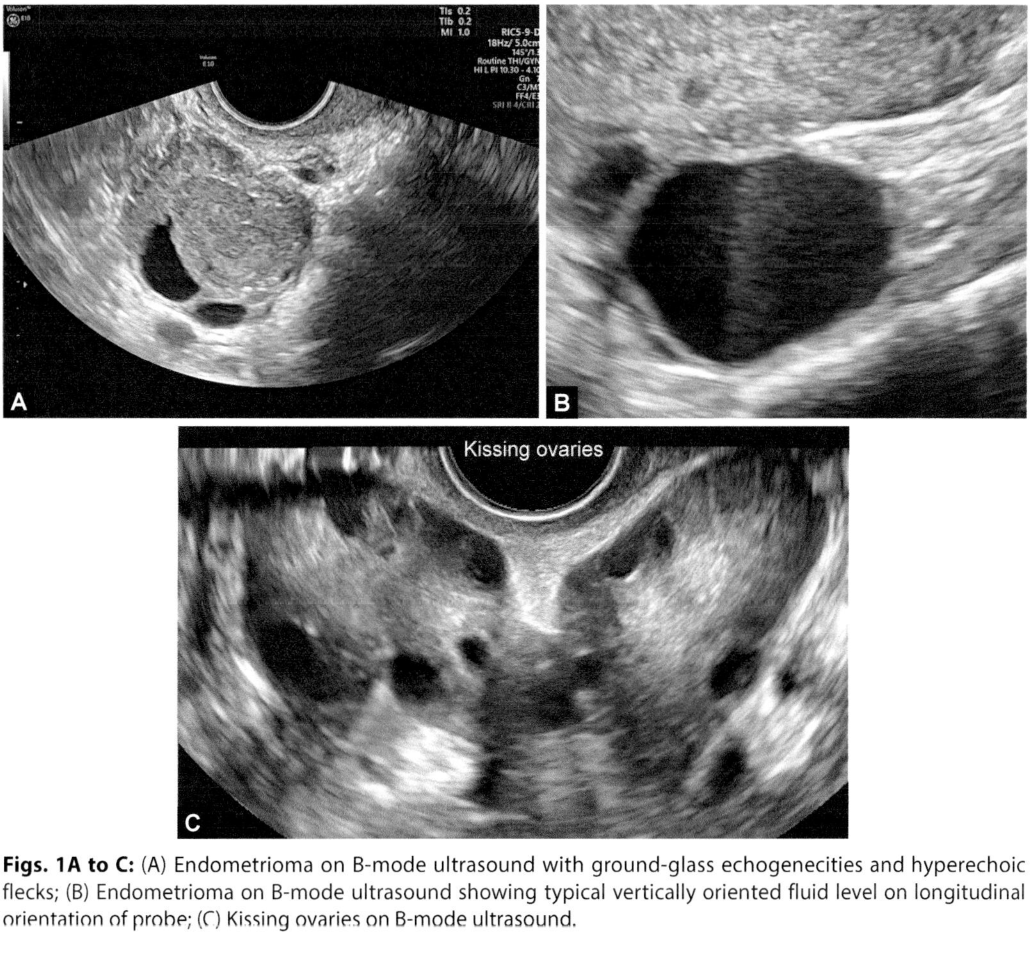

Figs. 1A to C: (A) Endometrioma on B-mode ultrasound with ground-glass echogenecities and hyperechoic flecks; (B) Endometrioma on B-mode ultrasound showing typical vertically oriented fluid level on longitudinal orientation of probe; (C) Kissing ovaries on B-mode ultrasound.

and therefore should be considered for surgical therapy.[5] Kurjak et al. have shown a sensitivity of 83.9%, specificity of 97.1%, positive predictive value (PPV) of 82%, and negative predictive value (NPV) of 97.5% on vaginal sonography for characterization of endometriomas. If cancer antigen (CA) 125 >35 IU/mL was added as a cut-off to these parameters, the sensitivity and specificity reached 99.04% and 99.64%, and PPV and NPV reached 98.10% and 99.82%, respectively.[5] Endometriomas typically show short-coursed vessels **(Fig. 2A)**. The vessels are seen approaching the endometrioma, but do not run along with the wall of the endometrioma. 3D power Doppler typically shows multiple short-coursed regularly separated pericystic vessels giving a typical bird's nest appearance **(Fig. 2B)**.[6]

Apart from endometriomas, endometriosis may also present as superficial or deep infiltrating endometriosis. Endometriosis when extends to >5 mm deep from the peritoneal surface is deep infiltrating endometriosis; otherwise, it is superficial endometriosis. The latter is difficult to diagnose on ultrasound.

The endometriotic patch typically leads to inflammation and fibrosis, leading to distortion of the surrounding anatomy. These generally appear as ill-defined irregular hypoechoic areas with some acoustic shadowing at times. These are tender on probe pressure and are typically hypovascular. Adhesions of involved surfaces are common. Transvaginal scan has shown 81.1% sensitivity and 94.2% specificity for the diagnosis of DIE.[7] Deep infiltrating endometriosis may involve bowel, bladder, uterosacral ligament, and vaginorectal septum, most commonly, but may also involve abdominal organs at times.

Rectosigmoid Deep Penetrating Endometriosis

It usually involves the anterior muscularis of the rectosigmoid part of the large bowel. It is known that the muscularis of the large bowel has an inner layer of circular and outer layer of longitudinal muscle fibers. The entire muscularis, which otherwise appears as a hypoechoic linear band, is seen being traversed by an echogenic line that separates these two layers. Discontinuity of this line due to a fusiform or elongated hypoechoic area indicates endometriosis. On the transverse section, this typically gives a signet ring appearance. When the submucosa is involved, fibrotic retraction of the lesion

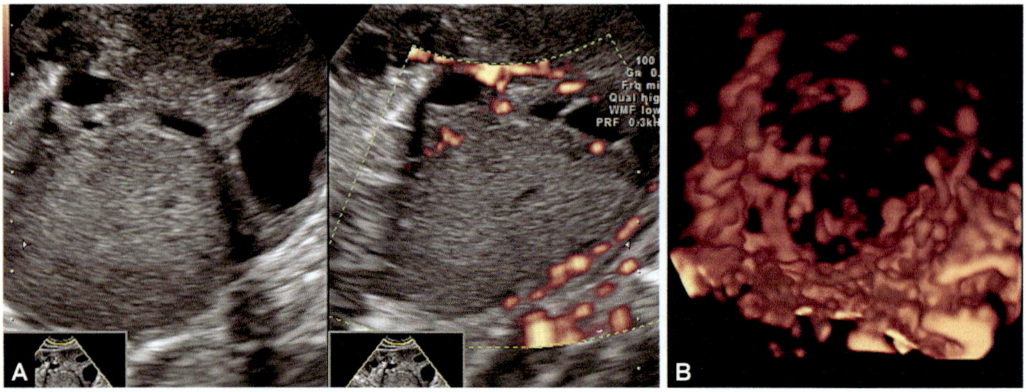

Figs. 2A and B: (A) Short coursed vessels of endometrioma, seen on power Doppler; (B) "Bird's nest sign" of endometrioma on 3D power Doppler angiomode rendering.

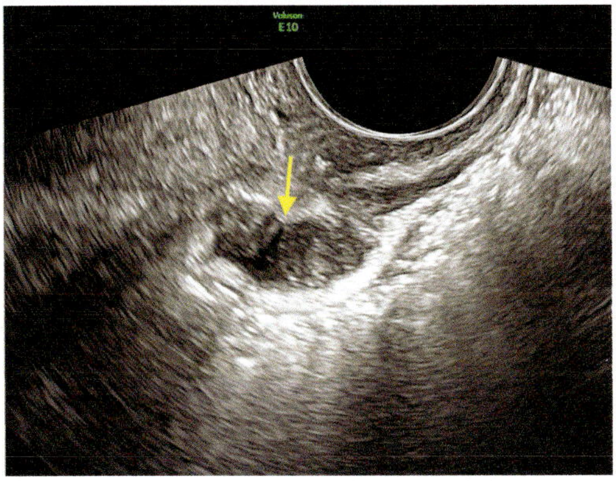

Fig. 3: B-mode ultrasound image of bowel endometriosis patch "Red Indian head" sign.

in the submucosa leads to a typical "Red Indian head" appearance **(Fig. 3)**. A negative sliding organ sign between the uterus and the bowel may be an additional sign. This has a likelihood ratio of 23.6 for rectal DIE.[8]

This lesion may extend into the posterior vaginal wall.

- *Vaginal DIE*: It is seen as localized hypoechoic thickening of the vaginal wall, though the margins are not well defined. When the lesion extends from the rectum, the rectovaginal septum is typically not continuous. The vaginal wall thickening can be more clearly appreciated if the scan is done with the probe placed only superficially in the vaginal canal when the vaginal cavity is filled with gel (gel vaginosonography).
- *Cervical DIE*: It is seen as a thick firm cervical wall that appears as the hypoechoic area on ultrasound with ill-defined margins and also at times associated with acoustic shadowing. Like all other endometriotic lesions, even these lesions are tender on probe pressure.
- *Uterosacral DIE*: It is the most difficult to image on ultrasound, unless when there is fluid around. If the uterosacral ligament is seen as a thick soft tissue mass instead of a string-like structure, it may indicate DIE.
- *Bladder DIE*: It may appear as localized thickening of bladder wall, hypoechoic and hypovascular on ultrasound. These may also sometimes appear like localized solid projections. Trigone is the area most commonly affected. When the lesion extends from the anterior vaginal wall as a penetrating lesion, and may involve the bladder diffusely, it gives a typical hourglass shape to the bladder.

Magnetic Resonance Imaging

Though endometriotic cysts are confidently diagnosed by transvaginal ultrasound, for rectovaginal endometriosis and deep infiltrating endometriosis at other sites in pelvis magnetic resonance imaging (MRI) may be a supplementary modality. With high-frequency probes and possibility of dynamic assessment by ultrasound, ultrasound is turning out to be more important for the diagnosis of DIE.

The state-of-the-art MRI protocol for the diagnosis of endometriosis includes T2- and fat-suppressed T1-weighted sequences.

T2-weighted sequences without fat suppression are the best sequences for detecting pelvic endometriosis,[9] in particular for the evaluation of fibrotic *fat-suppressed T1-weighted 3D gradient-echo LAVA sequence.* This pulse sequence improves the sensitivity of MRI in the detection of small lesions. It is the most sensitive for the detection of bloody foci, peritoneal endometriosis, and lesions.[10]

Contrast-enhanced fat-suppressed T1-weighted 3D gradient-echo LAVA sequence is useful in detection of enhancing mural nodules within adnexal masses, when atypical features on ultrasound or T2-weighted magnetic resonance sequences suggest potential malignancy.[9]

Pathologic appearance of endometriosis depends on the duration of the disease and depth of penetration of the lesions.[11]

At MRI, these small implants manifest as multiple round (cystic or nodular) lesions homogeneously hyperintense on fat-suppressed T1-weighted images, due to old hemorrhagic content, regardless of their signal intensity on T2-weighted images.[12]

At MRI, especially on T2-weighted images, retractile adhesions may be observed as spiculated hypointense peritoneal strands arranged in confluent angles. Tethering of pelvic structures and loss of the corresponding cleavage planes, without appreciable nodular lesions, maybe another imaging finding suggestive of adhesions.[13] At MRI, both fibrous tissue and smooth muscle show intermediate signal intensity on T1-weighted images and low signal intensity on T2-weighted images. Therefore, on T2-weighted images, solid endometriotic lesions appear as hypointense nodular structures with irregular or stellate margins due to fibrous tissue and smooth muscle proliferation. Within solid endometriotic masses, hyperintense foci on T2-weighted images may be seen, representing dilated ectopic endometrial glands.[10]

Micro intraovarian endometriomas are small-sized (<1 cm) implants within the ovaries. They show hyperintense signal on T1-weighted images and variable signal intensity on T2-weighted images. At MRI, the pathognomonic feature of endometriomas is the "shading" sign, which can be seen on T2-weighted images. It reflects the chronic nature of endometriomas and is the result of cyclic bleeding occurring over time. Endometriotic cysts show high signal intensity on T1-weighted images.

The most specific pathologic feature of endometrioma is the thick fibrous capsule containing a cluster of hemosiderin-laden macrophages due to repeated hemorrhage. In a recently published meta-analysis, the sensitivity and specificity of MRI for the diagnosis of endometrial cysts were 95% and 91%, respectively.[14]

CA 125: It is not used as a diagnostic criterion for endometriosis as it may or may not be raised in endometriosis and even if it is raised it is not a specific marker for endometriosis.

- *Diagnostic laparoscopy*:
  - Even if ultrasound is normal in suspected cases, diagnostic laparoscopy should be done in clinically suspected cases [National Institute of Care and Health Excellence (NICE) Guidelines, 2017].
  - Before operative laparoscopy, ultrasound and MRI assessment are recommended.
  - In all suspected cases, biopsy must be done to exclude malignancy.
- *Staging and classification*: American Society for Reproductive Medicine (ASRM) classification of endometriosis is shown in **Figure 4A**.[15]

Ignore endometriosis: In minimal and mild endometriosis, controlled ovarian hyperstimulation (COH) and intrauterine insemination (IUI) increase pregnancy rates and live birth rate as compared to expectant management.[18] It is to be treated as unexplained infertility.[19] Even after laparoscopic fulguration, COH with IUI should be done and that increases the conception rates.

When there is stage III and IV endometriosis, especially after the age of 35 years, assisted reproductive technology (ART) should be the first line of treatment.[18] Even if the surgery is done, spontaneous conception rates are very low and ART is the preferred option in all cases of advanced endometriosis. Systematic reporting method of endometriosis is shown in **Figures 4B and C**.

Revised American Society for Reproductive Medicine classification of endometriosis 1985

Patient's Name ______________________ Date: ______________________

Stage I (Minimal) 1–50 Laparoscopy ______ Laparotomy ______ Photography _______

Stage II (Mild) 6–15 Recommended treatment ______________________________

Stage III (Moderate) 16–40 ____

Stage IV (Severe) >40

Total __________ Prognosis ____________________________

	Endometriosis	<1 cm	1–3 cm	>3 cm
Peritoneum	Superficial	1	2	4
Peritoneum	Deep	2	4	6
Ovary	R superficial	1	2	4
Ovary	Deep	4	16	20
Ovary	L superficial	1	2	4
Ovary	Deep	4	16	20
	Posterior Cul-de-sac obliteration	Partial	Complete	
		4	40	
	Adhesions	<1/3 Enclosure	1/3–2/3 Enclosure	>2/3 Enclosure
Ovary	R Filmy	1	2	4
Ovary	Dense	4	8	16
Ovary	L Filmy	1	2	4
Ovary	Dense	4	8	16
Tube	R Filmy	1	2	4
Tube	Dense	4	8	16
Tube	L Filmy	1	2	4
Tube	Dense	4*	8*	16

*If the fimbriated end of the fallopian tube is completely enclosed, change the point assignment to 16.

Additional endometriosis: ______________ Associated pathology: ______________

To be used with normal tubes and ovaries **To be used with abnormal tubes and/or ovaries**

L R L R

Fig. 4A: Proposed toolbox for surgical classification for endometriosis.

MANAGEMENT IN RELATION TO INFERTILITY

Medical management: Medical management has no place in improving fertility (NICE guidelines, 2017). It suppresses ovulation and does not improve fertility. Waiting for the medical therapy to work on endometriosis may reduce ovarian reserve and anti-Müllerian hormone (AMH) further. All the drugs used for endometriosis such as gonadotropin-releasing hormone agonist (GnRHa), Danazol, progesterone compounds,

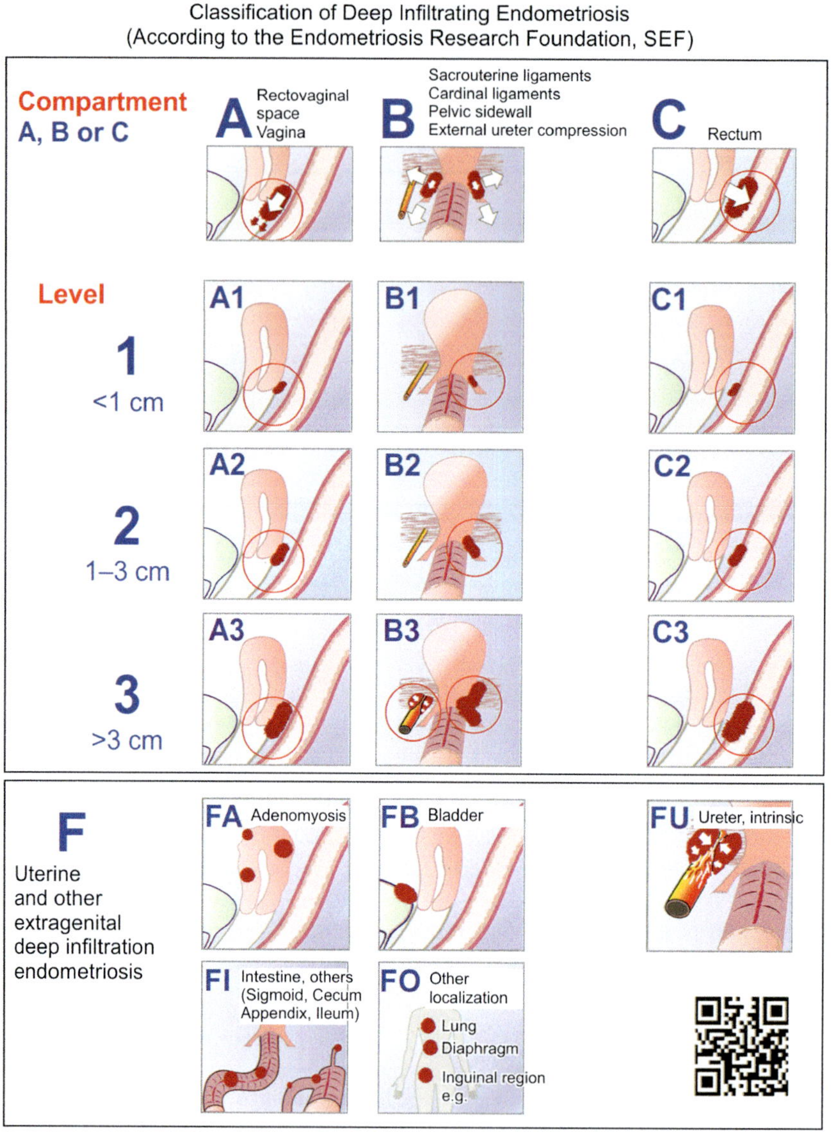

Fig. 4B: Classification of deep infiltrating endometriosis.

oral contraceptive (OC) pills, etc., only give symptomatic relief and suppress ovulation and so are not useful to improve fertility.[20]

GnRHa can be given for 3–6 months before ART and it increases the clinical pregnancy rate by four-fold.[21] After ovum picks up, GnRHa can be given for 2–3 months before the frozen embryo transfer and is more effective for improving pregnancy rates.

Surgical treatment for infertility:

- *During laparoscopy*: Incidental finding
- Laparoscopy for endometriosis
- *Endometrioma*: Cyst removal or repeat surgery

Diagnosis during laparoscopy:

- *Mild endometriosis*: It may be diagnosed as an incidental finding during laparoscopy done to investigate for infertility or

Endometriosis fertility index (EFI)
Surgery Form

Least function (LF) score at conclusion of surgery

Score		Description		Left	Right
4	=	Normal	Fallopian tube	☐	☐
3	=	Mild Dysfunction			
2	=	Moderate Dysfunction	Fimbria	☐	☐
1	=	Severe Dysfunction			
0	=	Absent or Nonfunctional	Ovary	☐	☐

To calculate the LF score, add together the lowest score for the left side and the lowest score for the right side. If an ovary is absent on one side, the LF score is obtained by doubling the lowest score on the side with the ovary

Lowest score ☐ + ☐ = ☐
Left Right LF score

Endometriosis fertility index (EFI)

Historical factors			Surgical factors		
Factor	**Description**	**Points**	**Factor**	**Description**	**Points**
Age			LF score		
	If age is ≤35 years	2		If LF score = 7 to 8 (high score)	3
	If age is 36 to 39 years	1		If LF score = 4 to 6 (moderate score)	2
	If age is ≥40 years	0		If LF score = 1 to 3 (low score)	0
Years infertile			AFS endometriosis score		
	If years infertile is ≤3	2		If AFS endometriosis lesion score is <16	1
	If years infertile is > 3	0		If AFS endometriosis lesion score is ≥ 16	0
Prior pregnancy			AFS Total score		
	If there is a history of a prior pregnancy	1		If AFS total score is <71	1
	If there is no history of a prior pregnancy	0		If AFS total score is ≥ 71	0
Total Historical Factors			**Total Surgical Factors**		

EFI = Total historical factors + Total surgical factors: ☐ + ☐ = ☐
Historical Surgical EFI score

Fig. 4C: Endometriosis fertility index—surgery form.

Source: Cook AS, Adamson GD. The role of the endometriosis fertility index (EFI) and endometriosis scoring systems in predicting infertility outcomes. Current Obstetrics and Gynecology Reports. 2013;2(3):186-94.

for tubal evaluation. Fulguration of endometriotic spots in these cases is believed to increase conception rate, though there are contradictory evidences also.[19,22] But if laparoscopy is already done, it may be a better idea to fulgurate those endometriotic spots instead of leaving those untreated. The European Society of Human Reproduction and Embryology (ESHRE) guidelines also claims that it improves conception rates.[19] The explanation given for this is that the women having mild to moderate endometriosis have higher incidence of endocrine abnormalities, anovulation, luteal phase defect, luteinized unruptured follicle, and hyperprolactinemia. Correction of these subtle hormonal abnormalities resulting due to fulguration of these lesions improves pregnancy rates.[23] So diagnostic laparoscopy should have a "see and treat" approach.

- *Moderate and severe endometriosis*: When laparoscopy shows moderate or severe endometriosis, it should be treated at the same time. If tubo-ovarian relations are not normal even after surgery in moderate endometriosis, ART is the only option for these females. In stages III and IV, ART is recommended directly. Even after surgery, ART does not increase the rate. GnRHa// and laser ablation are done for severe pain.[24]

Endometrioma and infertility: Ovulation induction does not increase the size of endometriomas.[25] It is found in 25–50% of cases with endometriosis. Endometriomas can be diagnosed confidently by ultrasound as mentioned earlier in this chapter.

Surgery

Removal of the endometriotic cyst is the greatest disadvantage in cases of infertility. During surgical removal of cyst wall ovarian tissue is also dissected and removed and that leads to marked decrease in ovarian reserve. A drastic reduction in AMH after the surgery confirms this. Surgery also increases the risk of adhesions, which may also involve the fimbrial end of the tube, damage tubo-ovarian relation, and cause infertility instead of treating it. Moreover, recurrence of endometriotic cysts is commonly documented. Therefore, unless the cyst causes severe pain, it is not removed before pick-up. The dose of gonadotropins required is less and the number of oocytes retrieved is more if oocyte retrieval is done before surgery. Conservative treatment is recommended if subfertility is the only problem as expectant and surgical treatment has almost the same live birth rates.[26] Cyst wall is attached to normal ovarian tissues containing primordial follicles and in >50% of endometriomas.[27] According to ESHRE guidelines also, there is no evidence that cystectomy before ART improves the pregnancy rate.[19,28,29] With regard to endometrioma, a recent Cochrane review for four trials concluded that surgery (aspiration or cystectomy) versus expectant management showed no evidence of a benefit for clinical pregnancy with either technique.[30] The only disadvantage is accidental rupture of cyst during pickup and that can cause infection. Higher antibiotics are to be given to these patients. Cyst is to be removed only when the size is large enough to prevent ovum pickup. But even if we puncture and aspirate the cyst, the result is not affected.

Disadvantages of in vitro fertilization (IVF) before surgery:
- Disease progression
- Undiagnosed malignancy
- Difficult aspiration, cyst puncture, and contamination
- Increased oxidation stress
- Infection and peritonitis

Disadvantages of surgery:
- Skilled operator is required.
- Diminished ovarian reserve
- Increases cost and delays fertility treatment
- Surgical complications may delay ART
- Incomplete surgery and recurrence

Thus, individualization is required in each case.

Treatment of Infertility with Endometriosis

Ovulation Induction with Intrauterine Insemination

Controlled ovarian stimulation (COS) with IUI increases the pregnancy rates with different causes of infertility but it decreases to half in patients with endometriosis.[31] Clomiphene with IUI in stages III and IV has a very low pregnancy rate.[32] There is no difference in the pregnancy rate with clomiphene or letrozole.[33] So ovulation induction with IUI is offered to the patients with mild or moderate endometriosis, particularly for young patients with no other cause of infertility.

Assisted Reproductive Technology and Endometriosis

In stages III and IV endometriosis, ART should be pursued sooner. As in ART, fertilization and early embryo development occur in the controlled environment of the lab, thus avoiding the exposure of gametes and embryo to the hostile environment.

Barnhart et al. in a meta-analysis found that in overall, patients with endometriosis have lower pregnancy rate, decreased fertilization, and decreased implantation rate.[34] In a recent meta-analysis, the above findings were confirmed but it documented similar live birth rate and so comparable success with IVF and intracytoplasmic sperm injection (ICSI).[35]

Endometriosis and oocyte retrieval: Several studies using GnRHa for downregulation and ovum pick-up found no differences in the number of oocytes obtained in patients with or without GnRHa.[36] GnRHa has definitely improved IVF outcome. Few studies have found that GnRHa for 3 months have higher oocyte retrieval[37] while Chedid et al. documented no difference in short- and long-protocol agonist protocols.[38] 6–8 weeks of continuous OCs when given to patients with endometriosis also give the same follicular growth and oocyte gain as for the patient without endometriosis.[39] Recently, agonist and antagonist protocols have given the same results in mild and moderate endometriosis.[40] But patients with agonists had a higher number of embryos for cryopreservation. So in nutshell, patients with endometriosis respond in a similar way with gonadotrophins like other etiologies. But it works better when GnRHa or OC pills are used.

Effect on Fertilization and Embryo Development

There are so many studies that indicate lower fertilization and embryo development in endometriosis. This is more severe in stages III and IV than in stages I and II.[41] Conversely there have been several large studies which have found equal fertilization rate with and without endometriosis.[36] Most of the studies show equal fertilization and early embryo development.[42]

Effect on implantation: Earlier studies have found a decrease in the implantation rate. But use of GnRHa and OCs has overcome this problem and pregnancy rates have been seen to improve with 3–6 months' treatment with GnRHa and OC pills.[43] The implantation rate is low in stages III and IV endometriosis than with stages I and II, and this can be reverted by GnRHa for 3-6 months. It has also been documented that oocytes from a donor without endometriosis had the same implantation rate as a recipient having endometriosis.[44] So it is suggested that the endometrium-associated impairment of implantation results from a compromise to the potential of the oocyte or embryo rather than the endometrium itself. Diaz et al. also found that there is no difference in pregnancy, implantation, miscarriage, and live birth rate.[45] This study suggests that endometrial receptivity and implantation rate may not be affected by stages III and IV endometriosis. There is no difference in the pregnancy rate when compared to the stage by stage endometriosis and also with another cause of infertility.[29,46] Earlier studies indicated that stages III and IV can have higher early pregnancy loss but recent studies do not agree with it.[29] Even after aspiration of cyst, pregnancy rates, embryo quality, and miscarriage rates are the same as those patients in whom no endometrioma was present.[47]

It is unclear as to the bad oocyte quality or poor endometrium is the cause of subfertility in these cases. Though endometriosis does not impact live-birth rates in frozen embryo transfers of euploid blastocysts.[48] This confirms that ART is the treatment of choice in patients with infertility. Though in cases opting for natural conception, the pregnancy results are quite poor. The results are poor when ovulation induction with IUI is done or fresh transfer is done in ART cycles.[49]

Future Plans for Management

- Letrozole may improve folliculogenesis and should be included in the stimulation protocol.
- Antagonist also shows a benefit in patients with endometriosis.
- Donor oocytes can be used in patients of endometriosis, particularly in failed IVF patients.
- ICSI may prove beneficial in patients of impaired fertilization due to endometriosis.
- Blastocyst transfer proves beneficial as early embryo development is hampered by endometriosis. So selected healthy blastocysts can be transferred.
- Assisted hatching may be useful to these patients.
- Preimplantation genetic screening (PGS) may increase the success of IVF.
- Endometrial receptivity assays can be useful before transfer.

CARRY HOME MESSAGE

- Infertility is due to increased damage to oocytes, sperm, and embryos along with diminished implantation and peritoneal factor.
- Ultrasound is an effective modality for diagnosis.
- Medical management has a limited role in infertility.
- GnRHa can be used for 3–6 months before ART or 2 months before the transfer of frozen embryo.
- Ignore endometrioma before pick-up.
- For stages III and IV endometriosis, ART is the only option.
- For stages I and II, ovulation induction with IUI should be tried.
- Recent studies indicate no difference in implantation with or without endometriosis.
- Letrozole, antagonists, ICSI, endometrial receptivity array (ERA), and PGS improve results.

REFERENCES

1. Ilangavan K, Kalu E. High prevalence of endometriosis in infertile women with normal ovulation and normo-spermic partners. Fertil Steril. 2010;93:e10.
2. Agarwal A, Gupta S, Sikka S. The role of free radicals and antioxidants in reproduction. Curr Opin Obstet Gynecol. 2006;18:325-32.
3. Mansour G, Goldberg J, Agarwal A, Sharma R, Mahfouz R, Falcone T. Correlation between sperm DNA damage, stage of endometriosis and duration of infertility (ASRM 63rd Annual Meeting). Fertil Steril. 2007;90:247-57.
4. Alcazar JL. Transvaginal colour Doppler in patients with ovarian endometriomas and pelvic pain. Hum Reprod. 2001;16: 2672-5.
5. Kurjak A, Kupesic S. Scoring system for prediction of ovarian endometriosis based on transvaginal colour and pulsed Doppler sonography. Fertil Steril. 1994;62:81-8.
6. Raine-Fenning N, Jayaprakasan K, Deb S. Three-dimensional ultrasonographic characteristics of endometriomata. Ultrasound Obstet Gynecol. 2008;31:718-24.
7. Vimercatti A, Achilarre MT, Scardapane A, Lorusso F, Ceci O, Mangiatordi G, Angelelli G, et al. Accuracy of transvaginal sonography and contrast enhanced magnetic resonance colonography for pre-surgical staging of deep infiltrating endometriosis. Ultrasound Obstet Gynecol. 2012;40(5):593-603.
8. Hudelist G, Fritzer N, Staettner S, Tammaa A, Tinelli A, Sparic R, et al. Uterine sliding sign: a simple sonographic predictor for presence of deep infiltrating endometriosis of the rectum. Ultrasound Obstet Gynecol. 2013;41:692-5.
9. Bazot M, Bharwani N, Huchon C, Kinkel K, Cunha TM, Guerra A, et al. European Society of Urogenital Radiology (ESUR) guidelines: MR imaging of pelvic endometriosis. Eur Radiol. 2017;27(7):2765-75.
10. Coutinho A, Jr, Bittencourt LK, Pires CE, Junqueira F, de Oliveira Lima CMA, Coutinho E, et al. MR imaging in deep pelvic endometriosis: a pictorial essay. Radiographics. 2011;31(2):549-67.
11. Woodward PJ, Sohaey R, Mezzetti TP, Jr. Endometriosis: radiologic-pathologic correlation. Radiographics. 2001;21(1): 193-216.
12. Bis KG, Vrachliotis TG, Agrawal R, Shetty AN, Maximovich A, Hricak H. Pelvic endometriosis: MR imaging spectrum with

laparoscopic correlation and diagnostic pitfalls. Radiographics. 1997;17(3):639-55.
13. Scardapane A, Lorusso F, Bettocchi S, Bettocchi S, Fascilla FD, Angelelli G, et al. Deep pelvic endometriosis: accuracy of pelvic MRI completed by MR colonography. Radiol Med. 2013;118(2):323-38.
14. American Society of Reproductive Medicine. Revised American Society of Reproductive medicine classification of endometriosis: 1996. Fertil Steril. 1997;67:817-21.
15. Enzian scoring system for women with deep endometriosis. Reprinted with permission from Professor Jörg Keckstein. [online] Available from www.endometriose-sef.de/dateien/ENZIAN_2013_web.pdf [Last accessed March, 2021].
16. Adamson GD, Pasta DJ. Endometriosis fertility index: the new, validated endometriosis staging system. Fertil Steril. 2010;94:1609-15.
17. Johnson NP, Hummelshoj L, David Adamson G, Keckstein J, Taylor HS, Abrao MS, et al. World Endometriosis Society consensus on the classification of endometriosis. Hum Reprod. 2017;32(2):315-24.
18. The Practice Committee of American Society for Reproductive Medicine. Endometriosis and infertility: a committee opinion. Fertil Steril. 2012;98:591-8.
19. Dunselman GAJ, Vermeulen N, Becker C, Calhaz-Jorge C, D'Hooghe T, De Bie B, et al. ESHRE guideline: management of women with endometriosis. Hum Reprod. 2014:29:4000-12.
20. Hughes E, Brown J, Collins JJ, Farquhar C, Fedorkow DM, Vandekerckhove P. Ovulation suppression for endometriosis. Cochrane Database Syst Rev. 2007;(3):CD000155.
21. Sallam HN, Garcia-Valesco JA, Dias S, Arici A. Long term pituitary down regulation before in vitro fertilization (IVF) for women with endometriosis. Cochrane Database Syst Rev. 2006;(1):CD004635
22. Parazzini F. Ablation of lesions or no treatment in minimal-mild endometriosis in infertile women: a randomized trial. Gruppo Italiano per lo Studio dell' Endometriosi. Hum Reprod. 1999;14:1332-4.
23. MarcouxS, MaheuxR, BerubeS. The Canadian Collaborative group on Endometriosis. Laparoscopic surgery in infertile women with minimal or mild endometriosis. N Engl J Med. 1997;336:217-22.
24. Benalgia L, Somigliana E, Santi G, Scarduelli C, Ragni G, Fedele L. IVF and endometriosis-related symptom progression: insights from a prospective study. Hum Reprod. 2011;26:2368-72.
25. Koch J, Rowan K, Rombatus L, Yazdani A, Chapman M, Johnson N. Endometriosis and fertility—a consensus statement from a ACCEPT. Aust NZ J Obstet Gynecol. 2012;52:513-22.
26. Laursen JB, Schroll JB, Macklon KT, Rudnicki M. Surgery versus conservative management of endometriomas in subfertile women. A systematic review. Acta Obstet Gynecol Scand. 2017;96:727-35.
27. Muzii L, Bianchi A, Croce C, Manci N, Panici PB. Laparoscopic excision of ovarian cysts: is the stripping technique a tissue-sparing procedure? Fertil Steril. 2002;77:609-14.
28. Marcus FS, Edwards RG. High rates of pregnancy after long-term down-regulation of women with severe endometriosis. Am J Obstet Gynecol. 1994;171:812-7.
29. Bergedal A, Naffah S, Nagy C, Bergqvist A, Sjöblom P, Hillensjö T. Outcome of IVF in patients with endometriosis in comparison with tubal factor infertility. J Assist Reprod Genet. 1998;15:530-4.
30. Benschop L, Farquhar C, van der Poel N, Heineman MJ. Interventions for women with endometrioma prior to assisted reproductive technology. Cochrane Database Syst Rev. 2010;11:CD008571.
31. Hughes EG. The effectiveness of ovulation induction and intrauterine insemination in the treatment of persistent infertility: a meta-analysis. Hum Reprod. 1997;12:1865-72.
32. Capelo F, Kumar A, Steinkampf M, Azziz R. Laparoscopic evaluation following failure to achieve pregnancy after ovulation induction with clomiphene citrate. Fertil Steril. 2003;80:1450-3.

33. Abu Hashim H, El Rakhawy M, Abd Elaal I. Randomized comparison of superovulation with letrozole vs clomiphene citrate in an IUI program for women with recently surgically treated minimal to mild endometriosis. Acta Obstet Gynecol Scand. 2012;91:338-45.
34. Barnhart K, Dunsmoor-SU R, Coutifaris C. Effect of endometriosis on in vitro fertilization. Fertil Steril. 2002;77:1148-55.
35. Hamdan M, Omar SZ, Dunselman G, Cheong Y. Influence of endometriosis on assisted reproductive technology outcomes: a systematic review and meta-analysis. Obstet Gynecol. 2015;125:79-88.
36. Dmowski WP, Rana N, Michalowska J, Friberg J, Papierniak C, El-Roeiy A, et al. The effect of endometriosis, its stage and activity and of auto-antibodies on in vitro fertilization and embryo transfer success rates. Fertil Steril. 1995;63:555-62.
37. Surrey ES, Silverberg KM, Surrey MW, Schoolcraft WB. Effect of prolonged gonadotrophin releasing hormone agonist therapy on the outcome of in vitro fertilization - embryo transfer in patients with endometriosis. Fertil Steril. 2002;78:699-704.
38. Chedid S, Camus M, Smitz J, Van Steirteghem AC, Devroey P. Comparison among different ovarian stimulation regimens for assisted procreation procedures in patients with endometriosis. Hum Reprod. 1995;10:2406-11.
39. De Zeighler D, Gayet V, Aubriot PF, Fauque P, Streuli I, Wolf JP, et al. Use of oral contraceptives in women with endometriosis before assisted reproduction treatment improves outcomes. Fertil Steril. 2010;94:1796-9.
40. Recai P, Onalan G, Kaya C. GnRH agonist and antagonist protocols for stage I - II endometriosis and endometrioma in in vitro fertilization/intracytoplasmic sperm injection cycles. Fertil Steril. 2007;88:832-8.
41. Tanbo T, Omland A, Dale PO, Abyholm T. Transfer in in vitro fertilization/embryo transfer in unexplained infertility and minimal peritoneal endometriosis. Acta Obstet Gynecol Scand. 1995;74;539-43.
42. Suzuki T, Izumi SI, Matsubayashi H, Awazi H. Impact of ovarian endometrioma on oocyte and pregnancy outcome in in vitro fertilization. Fertil Steril. 2005;83:908-13.
43. Niu Z, Chen Q, Sun Y, Feng Y. Long term pituitary down regulation before frozen embryo transfer could improve pregnancy outcomes in women with adenomyosis. Gynecol Endocrinol. 2013;29:1026-30.
44. Sung L, Mukherjee T, Takeshige T, Bustillo M, Copperman AB. Endometriosis is not detrimental to embryo implantation in oocyte recipients. J Assist Reprod Genet. 1997;14:152-6.
45. Diaz I, Navarro J, Blasco L, Simon C, Pellicer A, Remohi J. Impact of stage III-IV endometriosis on recipients of sibling oocytes: Matched case-control study. Fertil Steril. 2000;74:31-4.
46. Olivennes F, Feldberg D, Liu HC, Cohen J, Moy F, Rosenwaks Z. Endometriosis: A stage by stage analysis—the role of in vitro fertilization. Fertil Steril. 1995;64:392-8.
47. Isaacs JD Jr, Hines RS, Sopelak VM, Cowan BD. Ovarian endometriomas do not adversely affect pregnancy success following treatment with in vitro fertilization. J Assist Reprod Genet. 1997;14:551-3.
48. Bishop LA, Gunn J, Jahandideh S, Devine K, Decherney AH, Hill MJ. Endometriosis does not impact live-birth rates in frozen embryo transfers of euploid blastocysts. Fertil Steril. 2021;115(2):416-22.
49. Pirtea P, de Ziegler D, Ayoubi JM. Effects of endometriosis on assisted reproductive technology: gone with the wind. Fertil Steril. 2021;115(2):321-2.

21 Chapter

Myomas

INTRODUCTION

Myomas are commonly known as fibroids or leiomyomas. These lesions arise from the smooth muscle of the uterus. These are usually benign tumors, more commonly seen in childbearing age. Their exact incidence is difficult to find as many are diagnosed only as an incidental finding in patients presenting for a routine health check-up or infertility. But evidently, their incidence appears to be increased due to late marriages and delayed child birth.[1] When symptomatic, fibroid may present as dysmenorrhea, menorrhagia, infertility, etc. There is a significant difference in the pregnancy rates in infertile women presenting with fibroid (11%) and without fibroid (25%). Removal of fibroid increases pregnancy rate from 25 to 42%.[2]

PATHOGENESIS

Estrogen is suspected as a causative factor for the fibroid. It is common in nulliparous women as there is unopposed action of estrogen uninterrupted by progesterone which is very high during pregnancy. But the authors have practiced also in the era when there was no ultrasound and no operative laparoscopy. We have seen fibroids as an incidental finding in many multiparous women during hysterectomy for different causes. So apart from estrogen, there must be some other cause of fibroids. Estrogen may increase the growth and size decreases after menopause or artificial hypoestrinism.

INCIDENCE

Most of the fibroids are diagnosed incidentally during routine gynecological examination and pelvic ultrasound scan for a routine checkup or for other reasons. Fibroids are diagnosed in 20–40% of women during the reproductive age and are reduced to half in the perimenopausal age. The incidence may be high as they go unnoticed when there are no symptoms.

DIAGNOSIS

Clinical Ultrasound

- Diagnosis is always confirmed by ultrasound. Ultrasound can give exact size, location, and relation with other organs.

  On ultrasound, the fibroid is identified as a round or an oval well-defined homogenously hypoechoic mass lesion **(Fig. 1A)**. Fibroids may cast alternate hyperechoic and hypoechoic coarse shadows deep to themselves **(Fig. 1A)**. These are fan shadows. However, fibroids cast bold acoustic shadows from their edges and these are called edge shadows **(Fig. 1B)**.

  If fibroids are large, these may distort the serosal or endometrial contour depending on their location. Fibroids, though arise from the myometrium, may penetrate into the endometrium or protrude out of the serosa, and depending on the penetration fibroids can be divided

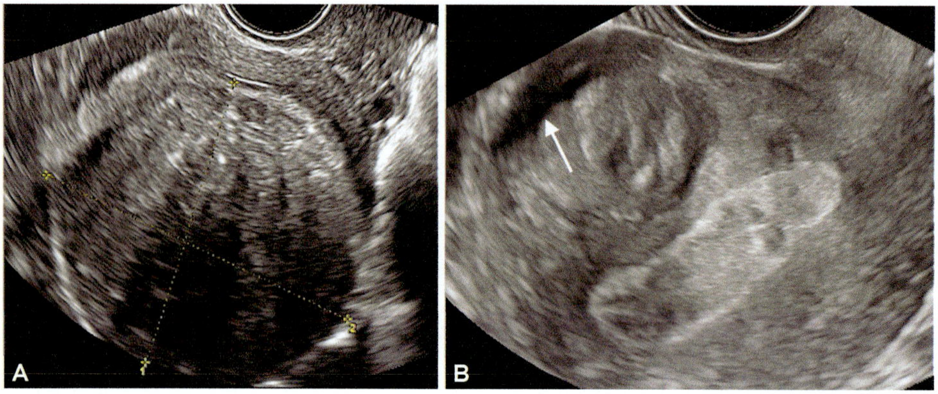

Figs. 1A and B: (A) B-mode ultrasound image of a large posterior fibroid, distorting the serosal contour and showing coarse fan shadows; (B) Anterior intramural fibroid with mildly heterogeneous echogenicity but shows edge shadows (arrow).

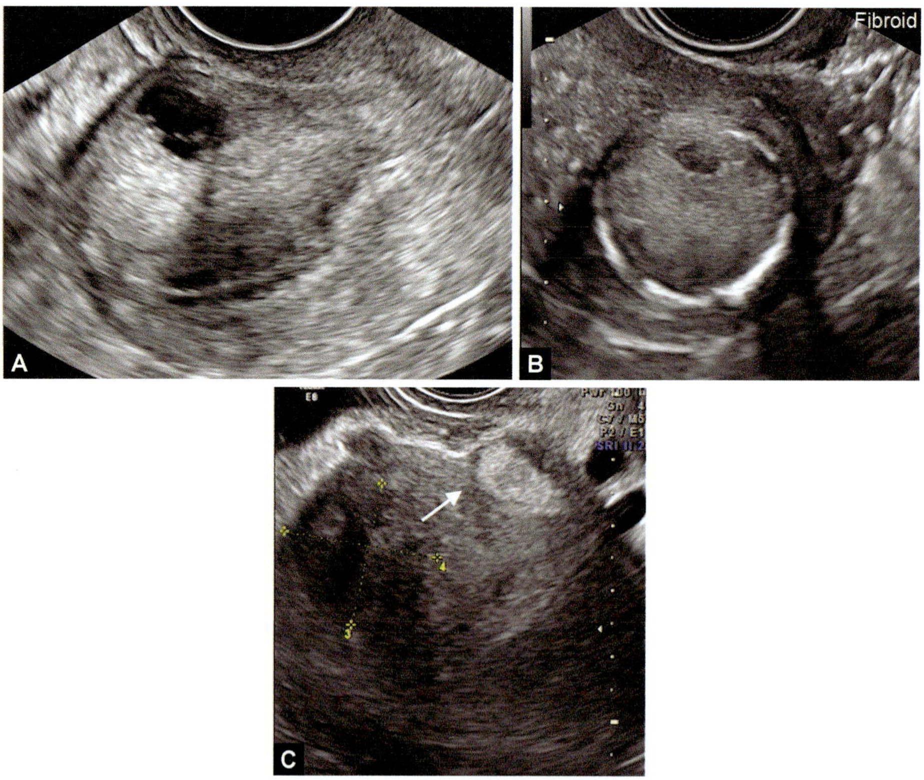

Figs. 2A to C: (A) Degenerated fibroid with cystic area; (B) Degenerated fibroid with a calcified rim; (C) Degenerated hyperechoic fibroid (arrow).

into subendometrial, intramural, or subserosal or can be divided according to Palm-Coein classification as described later in this chapter.

When degenerated fibroids become heterogenous, these may then show calcification, anechoic, or hyperechoic areas **(Figs. 2A to C)**.

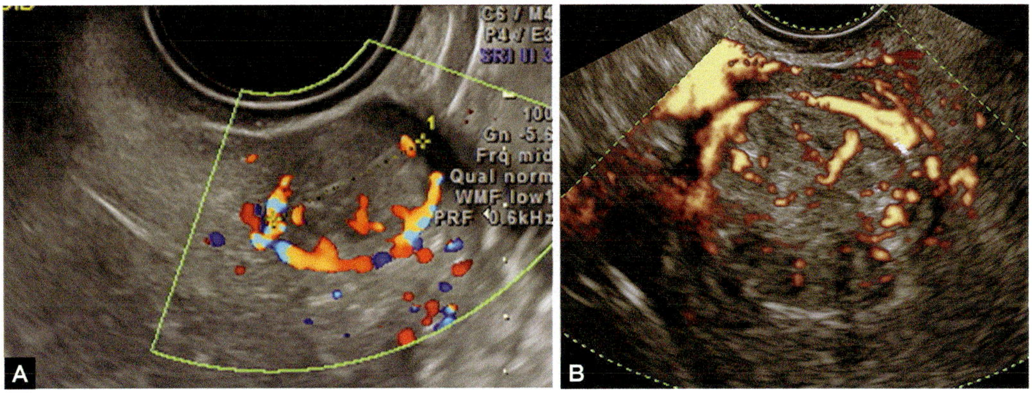

Figs. 3A and B: (A) Color Doppler image of fibroid with peripheral vascularity; (B) Power Doppler image of degenerated fibroid showing peripheral and intralesional vascularity.

On Doppler, fibroids always show peripheral vascularity **(Figs. 3A and B)** but when degenerated these also show intralesional vascularity.

- *Magnetic resonance imaging (MRI)*: Rarely, MRI is required when there are multiple fibroids and to understand their relation to other organs before surgery. It also rules out leiomyosarcoma.

  Today, in the era of endoscopy, it is extremely important not to touch the fibroid when it is not causing infertility or other symptoms. Unnecessary removal of fibroid can cause iatrogenic infertility because of adhesions and disturbing tubo-ovarian relations. So when the fibroid is an incidental finding on laparoscopy of an infertile patient, whether to operate or not is usually a dilemma. Ultrasound may help to sort out this dilemma.

  Many a times, it may be an incidental finding on ultrasound with no symptoms and in these cases, unnecessary intervention and overenthusiastic management should be avoided.

CLASSIFICATION OF FIBROIDS

- *Conventional classification*:
  - *Submucous fibroid*: When it is projecting inside the cavity
  - *Intramural fibroids*: When it is inside the myometrium
  - *Subserous fibroids*: When it projects on the peritoneal surface of the uterus

These were classified by Wamstekar et al.[3] based on the penetration in myometrium. Later on, it was adopted by the European Society for Gynecological Endoscopy (ESGE).

G0: Fibroid in the cavity with pedicle attached to the cavity

G1: >50% in the cavity

G2: >50% in the myometrium, <50% in the endometrial cavity

But Lasmar et al.,[4] in 2005, proposed a classification for surgical management of fibroid. According to this classification, fibroids are scored based on the size, topographic position of the fibroid, depth of the fibroid, extension in relation to the endometrial cavity, and involvement of the lateral wall **(Fig. 4)**.

In 2011, the International Federation of Gynecologists and Obstetricians proposed another classification as shown in **Figure 5**.[5]

Let us now discuss the signs and symptoms of infertility according to this classification.

Submucous Fibroids

Submucous fibroids are types 0, 1, and 2.

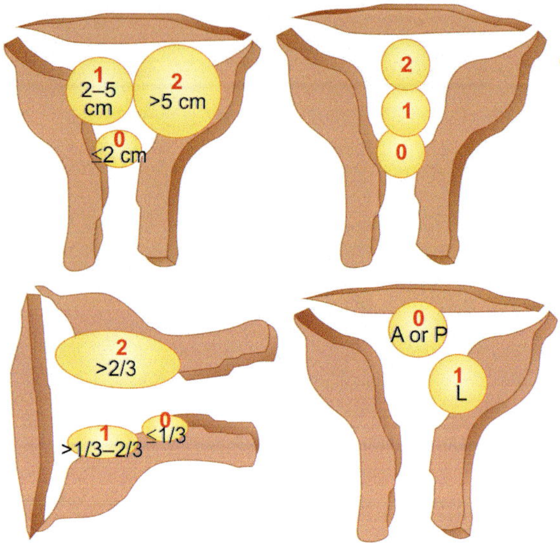

Parameters	*E-score*	*0*	*1*	*2*
Size		≤2	2–5	>5
Topography		Inf.	Mid.	Upper
Extension of the base		≤1/3	1/3–2/3	>2/3
Penetration		0	≤50%	>50%
Wall		Anterior/p	Lateral	

Score	*Group*	*Indication*
0–4	I	Low complexity hysteroscopic myomectomy
5–6	II	High complexity hysteroscopic myomectomy. GnRH? Two-step hysteroscopic myomectomy
7–9	III	Hysteroscopic myomectomy is not indicated

Fig. 4: Classification for surgical management of fibroid (STEP-W classification).[4]

Leiomyoma subclassification system

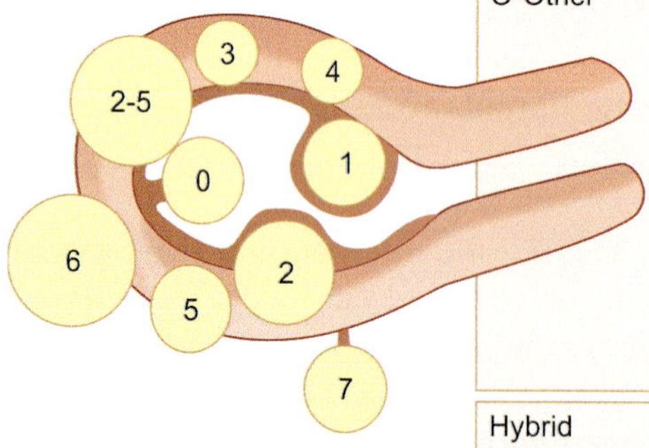

SM-Submucosal	0	Pedunculated intracavitary
	1	>50% intramural
	2	≥50% intramural
O-Other	3	Contacts endometrium; 100% intramural
	4	Intramural
	5	Subserosal ≥50% intramural
	6	Subserosal <50% intramural
	7	Subserosal pedunculated
	8	Other (specify, e.g., cervical, parasitic)
Hybrid leiomyomas (impact both endometrium and serosa)	2-5	Two numbers are listed separated by a hyphen. By convention, the first refers to the relationship with the endometrium while the second refers to the relationship to the serosa. One example is below Submucosal and subserosal, each with less than half the diameter in the endometrial and peritoneal cavities, respectively

Fig. 5: Classification of fibroids by the International Federation of Gynecologists and Obstetricians.[5]

Symptoms

Patients with submucous fibroids typically present with dysmenorrhea, menorrhagia if it is large and some portion in myometrium, intermenstrual bleeding because of ulceration in submucous fibroids, and discharge because of infection. If it is a pedunculated fibroid, a single feeding vessel can be seen on ultrasound. The size and location can be evaluated by ultrasound.

Relation to Infertility

Submucous fibroid is one of the most common causes of infertility, recurrent implantation failure, and recurrent pregnancy loss.

- It may be a mechanical obstacle for the passage of sperm, ovum, and embryo.
- It causes inflammatory reaction and impairs implantation. So many cytokines and growth factors are found that increase uterine contractions and can cause infertility.
- *Implantation*:
  - Cytokines such as interleukin-10 (IL-10) and glycodelin are reduced in the endometrium, which are necessary for implantation. This causes a low implantation rate in females with submucosal fibroids.[6]
  - There is a reduction in *HOXA10* and other genes' expression. These lead to implantation failure.[7]
  - There is a decrease in uterine NK cells and macrophages at endometrial–myometrial junction, which decreases the implantation rate.[8] So submucous fibroids distort the endometrial cavity and cause difficulty in conception and also increase the abortion rate **(Fig. 4)**.[9,10]

Treatment of Submucous Fibroids

Hysteroscopic myomectomy:

- It can be done in a single or double setting.
- In monopolar resection, glycine is used but the complication because of abortion of fluids is high.
- In bipolar resection, normal saline and Ringer's lactate solution are used having less electrolyte disturbances.
- The patient can go for vaginal delivery and uterine rupture is not reported.[11]
- Large type 1 and 2 fibroids between 3 and 5 cm can be removed by a skilled surgeon.
- Multiple submucous myoma should be removed laparoscopically.
- Fibroid of size > 5 cm should be removed abdominally by laparoscopic surgery, otherwise it will damage a large area of the endometrium and perforation will be very high because of thin myometrium **(Fig. 4)**.[12]
- Submucous myoma extended to serosa is removed abdominally.
- Mechanical hysteroscopic morcellation and laser ablation can be done.
- Vaporizing electrodes can be used.
- Hysteroscopic morcellation of myoma can be done.

Intramural Fibroids

Intramural fibroids are of types 3, 4, 5, 6 as shown in respective figures.

Symptoms

Patients with intramural fibroids may be asymptomatic and may have incidental findings. Few patients may complain of menorrhea and congestive dysmenorrhea. Larger fibroids can cause infertility and it may be the only presenting symptom.

Intramural fibroids can be diagnosed accurately by ultrasound for size and location. Sometimes MRI may be required in large, multiple fibroids to understand their relation to adjacent organs.

Intramural Fibroids and Infertility (Fig. 5)

- Mechanical distortion of the cavity due to intramural fibroid can cause infertility because of transport of sperm, ova, and embryo.

- It alters uterine contractions and impairs implantation.
- Fibroids touching the endometrium even if they are <4 cm can cause a decrease in cytokines and gene which are required for implantation. So it can cause a decrease in implantation rate due to deficiency of IL-10, glycodelin, HOXA10, etc.[7] When it touches the endometrial–myometrial junction, it can cause a decrease in uNK cells which decreases implantation.[7,8]
- But there is always a controversy whether intramural fibroids cause infertility or not. Buttram et al. reviewed 1,699 cases of myomectomy and found out that 27% of these women had infertility.[13]

When all other causes of infertility were ruled out, myomas were found to play a role in 2.4% of the cases. Hence, it was concluded that although myomas may be co-incidentally present in 25% of the cases of infertility, myomectomy would directly benefit only 2.4% of these women, when all other infertility factors have been ruled out. The rest will conceive following treatment of an identifiable cause rather than myomectomy.[9,10,13] Myomectomy does not always enhance fertility in all patients with myomas. On the contrary, it may lead to peritoneal adhesions and disturbs tubo-ovarian relations. It may reduce the uterine cavity, further reducing fertility potential, so because of myomectomy, IVF remains the only option in some of the patients.

Hence, the decision of myomectomy is a crucial one and should be tried only when there is no other cause for infertility and enough has been tried for unexplained infertility, e.g., three to six cycles of intrauterine insemination (IUI). Recurrent implantation failure (RIF) and intramural myoma of >5 cm size should be operated. The meta-analysis by Benecke et al.[14] and Sunkara et al.[15] concluded that the presence of myoma without cavity involvement can reduce the success rate in assisted reproductive technology (ART) cycles.

A study by Eldar-Geva et al. in 1998[16] found lower implantation and clinical pregnancy rate in a woman with intramural and submucosal fibroids even when there was no compromise of the uterine cavity.[17]

When the size of the fibroids is <4 cm, not encroaching the endometrial cavity, results are not affected. Results are not affected in small asymptomatic fibroids. So, myomectomy is done only in patients with fibroids of 4 cm.[18-20] So the conclusion is that even if the fibroid is not distorting the endometrial cavity but is >4 cm in diameter, it should be operated.

Management of Infertility

- *Laparoscopic myomectomy*: It is always done in all subserous, intramural, and sometimes in type 2, 3 fibroids. Meticulous suturing is required after laparoscopic myomectomy to reduce the incidence of rupture during pregnancy. Multilayer suturing reduces the rupture in pregnancy.
  All the complications of laparoscopy, as well as morcellation, should be explained to the patient. Ideally, morcellation should be done in the bag which ensures complete removal without bowel injury.
  A clinical pregnancy rate of 33% is reported after myomectomy for fibroids > 5 cm compared to 15% in nonoperated patients.
- *Abdominal myomectomy*: Large fibroids like those >7–10 cm should be removed by laparotomy. It takes very little time and meticulous suturing can also be done. The introduction of vasopressin has reduced blood loss. It is done under spinal anesthesia when general anesthesia is contraindicated in certain medical

conditions for laparoscopic myomectomy. Large fibroids should be operated by laparoscopy only by an experienced surgeon, otherwise complication rates are very high. There is a good proverb that every laparoscopic surgeon has to be a good laparotomy surgeon. The incidence of rupture uterus is less with abdominal myomectomy.

- *Uterine artery embolization*: It is contraindicated in infertile patients. It aggravates infertility by hampering blood supply to the endometrium. Even if conception occurs, the abortion rate is very high.[21]
- *MRI-guided focused ultrasound or high-intensity focused ultrasound (HIFU)*: It is not suitable for infertile patients. It is for the relief of symptoms in patients with large fibroids, who have finished childbearing. Patients who conceived after this treatment showed a higher incidence of abortion, preterm births, and ruptured uterus.[22]
  The rupture can be avoided and full-term delivery is possible provided the endometrium is spared from the coagulation and fibroid is away by doing transvaginal radiofrequency (RF) myolysis. It is an outpatient procedure.[23]
- *Cryomyolysis*: Ultrasound-assisted laparoscopic cryomyolysis is a commonly published technique for cryosurgery. Long-term studies are required for its applicability in infertile patients.
- *Doppler-guided uterine artery occlusion*: It is under trial and the effect on fertility is not clear.

MEDICAL MANAGEMENT OF MYOMAS

- *Nonsteroidal anti-inflammatory drugs (NSAIDs)*: These are not much useful in myomas. These do not decrease blood loss and do not help in infertility management. Surgery is advocated.
- *Gonadotrophin-releasing hormone agonist (GnRhA)*: It reduces the volume of the uterus and myomas as it reduces estrogen and progesterone. This in turn decreases the blood flow and reduces cytokines and growth factors. GnRhA are therefore used to reduce the size of the myoma, but that does not help improve fertility. Pretreatment of myoma with GnRhA is controversial because it causes difficulty in dissecting the cleavage plane during myoma surgery.[24] It is useful in building up the patient and in large solitary myoma to reduce the size before surgery.
- *GnRh antagonist*: It rapidly decreases uterine and myoma volume.[25]
- *Mifepristone (RU 486)*: Long-term treatment for 6 months can reduce the size of the myomas to 50%.[26] Ulipristal is also very useful in controlling bleeding and reducing the size of fibroid. The effect is better than the GnRhA depot.[27] Ulipristal in a dose of 5–10 mg for 3 months intermittently for 4 courses dramatically reduces the size of fibroid. The reduction can be sustained for 6 months. Reduction in the size helps to correct the cavity distortion and surgery may not be required in some cases. Another option is to give two courses which will reduce the size, and myomectomy can be done following that depending on the residual size and location. In Pearl I, II, and III studies, out of 21 patients, 15 had conceived after myomectomy or natural conception after reduction in the size of fibroid post Ulipristal treatment.[27,28] The author believes that the size of the fibroid does not matter if surgery is done by an experienced operator. Infertility treatment can be started soon after that.

Medical management is required for small fibroids near the endometrium or when one wants to build up the patient.

- *Progestins*: These are not useful for tumor reduction. These may be used for thinning the endometrium, but GnRhA and Danazol are better.
- *Levonorgestrel (LNG) intrauterine contraceptive device (IUCD)*: It is for menorrhagia, but does not reduce the tumor size.
- *Selective estrogen receptor modulator (SERM)*: Raloxifene is not useful in all patients and does not reduce the tumor size. Tamoxifen is also not much useful.
- *Asoprisnil*: It is for reduction in myoma size. The advantage of selective progesterone receptor modulator (SPRM) is that it does not cause hypoestrinism.
- *Pirfenidone*: It is an antifibrinolytic compound and is under trial.
- *Letrozole*: Letrozole 2.5 mg/day reduced fibroid size by 45.6% compared to GnRhA which reduced fibroid size by 33.2%.[29] So letrozole is useful and convenient for the patient. But clinical data is too limited to be used in clinical practice.
- Herbal therapies are under trial.
- Vitamin D can cause shrinkage of the fibroid and is under trial.

CARRY HOME MESSAGE

- Myoma is common in childbearing age and occurs due to the unopposed action of estrogen.
- Ultrasound helps for diagnosis and to plan management.
- Submucous fibroids should always be removed in infertile patients.
- Intramural fibroids of >4 cm can cause infertility due to implantation failure. These should be removed in infertile patients.
- Larger fibroids should be removed by laparotomy.
- Uterine artery embolization and magnetic resonance-guided HIFU are not used in infertile patients.
- Medical management can be used to build up the patient before surgery. Otherwise, these are used for symptomatic relief rather than infertility.

REFERENCES

1. Somigliana E, Vercellini P, Daguati R, Pasin R, De Giorgi O, Crosignani PG. Fibroids and female reproduction: a critical analysis of the evidence. Hum Reprod Update. 2007; 13(5):465-76.
2. Bulletti C, De Zeigler D, Polli V, Flamigni C. The role of leiomyomas in infertility. J Am Assoc Gynecol Laparosc. 1999;6:441-5.
3. Wamstekar K, Emanuel MH, de Kruif JH. Transcervical hysteroscopic resection of submucous fibroids for abnormal uterine bleeding: results regarding the degree of intramural extension. Obstet Gynecol. 1993;82(5):736-80.
4. Lasmar RB, Barrozo PRM, Dias R, de Oliveira MAP (2005). Submucous myomas: a new presurgical classification to evaluate the viability of hysteroscopic surgical treatment—preliminary report. J Minim Invasive Gynecol. 2005;12(4):308-11.
5. Munro MG, Critchley HOD, Broder MS, Fraser IS, FIGO Working Group on Menstrual Disorders. FIGO classification system (PALM-COEIN) for causes of abnormal uterine bleeding in nongravid women of reproductive age. Int J Gynaecol Obstet. 2011;113:3-13.
6. Ben-Nagi J, Miell J, Mavrelos D, Naftalin J, Lee C, Jurkovic D. Endometrial implantation factors in women with submucous uterine fibroids. Reprod Biomed Online. 2010; 21(5):610-5.
7. Cakmak H, Taylor HS. Implantation failure: Molecular mechanisms and clinical treatment. Hum Reprod Update. 2011;17(2): 242-53.
8. Kitaya K, Yasuo Y. Leukocyte density and composition in human cycling endometrium with uterine fibroids. J Hum Immunol. 2010;17(2):158-63.
9. Klatsky PC, Tran ND, Caughey AB, Fujimoto VY. Fibroids and reproductive outcomes: a systematic literature review from conception to delivery. Am J Obstet Gynecol. 2008; 198:35.
10. Falcone T, Parker WH. Surgical management of leiomyomas for fertility or uterine

preservation. Obstet Gynecol. 2013;121: 856-68.
11. Stewart E. Uterine fibroids. Lancet. 2001;357: 293-8.
12. American Association of Gynecological Laparoscopists, Advancing minimally invasive Gynecology worldwide. AAGL practice report: Practice guidelines for diagnosis and management of submucous leiomyomas. J Minim Invasive Gynecol. 2012;19(2):152-71.
13. Buttram VC Jr, Reiter RC. Uterine leiomyomata: etiology, symptomatology and management. Fertil Steril. 1981;36:433-45.
14. Benecke C, Kruger TF, Siebert TI, van der Merwe JP, Steyn DW. Effect of fibroid on fertility in patients undergoing assisted reproduction. Gynecol Obstet Invest. 2005;59:225-30.
15. Sunkara SK, Khairy M, Toukhy TE, Khalaf Y, Coomarasamy A. The effect of intramural fibroids without uterine cavity involvement on the outcome of IVF treatment: A systematic review and meta-analysis. Hum Reprod. 2010;25(2):418-29
16. Eldar-Geva T, Meagher S, Healy DL, MacLachlan V, Breheny S, Wood C. Effect of intramural, subserosal and submucosal uterine fibroids on the outcome of assisted reproductive technology treatment. Fertil Steril. 1998;70(4):687-91.
17. Practice Committee of American Society for reproductive medicine. Myomas and reproductive function. Fertil Steril. 2004; 82(Suppl 1):111-6.
18. Olivera FG, Abdelmassih VG, Diamond MP, Dozortsev D, Melo NR, Abdelmassih R. Impact of subserosal and intramural uterine fibroids that do not distort the endometrial cavity in the outcome of in vitro fertilization-intracytoplasmic sperm injection. Fertil Steril. 2004;81(3):582-7.
19. Vimercati A, Scioscia M, Lorusso F, Laera AF, Lamanna G, Alfredo Coluccia A, et al. Do uterine fibroids affect IVF outcomes? Reprod Biomed Online. 2007;15(6):686-91.
20. Somigliana E, De Benedicits S, Vercellini P, Nicolosi AE, Benaglia L, Scarduelli C, et al. Fibroids not encroaching the endometrial cavity and IVF success rate: a prospective study. Hum Reprod. 2011;26(4):834-9.
21. Goldberg J, Pereira L, Berghella V, Diamond J, DaraïE, Seinera P, et al. Pregnancy outcomes after treatment for fibromyomata: uterine artery embolization versus laparoscopic myomectomy. Am J Obstet Gynecol. 2004; 191:18-21.
22. Rabinivici J, David M, Fukunishi H, Morita Y, Gostout BS, Stewart EA, et al. Pregnancy outcome after magnetic resonance guided focused ultrasound surgery (MRgFUS) for conservative treatment of uterine fibroids. Fertil Steril. 2010;93(1):199-209.
23. Kim CH, Kim SR, Lee HA, Kim SH, Chae AD, Kang BM. Transvaginal ultrasound-guided radiofrequency myolysis for uterine myomas. Hum Reprod. 2011;26(3):559-63.
24. Campo S, Garcea N. Laparoscopic myomectomy in premenopausal women with and without preoperative treatment using gonadotrophin releasing hormone analogues. Hum Reprod. 1999;14:44-8.
25. Flierman PA, Oberye JJ, van der Hulst VP, de Blok S. Rapid reduction of leiomyoma volume during treatment with GnRh antagonist ganirelix. BJOG. 2005;112:638-42.
26. Murphy AA, Morales AJ, Kettel LM, Yen SS. Regression of uterine leiomyomata to antiprogesterone RU 486: dose-response effect. Fertil Steril. 1995;64:187-90.
27. Donnez J, Tomaszewski J, Vazquez F, Bouchard P, Lemieszczuk B, Baró F, et al. Ulipristal acetate versus leuprolide acetate for uterine fibroids. N Engl J Med. 2012; 366:421-32.
28. Donnez J, Tatarchuk T, Bouchard P, Puscasiu L, Zakharenko NF, Ivanova T, et al. Ulipristal acetate versus placebo for fibroid treatment before surgery. N Engl J Med. 2012;366:409-20.
29. Parsanezhad ME, Azmoon M, Alborzi S, Rajaeefard A, Zarei A, Kazerooni T, et al. A randomized, controlled clinical trial comparing the effects of aromatase inhibitor (letrozole) and gonadotrophin-releasing hormone agonist(Triptorelin) on uterine leiomyoma volume and hormonal status. Fertil Steril. 2010;93:192-8.

22 Chapter

Tuberculosis

INTRODUCTION

Tuberculosis remains a major public health problem. About 95% of cases of tuberculosis occur in developing countries and death rate due to tuberculosis is very high, reported as 2 million in 2016.[1] India has the highest incidence of tuberculosis in the world.

Genital tuberculosis is one of the common causes of infertility, particularly in the lower socioeconomic class of people, and the incidence is reported as high as 19% in some studies.[2]

More liberal immigration has increased the risk in the developed world also. Because of poor management in rural areas, multidrug resistant (MDR) and extreme drug-resistant (EDR) cases are increasing. This is a cause of serious global concern.[1]

EPIDEMIOLOGY OF GENITAL TUBERCULOSIS

- Most of the cases are asymptomatic and remain undiagnosed, particularly before marriage or adolescent age.
- Primary genital tuberculosis is extremely rare and it is secondary to pulmonary or intestinal tuberculosis.
- Infertility is the most common presentation along with chronic pelvic pain and menstrual irregularities. It may be an incidental finding in diagnostic laparoscopy for infertility.[3]

ETIOPATHOGENESIS[4,5]

The genital organs involved in female genital tuberculosis (FGTB) are as follows:

- *Fallopian tubes*: 90–100%
- *Uterus*: 50–80%
- *Ovaries*: 20–30%
- *Cervix*: 5–15%
- *Vagina and vulva*: 1–2%

It is mostly secondary to pulmonary tuberculosis but it may be due to extrapulmonary sites such as gastrointestinal tract or may be due to renal, skeletal, or miliary tuberculosis. The spread may be lymphatic or hematogenous. The primary FGTB may be from the vulva, vagina, or cervix. Thus, primary or secondary infertility is common because of FGTB.

Tubal Factors

- FGTB can cause blockage of the tubes (beaded appearance).
- The functional aspect of the tube is damaged as cilia are damaged and cause infertility or result in ectopic pregnancy.
- Tubo-ovarian mass formation takes place.
- Unilateral or bilateral hydrosalpinx can occur in 46% of cases affecting fertilization and implantation.[6,7]
- Thus, we get endosalpingitis, interstitial salpingitis, or salpingitis isthmica nodosa.

Ovarian Factors

- Tubo-ovarian mass formation leads to adhesions and poor ovarian reserve because of damage. Thus, higher doses of gonadotropins are required.

- Because of the direct effect of toxins or bacteria, FGTB (female genital tract tuberculosis) affects the quality of oocytes.
- FGTB may cause harmful luteinization by immune modulation.[8]

Uterine Factors

- FGTB causes endometrial damage. It may distort the cavity by caseation, adhesions, and Asherman's syndrome.
- It may cause secondary amenorrhea and infertility and the prognosis is very poor for infertility treatment.[4,9,10]
- In spite of all treatments, results are very poor as it adversely affects all endometrial biomarkers essential for implantation.[6]
- There is no vascularity in zones 3 and 4 of the endometrium and so implantation is poor.
- Dam et al. observed latent FGTB to be an important cause of repeat in vitro fertilization (IVF) failure in their settings.[11]

SYMPTOMS

- Asymptomatic
- *General symptoms*:
  - Evening rise of temperature (low grade)
  - Loss of weight and anorexia
  - Poor and debilitated general condition
  - Pain in abdomen
- *Menstrual symptoms*:
  - Menorrhagia
  - Followed by oligomenorrhea and amenorrhea
  - Dysmenorrhea
- *Infertility*:
  - Dyspareunia
  - Abnormal vaginal discharge

SIGNS

- Abdominal lump
- Restricted mobility of the uterus
- Acute abdomen if tubo-ovarian mass ruptures

INVESTIGATIONS

- *Mantoux test (tuberculin test)*: Extremely poor sensitivity and specificity
- Serological tests, such as ELISA (enzyme-linked immunosorbent assay), are banned by the government in India.
- X-ray of chest for pulmonary tuberculosis and blood complete.
- Ultrasound

The most common cause of chronic endometritis in our subcontinent is tuberculous endometritis, and it is a diagnostic enigma. May it be imaging criteria or laboratory criteria, none has been conclusive or foolproof for the diagnosis of tuberculosis. But certain ultrasound criteria have been found to be more commonly associated with tuberculosis which are as follows:

- Persistently thin endometrium **(Fig. 1A)**
- Disrupted endometrial–myometrial junction **(Fig. 1A)**
- Echogenic flecks in the endometrium
- Echogenic flecks in the myometrium
- Avascular myometrial cysts
- Fluid in the endometrial cavity in the mid-prolifcrativc phase (Day 6–10) **(Fig. 1B)**
- Echogenic inner layer of the endometrium **(Fig. 1B)**
- Vertically oriented interstitial part of the tube **(Fig. 1C)**
- Narrow contracted endometrial cavity **(Fig. 1D)**
- Micropolyposis **(Fig. 1E)**

Apart from these findings in the uterus, genital tuberculosis may also present with

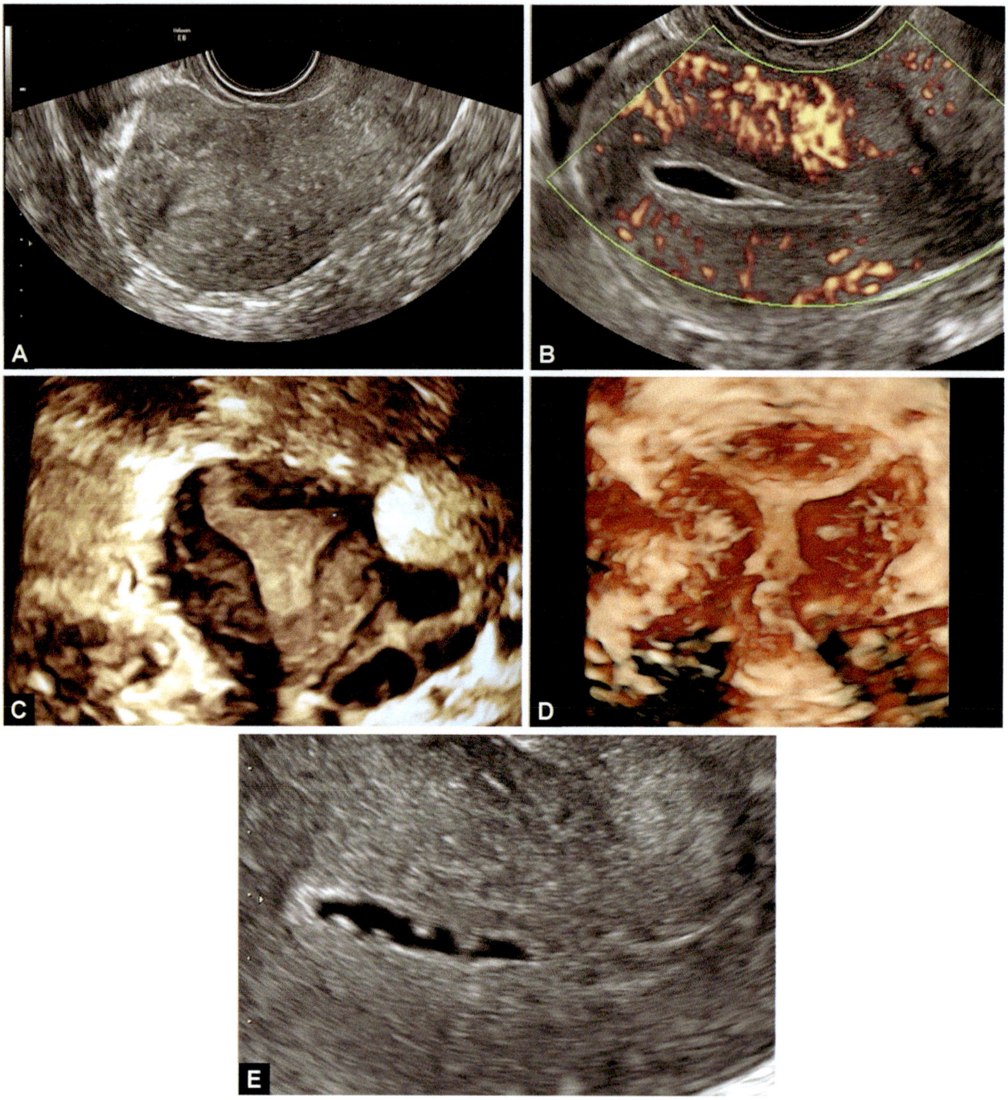

Figs. 1A to E: (A) Thin endometrium with ill-defined junctional zone; (B) Fluid in endometrial cavity with hyperechoic endometrial line; (C) Vertical orientation of interstitial part of the tube; (D) Contracted endometrial cavity; (E) Micropolyposis.

free fluid in pelvis with or without septa, hyperechoic spots in the ovary, hydrosalpinx, tubo-ovarian masses, and adhesions.

Calcified pelvic lymph nodes or calcified spots in the adnexa are also seen in tuberculous or nontuberculous chronic inflammatory lesions.

- *Computed tomographic scan*:
  - *Pelvic mass*: Unilateral or bilateral, commonly multilocular caseous necrotic material
  - Ascites
  - Thickening and enhancement of peritoneum—nodulous or smooth

- Adhesion in the abdominopelvic cavity
- Low attenuation necrotic lymph nodes with ring enhancement
- Thickening and enhancement of bowel wall

- *Magnetic resonance imaging (MRI)*: It has a higher resolution and may show tubo-ovarian masses. Unilateral or bilateral tubo-ovarian masses, hydrosalpinx, adnexal cysts, or tuberculous deposits on the peritoneum or liver have been reported in our study.[12]

Computed tomography and MRI are employed in FGTB in the presence of an abdominal or pelvic mass.[13]

- *Positron emission tomography (PET)*: PET-scan shows unilateral or bilateral tubo-ovarian masses with increased fluorodeoxyglucose (FDG) uptake by a TB lesion.[14,15] Increased FDG uptake by TB lesions has been observed in tubercular tubo-ovarian masses. It also helps in differentiating between carcinoma ovary and abdominopelvic TB.
- *Hysterosalpingography (HSG)*: Blocked tubes, beaded appearance, adhesions, T-shaped or distorted uterus
- *Endometrial biopsy and curettage*: Histopathology demonstrates epithelial granuloma. Staining with Ziehl–Neelsen stain for acid-fast bacilli is the gold standard.
- Mycobacterial culture in Lowenstein Jensen medium (LJ) and other media like Agar or Middlebrook 7H9 Broth. Growth in culture is the surest sign of tuberculosis. The disadvantage of culture is that it takes up to 4 weeks for growth, and another 4 weeks are required to test the drug sensitivity. So the treatment is delayed and the disease may progress further.
- Antitubercular treatment (ATT) should not be started on only polymerase chain reaction (PCR), but other clinical or laboratory findings should also be positive. PCR can be positive in cases of old infection, subclinical infection, or latent infection.

Modern Rapid Tests

- Reverse transcription polymerase chain reaction (RT-PCR) is positive in presence of live bacilli.
- Microcolony detection on solid media (rapid slide culture technique)
- Septi-Chek AFB method
- BACTEC 460 radiometric method

All these have higher sensitivity of 80–90% with quicker results in 5–10 days.

Serological Tests

QuantiFERON-TB Gold has been banned by the government of India due to its low specificity.

GeneExpert

GeneExpert of cartridge-based nucleic acid amplification test (CB-NAAT), if positive on endometrial biopsy, is a reliable test for FGTB and treatment can be started.[16]

Endoscopy

Hysteroscopy

There are pale tubercular nodules and caseation may be seen. The cavity may be partially or completely obliterated.

Laparoscopy

This is the most reliable modality to diagnose FGTB, especially for tubal, ovarian, and peritoneal diseases. Adhesions, tubercles, pyosalpinx, and frozen pelvis are very common. When FGTB is suspected even with negative polymerase chain reaction (PCR), laparoscopy must be done.

TREATMENT: FROM INFERTILITY PERSPECTIVE (FLOWCHART 1)

- Treatment of latent genital tuberculosis detected only by PCR is controversial due to high false-positive rates. Now PCR is not considered valid for the diagnosis of tuberculosis.
- The argument in favor of positive PCR with negative conventional tests may indicate subclinical infection and early treatment may prevent further progress of disease and irreversible damage.[17]
- Jindal et al. observed a 30% pregnancy rate in PCR positive women with antituberculosis treatment (ATT). Kulshrestha et al. also claimed a 31% pregnancy rate in patients with positive RT-PCR and on ATT.[18] Dam et al.

Flowchart 1: Treatment regimens for female genital tuberculosis (FGTB).

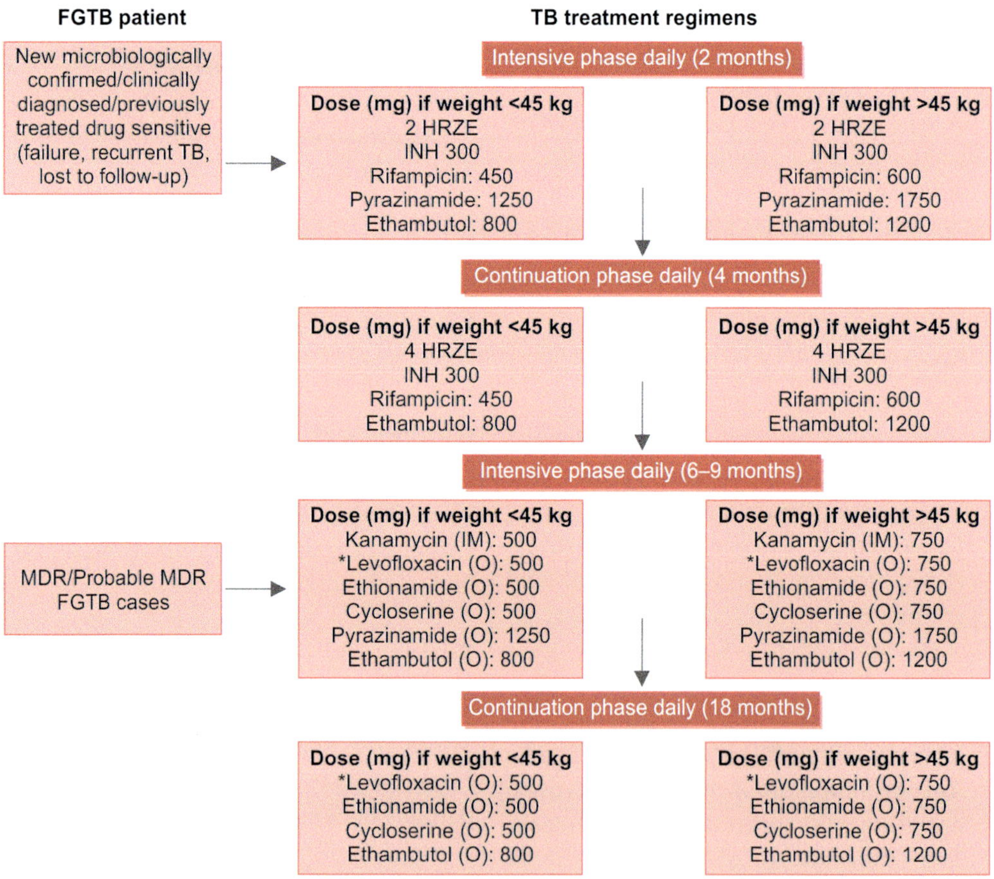

*Moxifloxacin to be given, if resistance to levofloxacin. Recently, 4 drug fixed dose combination (FDC) HRZE (75, 150, 400, 275) has been introduced.

(HRZE: isoniazid, rifampicin, pyrazinamide and ethambutol; INH: isoniazid; MDR: multi-drug resistant; IM: intramuscular; O: oral)

Source: Reproduced from Sharma JB, Sharma E, Sharma S, Dharmendra S. Female genital tuberculosis: revisited. Indian J Med Res. 2018;148(Suppl):71-83.

documented a better pregnancy rate with recurrent implantation failure patients with ATT, and lesser doses of gonadotropins were required.[11]

- Repeated IVF failures may be associated with latent tuberculosis and ATT may be tried on these patients.[6]
- However, treating women with positive PCR is associated with the risk of over-treatment as many women without FGTB are treated, and delay for fertility treatment occurs. But if endoscopy findings are suggestive of latent infection in association with positive PCR, ATT should be given.

  A short course of chemotherapy for 6–9 months has been found to be effective for medical treatment of FGTB.[4]
- Directly observed treatment, short course (DOTS) is found by the World Health Organization (WHO).
  - Daily therapy of Rifampicin (R), Isoniazid (H), Pyrazinamide (Z), and Ethambutol (E). RHZE fixed-dose combo-pack for 2 months is available. It is known as the intensive phase of treatment.
  - It is followed by rifampicin, isoniazid, and ethambutol (RHE) for 4 months. A combination blister pack of the same is available. It is known as continuous phase treatment.
- Revised National TB Control Programme (RNTCP) of India has also revised the guidelines to treat tuberculosis in 2017 and recommends daily treatment.[19]

Genital tuberculosis is classified as category I—seriously ill extrapulmonary disease. Sometimes, FGTB relapses after treatment or fails to respond to the above-said treatment and then it is categorized as category II. For its treatment, injection streptomycin is added daily along with the RHZE protocol for 2 months. This is followed by 1 month of RHZE regimen and then by RZE for 5 months as a continuous phase. So, the total treatment lasts for 8 months.[20]

Convenient and economic market packs are available.

Surgery

- Prior to IVF, hydrosalpinx or pyosalpinx is to be surgically removed.
- If removal is not possible, tubal occlusion with clip or bipolar coagulation should be done.

Hysteroscopy

It is done in mild-to-moderate intrauterine adhesions. But in tuberculosis, usually vascularity is affected due to endarteritis and so in spite of clearing adhesions, implantation rates might not improve. In cases with a contracted endometrial cavity (the so-called T-shaped uterus), lateral metroplasty may improve the endometrial volume but it is controversial.

Laparoscopy or Laparotomy

Complication rates are very high during the surgery.[21,22] Tuboplasty should never be done in these cases as results are extremely poor. Surgical procedures should be avoided as intestinal complications are very high and do not improve pregnancy rates.

ROLE OF IN VITRO FERTILIZATION

- Assisted reproductive technology (ART) is the only option left for patients whose fallopian tubes are damaged due to tuberculosis.
- When the ovarian reserve is decreased, ART demands very high doses of gonadotropins.

- When the endometrium is grossly damaged and there is a thin endometrium without vascularity in the endometrium, surrogacy remains the only option.
- Pre-IVF evaluation does not differ much from regular IVF patients. But endometrium and vascularity should be assessed thoroughly before ART.
- Only on positive PCR, ATT should not be started. Endoscopy and culture are required for confirmation.
- In severe Asherman's syndrome, stem cell therapy can be tried but results are not as good as in patients with nontuberculous Asherman's syndrome.
- Surrogacy or adoption remains the only option in majority of advanced cases.

CARRY HOME MESSAGE

- FGTB is a common cause of infertility.
- Tubes and endometrium are damaged commonly after pulmonary involvement.
- Endometrial culture and GeneXpert are surest signs of positive tuberculosis.
- Laparoscopy is also a highly reliable modality for the diagnosis of genital tuberculosis in females.
- PCR should not be done for diagnosis.
- Empirical ATT has no role in unexplained infertility.
- Endometrial damage is extremely difficult to treat and surrogacy may be the only option left.
- Tuboplasty should never be done in cases with FGTB.

REFERENCES

1. World Health Organization. Global tuberculosis report 2017. [online] Available from https://www.who.int/tb/publications/global_report/gtbr2017_main_text.pdf [Last accessed March, 2021]
2. Parikh FR, Nadkarni SG, Kamat SA, Naik N, Soonawala SB, Parikh RM. Genital tuberculosis: a major pelvic factor causing infertility in Indian women. Fertil Steril. 1997;67:497-500.
3. Singh N, Sumana G, Mittal S. Genital tuberculosis: a leading cause for infertility in women seeking assisted conception in North India. Arch Gynecol Obstet. 2008;278:325-7.
4. Sharma JB. Tuberculosis and gynecological practice. In: Studd J, Tan SL, Chervanak FA (Eds). Current Progress in Obstetrics and Gynecology, 1st edition. Mumbai: Tree Life India; 2012. pp. 304-27.
5. Schaefer G. Female genital tuberculosis. Clin Obstet Gynecol. 1976;19:223-39.
6. Chakravarty BN. Genital Tuberculosis-ovarian function and endometrial receptivity. In: Mukherjee GG, Tripathy SN, Tripathy SN (Eds). Genital Tuberculosis, 1st edition. New Delhi: Jaypee Brothers Medical Publishers; 2010. pp. 27–42.
7. Chen CD, Yang JH, Lin KC, Chao KH, Ho HN, Yang YS. The significance of cytokines, chemical composition and murine embryo development in hydrosalpinx fluid for predicting the IVF outcome in women with hydrosalpinx. Hum Reprod. 2002;17(1):128-33.
8. Caliskan E, Cakiroglu Y, Sofuoglu K, Doger E, Akar ME, Ozkan SO. Effects of salpingectomy and antituberculous treatments in fertility results in patients with genital tuberculosis. J Obstet Gynecol Res. 2014;40:2104-9.
9. Neonakis IK, Spandidos DA, Petinak E. Female Genital tuberculosis: a review. Scand J Infect Dis. 2011;43:564-72.
10. Sharma JB, Roy KK, Pushparaj M, Gupta N, Jain SK, Malhotra N, et al. Genital tuberculosis: an important cause of Asherman's syndrome in India. Arch Gynecol Obstet. 2008;277:37-41.
11. Dam P, Shirazee HH, Goswami SK, Ghosh S, Ganesh A, Chaudhury K, et al. Role of latent genital tuberculosis in repeated IVF failure in Indian clinical settings. Gynecol Obstet Invest. 2006;61:223-7.
12. Sharma JB, Karmakar D, Hari S, Singh N, Singh SP, Kumar S, et al. Magnetic resonance imaging findings among women with tubercular tubo-ovarian masses. Int J Gynaecol Obstet. 2011;113:76-80.
13. Gatongi DK, Gitau G, Kay V, Ngwenya S, Lafong C, Hasan A. Female genital tuberculosis. Obstet Gynaecol. 2005;7:75-9.

14. Sharma JB, Karmakar D, Kumar R, Shamim SA, Kumar S, Singh N, et al. Comparison of PET/CT with other imaging modalities in women with genital tuberculosis. Int J Gynaecol Obstet. 2012;118:123-8.
15. Jeffry L, Kerrou K, Camatte S, Lelievre L, Metzger U, Robin F, et al. Peritoneal tuberculosis revealed by carcinomatosis on CT scan and uptake at FDG-PET. BJOG. 2003; 110:1129-31.
16. Sharma JB, Kriplani A, Dharmendra S, Chaubey J, Kumar S, Sharma SK. Role of Gene Xpert in the diagnosis of female genital tuberculosis: a preliminary report. Eur J Obstet Gynecol Reprod Biol. 2016;207: 237-8.
17. Jindal UN, Verma S, Bala Y. Favourable infertility outcomes following anti-tubercular treatment prescribed on the sole basis of positive polymerase chain reaction test for endometrial tuberculosis. Hum Reprod. 2012;27:1368-74.
18. Kulshrestha V, Kriplani A, Agarwal N, Singh UB, Rana T. Genital tuberculosis among infertile women and fertility outcome after antitubercular therapy. Int J Gynecol Obstet. 2011;113:229-34.
19. Sharma JB, Kriplani A, Dharmendra S, Singh UB, Vanamail P, Kumar S, et al. Six months versus nine months anti-tuberculous therapy for female genital tuberculosis: a randomized controlled trial. Eur J Obstet Gynecol Reprod Biol. 2017;210:108-15.
20. Sharma JB, Sharma E, Sharma S, Dharmendra S. Female genital tuberculosis: revisited. Indian J Med Res. 2018;148(Suppl):71-83.
21. Sharma JB, Mohanraj P, Roy KK, Jain SK. Increased complication rates associated with laparoscopic surgery among patients with genital tuberculosis. Int J Gynecol Obstet. 2010;109:242-4.
22. Sharma JB, Mohanraj P, Jain SK, Roy KK. Surgical complications during laparotomy in patients with abdomino-pelvic tuberculosis. Int J Gynecol Obstet. 2010;110:157-8.

23

Chapter

Luteal Phase Defect

INTRODUCTION

Luteal phase starts from ovulation and ends at the onset of menstruation or when the pregnancy is diagnosed. The dominant follicle after ovulation is converted into corpus luteum (CL) and it is one of the most hormonally active glands in the body. Progesterone secretion from CL is the hallmark of luteal phase.

Luteal phase defect (LPD) is defined as inadequate corpus luteal function in the latter half of the ovulatory cycle. It is due to insufficient endogenous progesterone production or suboptimal response of endometrium to normal progesterone (P4) level. LPD is also known as luteal phase insufficiency or CL insufficiency or inadequate luteal phase. LPD is associated with infertility, early pregnancy loss, short cycles, and premenstrual spotting **(Box 1)**.

Box 1: Role of progesterone in luteal phase.

- Brings about secretory changes for implantation
- Vasodilatation for improved flow in endometrium
- Downregulates estrogen receptors (ERs), leukemia inhibitory factor (LIF) and β-integrin
- Decidualization with pinopode formation
- Upregulation of insulin-like growth factor 1 (IGF1), interleukin, *HOXA* genes, cytokines, epidermal growth factor (EGF), transforming growth factor (TGF), vascular endothelial growth factor (VEGF), mucin I, integrins, selectins and immunoglobulins, etc.
- Relaxes uterine musculature
- Improves endometrial receptivity

LUTEAL PHASE PHYSIOLOGY

Preovulation luteinizing hormone (LH) surge is the stimulus for the luteinization. LH from pituitary continues to act through endocrine feedback during entire luteinization process. In patients with luteal phase <10 days, lower levels of follicle-stimulating hormone (FSH) and LH are found in proliferative phase. Long follicular phase cycles do not have short luteal phase in majority of cases. Day 3 high estrone-3-glucuronide (ETT) and pregnanediol 3-alpha glucuronide (PDG) are predictors of short early luteal phase. Here LH is increased in about half the cycles. Luteal phase has three phases. The first is a modulated luteinization process whereas second and third are relatively less modulated processes of progesterone and luteolysis.

- Duration is 12–14 days.
- Progesterone peak is 6–8 days after ovulation.
- Progesterone is secreted in pulses.
- Luteinizing hormone peak decides the quality of CL.
- Pulsatile LH is necessary for CL function.
- Steroidogenic acute regulatory (StAR) protein governs cholesterol transport for progesterone production
- Corpus luteum is refractory to LH in the later half.
- Human chorionic gonadotropin (hCG) can rescue CL by StAR and vascular endothelial growth factor (VEGF) after implantation.

Flowchart 1: Production and function of progesterone.

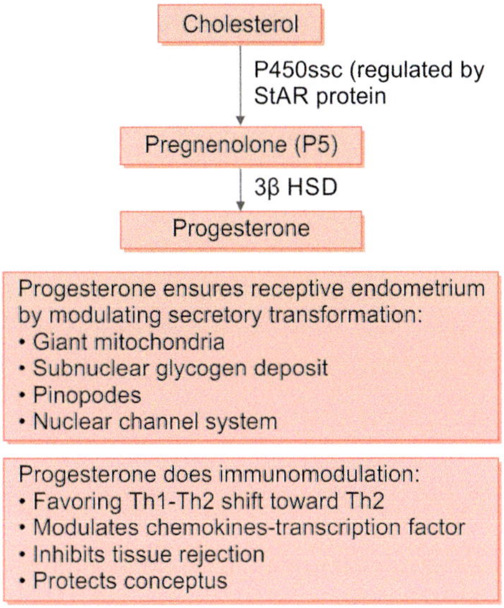

- Minimum required levels of P4 are not confirmed.
- Luteal phase estradiol (E2) is LH dependent and not FSH dependent.[1]
- Decline in StAR protein expression decreases steroidogenesis and leuteolysis.[1]

This StAR protein is not present in granulosa cells and appears after LH peak only. Before preovulatory period, this protein expression is on the theca cells and converts cholesterol into androgen **(Flowchart 1)**.

PATHOPHYSIOLOGY OF LUTEAL PHASE DEFECT

- Deficient P4 secretion from CL can be due to abnormal folliculogenesis, leading to unhealthy follicle, that secrets low levels of E2, therefore inadequate LH surge. Inadequate LH surge may cause luteinization but ovulation might not occur and produces unhealthy CL, producing low-level progesterone.
- So, LH surge is a must for a healthy CL. It is the most vascular organ. Blood flow to the CL is 6–10 mL/g/mt.[2] Daily P4 production from CL is 25–50 mg, and is secreted in pulses, every 90 minutes. P4 and E2 secretion from CL correlates with LH pulse. Average E2 production is 0.6 mg/day in luteal phase. CL secretes estrogen under the influence of LH and insulin-like growth factor-1 (IGF-1) and not FSH.
- Corpus luteum has two types of cells. The large cells develop from granulosa cells and secrete P4 in the first half of luteal phase under the influence of LH pulse. The small cells develop from theca internal and produce P4 after the stimulation of hCG.[3,4]
- Estrogen induces progesterone receptors.
- Progesterone acts through its own receptors and produces mediator protein known as progesterone-induced blocking factor (PIBF). PIBF produces asymmetrical antibodies, i.e., Th2 and natural killer (NK) cells for protection.

If PIBF is inadequate, Th1 and lymphokine-activated killer cell (LAK) cells are produced which are cytotoxic and rejects the embryo.[5] So the acceptance or rejection depends on the estrogen and progesterone.

RESCUE OF CORPUS LUTEUM IN INFERTILE PATIENT

Human chorionic gonadotropin from embryo restores StAR protein expression to late CL and induces progesterone production and production of VEGF that cause angiogenesis.

Implantation occurs between Day 8 and 10 after LH surge. Miscarriage rate is very high if implantation is late because unhealthy embryo produces less hCG and inadequate rescue signals in spite of normal CL. So low P4 in early pregnancy is because of low hCG produced by unhealthy embryo and progesterone supplementation does not work.[6] Placental steroidogenesis starts at 7 weeks. CL starts reducing after 5 weeks of pregnancy but remains active up to 11 weeks. 17-OHP is secreted by CL only which starts regressing after 5 weeks along with regressing vascularity.

After 5 weeks even hCG does not increase neoangiogenesis and this indicates that hCG-induced rescue for CL is temporary.[7]

DIAGNOSIS OF LUTEAL PHASE DEFECT

- *History*: Short luteal phase of <13 days from the LH surge to menstruation may be indicative of luteal phase defect. Patient may have premenstrual spotting, infertility, and early abortions. But history is not conclusive, for diagnosis of LPD.
- *Basal body temperature (BBT) chart*: Absence or inadequate thermogenic shift in BBT chart indicates LPD. Its utility is questioned and presently it has no place in the diagnosis of luteal phase abnormality.
- *Endometrial biopsy (EB)*: Noyce criteria for dating of endometrium are very popular for six decades. Though endometrial histology is an indirect marker of progesterone action. There is interobserver variation and also intercycle variability. There is no consensus whether biopsy should be taken in one or two or three cycles. Biopsy taken in the latter half of the luteal phase, indicates total progesterone effect rather than progesterone secretion on that day. The most interesting thing is that out of phase endometrial histology is also seen in fertile patients and patients who conceive.[8] So endometrial histology is not used as a criterion for diagnosis of LPD.
- *Serum progesterone*: Progesterone secretion starts after 30 minutes of LH surge. In early luteal phase, P4 secretion is nonpulsatile but in mid- and late luteal phase, its secretion becomes pulsatile. Therefore, single assessment does not reflect the actual progesterone secretion. It was reported that three readings between Day 5 and 9 postovulatory should be taken and cut off of 30 ng/mL was thought to have a sensitivity of 100% and specificity of 80%.[9] Normal P4 level in mid-luteal phase is 10 ng/mL. But there are no studies to confirm these findings. Histology of the endometrium does not correlate with progesterone level. So P4 does not differentiate normal and defective luteal phase. Serum progesterone > 3 ng/mL only documents ovulation. But it is not used for the diagnosis of luteal phase defect.
- *Ultrasound*:
  - Correlation of corpus luteum-resistance index (CL-RI), and serum progesterone
  - Corpus luteum Doppler shows high resistance flow (RI: 0.58 + 0.4) **(Figs. 1A and B)**.
  - Bilateral high resistance intraovarian flow, and same in both ovaries, unlike normal luteal phase that shows low resistance in the dominant ovary.
  - Increased resistance in spiral artery RI (0.72 + 0.065) **(Figs. 2A and B)**
- *New promising tests*:
  - Daily salivary progesterone measurement
  - Progesterone-induced blocking factor measurement

Currently, no tests can stamp the diagnosis of LPD and differentiate fertile from infertile patients.[6]

Etiological factors beyond P4 may be pinopodes development, insulin-like growth factor binding proteins (IGFBP), integrins, cytokines, etc. Tests to detect these abnormalities are experimental and not useful in clinical practice.

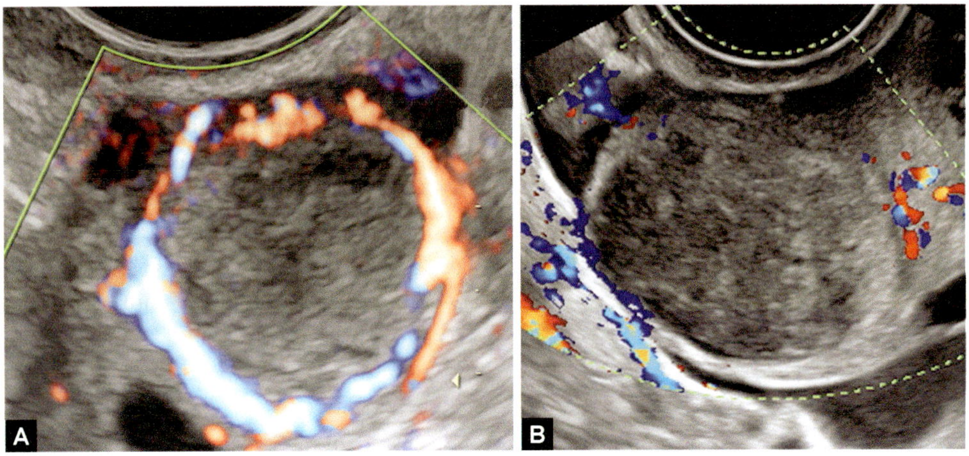

Figs. 1A and B: (A) Normal corpus luteal flow as complete ring of color; (B) Scanty corpus luteal flow of corpus luteal inadequacy—luteal phase defect.

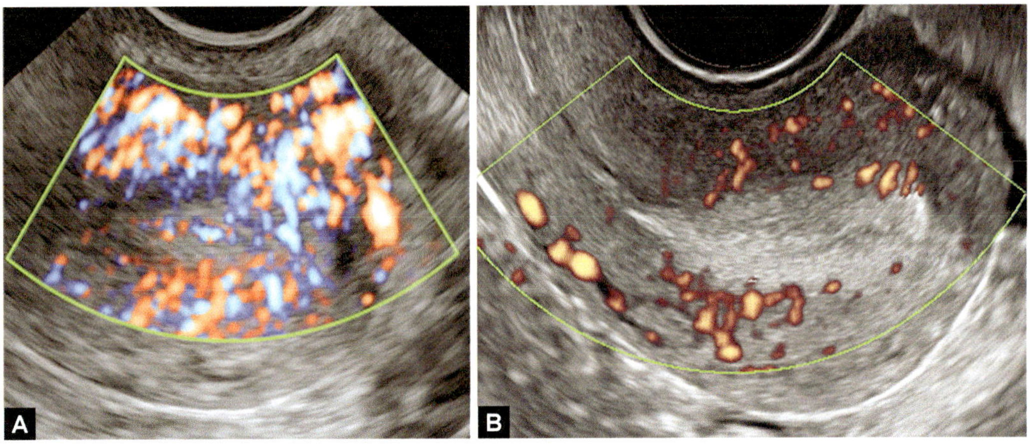

Figs. 2A and B: (A) Normal secretory endometrial flow; (B) Scanty secretory endometrial flow—luteal phase defect.

Controversies in Diagnosis

- Luteal phase defect can exist with normal progesterone levels.[10]
- There may be no correlation between endometrial histology and serum progesterone.
- Pregnancy can continue with lower serum progesterone levels.
- Serum progesterone and EB are not related tests.
- Some papers say that E2:P ratio is more important than only progesterone levels.[11]
- No tests can stamp the diagnosis.

The timing of embryo transfer depends on the duration of exposure rather than blood levels.[12]

LUTEAL PHASE SUPPORT

There are two dilemmas:

1. What to use for luteal support?
2. When to use luteal support?

What to Use for Luteal Support?

- Progesterone
- Human chorionic gonadotropin
- Gonadotropin-releasing hormone agonist (GnRHa)
- Addition of E2

Different Progesterone Preparations

Natural progesterone:

- *Not commonly used routes*:
  - Intranasal
  - Sublingual
  - Rectal
- *Commonly used routes*:
  - Oral
  - Injectable
  - Vaginal routes

Oral progesterones:

- It is available as soft gelatin capsules or tablet form and as sustained-release tablets.
- It causes drowsiness, flushing, and nausea and it has selective and hypnotic effect because of metabolites.
- It causes fluid retention.
- Efficacy changes with food particle size and its vehicle. Bioavailability is only 10% when taken orally.
- Extensive first-pass hepatic metabolism and therefore multiple doses required. It has poor intestinal absorption.
- It is ineffective in inducing an in-phase secretory endometrium.[13]
- It has lower pregnancy rate.

Oral sustained-release tablets: Slow-release (SR) EROMAT is a new technology. The drug is released gradually in a controlled manner over a span of 16–24 hours in the distal part of the gastrointestinal (GI) tract allowing lymphatic absorption of intact drug into systematic circulation and direct entry of the drug through the mucosal lining of colon into systemic circulation. The dose of sustained-release progesterone capsule is 200–400 mg daily. This has less side effects compared to conventional oral preparation. Only 20% of the drug is released in first 4 hours and minimizes hepatic and prehepatic metabolism. Rest of the drug is released in distal GI tract. The serum P level should be >14 ng/mL for threatened abortion and LPD. Oral SR preparations, 400/300/200 mg/day gives blood levels up to 46.2/36.2/20.6 ng/mL, respectively.

The drug at present is available in very few countries and there are not many international trials available to prove its role. The sole application of this drug is not recommended by majority of the assisted reproductive technology (ART) clinics. It is always used in combination of other progesterones. This drug still requires further studies in spite of its wide availability.

Injectable progesterone:

- *Intramuscular (IM) progesterone*:
  - It gives high serum concentrations, adequate endometrial secretory features, and satisfactory pregnancy rates, comparable to vaginal progesterone.
  - Daily injections are uncomfortable and very painful and may result in inferior secretory endometrial histology.
  - It can cause inflammation at injection site leading to redness, pain, and even sterile abscess at injection site because of the preservative (Benzyl alcohol) used.
  - Rarely it may also cause acute eosinophilic pneumonia.
  - It is not preferred in favor of vaginal progesterone or subcutaneous progesterone injection.

- Subcutaneous aqueous progesterone preparations are also available now, in which progesterone is combined with cyclodextrin, a starch residue, and is given as 25 mg or 50 mg doses a day and has shown results compatible with IM progesterone.[14] Gillian et al. have proved that subcutaneous injection of water-soluble progesterone 25 mg is safe and as effective as vaginal progesterone gel and remains an option for those, who do not want vaginal progesterone for cultural, personal, or medical reasons.[15]

  Transdermal progesterone is not the option because the skin is rich in five reductase, which will inactivate progesterone. Another reason is that daily E2 production is 0.5 mg/day, while that of progesterone is 25 mg/day. Such large doses are difficult to deliver by transdermal patches.
- *Vaginal progesterone*: Vaginal suppositories: Vaginal application is the most accepted route for progesterone administration **(Box 2)**. It has several advantages:
  - It avoids all GI side effects, sedative and hypnotic effect.
  - *The first uterine pass effect (FUPE)* ***(Fig. 3)*** *is another major advantage*: From the vagina, the drug is directly transported to the uterus. So in spite of low blood levels of progesterone, its level in uterus is high. Migration of the drug occurs from cervix and lower segment of uterus to the fundus of the uterus.[16] A countercurrent exchange **(Figs. 4A and B)** also occurs in the upper third of the vagina. The drug is absorbed in the veins of the vagina and from there directly goes to the arteries of the uterus, without entering into the general circulation. This leads to low serum level but high concentrations in the uterus.[17-19]

These mechanisms lead to consistent tissue level of progesterone with vaginal application.[16] In spite of low blood levels.

Box 2: Natural micronized progesterone.

- Reduced size
- Enhances dissolution
- Maximum serum concentration
- Reduced destruction
- Increases half life

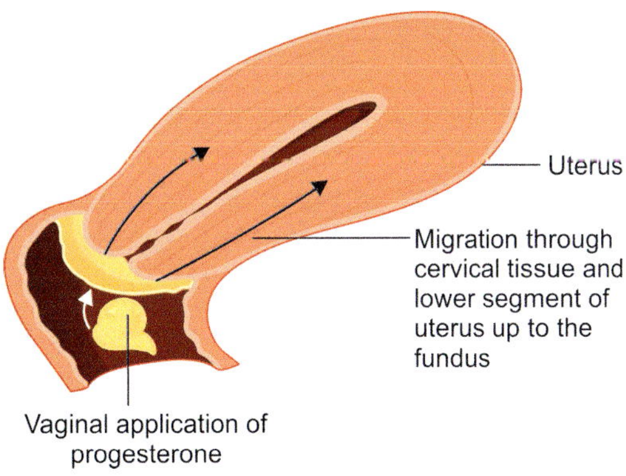

Fig. 3: Diagrammatic representation of uterine first-pass effect.

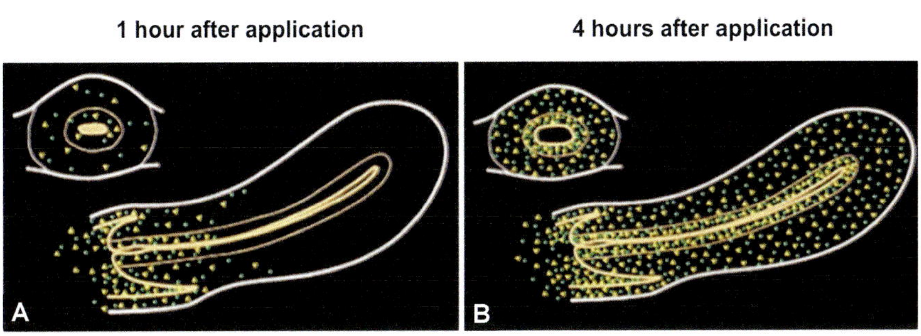

Figs. 4A and B: Progressive diffusion of progesterone from the cervix to the fundus of the uterus.

This improves implantation rates and decreases early pregnancy loss.[20]

Czajkowski et al. proved that vaginal progesterone 300 mg is effective in reducing spiral artery pulsatility, pulsatility index (PI), and systolic/diastolic (S/D) ratio as compared to 30 mg of oral dyhydrogestone.[21] Mohammed A et al. have found in their study that vaginal versus IM progesterone for luteal support in ART in systematic review and meta-analysis of randomized controlled trial (RCT) that vaginal progesterone has same results as IM progesterone in ART and is more satisfactory.[22]

- *Progesterone vaginal effervescent tablets*: This is a new delivery system of progesterone. Disintegration of tablet occurs in 7–10 minutes. It increases absorption. Twice a day dosage can achieve higher concentration of progesterone and reach steady state within 24–32 hours and maintain mean concentration above 10 ng/mL.[23]

  As explained in **Figure 5**, the absorption of progesterone occurs by passive diffusion as well as paracellular transport which results in greater concentration and prolonged blood levels. CO_2 opens up tight junctions of the cells and so paracervical absorption is increased.

  Advantages of effervescent tablet:
  - Greater bioavailability
  - Effective systemic absorption
  - Avoids hepatic first-pass metabolism
  - Higher concentration in endometrium
  - Lower doses are required
  - Less fluctuation in serum levels
  - Healthy vaginal environment because of acidic pH
  - As efficient as other vaginal progesterone
  - Less irritation and discharge
- Vaginal progesterone rings are also available now. These rings once inserted would release 10–20 nmol/L for 90 days. Compared to 50 mg/day IM progesterone, this product has shown comparable or better implantation rate.[24]
- *Progesterone gel*: It contains 90 mg (8%) of progesterone. It contains micronized progesterone in emulsion system which also contains water-insoluble polymer,

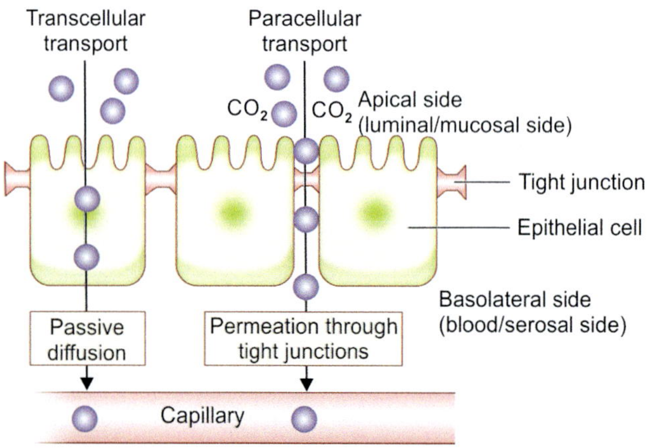

Fig. 5: Diagrammatic explanation of the vaginal absorption of effervescent progesterone vaginal tablets (from monogram Susten VT).

"Polycarbophil" having mucin-like actions. It is as effective as vaginal tablets. There is no substantial difference in the ongoing pregnancy rate between vaginal progesterone gel and vaginal micronized progesterone tablets.[25] But vaginal gel has given higher pregnancy rates than IM progesterone below the age of 35 years in in vitro fertilization (IVF) patients and after the age of 35 years, pregnancy rates were same for both the gel and the IM progesterone group.[26] Its dosage schedule is once a day, so acceptance is very good. The only disadvantage of this preparation is its high cost. Gel preparation is always used in the morning and the patient is advised not to rest after that. Because of the movements, friction occurs between the vaginal walls and that helps to separate progesterone and facilitate its absorption. Absorption will be poor if it is applied at night. If it is to be applied twice a day, the evening application should be at least 3–4 hours before bedtime.

- *Progesterone combinations*:
  - *P + E2*: No role except in long protocol where it may improve implantation.[27]
  - *P + Ascorbic acid*: No role[28]
  - *P + Prednisolone*: No role[29]
  - *P + Aspirin*: No role[30]
  - Prednisolone and aspirin might have a role in recurrent IVF failures.

Synthetic progesterones: Dydrogesterone is the drug which is available since 60 years. In spite of that much RCTs are not available in the literature. Formerly drug was marketed for its use in recurrent pregnancy loss (RPL) and early pregnancy loss. But since last few years, few workers have tried and documented it for luteal phase support.

Former studies by Fatemi et al.[31] documented that all oral progesterones including dydrogesterone do not give "in phase" endometrium, when used as luteal phase support. Other trials also advocated vaginal progesterone for better pregnancy rates, when compared with oral progesterones.

But recently LOTUS I and LOTUS II trial compared dydrogesterone 30 mg with 600 mg vaginal progesterone or 8% micronized vaginal progesterone (MVP) gel. In these studies, the pregnancy rates and the live birth rates were the same.[32,33]

Infant safety data are similar in these studies and maternal safety profile is also normal with both the drugs. It is recommended as the drug can be taken orally.

LOTUS are the only trials available at present, and are supported by the pharma.[32,33] Though this drug is available for many years, very few studies are available. More RCTs are required for further research that can give the correct idea about the role of this drug in luteal support. As mentioned earlier, these studies have compared the effect of dydrogesterone with 600 mg of MVP, but in most ART clinics, the dose of MVP used is 800–1200 mg/day. So studies with higher dose of MVP are recommended. Most centers do not use dydrogesterone alone as luteal support in ART cycles. It is used in combination with other progesterone supplement. Therefore, its efficacy cannot be clearly established. There better planned and larger studies are required to evaluate the effect of dydrogesterone as luteal phase support.

Two Indian studies compared 20 mg and 30 mg of dydrogesterone with 600 mg of MVP and claimed superiority of dydrogesterone between 2005 and 2007.[34,35] But these were single-center studies and to prove the efficacy of the drug, larger multicentric studies are required.

A study by Fatemi et al.[36] concluded that dydrogesterone has not proved its efficacy in absence of endogenous progesterone and therefore in presence of endogenous progesterone (as in natural cycle) the efficacy of dydrogesterone is difficult to establish. In frozen embryo transfer (FET) cycles effect of dydrogesterone is not much studied. As mentioned earlier also, in these cases dydrogesterone is used with other progesterone also since endogenous progesterone is absent.

European Society of Human Reproduction and Embryology (ESHRE) 2017 guidelines also are for RPL and not for luteal phase support (LPS). So, though LOTUS trial shows promising results for dydrogesterone for LPS, further larger and independent trials are required.

Human Chorionic Gonadotropin Supplementation

In a normo-ovulatory female, in unstimulated cycle, administration of hCG in luteal phase does not downregulate LH secretion in luteal phase.[37] It stimulates theca lutein cells to produce more progesterone and other steroids that are required for the maintenance of normal pregnancy. hCG also increases the placental protein 4 and relaxing that is required for implantation. It is administered every 3–4 days. It is given in the dosage of 2,000 IU on Day 3, 7, 10, or 5,000 IU on Day 5–9 postovulatory. It is an excellent drug in non-IVF patients and in poor responders in IVF also. But if the pre-trigger E2 is more than 1,600 IUI intrauterine insemination (IUI) cycle and more than 4,000 IU in IVF cycle, hCG is not given as a trigger for the risk of ovarian hyperstimulation syndrome (OHSS). In these cases, agonist is given as a trigger. In these cases, hCG 1,500 IU is given at the time of IUI or at the time of ovum pick-up (OPU) to rescue the CL, if the number of follicles are not more than 25 of more than 11 mm in diameter. It gives equal pregnancy rates as hCG trigger and avoids OHSS.[38,39]

It can be used safely even in IVF cycles especially in poor responders. But now since antagonist can be used to suppress LH surge and agonist can be used for ovulation trigger, hCG in these patients can be used in the dose of 1,500 IU every fourth day as a luteal phase support.

Disadvantages of hCG:

- It should not be given when E2 is >1,600 pg/mL in IUI cycles and >4,000 pg/mL in IVF cycles because of development of OHSS and multiple pregnancies.
- When there are more follicles, it will increase E2 and may change E2:P which may decrease implantation but this is only a theoretical assumption.
- Even the low dose of hCG as 1,500 IU is given, every 3 days after agonist trigger, can cause OHSS.[38]
- Prolonged hCG exposure in proliferative phase may affect endometrial receptivity.[40] During natural menstrual cycle, LH in luteal phase seldom exceeds 5–10 IU/mL, which is capable of eliciting progesterone level in excess of 25–35 nmol/L. So supraphysiological levels of LH/hCG are not required in luteal phase. Endogenous progesterone is very high due to multiple corpus lutea and exogenous progesterone results in concentration of <75 nmol/L only.
- Microdose supplement 100–150 IU/day of hCG throughout the luteal phase without using any exogenous progesterone is sufficient. The progesterone level thus achieved is similar to that achieved when ovulation trigger is given by 6,500 IU

hCG and progesterone support. When this microdose hCG is used with agonist trigger, hCG levels remain within physiological limits, i.e., 5–10 IU/mL. The only difficulty is the delivery of microdose.[41]

Gonadotropin-releasing Hormone Agonist as Luteal Phase Support

Gonadotropin-releasing hormone agonist increases LH secretion from pituitary. It acts directly on endometrium through locally expressed GnRH receptors.[42]

- Agonist increases serum hCG, by acting on embryos, E2, and progesterone levels in luteal phase of agonist and antagonist cycles.[43]
- But adverse effects on oocytes and embryos need evaluation by larger studies.

Gonadotropin-releasing hormone agonist is used for luteal support as it stimulates to release LH from the pituitary. It is used in combination with progesterone. It is given after 6 days after oocyte retrieval or 3 days after embryo transfer. It increases implantation and pregnancy rate in ART.[44] Pirard et al. introduced daily injection of GnRHa (Nafarelin 200 µg twice a day) for 14 days for luteal support giving similar results.[42] Cochrane meta-analysis demonstrated significantly higher pregnancy rate when progesterone luteal support was combined with GnRHa compared with progesterone alone without influencing the miscarriage rate or multiple pregnancy rate.[45] GnRHa acts on CL, endometrium, and embryo by secretion of LH. Buserelin 200 µg twice a day or leuprolide acetate 1 mg as a single or multiple diseases can be given as a luteal support. It avoids OHSS in hyper-responders.

Estradiol Supplementation in Luteal Phase

Estradiol supplementation is mandatory to prepare the endometrium for the embryo recipient model. But several papers show that E2 supplementation is not necessary in luteal phase. In an IVF cycle, levels of estrogen and progesterone drop in mid- to late luteal phase. It has not been proved that this drop has an effect on clinical pregnancy rates in a meta-analysis conducted by Fatemi et al., whether only progesterone or estrogen plus progesterone were added in luteal phase.[46] Low E2 depletes the progesterone receptors and changes the endometrial receptor dynamics. E2 inhibits reactive oxygen species (ROS)-induced apoptosis of CL cells. It decreases HOXA-10 expression. Pregnancy rate is decreased in long protocol because increased E2 in the proliferative phase gives negative feedback and decreases LH secretion that prevents E2 and progesterone production from CL. So estrogen supplementation (4 mg E2 valerate) is useful in long protocols for a higher pregnancy rate.[47] E2 production in luteal phase is dependent on LH or hCG and not on FSH and so serum LH level assessment is a must and beta hCG helps in production of E2 in pregnancy. Addition of E2 is different when GnRHa is used as trigger. Here it is always necessary as there is deficiency of LH and CL is not at all stimulated to produce E2 and progesterone.

When to Use Luteal Support?

- Natural cycle
- Clomiphene citrate (CC)
- Letrozole
- Gonadotropin stimulation
- hCG trigger
- GnRH agonist in the long protocol
- GnRH antagonist protocol

- GnRH agonist trigger
- FET cycles

These are the clinical situations when luteal support is used. Let us now evaluate the role of luteal support in each particular situation and also understand why this support is required.

Luteal Support in Natural Cycle

In natural cycle when follicle develops, E2 is >150 pg/mL/follicle. This E2 is sufficient to develop progesterone receptors and to cause positive feedback for LH release. This high LH lasts for more than 48 hours and is enough to rescue the corpus luteal function. These FSH and LH surge last for about 48 hours. The LH surge has a short ascending phase of 14 hours, a peak plateau of 20 hours, and descending phase of 20 hours. This LH surge is sufficient to maintain luteal phase and so routine use of progesterone in luteal phase is not justified in natural unstimulated cycles.[1] So routine use of progesterone is not justified in natural cycle. Progesterone is therefore not routinely started after spontaneous rupture of the follicle.

The cause of LPD in natural non-ART cycles is abnormal folliculogenesis. Unhealthy follicle produces less E2, leading to less progesterone receptors and lower peak of LH. This lower LH peak will give unhealthy CL and low progesterone levels. The clinical situations when LH surge is inadequate are:

- Hypoprolactinemia
- Extremes of age
- Stress
- Polycystic ovarian syndrome (PCOS)
- Endometriosis
- Obesity
- Anorexia
- Athletes
- Postpartum
- Infections

Hypothalamo-pituitary dysfunction disturbs GnRH pulsatility, which in turn disturbs FSH and LH secretion which leads to abnormal folliculogenesis and LPD. So, all these patients require ovulation induction to improve quality of the follicle.

Luteal phase support with CC: Clomiphene acts on hypothalamus and pituitary to secrete FSH and LH that leads to development of follicles and secretes more estrogen. High estrogen causes upregulation of LH and progesterone receptors. Therefore, in clomiphene-stimulated cycles, LPD is not common. In spite of estrogen receptors being occupied by CC, multiple follicles develop and there is no abnormality of LH or progesterone secretion because of high E2 level. LPD found in CC cycle is due to high LH, particularly in PCOS patients, that is detrimental to ovum leading to abnormal folliculogenesis, and is responsible for LPD. Adding estrogen to clomiphene is not proved to improve the pregnancy rate. So, luteal phase support is not justified in clomiphene cycles.

Luteal phase support in letrozole stimulated cycle: Letrozole prevents aromatization of androgen to estrogen leading to estrogen deficiency. This E2 deficiency has negative feedback to pituitary causing the release of FSH and LH which develops follicle. E2 from developed follicle goes to pituitary and decreases FSH and LH to give monofollicular development. This decrease in LH may cause LPD and a decrease in E2 may lead to poor development of progesterone receptors. Therefore when letrozole is used for ovulation induction luteal phase support is indicated, though sufficient literature on the same is still not available. Luteal support with vaginal progesterone increases clinical pregnancy rate in women with PCOS using letrozole for ovulation induction.[48]

Luteal phase support in gonadotropin-stimulated cycles: Exogenous gonadotropins affect the ovaries to produce more E2. This leads to negative feedback to hypothalamo-pituitary ovarian (HPO) axis and may lead to abnormal LH pulsatility and abnormal progesterone secretion from CL.[49] Though progesterone is important for pregnancy, elevated progesterone level on the day of trigger, affects pregnancy rates adversely. Progesterone level of 1.5 ng/mL is a threshold for poor ovarian responders, greater than 1.75 ng/mL is associated with low ongoing pregnancy rates for intermediate responders and 2.25 ng/mL can be applied for high responders.[50] This progesterone level is elevated in superovulated cycles as each mature follicle secretes a trace of progesterone. Endometrium is exposed to progesterone before hCG injection leads to decreased endometrial receptivity.[51] A systematic review and meta-analysis suggest that luteal phase support improved the likelihood of clinical pregnancy and live birth in gonadotropin stimulated IUI cycles.[52]

It is an established fact that luteal phase is defective in all stimulated cycles.[38] In controlled ovarian stimulation, there are multiple follicles which grow giving supraphysiological levels of E2 and progesterone which inhibits LH secretion by the pituitary by negative feedback at hypothalamo-pituitary axis level for LH release which causes early demise of CL and fall in progesterone level.[53] Moreover, agonist or antagonist has already suppressed LH in follicular phase and therefore endogenous LH is very low. Adequate LH is important for maintenance of CL. So, luteal phase support is required in all the patients when agonists or antagonists are used. Endogenous LH is also important for secretion of other growth factors and cytokines and leukemia inhibitory factor (LIF) for implantation. Exogenous hCG helps to rescue CL. In gonadotropin stimulation, there is advancement of histology in late proliferative phase, earlier shift into implantation window and asynchrony if the maturation of mid and late luteal phase due to high E2, i.e., altered E2:P ratio.[54] So in all gonadotropin-stimulated cycles, luteal phase support is mandatory.

Luteal phase support with hCG trigger: In follicular phase, LH is low because of agonist or antagonist as well as high E2 and progesterone giving negative feedback to pituitary for LH. However, early luteal phase function of LH is covered by bolus of hCG (5,000–10,000 IU), which is routinely used for trigger. hCG also secures growth factors and cytokines for implantation. Normally 500 IU of hCG is required for completion of meiosis and 9,500 IU of hCG is required for follicular rupture. Therefore in IUI cycles usually 10,000 IU of hCG is given. But this dose may be too large for ART cycles. But this large dose takes care of the CL in the early luteal phase and maintains progesterone secretion from CL. The hCG supports corpus luteum only for 5 days and the embryo starts producing hCG after the 8th day after ovulation, that will again support the CL. So from 5th till 8th day, CL is not supported and there is progesterone deficiency and is known as "luteal gap" and leads to implantation failure or early abortions.[55]

After Day 5, endogenous LH levels are also low due to high surrogate LH and high progesterone.[56] It is crucial to have a certain amplitude and frequency of LH during the luteal phase. Progesterone supplement is therefore essential for the luteal phase support when hCG trigger is given.[45]

Luteal phase support with GnRHa downregulation: Downregulation in ART cycles is started from Day 21 of the previous cycle. GnRHa is given daily till menstruation starts and after menstruation starts the dose of GnRHa is reduced to half. The purpose of giving GnRHa is to prevent premature LH surge. This happens because GnRHa reduces LH pulsatility and very low levels of LH are present right from Day 21 of the previous cycle till the day of ovulation trigger. These low LH levels continue during the luteal phase also, do not support the CL and cause severe LPD. Due to prolonged suppression of FSH and LH, all agonist downregulated cycles require judicious luteal support.[57] Though in most centers now GnRHa cycles are replaced by GnRH antagonist cycles, these are still used in the centers where group IVF is practiced. Pituitary gonadotropins remain suppressed for 2–3 weeks after discontinuation of agonist and luteal phase support is necessary because of low E2 and P.[58]

Luteal phase support when using antagonist: Antagonist downregulation is now a preferred protocol in majority of the ART centers instead of agonist downregulation. Antagonist is started from Day 5 to 6 of the start of stimulation in the fixed antagonist protocol or from the day the lead follicle reaches 14 mm, if using the flexible protocol. It suppresses the LH level temporarily before ovulation triggers.

It was formerly believed that antagonist cycles do not require luteal phase support and so lots of pregnancies were wasted. But then it was understood that suppression of LH by antagonist also continues in the luteal phase and it reduces luteal phase length and compromises pregnancy rate. So luteal phase support is always required after the OPU in cases when fresh transfer is planned.[59]

Antagonist downregulation decreases the risk of OHSS and does allow the use of agonist as a trigger, thus almost abolishing the risk of OHSS.

GnRHa trigger and luteal phase support: GnRHa trigger is preferred to hCG trigger when:

- There is a risk of OHSS.
- When preimplantation genetic diagnosis/ preimplantation genetic screening (PGD/ PGS) is to be done.
- In donor cycles
- When fresh transfers are not to be done.

Gonadotropin-releasing hormone agonist causes FSH and LH surge, while hCG causes only LH surge. FSH surge is a must in animals for completion of meiosis of the ovum and rupture of the follicle, but its role in human being is not yet fully understood. LH surge that occurs after GnRHa trigger completes meiosis but is inadequate for the luteal support and thus leads to LPD. LH surge that occurs after GnRHa has only 4 hours of ascending limb and 14 hours of descending limb, whereas the natural LH surge has an ascending limb of 14 hours, the plateau of 20 hours, and descending limb of 20 hours. This gap between the two cannot be bridged by increasing the dose of GnRHa as the defect is because of low LH. The normal progesterone level on OPU + Day 5 of 11 ng/mL was only achieved after 600 mg/day of exogenous progesterone which indicates complete luteal phase insufficiency after agonist trigger.

Strategies for supporting luteal phase after GnRHa trigger:

- Exogenous E2 + P support with close monitoring
- *Dual trigger*: Agonist + hCG (1,000–2,500 IU)
- hCG 1,500 IU at the time of oocyte retrieval
- Low-dose hCG in luteal phase
- Luteal phase LH administration

Strategies are used for fresh embryo transfers:

- *Intensive luteal support*: IM progesterone 25–75 mg/day or micronized progesterone 800 mg/day vaginally with E2 patch 0.1 mg, 3–4, on alternate days or 2–8 mg with oral E2 valerate is given. Adjust the dose to keep serum E2 level above 200 pg/mL and progesterone level 20 ng/mL by frequent testing. The results are similar to those of hCG trigger and progesterone support.[60]
- *Dual trigger*: Agonist + hCG (1,000–2,500 IU): Along with GnRHa trigger, hCG 1,000–2,500 IU is added for rescuing CL by providing additional signal for adequate luteinization. It has given pregnancy rate up to 53% with one case of OHSS.[46] If serum E2 is < 4000 pg/mL, GnRHa trigger with 1,000–2,500 IU of hCG gives pregnancy rates as high as 53% with almost no risk of OHSS.

  So, hCG at the time of ovulation trigger gives excellent pregnancy rates with very low OHSS risk. The other advantage of dual trigger is that sometimes LH peak may not be sufficient with agonist trigger and if it is <9 IU/mL, meiosis may not occur and on OPU no ova will be retrieved, as it may occur in empty follicle syndrome. Adding low-dose hCG with agonist assures meiosis and is therefore preferred compared to low-dose hCG at the time of OPU.
- *Human chorionic gonadotropin at the time of OPU*: When pretrigger E2 is <4,000 pg/mL or when there are less than 25 follicles of >11 mm in diameter, hCG 1,500 IU is given at the time of oocyte retrieval to rescue the CL and achieve comparable pregnancy rates to hCG trigger. Second bolus is not given as it may increase the risk of OHSS.[61]

  So, modified luteal phase support may be—GnRHa trigger, hCG 1,500 IU after IUI or OPU, vaginal micronized progesterone 400 mg BD, and E2 2 mg BD supplementation. This regimen reduces OHSS and gives more eggs with equal live birth rates.[61]
- *Low-dose beta hCG*: 100–150 IU hCG as luteal support is enough to rescue the CL and produce sufficient progesterone for adequate luteal support.[62] In the same paper, it has also been mentioned that it cause blood levels of progesterone as high as 10–15 IU/L, which is sufficient for mid-luteal phase and is similar to 6,500 IU of hCG for ovulation trigger and vaginal progesterone. But the delivery of this small dose of hCG is difficult at present. This might prove to be a choice of luteal phase support if hCG becomes available in Pen device.
- *Recombinant LH*: It is very useful as it lowers the incidence of OHSS for fresh cycle transfer. But it is very expensive and therefore its usage is not accepted in clinical practice.

Luteal phase support in FET cycles:

- *Frozen embryo transfers is indicated for*:
  - *Prevention of OHSS*: When PGS or PGD is required.
  - When progesterone rises >1.5 ng/mL in proliferative phase.
  - Fluid in uterine cavity
  - Patient's choice
  - Clinician's preference, as freezing of embryos and transfer later has shown better results.
- *Physiology of implantation*:
  - Window of implantation is the time when endometrium supports trophoblast-endometrial interaction occurs around 22–24 days of 28 days

cycle,[63] i.e., 3–4 days after ovulation and opens for 4–5 days.
  - Endometrium is unchanged in thickness in secretory phase but epithelium and vasculature continue to grow and result in dense endometrium.
  - During the window of implantation, a number of specific proteins and biochemical markers are present that can be known by microarrays.
  - Subendometrial wave activity reduces implantation and may cause ectopic pregnancy. These are due to high estrogen levels.
  - Progesterone > 20 ng/mL on the day of transfer in FET cycle gives lower pregnancy rate.
  - High pregnancy rates in FET cycle teach that all the substances secreted from the ovary except estrogen and progesterone such as androgen, peptides are harmful for good endometrial receptivity.
- *Frozen embryo transfer can be done in*:
  - Natural cycle FET (NC-FET)
  - Modified natural cycle FET (mNC-FET)
  - Artificial cycle FET (AC-FET)
  - Agonist cycle
  - Natural cycle transfer
- *Natural cycle FET*:
  - In NC-FET cycle, E2 and progesterone are derived from spontaneous follicular development and ovulation. So this method is to be offered to the patient with ovulatory cycles.
  - In natural cycle, by urinary LH kit, LH surge is detected and progesterone is started. But in several cases endometrium may be out of phase.[64]
  - This may be due to inaccurate determination of ovulation and also due to cycle-to-cycle variation.
  - Embryo transfer is done on LH + Day 6.
  - So they may benefit from progesterone supplementation.[64]
- *Modified natural cycle with hCG*:
  - Give hCG when follicle is 17–18 mm in size.
  - Progesterone support is not required.
  - Embryo transfer is done on hCG + Day 7.
  - Results of NC-FET and mNC-FET are the same.
  - Premature LH or progesterone rise is possible and should be measured. But progesterone rise does not change the pregnancy rate in FET cycle and cancellation of cycle because of elevated LH is not done.[65]
- *Artificial cycle FET (AC-FET)*:
  - E2, 4–12 mg for 2–3 weeks, till endometrium becomes 8 mm with vascularity in zone 3–4.
  - Abortion rate is increased when E2 is given for <12 or >28 days.
  - Transdermal or oral drugs have the same results.
  - E2 4–6 mg in early stage prevents follicular growth.
  - High E2 prevents follicular development.
  - Progesterone is given for 3–5 days according to the day of transfer.
  - Day 5 transfer gives better results than Day 6 transfer.[66]
  - As CL is not there, luteal support is given for 12 weeks.

If endometrial peristalsis is <5/min on the previous day than the embryo transfer (FET) should be done, otherwise, review progesterone dosage. Personalized embryo transfer is useful by adding progesterone for 1–3 days in cases of delayed endometrial maturity.

Luteal support with progesterone 800 mg/day in FET cycles may give blood progesterone levels of 9.2 ng/mL in 25% of cases. This reduces the ongoing pregnancy rate and pregnancies are sacrificed. So IM progesterone is recommended every third day.[67]

Therefore, apart from vaginal progesterone, if aqueous progesterone is also given subcutaneously, it improves on-going pregnancy rates in FET cycles.

Gonadotropin-releasing hormone agonist downregulation (programmed FET regimen): It prevents spontaneous follicular development and ovulation. After 5 days of progesterone, endometrium mimics that of the 20th day of 28 days cycle.

In 25%, there is a delay of endometrial development; so, a mock cycle with microarray or biopsy may be preferred. Routinely agonists are not used in FET cycle as it does not have much benefit.

- *Additional luteal support in FET cycles*:
  - Serum progesterone level on Day 7 after 800 mg progesterone per day in woman for FET cycle, 25% of women had P level of <9.2 ng/mL and ongoing pregnancy rate was markedly reduced. So, if these findings are correct, we must be sacrificing numerous pregnancies when we use only vaginal progesterone as luteal support.[68]
  - In FET cycles apart from vaginal progesterone twice a day, IM progesterone is recommended every third day for better results.[69]
  - In natural cycle FET, hCG used as luteal support, does not improve the pregnancy rates.[70]
  - NC-FET, mNC-FET, and AC-FET give the same results.

PROGESTERONE RESISTANCE

- Endometriosis
- Polycystic ovarian syndrome with androgen elevation

Progesterone resistance is because of inhibitor progesterone receptor isoform (PR-A) and the absence of the stimulation isoform PRB.[71] There is pituitary ovarian dysfunction.[72] This is because of impaired follicular growth giving low FSH and LH because of low E2 and causing LPD. It causes abnormal expression of endometrial biomarkers of implantation.[73] But this is a controversial issue. In case of progesterone resistance, luteal support will not be efficient until the resistance is removed. So before initiating the treatment, progesterone resistance must be dealt with. In endometriosis, ART outcome was improved by 3–6 months of ovarian suppression by GnRHa.[74] Recently it has been shown that 6–8 weeks with oral contraceptive (OC) pills normalized implantation and pregnancy rates in women suffering from endometriosis.[75] It is doubtful if similar treatment is helpful in PCOS. This is because of androgen excess. OC pills lower the LH and in turn androgen. Whether higher levels of progesterone can counter progesterone resistance or not, is also not proved.

ONSET OF LUTEAL SUPPORT

Progesterone started on the day of oocyte retrieval decreases uterine contractility on the day of transfer rather than started late. Uterine contractility was higher 4 days after hCG administration than the natural cycle LH surge. Higher E2 level increases uterine contractility and this high E2 causes uterine resistance to the uterine relaxing property of progesterone.[76] The vaginal progesterone causes selective tissue concentration in the uterus through direct transport. There is no harm in starting the luteal support from the day of oocyte retrieval.[47] There is no difference when luteal support is started on the day of hCG, on the day of ovum retrieval or the day of embryo transfer.[77] The onset of luteal phase support should not be later than Day 3 after ovum retrieval. But if it is started before OPU or at the time of trigger, it closes the window of receptivity earlier. There is endometrial advancement because of increased E2 and progesterone in the proliferative phase. Increased E2 is because of high androgen secreted from theca cells, where granulosa cells convert it into estrogen. So progesterone being an intermediate product, always is high whenever E2 is high in proliferative phase. So even normal progesterone level will appear early and initiate premature secretory changes. This leads to advancement of endometrium. Therefore, whether the progesterone is started on the day of hCG or day of OPU or within 3 days of OPU, pregnancy rates are the same.[77]

Vaginal progesterone if it is delayed for a day or two, gives good results as compared to IM progesterone which is given on the day of oocyte retrieval. So the route of administration is also important along with the starting day of the luteal support.[26]

DURATION OF LUTEAL SUPPORT

Prospective RCT[78] indicated that prolongation of progesterone supplementation in early pregnancy had no influence on miscarriage rate. Theoretically, we can stop progesterone support once beta hCG is positive, but most of the IVF specialists continue till 10–12 weeks of pregnancy. Caspo et al. have shown that continuation of pregnancy is independent of CL function as early as 8–10 weeks of pregnancy.[79] The function is taken over by the placenta.[80] It has shown that vaginal progesterone supplementation after ART can be safely withdrawn at 5 weeks of gestation because cycle outcome was similar to conventional luteal support that is given till 8 weeks of gestation.[77] At 5 weeks, hCG level is >1,000 IU/L and that is sufficient to support CL. The circulating level of progesterone is >8 ng/mL at 5 weeks of pregnancy. But in FET cycle, it is continued till the luteo-placental shift, i.e., 9–10 weeks of pregnancy.

CARRY HOME MESSAGE

- Luteal phase defect is because of low progesterone or suboptimal response with normal progesterone.
- Low progesterone may be due to abnormal folliculogenesis in non-IVF patients.
- Low LH is mainly responsible for LPD in IVF cycles.
- No laboratory tests are reliable for the diagnosis of LPD.
- Corpus luteum rescue is because of hCG.
- Low progesterone is because of low hCG in unhealthy embryo.
- Duration of exposure to progesterone is important than blood levels.
- Ovulation induction is a very useful luteal support.
- Human chorionic gonadotropin is also an effective luteal support. 100–150 IU of hCG may prove to be a good alternative to luteal support.
- Micronized progesterone is the best.
- Vaginal route is the best route.
- Subcutaneous route has replaced IM route.
- Luteal support in natural cycle is not justified.
- Progesterone support in CC cycle is not of much benefit.
- Progesterone support is required in letrozole-stimulated cycle.
- Dyhydrogestone and SR tablets are undertrial.
- All superovulated cycles require luteal support.
- Agonist and antagonist cycles cause LPD.
- With GnRHa trigger luteal support is always required.
- Judicious use of E2 + P, dual trigger or 1,500 IU of hCG at the time of pick up are remedies for fresh transfer.
- "Freeze all" can avoid OHSS.
- Results of NC-FET, mNC-FET, and AC-FET are the same.
- E2 supplementation is given for LPS in long protocol and agonist trigger.

Contd...

Contd...

- Endometriosis and PCOS have progesterone resistance.
- Luteal support should not be started later than 3 days after ovum retrieval.
- Duration of progesterone after positive beta hCG is controversial.
- All FET cycles should be given luteal phase support for 10–12 weeks.

REFERENCES

1. Speroff L, Fritz MA. Clinical Gynecologic Endocrinology and Infertility, 7th re-edition. Philadelphia: Lippincott Williams and Wilkins; 2005. pp. 199-242.
2. Niswender GD, Juengel JL, Silva PJ, Rollyson MK, McIntush EW. Mechanisms controlling the function and lifespan of the corpus luteum. Physiol Rev. 2000;80:1-29.
3. Hinney B, Henze C, Kuhn W, Wuttke W. The corpus luteum insufficiency: a multifactorial disease. J Clin Endocrinol Metab. 1996; 81:565-70.
4. Kiriakidou M, McAllister JM, Sugawara T, Strauss JF. Expression of steroidogenic acute regulatory protein (StAR) in the human ovary. J Clin Endocrinol Metab. 1996;814:122-8.
5. Daya S. Habitual abortion. In: Copeland LJ (Ed). Textbook of Gynecology. Philadelphia: WB Saunders; 2000.
6. The Practice Committee of the American Society of Reproductive Medicine. The clinical relevance of luteal phase deficiency: a committee opinion. Fertil Steril. 2012; 98(5):1112-7.
7. Jarvela IY, Ruokonen A, Tekay A. Effect of rising hCG levels in the human corpus luteum during early pregnancy. Hum Reprod. 2008;23(12):2275-81.
8. Balasch J, Vanrell JA. Corpus luteum insufficiency and fertility: a matter of controversy. Hum Reprod. 1987;2:557-67.
9. Jordan J, Craig K, Clifton D, Soules MR. Luteal phase defect: the sensitivity and specificity of diagnostic methods in common clinical use. Fertil Steril. 1994;62:54.
10. Check JH, Levin E, Bollendorf A, Locuniak J. Miscarriage in the first trimester according to the presence or absence of the progesterone induced blocking factor at three to five weeks from conception in progesterone supplemented women. Clin Exp Obstet Gynecol. 2005;32(1):13-4.
11. Maclin VM, Padwanska E, Binor Z, Dmowski WP. Progesterone:estradiol ratios at implantation in ongoing pregnancies, abortion, nonconception cycles resulting from ovulation induction. Fertil Steril. 1990;54:238-44.
12. De Ziegher D. Hormonal control of endometrial receptivity. Hum Reprod. 1995;10:4-7.
13. Devroey P, Braekmans P, Camus M, Khan I, Smitz J, Staessen C, et al. Embryo donation in patients with primary ovarian failure. Hum Reprod. 1988;3(Suppl 2):85-7.
14. De Zeigler D, Sator M, Binelli D, Leuratti C, Cometti B, Bourgain C, et al. A randomized trial comparing the endometrial effects of daily subcutaneous administration of 25 mg and 50 mg progesterone on aqueous preparation. Fertil Steril. 2013;100(3):860-6.
15. Lockwood G, Griesinger G, Comett B, 13 European Centers Collaborators. Subcutaneous progesterone versus vaginal progesterone gel for luteal phase support in invitro fertilization: a noninferiority randomized controlled study. Fertil Steril. 2014;101:112-9.
16. Balasch J, Fabregues F, Ordi J, Creus M, Peñarrubia J, Casamitjana R, et al. Further data favoring the hypothesis of the uterine first-pass effect of vaginally administered micronized progesterone. Gynecol Endocrinol. 1996;10:421-6.
17. Cicinelli E, de Ziegler D. Transvaginal progesterone: evidence for a new functional 'portal system' flowing from vaginal to the uterus. Hum Reprod Update. 1999;5:365-72.
18. Cicinelli E, de Ziegler D, Morgese S, Bulletti C, Luisi D, Schonauer LM. First uterine pass effect is observed when E2 is placed in the upper but not lower third of the vagina. Fertil Steril. 2004;81:1414-6.
19. Atrini PG, Volpe A, Angioni S, Galassi MC, Battaglia C, Genazzani AR. A comparative

randomized study of three different progesterone support of the luteal phase following IVF/ET program. J Endocrinol Invest. 1995;18:51-6.
20. Miles RA, Paulson RJ, Lobo RA, Press MF, Dahmoush L, Sauer MV. Pharmacokinetics and endometrial tissue levels of progesterone after administration by intramuscular and vaginal routes: a comparative study. Fertil Steril. 1994;62:485-90.
21. Czajkowski K, Seinko J, Mogilinski M, Bros M, Szczenia R, Czajkowski A. Uteroplacental circulation in early pregnancy complicated by threatened abortion supplemented with vaginal micronized progesterone or oral dydrogesterone. Fertil Steril. 2007; 87(3):613-8.
22. Abdelhakim AM, Abd-EIGawad M, Hussein RS, Abbas AM. Vaginal versus intramuscular progesterone for luteal phase support in assisted reproductive techniques: a systematic review and meta-analysis of randomized controlled trial. Gynecol Endocrinol. 2020;36(5):389-97.
23. Fanchin R, Righini C, Olivennes F, Taylor S, de Ziegler D, Frydman R. Uterine contractions at the time of embryo transfer alter pregnancy rates after in vitro fertilization. Hum Reprod. 1998;13:1968-74.
24. Zegers-Hochschild F, Balmaceda JP, Fabres C, Alam V, Mackenna A, Fernández E, et al. Prospective randomized trial to evaluate the efficacy of vaginal ring releasing progesterone for IVF and oocyte donation. Hum Reprod. 2000;15:2093-7.
25. Bergh C, Lindenberg S; Nordic Crinone Study Group. A prospective randomized, multicenter study comparing vaginal progesterone gel and vaginal micronized progesterone tablets for luteal phase support after IVF/ICSI. Hum Reprod. 2012; 27:3467-73.
26. Silverberg KM, Vaughn TC, Hansard LJ, Burger NZ, Minter T. Vaginal (Crinone 8%) gel versus intramuscular progesterone in oil for luteal phase support in in vitro fertilization: a large prospective trial. Fertil Steril. 2012;97:344-8.
27. Farhi J, Weissman A, Steinfeld Z, Shorer M, Nahum H, Levran D. Estradiol supplementation during the luteal phase may improve the pregnancy rates in patients undergoing in vitro fertilization-embryo transfer cycles. Fertil Steril. 2000;73:761-6.
28. Griesinger G, Franke K, Kinast C, Kutzelnigg A, Riedinger S, Kulin S, et al. Ascorbic acid supplement during luteal phase in IVF. J Assist Reprod Genet. 2002;19:164-8.
29. Ubaldi F, Reinzi I, Ferrero S, Anniballo R, Iacobelli M, Cobellis L, et al. Low dose prednisolone administration in routine ICSI patients does not improve pregnancy and implantation rates. Hum Reprod. 2002;17:1544-7.
30. Urman B, Meran R, Alatas C, Balaban B, Isiklar A, Nuhoglu A. Low dose aspirin does not increase implantation rates in patients undergoing intracytoplasmic sperm injection: a prospective randomized study. J Assist Reprod Genet. 2000;17:586-90.
31. Fatemi HM, Bourgain C, Donoso P, Blockeel C, Papanikolaou EG, Popovic-Todorovic B, Devroey P. Effect of oral administration of dydrogesterone versus vaginal administration of natural micronized progesterone on the secretory transformation of endometrium and luteal endocrine profile in patients with premature ovarian failure: a proof of concept. Hum Reprod. 2007;22(5):1260-3.
32. Tournaye H, Sukhikh GT, Kahler E, Griesinger G. Phase 3 randomized controlled trial comparing efficacy, safety and tolerability of oral dydrogesterone versus micronized vaginal progesterone for luteal support in IVF. Hum Reprod. 2017;32(5):1019-27.
33. Griesinger G, Blockeel C, Sukhikh GT; Patki A, Dhorepatil B, Yang DZ, et al. Oral dydrogesterone versus intravaginal micronized progesterone gel for luteal support in IVF. A randomized clinical trial. Hum Reprod. 2018;33(12):2212-21.
34. Chakravarti BN, Shirazee HH, Dam P, Goswami SK, Chatterjee R, Ghosh S. Oral dydrogesterone versus intravaginal micronized progesterone as luteal phase

support in assisted reproductive technology (ART) cycles: results of randomized study. J Steroid Biochem Mol Biol. 2005;97(5):416-20.
35. Patki A, Pawar VC. Modulating fertility outcome in assisted reproductive technologies by the use of dydrogesterone. Gynecol Endocrinol. 2007;23(Suppl 1):68-72.
36. Fatemi HM, Popovic-Todorovic B, Papnikolaou E, Donoso P, Devroey P. An update of luteal phase support in stimulated IVF cycles. Hum Reprod Update. 2007; 13:581-90.
37. Tavaniotou A, Devroey P. Effect of human chorionic gonadotropins on luteal luteinizing hormone concentrations in natural cycles. Fertil Steril. 2003;80:654-5.
38. Humaidan P, Ejdrup Bredkjaer H, Westergard LG, Andersen CY. 1,500 IU human chorionic gonadotropins administered at oocyte retrieval rescues the luteal phase when gonadotropin-releasing hormone agonist is used for ovulation induction: a prospective, randomized, controlled study. Fertil Steril. 2010;93:847-54.
39. Kummer N, Benadiva C, Feinn R, Mann J, Nulsen J, Engmann L. Factors that predict the probability of successful clinical outcome after induction of oocyte maturation with gonadotropin-releasing hormone agonist. Fertil Steril. 2011;96:63-8.
40. Evans J, Salamonsen LA. Too much of a good thing? Experimental evidence suggests prolonged exposure to hCG is detrimental to endometrial receptivity. Hum Reprod. 2013;28(6):1610-9.
41. Anderson Y, Fisher R, Giorgione V, Kelsey TW. Microdose hCG as luteal support without exogenous progesterone administration. Mathematical model of hCG concentration in circulation and initial experience. J Assist Reprod Genet. 2016;33:1311-8.
42. Pirard C, Donnez J, Loumaye E. GnRH agonist as novel luteal support: results of a randomized, parallel group, feasibility study using intranasal administration of buserelin. Hum Reprod. 2005;20:1798-804.
43. Tesarik J, Hazout A, Mendoza-Tesarik R, Mendoza N, Mendoza C. Beneficial effect of luteal phase GnRH agonist administration on embryo implantation after ICSI in both GnRH agonist and antagonist treated ovarian stimulation cycles. Hum Reprod. 2006;21: 2572-9.
44. Brigante CMM, Renzinin M, Dal Canto M, Coticchio G, Comi R, Fadini R. Efficacy of luteal phase support with GnRH agonist: a preliminary comparative study. Fertil Steril. 2013;100(3):299.
45. Vander Linden H, Buckingham K, Farquhar C, Kremer JA, Metwally M. Luteal support for assisted reproduction cycles. Cochrane Database Syst Rev. 2011;(10):CD009154.
46. Fatemi HM, Kolibianakis EM, Camus M, Tournaye H, Donoso P, Papanikolaou E, et al. Addition of estradiol to progesterone for luteal supplementation in patients stimulated with GnRH antagonists/rFSH for IVF: a randomized controlled trial. Hum Reprod. 2006;21:2628-32.
47. Lukaszuk K, Liss J, Lukaszuk M, Maj B. Optimization of estradiol supplementation during the luteal phase improves the pregnancy rate in women undergoing IVF-ET cycles. Fertil Steril. 2005;83:1372-6.
48. Montville CP, Khabba M, Aubuchon M, Williams DB, Thomas MA. Luteal support with intravaginal progesterone increases clinical pregnancy rates in women with polycystic ovary syndrome using letrozole for ovulation induction. Fertil Steril. 2010;94(2):678-83.
49. Tavaniotou A, Albano C, Smitz J, Devroey P. Impact of ovarian stimulation on corpus luteum function and embryonic implantation. J Reprod Immunol. 2002;55(1-2): 123-30.
50. Xu B, Li Z, Zhang H, Jin L, Li Y, Ai J, et al. Serum progesterone level effects on the outcome of in vitro fertilization in patients with different ovarian response: an analysis of more than 10,000 cycles. Fertil Steril. 2012;97(6):1321-7.
51. Doldi N, Marsiglio E, Destefanu A, Gessi A, Merati G, Ferrari A. Elevated serum P on the day of hCG administration in IVF is associated with a higher pregnancy rate in polycystic ovary syndrome. Hum Reprod. 1999;14:1601-5.

52. Hill MJ, Whitcomg BW, Lewis TD, Wu M, Terry N, DeCherney AH, et al. Progesterone luteal support after ovulation induction and intrauterine insemination: a systematic review and meta-analysis. Fertil Steril. 2013;100(5):1373-80.
53. Fatemi HM. The luteal phase after 3 decades of IVF: what do we know? Reprod Biomed Online. 2009;19(Suppl 4):4331.
54. Devroey P, Bourgain C, Macklon NS, Fauser BCJM. Reproductive biology and IVF: ovarian stimulation and endometrial receptivity. Trends Endocrinol Metab. 2004; 15(2):84-90.
55. Humaidan P, Papnikolaou EG, Kyrou D, Alsbjerg B, Polyzos NP, Devroey P, et al. The luteal phase after GnRH agonist triggering of ovulation: present and future perspectives. Reprod Biomed Online. 2012;24:134-41.
56. Miyake A, Aono T, Kinugasa T, Tanizawa O, Kurachi K. Suppression of serum levels of luteinizing hormone by short and long-loop negative feedback in ovariectomized women. J Endocrinol. 1979;80:353-6.
57. Smitz J, Devroey P, Faguer B, Bourgain C, Camus M, Van Steirteghem AC. A prospective randomized comparison of intramuscular or intravaginal natural progesterone as a luteal phase and early pregnancy supplement. Hum Reprod. 1992;7:168-75.
58. Daya S, Gunby J. Luteal phase support in assisted reproductive cycles. Cochrane Database Syst Rev. 2004;(3):CD004830.
59. Beckers NGM, Macklon NS, Eijkemans MJ, Ludwig M, Felberbaum RE, Diedrich K, et al. Non-supplemented luteal phase characteristics after the administration of recombinant human chorionic gonadotropin, recombinant luteinizing hormone, or gonadotropin releasing hormone (GnRH) agonist to induce final oocyte maturation in in vitro fertilization patients after ovarian stimulation with recombinant follicle stimulating hormone and GnRH antagonist co-treatment. J Clin Endocrinol Metab. 2003;88:4186-92.
60. Papanikolaou EG, Verpoest W, Fatemi H, Tarlatzis B, Devroey P, Tournaye H. A novel method of luteal supplementation with recombinant luteinizing hormone when a gonadotropin releasing hormone agonist issued instead of human chorionic gonadotropin for ovulation trigger: a randomized prospective proof of concept study. Fertil Steril. 2011;95:1174-7.
61. Humaidan P, Bredkjaer HE, Westergard LG, Andersen CY. 1,500 IU human chorionic gonadotropins administered at oocyte retrieval rescues the luteal phase when gonadotropin-releasing hormone agonist is used for ovulation induction: a prospective, randomized, controlled study. Fertil Steril. 2010;93:847-54.
62. Anderson CY, Elbaek HO, Alsbjerg B, Laursen RJ, Povisen BB, Thomsen L, Humaidan P. Hum Reprod. 2015;30(10): 2387-95.
63. Berg PA, Navot D. The impact of embryonic development and endometrial maturity on the timing of implantation. Fertil Steril. 1992;58:537-42.
64. Jawar MP, Deshpande MM, Gadgil PA, Mahanta AA. Histopathological study of endometrium in infertility. Indian J Pathol Microbiol. 2003;46:630-6.
65. Groenewound ER, Macklon NS, Cohlen BJ, ANTARCTICA study group. The effect of elevated progesterone levels before hCG triggering in modified natural cycle frozen thawed embryo transfer cycles. Reprod Biomed Online. 2017;34:546-54.
66. Polyzos NP, Drakopoulos P, Toumaye H. Modified natural cycle IVF for poor ovarian responders: rethink before concluding. Hum Reprod. 2016;31(1):221-2.
67. Labrata E, Mariani G, Holtmann N, Celada P, Remohi J, Bosch E. Hum Reprod. 2017;32(12):2437-42.
68. Labarta E, Mariani G, Holtman N, Celada P, Remohí J, Bosch E. Low serum progesterone on the day of embryo transfer is associated with diminished on going pregnancy rate in oocyte donation cycles after artificial endometrial preparation: a prospective study. Hum Reprod. 2017;32:2437-42.
69. Devine K, Richter KS, Widra EA, McKeeby JL. Vitrified blastocyst transfer cycles with the use of only vaginal progesterone replacement

with endometrium have inferior ongoing pregnancy rates: results from planned interim analysis of a three arm randomized controlled noninferiority trial. Fertil Steril. 2018:109:266-75.

70. Lee VYC, Li RH, Yeung WS, Chung HOP, Ng EHY. A randomized double-blinded controlled trial of hCG as luteal support in natural cycle frozen embryo transfer. Hum Reprod. 2017;32:1130-7.
71. Attia GR, Zeitoun K, Edwards D, Johns A, Carr BR, Bulun SE. Progesterone receptor isoform A but not B is expressed in endometriosis. J Clin Endocrinol Metab. 2000;85:2897-902.
72. Cahill DJ, Hull MG. Pituitary-ovarian dysfunction and endometriosis. Hum Reprod Update. 2000;6:56-66.
73. Donaghay M, Lessey BA. Uterine receptivity: alterations associated with benign gynecological disease. Semin Reprod Med. 2007;25:461-75.
74. Surrey ES, Silverberg KM, Surrey MW, Schoolcraft WB. Effect of prolonged gonadotropin-releasing hormone agonist therapy on the outcome of in vitro fertilization-embryo transfer in patients with endometriosis. Fertil Steril. 2002;78:699-704.
75. De Ziegler D, Gayet V, Aubriot FX, Fauque P, Streuli I, Wolf JP, et al. Use of oral contraceptives in women with endometriosis before assisted reproduction treatment improves outcomes. Fertil Steril. 2010;94:2796-9.
76. Ayoubi JM, Epiney M, Brioschi PA, Fanchin R, Chardonnens D, de Ziegler D. Comparison of changes in uterine contraction frequency after ovulation in menstrual cycle and in in vitro fertilization cycles. Fertil Steril. 2003;79:1101-5.
77. Mochtar MH, Van Wely M, Van der Veen F. Timing luteal phase support in GnRH agonist down-regulated IVF/embryo transfer cycles. Hum Reprod. 2006;21:905-8.
78. Nyboe AA, Popovic-Todorovic B, Schmidt KT, Loft A, Lindhard A, Højgaard A, et al. Progesterone supplementation during early gestations after IVF and ICSI has no effect on the delivery rates: a randomized controlled trial. Hum Reprod. 2002;17:357-61.
79. Caspo AI, Pulkkinen MO, Wiest WG. Effects of lutectomy and progesterone replacement therapy in early pregnant patients. Am J Obstet Gynecol. 1973;115:759-65.
80. Schmidt KL, Ziebe S, Popovic B, Lindhard A, Loft A, Andersen AN. Progesterone supplementation during early gestation after in vitro fertilization has no effect on delivery rate. Fertil Steril. 2001;75:337-41.

24 Chapter

Ovarian Hyperstimulation Syndrome

INTRODUCTION

Ovarian hyperstimulation syndrome (OHSS) is the most serious and life-threatening complication of ovulation induction. The incidence of moderate OHSS is 3–6% and severe OHSS is 0.1–2%.[1] Fortunately, with acceptance of antagonist used for downregulation with agonist being used as a trigger and "freeze all" policy, the incidence has markedly decreased and has become almost zero in some centers.

The OHSS is due to the overproduction of ovarian hormones and vasoactive substances that are secreted as a result of uncontrolled ovarian stimulation. These substances increase the permeability allowing the fluids to go to the third space. This accumulation of fluid in the third space is responsible for the signs, symptoms, and complications of OHSS.

TYPES OF OVARIAN HYPERSTIMULATION SYNDROME

The OHSS may be *early-onset* or *late-onset.*

Early-onset OHSS is detected from Day 3–7 after ovulation trigger with human chorionic gonadotropin (hCG). But late-onset OHSS appears after 10–12 days following the hCG trigger. Early OHSS is because of excessive drug (gonadotropins) dosages for that particular ovary. Very rarely, mutations in follicle-stimulating hormone (FSH) receptor may be stimulated by endogenous hCG and spontaneous OHSS may occur. Late-onset OHSS is because of endogenous hCG secreted by the embryo and as the embryo grows and hCG secretion increases, the OHSS becomes more severe. Late OHSS is present in almost 70% of the patients who had severe OHSS. It cannot be predicted, unlike early OHSS. Moreover, it has equal association with singleton as with multiple pregnancies.[2]

CLASSIFICATION OF OVARIAN HYPERSTIMULATION SYNDROME

Classification is extremely useful for the clinician to decide the severity of the condition and also to decide if the patient requires hospitalization and medical or surgical line of treatment. Various classification systems have been described in the literature stating mild, moderate, and severe variety. But mild OHSS is very common and does not require any treatment. So, the most accepted recent classification introduced by Rizk and Aboulghar stated only two categories: (1) moderate and (2) severe.[3] This classification is useful in defining clinical groups in relation to prognosis and treatment protocols.

Moderate Ovarian Hyperstimulation Syndrome

- The patient presents with discomfort, pain, nausea, and abdominal distention but no clinical ascites.

- Though ultrasound shows enlarged ovaries with ascites.
- Hematological and biological profiles are normal.
- The patient can be treated on an outdoor basis, provided she can come for the follow-up as and when required, depending on her symptoms.

Severe Ovarian Hyperstimulation Syndrome

Severe OHSS is divided into grades depending on its severity.

Grade A

- The patient presents with dyspnea, nausea, vomiting, diarrhea, and abdominal pain with marked distention.
- Oliguria, ascites, and hydrothorax may be clinically detected.
- Ultrasound shows large ovaries and ascites.
- The biochemical profile is normal.
- These patients can be treated as outpatients or may require admission depending on the patient's or consultant's comfort.

Grade B

- All signs and symptoms of grade A with increased severity
- Marked oliguria
- Increased hematocrit, elevated urea and creatinine, and abnormal liver function tests (LFTs)
- Requires admission and vigilant supervision

Grade C

- Apart from all the signs and symptoms of grade B, acute respiratory distress syndrome (ARDS)
- Renal shutdown
- Venous thrombosis
- Requires intensive care unit (ICU) support

PATHOPHYSIOLOGY OF OVARIAN HYPERSTIMULATION SYNDROME

It is extremely important to understand the pathophysiology for the prevention and treatment of the disease. It is characterized by ovarian enhancement and shifting of fluid rich in protein, especially albumin in the third space, causing ascites and effusion. The severity of OHSS is directly related to capillary permeability **(Flowchart 1)**.

Changes in Ovary

- Bilateral cystic enlargement of the ovary
- Increased stromal edema
- Multiple corpora lutea
- Neovascularization
- Secretion of vascular endothelial growth factor (VEGF), prorenin, active renin, interleukins, N680, interleukin-1β, 2 and 6, prostaglandins, tumor necrosis factor-α (TNF-α), transforming growth

Flowchart 1: Clinical pathology of ovarian hyperstimulation syndrome.

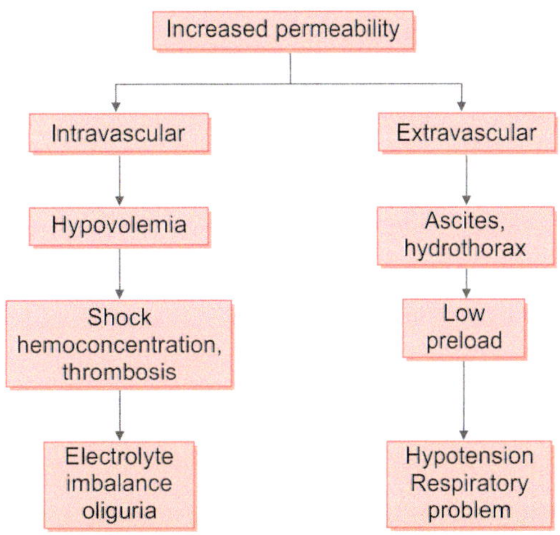

factor-1 (TGF-1), TGF, etc. Most of these substances are angiogenic and are responsible for neovascularization during folliculogenesis and luteinization in the ovary and act through VEGF.

Third Space

There is collection of fluid in the third space presenting as ascites and hydrothorax with massive pleural effusion. This fluid shift is due to increased capillary permeability. The shift starts after hCG injection and even before ovum aspiration. VEGF is responsible for increased capillary permeability and fluid shift.[4] Production of VEGF is dependent on hCG, which is given for trigger or on endogenous hCG from embryo. VEGF is secreted by granulosa cells. Intraperitoneal pressure increases beyond the intraluminal pressure of the inferior vena cava (IVC). Therefore, blood flow in IVC decreases, leading to decreased preload in the heart and decreased cardiac output causing impairment of respiratory and renal functions. Antidiuretic hormone (ADH) is also increased because of activation of the renin-angiotensin mechanism and secretes ADH. This causes oliguria and hemoconcentration. Hypovolemia and hypotension cause arterial constriction. OHSS may be more common in intrauterine insemination (IUI) cycles rather than in vitro fertilization (IVF) as in IVF, all the follicular fluid containing the causative ingredients of OHSS are extracted out during follicular aspiration.

Vascular permeability factor (VPF): It is similar to VEGF. This causes vascular leakage and is present in corpus luteum. The concentration of VPF is very high in follicular fluid, serum, and peritoneal fluid, in patients in whom OHSS develops.[5] It is two times higher in follicular fluid and that indicates ovarian origin. When pregnancy occurs, hCG rescues the corpus luteum and there is an increase in VPF secretion.

Familial mutations in FSH receptors increase their sensitivity to trophoblastic hCG and can cause OHSS with spontaneous pregnancy. High estradiol (E2) is not responsible for OHSS as when hCG is withheld, high E2 cannot cause OHSS. So, estrogen is not having vasoactivity and cannot cause vascular dysfunction.

PREDICTION OF OVARIAN HYPERSTIMULATION SYNDROME

Prediction is extremely important for treating the patient and should be done as early as possible. This can be done:

- Before stimulation
- During stimulation
- Before trigger
- During pregnancy

Before Stimulation

Clinical

- Young patient
- Polycystic ovarian syndrome (PCOS)—antral follicle count (AFC) > 26, increased stromal vascularity
- Low body mass index (BMI)—thin, lean PCOS
- History of OHSS in the previous pregnancy
- High anti-Müllerian hormone (AMH) > 30 pmol/mL or > 7 ng/mL. In one study, all cycles were canceled in this scenario.[6]
- AMH > 3.36 ng/mL has 90.5% sensitivity and 81.3% specificity for subsequent development of OHSS.[7]

Ultrasound Based

- Follicle number per ovary (FNPO) > 15
- Stromal vessels resistance index (RI) < 0.5
- Stromal peak systolic velocity (PSV) > 10 cm/s

- Ovarian volume > 10 cc
- Stromal flow index (FI) > 15
- More follicles of 6–9 mm size

Follicle-stimulating Hormone Receptor Genotype

Follicle-stimulating hormone receptor mutations and polymorphisms can cause OHSS when they are activated.[8] To date, 744 single nucleotide polymorphisms have been identified in the FSH receptor gene. The N680 allele can be associated with hyper-responders who are more prone to OHSS. A significant increase in N680 allele is observed as the severity of OHSS increases. So it is concluded that a genotype in the position of N680 of FSH receptor cannot predict which patient will develop OHSS but it can predict the severity of OHSS among the patients who develop OHSS.[9]

Prediction by Bone Morphogenetic Protein-15 Gene

Bone morphogenetic protein (BMP)-15 is related to OHSS which is dose-dependent. It is a member of TGF-β. It helps to predict which patients are at a risk of developing OHSS.[10]

Cystic Fibrosis Transmembrane Conductance Regulator

Estradiol upregulates cystic fibrosis transmembrane regulator (CFTR) expression and this phenomenon can cause an increase in fluid in the peritoneal cavity. So it may provide a causative link between hyperestrinism and OHSS.[11]

During Treatment

- Long protocol favors the development of OHSS.
- The number of days of gonadotropin stimulation is very important for the development of OHSS. These days are always more in downregulated cycles and so these cycles are more prone to OHSS.
- hCG as luteal support
- *Ultrasound prediction*:
  - There is a positive correlation between the mean number of immature follicles and OHSS.
  - During stimulation, an increase in immature follicles and a decrease in mature follicles favor severe OHSS (>9 mm follicles, >20 in number).[12]
  - The risk of OHSS increases sharply with an increase in the volume of the ovary.
  - Stromal volume is important in predicting the risk of OHSS.
- The type of gonadotropin used did not show any significant difference in the risk of development of OHSS. Its incidence is the same with recombinant FSH (rFSH), urinary FSH, and purified human menopausal gonadotropin (hMG).[13] More important is the type of protocol used (chronic low-dose, step-up, or step-down protocol). The chronic low-dose protocol has a very low incidence of OHSS.

Before Trigger

- *Estradiol level*: E2 > 4,000 pg/mL in assisted reproductive technology (ART) and > 1,700 pg/mL in IUI is considered high risk for development of OHSS.
- *Ultrasound findings*: Even when the age of the patient and the total number of follicles are similar, the ovarian volume was significantly higher in the patients who developed OHSS (271 ± 87 vs. 157.30 ± 54.20 mL).[14] The presence of medium-sized follicles (11–14 mm) > 5–7 on either side is thought to be a risk factor for the development of OHSS. ≥25 follicles larger than 11 mm in size or ≥25 oocytes retrieved is a risk factor for OHSS.

Pregnancy

Pregnancy itself is considered a risk factor for the development of OHSS.

PREVENTION OF OVARIAN HYPERSTIMULATION SYNDROME

- Primary prevention **(Box 1)**
- Secondary prevention **(Box 2)**

Primary Prevention of Ovarian Hyperstimulation Syndrome

It is by the selection of stimulation protocols and drugs that decrease the risk of OHSS.

- *Gonadotropin-releasing hormone (GnRH) antagonist protocol*: Initial studies showed no difference in severe OHSS in antagonist or long protocols. In antagonist protocols, the pregnancy rate was also found to be lower.[15] But the two recent meta-analyses comparing agonist and antagonist protocols showed significantly reduced OHSS and also less severity if it occurs with the antagonist protocol.[16,17]
- *Laparoscopic ovarian drilling*: Both ovarian diathermy and laser vaporization performed prior to stimulation reduce the incidence of OHSS. The transvaginal ovarian diathermy can be used in difficult cases. The best results are obtained in thin, lean PCOS. Ovarian diathermy should be reserved for young patients with severe PCOS who tend to hyperstimulation even on a prolonged low-dose FSH regimen.
- *Metformin*: The short-term course of metformin 850 mg BD in PCOS given before the ovum stimulation up to the day of oocyte collection decreases the incidence of OHSS and improves the pregnancy rate.[18,19] But some studies recommend metformin for 2–3 months prior to IVF.
  - *In vitro maturation of immature oocytes*: This is an alternative management for patients having a high risk of OHSS. It totally avoids OHSS.[20]
  - *Low-dose gonadotropins*: Low dose with the step-up protocol should be used to avoid OHSS. 150 IU urinary FSH should be the starting dose.[21]
  - *Natural cycle ART*: IT completely eliminates OHSS but has a low pregnancy rate.
  - Avoid hCG as a luteal phase support.

Box 1: Primary prevention of ovarian hyperstimulation syndrome.

- GnRH antagonist protocol
- Laparoscopic ovarian drilling
- Insulin sensitizers
- In vitro maturation of ova
- Low-dose gonadotropin protocol
- Natural cycle ART
- Avoid hCG in the luteal phase

(ART: assisted reproductive technology; GnRH: gonadotropin-releasing hormone; hCG: human chorionic gonadotropin)

Box 2: Secondary prevention of ovarian hyperstimulation syndrome.

- Withholding hCG
- Coasting
- Reducing the dose of hCG
- GnRH agonist trigger
- Recombinant LH as a trigger
- Intravenous albumin
- Intravenous HES
- Glucocorticoids
- Ovarian suppression
- Dopamine agonist
- Freeze all
- Aspirate all follicles
- Intravenous calcium

(GnRH: gonadotropin-releasing hormone; hCG: human chorionic gonadotropin; HES: hydroxyethyl starch; LH: luteinizing hormone)

Secondary Prevention of Ovarian Hyperstimulation Syndrome

- *Withholding hCG*: Withholding hCG and canceling the cycle when the E2 level is

>4,000 pg/mL can avoid OHSS. Its values are doubling or increasing every 2–3 days. It is a warning sign of OHSS. This is a common method used to avoid OHSS but there is a financial burden on the patient and the patient is never happy in spite of explanations. hCG is the main culprit for OHSS as it promotes secretions of VEGF. Luteinizing hormone (LH) receptors are present on a follicle of 8–10 mm size. Thus, more the medium sized follicles more is the risk of OHSS.

- *Coasting*: It is delaying the administration of hCG. It was once the most popular method in long protocol to prevent OHSS as it does not require cancellation of the cycle. Ideally, coasting starts when the lead follicle is <15 mm and the E2 level is >1,500 pg/mL. The lead follicle continues to grow as it already has LH receptors. No further FSH is given for stimulation. Normally, the follicle continues to grow for 4 days. Coasting should not be done for >4 days as it grossly reduces the E2 level and pregnancy rates. hCG is given when E2 decreases to <3,000 pg/mL, as it reduces OHSS without affecting pregnancy.[16] In an agonist cycle, withdrawing agonist and replacing it by antagonist and then giving agonist trigger can reduce OHSS.[22] Antagonist can be continued in high-risk OHSS patients who were downregulated by GnRHa. Coasting with GnRHa has no beneficial role in preventing OHSS as discussed in a Cochrane review.[23]

  Mechanism of coasting: It diminishes functioning of granulosa cell cohort, atresia of smaller follicles, and reduces VEGF secretion and gene expression. But there is insufficient evidence to recommend coasting for prevention of OHSS according to the practice committee of the American Society for Reproductive Medicine (ASRM).
- *Reducing the dose of hCG*: There are not much data available on decreasing dose of hCG but there is general consensus that when E2 is >3,000 µg/mL the dose should be halved. The dose between 3,300 and 5,000 U decreases the risk.[24]
- *GnRHa trigger*: In an antagonist protocol, GnRHa can be used as the ovulation trigger. The quality of the oocytes is the same as of hCG trigger and fertilization and cleavage rates are same. But ongoing pregnancy rates are very low because of luteal phase defects. Though it definitely abolishes the occurrence of OHSS. hCG 1,500 IU, on the day of ovum pick-up, can be given to rescue the corpus luteum, if there are <24 follicles, which gives a good pregnancy rate with an extremely low OHSS rate as suggested by Humaidan et al.[25] Griesinger et al. proposed to freeze all embryos and transfer in the subsequent cycle after GnRHa trigger. This gives higher cumulative pregnancy rates.[26] Occasionally, moderate OHSS may occur particularly when a patient conceives but severe OHSS is not reported with GnRHa trigger.
- *Recombinant LH for ovulation*: Triggering the ovulation with recombinant LH (rLH) decreases OHSS because it does not produce VEGF and so vascular permeability is not increased. But pregnancy rates are low and so optimum dose is under research which would maintain the pregnancy rates along with low risk of OHSS. The ovulating dose is very high and so it is an expensive treatment as multiple doses are required because of its short half-life (20 minutes).[27] rLH is safer than hCG and has a long half-life than native LH. So a single peak can cause final maturation. The dose is between 5,000 and 30,000 IU of rLH.

- *Intravenous (IV) albumin*: IV albumin prevents third space fluid accumulation and corrects hemodynamic instability by increasing colloidal oncotic pressure. There are various reports in favor of and against the use of albumin for the prevention of OHSS. Albumin maintains intravascular volume and prevents hypovolemia, ascites, and hemoconcentration. It counters the vasoactive substance released from corpus lutea. In a Cochrane review, there is a significant reduction in OHSS in the albumin group. It is to be given at the time of oocyte retrieval and 48 hours after oocyte retrieval.[28] In established OHSS, albumin always helps to prevent complications that are due to hemoconcentration. But oncotic pressure lasts for only 36 hours and so repeat therapy is needed.
- *IV hydroxyethyl starch (HES) solution*: HES is the volume expander. 6% HES is used in a dose of 1,000 mL at the time of ovum pick-up and 500 mL is given 48 hours after the first one. HES decreases the incidence of moderate and severe OHSS. A recent Cochrane review states that better results are seen with HES than albumin.[29]
- *Glucocorticoids*: They were thought to be useful because of their anti-inflammatory action during the development of OHSS. But most of the papers have found no protective effect with corticosteroids. They may have an inhibitory effect on VEGF gene expression.[30] Aspirin reduces the incidence of OHSS and has grade B evidence according to the practice committee of ASRM. The ASRM practice committee has also shown that Aspirin + glucocorticoids are also beneficial from stimulation to positive beta-hCG.[31,32]
- *Ovarian suppression*:
  - *GnRHa*: Continuous GnRHa after hCG also decreases LH surge and diminishes the occurrence of OHSS. All the embryos are cryopreserved in this case. This is very useful in donation cycles.
  - E2 and hydroxyl progesterone IM after embryo transfer also prevent ovarian secretion and prevent OHSS but it is experimental.
  - Aromatase inhibitors in the luteal phase are promising. It decreases luteal E2 concentration and decreases OHSS. It is very useful in donor cycles.
- *Dopamine agonist*: VEGF increases vascular permeability. VEGF acts by VEGF receptor 2 specific. Inhibition of this receptor can prevent increased vascular permeability which is done by cabergoline or bromocriptine or quinagolide. There are gene expressions of 80 upregulated and 7 downregulated genes in OHSS as compared to controls. Tyrosine hydroxylase is downregulated. So it is the natural inhibitor for the angiogenic process. This suggests that dopamine can be an antiangiogenic factor and deficit or it can cause OHSS. Dopamine decreases vascular permeability by decreasing VEGF-2 phosphorylation. Dopamine receptor-2 agonist (cabergoline) inhibits VEGF receptor 2-dependent vascular permeability without affecting luteal angiogenesis. It has no luteolytic effect.[27] The recommended dose is 0.5 mg cabergoline from the day of hCG up to 8 days. It does not affect fertilization, cleavage, or implantation. The reproductive outcome is not changed.[33] The study of Alvarez et al. showed marked improvement in moderate OHSS but there is no difference in severe OHSS and E2 level also. The non-ergot-derived dopamine agonist quinagolide is promoted now as cabergoline causes vascular disorders in Parkinson's disease.

The dose is 50–100–200 μg/daily for 17-21 days till β-hCG is done.

- *Freeze all*: Effective cryopreservation is done in all embryos and so we can avoid late OHSS which is due to pregnancy. The results of fresh transfer and cryopreserved embryos used in the next cycle are the same.[34] But the advantage of avoiding pregnancy-induced OHSS is beneficial to the patient. Though still there is insufficient data for this policy and the Cochrane review does not support this.[35] OHSS-free clinic will be a reality with embryo freezing. The entire IVF procedure is divided into segments.
  - *Segment A*: Ovarian stimulation with antagonist protocol and agonist trigger
  - *Segment B*: Cryopreservation of embryos and vitrification
  - *Segment C*: Embryo transfer after thawing and endometrial preparation by hormone replacement therapy.
- *Aspirate all follicles*: All the follicles, larger or smaller, should be aspirated to decrease the incidence of OHSS.[36] Aspiration of all the follicles from one ovary before hCG was recommended before, but much better solutions are available now and so aspiration before hCG is not practiced.
- *IV calcium*: 10%, 10 mL of calcium gluconate is given IV in 30 minutes or 200 mL of normal saline at 1.5 mL/min on the day of oocyte retrieval and repeated on Day 1, 2, and 3 postoocyte retrieval.[37,38] The difference in the severity of clinical symptoms is significant. Ascitic fluid volume decreases from Day 3 post oocyte retrieval and ovarian size decreases after Day 10 of oocyte retrieval. It has no detrimental effects on pregnancy rates. IV calcium reduces the fluid transfer to the third space. IV calcium is better than HES in reducing ascites. It prevents damage and repairs the endothelial cell membrane. It is an inexpensive and nontoxic approach that reduces ascites and hematocrit. hCG causes mobilization of calcium from intracellular stores. This is influenced by granulosa cells. hCG and LH receptors are members of a protein-coupled receptor family whose transducers are represented by calcium-dependent kinases and so calcium action in OHSS can be linked to hCG.
- OHSS-free clinic by segmentation of IVF treatment.[39]
  - *Segment A*: Optimizing ovarian stimulation with antagonist cycle and agonist trigger
  - *Segment B*: Optimum cryopreservation method or vitrification
  - *Segment C*: Embryo replacement in nonstimulated, receptive endometrium

TREATMENT (TABLES 1 AND 2)

The patient is treated according to the severity of the condition.

Outpatient Management of Moderate Ovarian Hyperstimulation Syndrome

The patient should give a telephonic report of her condition every day and she should be called twice a week for assessment.

Assessment:

- *Symptoms*: Vomiting, pain, distention.
- Weight and abdominal girth, vital data
- Pelvic ultrasound for ovarian size, ascites
- Urine output, blood tests [blood count, LFT, renal function test (RFT) and coagulation profile, electrolytes]
- The patient should be educated to report for dyspnea, oliguria, or neurological symptoms.

TABLE 1: Monitoring in OHSS.

Clinical monitoring	*Biochemical monitoring*	*Ultrasound monitoring*
Blood pressure	Blood count	Ovarian size
Heart rate	Hematocrit	Ascites
Respiratory rate	LFT	Pleural effusion
Weight	RFT	Pericardial effusion
Abdominal girth	Electrolytes	Pregnancy status
Intake output chart	Coagulation profile	Chest X-ray
	Blood gases	
	β-hCG	

(hCG: human chorionic gonadotropin; LFT: liver function tests; RFT: renal function test)

TABLE 2: Grading of OHSS based on symptoms and signs.

	Moderate OHSS	*Severe OHSS Grade A*	*Severe OHSS Grade B*	*Severe OHSS Grade C*
Symptoms				
Discomfort	+	+	+	+
Abdominal pain	+	+	+	+
Nausea	+	+	+	+
Distention	+	+	+	+
Dyspnea	–	+	+	+
Oliguria	–	+	+ <500 cc	+ <500 cc
Vomiting	–	+	+	+
Diarrhea	–	+	+	+
Signs				
Ascites	–ve	+	++	+++
Urine output	Normal	Oliguria	++	+++
Hydrothorax	–ve	+	++	+++
Ultrasound				
Ascites	+	+ve	++	+++
Large ovary	+>5 cm	+ve	++>8 cm	+++>8 cm
Investigations				
Hematocrit	<45	Normal	>45	>55
Blood comp	Normal	Normal	WBC > 15,000	WBC > 25,000
LFT	Normal	Normal	Abnormal	Abnormal
RFT	Normal	Normal	Creatinine >1.5	Creatinine >1.5
Coagulation profile	Normal	Normal		Abnormal
Electrolytes	Normal	Normal		Abnormal

Contd...

Contd...

	Moderate OHSS	*Severe OHSS Grade A*	*Severe OHSS Grade B*	*Severe OHSS Grade C*
Complications				
Renal failure	–			
Venous thrombosis	–			
ARDS	–			
Treatment		Indoor/outdoor	Indoor	ICU
	Outdoor	Depends on patient condition	Expectant management	
		Doctor's convenience		
		Facility		

(ARDS: acute respiratory distress syndrome; LFT: liver function tests; RFT: renal function test; ICU: intensive care unit; OHSS: ovarian hyperstimulation syndrome)

The patient should be clearly instructed for:

- No sexual intercourse
- No strenuous activity
- Oral intake of at least 1 L
- Leg exercises should be done to avoid thromboembolism.

Management of Severe Ovarian Hyperstimulation Syndrome

Outpatient management of severe OHSS can be done for only patients having grade A severe OHSS. Its feasibility depends on the comfort of the physician and the reliability of the patient. Early and frequent paracentesis is more effective and the patient can be treated on an outpatient basis.

Hospital Management

All the patients with grades B and C should be admitted. You have to be vigilant as a complication can occur at any time.

Clinical Management

- *General condition with all vital signs*: Hypotension, tachycardia due to decreased preload
- Daily weight assessment and an abdominal girth measurement of the patient

Intake and output chart (urine output important). Activation of the renin-angiotensin mechanism causes increased antidiuretic hormone (ADH) which causes oliguria. Vascular permeability factor (VPF) plays an important role.

Biochemical Monitoring

- Blood count > 25,000 and hematocrit > 45% are seen in severe cases.
- Count of 25,000 usually causes a hematocrit of 55%.
- Liver function test
- Renal function test—creatinine > 1.2 mg
- *Serum electrolytes*: Na < 135 mEq/L, K > 5 mEq/L
- Coagulation profile
- Blood gases
- β-hCG
- The frequency of repetition of investigations would depend on the severity of the condition.

On Ultrasound

- Ovarian size
- Ascites
- Pleural and pericardial effusion
- Status of pregnancy

Chest X-ray

To exclude hydrothorax

Invasive Monitoring

Central venous pressure and pulmonary artery pressure assessment.

Medical Management of Ovarian Hyperstimulation Syndrome (Box 3)

After OHSS is diagnosed, drugs that are not effective are:

- Prostaglandin synthetase inhibitor
- Antihistamine
- Diuretics
- Danazol
- Volume expanders
- Dopamine
- Anticoagulant therapy
- Abdominal parameters

Antibiotic Therapy

Before doing any procedure like ascitic tapping or tapping of pleural effusion, antibiotic cover must be given. Hypoglobulinemia in severe cases may also predispose to infections.

Box 3: Medical management of ovarian hyperstimulation syndrome.

- Antibiotic therapy
- Volume correction
- Electrolyte replacement
- Anticoagulants
- Diuretics
- *Other drugs*:
  - Dopamine
  - GnRH antagonist
  - GnRH agonist

Volume Correction

High oral intake is advised in mild-to-moderate OHSS. Parental treatment includes IV fluids and plasma expanders in moderate and severe cases.

- *IV fluids*: The motto for IV fluids is to maintain the intravascular volume and electrolyte balance. There is hemoconcentration and to preserve normal renal function, adequate intravascular volume is a must. Fluid should be replaced as crystalline solutions, i.e., normal saline or Ringer's lactate, like in treating hypovolemia, but it should be titrated with urine output to avoid overload. It should be given at a rate of 125–150 mL/h and urine output of >20–30 mL/h should be monitored.
- *Plasma expanders*: These can be used but give temporary relief; however, may increase the third-space volume by increasing the intravascular osmotic pressure. Albumin or HES (6%) are the ones commonly used. Albumin should be given in a dose of 50–100 g at 25% concentration every 2–12 hourly till hematocrit falls below 45% and urine output increases. The risks of human blood products must be kept in mind. The reports for the efficacy of these compounds in treating established OHSS are varied in different studies. Though their role for the prevention of OHSS is more convincing and can be given at the time of ovum pick-up. Hematocrit should be repeatedly checked when these compounds are administered. The combination of albumin and furosemide works well in patients with oliguria. First, the plasma volume is increased by albumin and then if urine output is low, it adds furosemide.

Electrolyte Replacement

Electrolyte imbalance should be corrected. Salt and water restrictions are not required during the treatment.[40] Though in cases with ARDS, fluid restriction and dopamine forced diuresis are required. It occurs after fluid overload and so fluids may have to be restricted in severe OHSS. Dextrose normal saline (DNS) is always preferred. It is important to avoid hypotonic solution such as Ringer's lactate that contains potassium.

Anticoagulants

Venous thrombosis is one of the most serious complications of OHSS and is best prevented. Preventive measures with heparin are extremely beneficial in hypercoagulable states or when there is a risk of thromboembolism. Immobilization, pressure on ovaries and ascites, hypercoagulable state due to pregnancy, and hyperestrinism all add to the risk of thromboembolism. Heparin as prophylaxis is extremely beneficial for the patient. Though there are diverse views for the use of heparin in severe OHSS, still it should be given in all the patients with congenital thrombophilia or with a family history of thrombotic disorders. Prophylaxis is continued for 12–20 weeks depending on the condition of the patient. Hyperestrinism is the precipitating factor along with hypovolemia and hypotension. Arterial thrombosis is more common than venous thrombosis, which occurs later on.

Diuretics

These are contraindicated as these will cause more hemoconcentration. These will increase blood viscosity and thromboembolism. The only indication of diuretics in OHSS is pulmonary edema. It may be given in patients with oliguria and only after sufficient hemodilution.

- Abdominal paracentesis may be helpful in these cases.
- GnRH antagonist on the 6th day of pick-up after 4 days of OHSS can reduce OHSS. Luteal support is given with estrogen and progesterone.[41]
- GnRHa will also help reduce OHSS.

Dopamine

Dopamine is extremely useful in OHSS patients with oliguria as it improves renal circulation. It is required for only 7 days in nonpregnant patients, but if the patient has conceived it may be required for 10–20 days depending on the rise in β-hCG. The recommended dose is 4.32 mg/kg/day.[42] A 750-mg tablet of dopamine 8 hourly can be a suitable dose to reduce the severity of OHSS.

Indomethacin

Prostaglandin inhibitors such as indomethacin do not cause any clinical improvement in the condition. Instead, it may be dangerous due to renal toxicity.[40]

Surgical Management of Ovarian Hyperstimulation Syndrome (Box 4)

Fluid Aspiration

Indications: Relief of the symptoms, oliguria, tense ascites, rising serum creatinine,

Box 4: Surgical management of ovarian hyperstimulation syndrome (OHSS).

- Aspiration of ascitic fluid and tapping of pleural effusion in severe OHSS
- *Dealing with surgical emergencies*:
  - Ovarian torsion
  - Ectopic pregnancy
  - Cyst rupture
  - Thromboembolism
  - Pregnancy termination

hemoconcentration not responding to medical line of treatment, respiratory symptoms are some of the indications. Acute distention of the abdomen, acute abdominal pain, dyspnea, deteriorating respiratory function tests, and oliguria are absolute indications.

- *Transvaginal (TVS) sonography-guided aspiration*: It is a safe and effective procedure. Injury to the ovaries can be avoided and maximum fluid can be aspirated from the dependent pocket. This reduces pressure on the kidney and improves renal perfusion and urine output. It relieves pain, improves respiration, and decreases distention. Early and frequent paracentesis is more effective, even on an outpatient basis.
- *Abdominal paracentesis*: It has the same advantages as TVS-guided aspiration, but there is a risk of occasional injury to the friable large ovary and may lead to hemoperitoneum. A percutaneous pigtail catheter can be placed to avoid repeated punctures for repeated aspirations. The amount of fluid to be aspirated depends on the severity of the symptoms and may vary from 500–4,000 cc. Albumin transfusion may be required to compensate for the protein loss in the aspirated fluid.
- *Autotransfusion of ascitic fluid*: This is a simple and safe procedure. Administration of exogenous fluid is not required. But the disadvantage is the reinjection of cytokines in the circulation that may aggravate OHSS. Peritoneovenous shunting in the antecubital vein is also recommended.[43]
- *Pleurocentesis*: This gives a dramatic improvement in symptoms. Pulmonary thrombosis needs to be excluded before pleurocentesis as a cause of severe pulmonary symptoms.
- Pericardial effusion tapping may be rarely required.

Cases where surgical treatment in patients with ovarian hyperstimulation syndrome is required are:

- *Ovarian torsion*: The patient complains of severe unilateral or bilateral abdominal pain. The diagnosis is by ultrasound with Doppler. Whirlpool sign and gradual loss of ovarian vascularity are the signs commonly found on ultrasound, though later they may not be seen in all cases or may be seen to a variable extent.[16] Early diagnosis can save the ovary. Ovarian unwinding is done by laparoscopy and this regains the ovarian vascularity and perfusion.
- *Ectopic pregnancy*: Due to large ovaries and ascites, the diagnosis is difficult. Rapid deterioration in a patient's clinical condition and falling hemoglobin may be indicative.
- *Surgery for a ruptured cyst*: Hemostasis is achieved by laparoscopy or open surgery depending on a surgeon's expertise. It needs to be differentiated from ectopic pregnancy.
- *Pregnancy termination*: This may be required in very severe cases with marked renal and respiratory symptoms.

RECENT ADVANCES

The VEGF is the critical modulator of the syndrome. Treatment with a VEGF receptor antagonist prevents the capillary permeability in OHSS in a rat model.[44] Similarly, treatment with *fms*-like tyrosine kinase which binds with VEGF and decreases its availability for endothelial effects have similar results in OHSS in a rat model.[45]

CARRY HOME MESSAGE[46]

- Women with PCOS, elevated AMH, and elevated AFC benefit from ovarian stimulation protocols that reduce the risk of OHSS.
- In women with a high risk of OHSS, the GnRH antagonist protocol is preferred by ovarian stimulation.
- Using GnRHa as an ovulation trigger reduces the risk of OHSS, if multiple follicles have developed or E2 levels are high with stimulation.
- When GnRHa is used as a trigger, hCG co-trigger, luteal hormonal support, or cryopreservation of embryos should be used to improve results.
- Dopamine agonist administration starting at the time of hCG trigger for several days may also reduce the risk of OHSS.
- Metformin, aspirin, or cryopreservation of embryos may be used as additional means to prevent OHSS.
- The mainstay of OHSS treatment includes fluid resuscitation and prophylactic anticoagulant. Paracentesis or culdocentesis may be recommended for management of OHSS when a large amount of ascites is present.

REFERENCES

1. Rizk B, Rizk CB, Nawar MG, Garcia-Velasco JA, Sallam HN. Ultrasonography in the prediction and management of ovarian hyperstimulation syndrome. In: Rizk B (Ed). Ultrasonography in Reproductive Medicine and Infertility. Cambridge, UK: Cambridge University Press; 2010. pp. 299-312.
2. De Neubourg D, Mangelschots K, Van Royen E, Vercruyssen M, Gerris J. Singleton pregnancies are as affected by ovarian hyperstimulation syndrome as twin pregnancies. Fertil Steril. 2004;82:1691-3.
3. Rizk B, Aboulghar MA. Classification, pathophysiology and management of ovarian hyperstimulation syndrome. In: Brinsden P (Ed). A textbook of in-vitro fertilization and assisted reproduction. 2nd edition. Carnforth, UK: The Parthenon Publishing Group; 1999. pp. 131-55.
4. Rizk B, Aboulghar M, Smitz J, Ron-El R. The role of vascular endothelial growth factor and interleukins in the pathogenesis of severe ovarian hyperstimulation syndrome. Hum Reprod Update. 1997;3:255-66.
5. Krasnow JS, Berga SL, Guzick DS, Zeleznik AJ, Yeo KT. Vascular permeability factor and vascular endothelial growth factor in ovarian hyperstimulation syndrome: a preliminary report. Fertil Steril. 1996;65(3):552-5.
6. La Marca A, Guilini S, Tirelli A, Bertucci E, Marsella T, Xella S, et al. Anti-Müllerian hormone measurement on any day of the menstrual cycle strongly predicts ovarian response in assisted reproductive technology. Hum Reprod. 2007;22:766-71.
7. Lee TH, Liu CH, Huang CC, Wu YL, Shih YT, Ho HN, et al. Serum anti-Mullerian hormone and estradiol levels as predictors of ovarian hyperstimulation syndrome in assisted reproductive technology cycles. Hum Reprod. 2008;23:160-7.
8. Rizk B. Genetics of ovarian hyperstimulation syndrome. Reprod Biomed Online. 2009;19:14-27.
9. Daelemans C, Smits G, de Maertelaer V, Costagliola S, Englert Y, Vassart G, et al. Prediction of severity of symptoms in iatrogenic ovarian hyperstimulation syndrome by follicle-stimulating hormone receptor Ser680Asn polymorphism. J Clin Endocrinol Metab. 2004;89:6310-5.
10. Moron FJ, de Castro F, Royo JL, Montoro L, Mira E, Sáez ME, et al. Bone morphogenetic protein 15 (BMP15) alleles predict over-response to recombinant follicle stimulation hormone and iatrogenic ovarian hyperstimulation syndrome (OHSS). Pharmacogenet Genomics. 2006;16:485-95.
11. Ajonuma LC, Tsang LL, Zhang GH, Wong CHY, Lau MC, Ho LS, et al. Estrogen-induced abnormally high cystic fibrosis transmembrane conductance regulator expression results in ovarian hyperstimulation syndrome. Mol Endocrinol. 2005;19:3038-44.
12. Blankstein J, Shalev J, Saadon T, Kukia EE, Rabinovici J, Pariente C, et al. Ovarian hyperstimulation syndrome: prediction by number and size of preovulatory ovarian follicles. Fertil Steril. 1987;47(4):597-602.
13. Bergh C, Howles CM, Borg K, Hamberger L, Josefsson B, Nilsson L, et al. Recombinant human follicle-stimulating hormone

(r-hFSH; Gonal F) versus highly purified urinary FSH (Metrodin HP): results of a randomized comparative study in women undergoing assisted reproductive techniques. Hum Reprod. 1997;12:2133-9.
14. Oyesanya OA, Parsons JH, Collins WP, Campbell S. Total ovarian volume before human chorionic gonadotrophin administration for ovulation induction may predict the hyperstimulation syndrome. Hum Reprod. 1995;10:3211-2.
15. Al-Inany H, Aboulghar M. GnRH antagonist in assisted reproduction: a Cochrane review. Hum Reprod. 2002;17:874-85.
16. Al-Inany HG, Abou-Setta AM, Aboulghar M. Gonadotropin-releasing hormone antagonists for assisted conception. Cochrane Database Syst Rev. 2006;(3):CD001750.
17. Kolibianakis EM, Collins J, Tarlatzis BC, Devroey P, Diedrich K, Griesinger G. Among patients treated for IVF with gonadotropins and GnRH analogues, is the probability of live birth dependent on the type of analogue used? A systematic review and meta-analysis. Hum Reprod Update. 2006;12:651-71.
18. Tang T, Glanville J, Orsi N, Barth JH, Balen AH. The use of metformin for women with PCOS undergoing IVF treatment. Hum Reprod. 2006;21:1416-25.
19. Moll E, van der Veen F, van Wely M. The role of metformin in polycystic ovarian syndrome: a systematic review. Hum Reprod Update. 2007;13:527-37.
20. Son WY, Yoon SH, Lee SW, Ko Y, Yoon HG, Lim JH. Blastocyst development and pregnancies after IVF of mature oocytes retrieved from unstimulated patients with PCOS after in-vivo hCG priming. Hum Reprod. 2002;17:134-6.
21. Polson DW, Mason HD, Saldahna MB, Franks S. Ovulation of a single dominant follicle during treatment with low-dose pulsatile FSH in women with PCOS. Clin Endocrinol (Oxf). 1987;26:205-12.
22. Martinez F, Rodriguez DB, Buxaderas R, Tur R, Mancini F, Coroleu B. GnRH antagonist rescue of a long-protocol IVF cycle and GnRH agonist trigger to avoid ovarian hyperstimulation syndrome: three case reports. Fertil Steril. 2011;95(7):2432.e17-9.
23. Aboulghar M. Agonist and antagonist coast. Fertil Steril. 2012; 97(3):523-6.
24. Chen D, Burmeister L, Goldschlag D, et al. Ovarian hyperstimulation syndrome: Strategies for prevention. Reprod Biomed Online. 2003;7:43-9.
25. Humaidan P, Bredkjaer HE, Westergaard LG, Andersen CY. 1,500 IU human chorionic gonadotropin administered at oocyte retrieval rescues the luteal phase when gonadotropin-releasing hormone agonist is used for ovulation induction: a prospective, randomized, controlled study. Fertil Steril. 2010;93:847-50.
26. Griesinger G, von Otte S, Schroer A, Ludwig AK, Diedrich K, Al-Hasani S, et al. Elective cryopreservation of all pronuclear oocytes after GnRH agonist triggering of final oocyte maturation in patients at risk of developing OHSS: a prospective, observational proof-of-concept study. Hum Reprod. 2007; 22:1348-52.
27. Ludwig M, Katalinic A, Diedrich K. Use of GnRH antagonists in ovarian stimulation for assisted reproductive technologies compared to long protocol. Meta-analysis. Arch Gynecol Obstet. 2001;265:175-82.
28. Aboulghar M, Evers JH, Al-Inany H. Intravenous albumin for preventing severe ovarian hyperstimulation syndrome. Cochrane Database Syst Rev. 2000;2: CD001302.
29. Youssef MA, Al-Inany HG, Evers JL, Aboulghar M. Intravenous fluids for the prevention of severe ovarian hyperstimulation syndrome. Cochrane Database Syst Rev. 2011;(2): CD001302.
30. Rizk B. Ovarian hyperstimulation syndrome. In: Studd J, (Ed). Progress in obstetrics and gynaecology. Edinburgh: Churchill Livingstone; 1993. pp. 31-49.
31. Varnagy A, Bodis J, Manfai Z, Wilhelm F, Busznyák C, Koppán M. Low-dose aspirin therapy to prevent ovarian hyperstimulation syndrome. Fertil Steril. 2010;93:2281-4.
32. Revelli A, Dolfin E, Gennarelli G, Lantieri T, Massobrio M, Holte JG, et al. Low-dose

acetylsalicylic acid plus prednisolone as an adjuvant treatment in IVF: a prospective, randomized study. Fertil Steril. 2008;90:1685-91.
33. Youssef MA, van Wely M, Hassan MA, Al-Inany HG, Mochtar M, Khattab S, et al. Can dopamine agonist reduce the incidence and severity of OHSS in IVF/ICSI treatment cycles? A systematic review and meta-analysis. Hum Reprod Update. 2010;16(5):459-66.
34. Griesinger G, Schultz L, Bauer T, Broessner A, Frambach T, Kissler S. Ovarian hyperstimulation syndrome prevention by gonadotropin-releasing hormone agonist triggering of final oocyte maturation in a gonadotropin-releasing hormone antagonist protocol in combination with 'freeze-all' strategy: a prospective multicentric study. Fertil Steril. 2011;95:2029-33.
35. D'angelo, Amso N. Embryo freezing for preventing ovarian hyperstimulation syndrome. Cochrane Database Syst Rev. 2007;(3):CD002806.
36. Zhu WJ, Li XM, Chen XM, Zhang L. Follicular aspiration during the selection phase prevents severe ovarian hyperstimulation in patients with polycystic ovary syndrome who are undergoing in vitro fertilization. Eur J Obstet Gynecol Reprod Biol. 2005; 122(1):79-84.
37. Yakovenko SA, Sivozhelezov VS, Zorina IV, Dmitrieva NV, Apryshko VP, Voznesenskaya JV. Prevention of OHSS by intravenous calcium. Hum Reprod. 2009;24(Suppl 1):i61.
38. Gurgan T, Demirol A, Guven S, Benkhalifa M, Girgin B, Li TC. Intravenous calcium infusion as a novel preventive therapy of ovarian hyperstimulation syndrome for patients with polycystic ovarian syndrome. Fertil Steril. 2011;96:53-7.
39. Devroey P, Polyzos N, Blockeel C. OHSS free clinic by segmentation of IVF treatment. Hum Reprod. 2011;26:2593-7.
40. Rizk B. Ovarian Hyperstimulation Syndrome: Epidemiology, Pathophysiology, Prevention and Management. Cambridge, UK: Cambridge University Press; 2006.
41. Lainas TG, Sfontouris IA, Zorzovilis IZ, Petsas GK, Lainas GT, Alexopoulou E, et al. Live births after management of severe OHSS by GnRH antagonist administration in the luteal phase. Reprod Biomed Online. 2009;19(6):789-95.
42. Aboulghar MA, Mansour RT, Serour GI, Amin A. Ultrasonically guided vaginal aspiration of ascites in the treatment of severe ovarian hyperstimulation syndrome. Fertil Steril. 1990;53:933-5.
43. Koike T, Araki S, Minakami H, Ogawa S, Sayama M, Shibahara H, et al. Clinical efficacy of peritoneovenous shunting for the treatment of severe OHSS. Hum Reprod. 2000;15:113-7.
44. Gomez R, Simon C, Remohi J, Pellicer A. Vascular endothelial growth factor receptor-2 activation induces vascular permeability in hyperstimulated rats, and this effect is prevented by receptor blockade. Endocrinology. 2002;143:4339-48.
45. McElhinney B, Ardill J, Caldwell C, McClure N. Preventing ovarian hyperstimulation syndrome by inhibiting the effects for vascular endothelial growth factor. J Reprod Med. 2003;48:243-6.
46. Practice Committee of the American Society for Reproductive Medicine. Prevention and treatment of moderate and severe ovarian hyperstimulation syndrome: a Guideline. Practice committee of the American Society for Reproductive medicine. Fertil Steril. 2016;106(7):1634-7.

25 Chapter
Intrauterine Insemination

INTRODUCTION

Intrauterine insemination (IUI) has attained a wide popularity in management of infertility. But it is still the least standardized procedure as far as infertility treatment is concerned. Optimal guideline adherence has substantial economic benefits when compared with suboptimal guideline adherence.[1] IUI is blamed for low pregnancy rates but meticulous patient selection, stimulation protocol, good ultrasound (US) monitoring, and good semen preparation if combined with IUI only then give good results.

In IUI, a bolus of sperms is placed in the uterus directly, bypassing the vaginal acidity and cervical hostility. This allows a safe quick access of the sperms to ova in the ampullary part of the oviduct. IUI must be done with the washed sample and never with the nit sample of semen. Using unwashed/nonprocessed semen leads to uterine cramps, infection, and collapse. Primary treatment with IUI is much more cost-effective than in vitro fertilization (IVF).[2]

INDICATIONS OF INTRAUTERINE INSEMINATION

Most Common Indications

- *Unexplained infertility*: It is the first in the list of indications of IUI. It is not at the top of the list in indications for IVF. We have documented a series of 189 patients who have conceived with IUI after three or more IVF cycles failed elsewhere. In this group, the majority of the patients had unexplained infertility.
- *Dysovulatory infertility*: Absolute pregnancy rate is higher with multifollicular compared to monofollicular growth.[3]
- *Male subfertility*: When the total motile sperm count before sperm preparation is <10 million, it is called mild male factor subfertility. Mild ovarian hyperstimulation with IUI is done in these cases.[4]
  Most clinics use a cutoff of 0.8–1.0 million. John Balasch recommends 2 million counts and 4% normal morphology postwash as eligible for IUI, but for male factor, double IUI, one IUI before ovulation and another at the time of ovulation, gives better conception rates compared with single IUI.[5]
- *Mild-to-moderate endometriosis*: These patients must be treated as those with unexplained subfertility and benefit from mild ovarian hyperstimulation with IUI, which results in two to three follicles.
  Ablation of endometriotic lesions rather than diagnostic laparoscopy improves spontaneous pregnancy rates. But stage III and IV endometriosis gives only a 2–3% pregnancy rate and for these patients, ART is recommended.

Other Uncommon Indications

- *Cervical hostility*: The cervix normally acts as a sperm reservoir.

Cervical factor is mostly affected due to multiple D and C (dilatation and curettage). Previous surgery on cervix, such as cauterization, conization, or Fothergill's surgery, also disturbs the cervical environment. As these operations are extremely rare nowadays, cervical factor is not commonly seen as a cause of infertility.

- *Immunological infertility*: IUI is the first choice before IVF/intracytoplasmic sperm injection (ICSI).[6]
- HIV positive male partner with HIV negative female partner
- Single patent tube

  At the time of ovulation, ovarian fimbria contracts: As it is attached to the ovary, the fimbrial end comes closer to the ovary and completely covers the ovarian surface at the site of the follicle. The ciliary movement of the columnar epithelium of the fallopian tube creates negative pressure of 1 mm of mercury. This negative pressure sucks the ova inside the tube. So, it is the tube that takes an ova rather than ova going inside the tube.

  So for successful IUI, tubo-ovarian relations should be normal and the ova enters the tube of the same side. Therefore, IUI should be done, if the tube is open on the side on which follicle develops.
- Ejaculatory failure
- Failed artificial insemination with donor sperm (AID)
- *Frozen samples*: When the husband is absent or on antineoplastic treatment

STEPS OF INTRAUTERINE INSEMINATION

The success of IUI depends on the following steps, each step having equal importance:

- Ovulation stimulation (superovulation)
- Ultrasound monitoring and timing of ovulation trigger
- Timing and method of IUI
- Semen preparation
- Luteal support

Superovulation

Advantages

- To increase the number of oocytes available for fertilization
- More oocytes, more chances of conception
- Increased steroids may improve chances of fertilization and implantation
- Subtle hormonal deficiencies are corrected
- Luteal phase defect (LPD) is corrected
- Increased fertilization window as several oocytes are released over a protracted period.

Both ovulation induction and IUI independently increase pregnancy rates.

Superovulation with IUI has higher pregnancy rates than after timed intercourse and clomiphene citrate (CC).[7]

This study shows:

- *No stimulation*: Pregnancy rates vary from 2 to 8% per cycle, but they are always lower than the stimulated cycle. As stimulated cycles have higher multiple pregnancy rates, many centers, including Bourn Hall Clinic, London, offer natural cycle IUI. In couples with cervical factor subfertility, IUI in natural cycles significantly increases the probability of conception.[8]
- *Clomiphene citrate*: It can be given from Days 5–9 in a dosage of 50–100 mg/day. Cycle fecundability in spontaneous and CC-induced cycle is the same (6–13%) as compared to gonadotropins (14–24%).[9] We do not prefer CC for IUI as pregnancy rates are extremely low.

  Ovarian stimulation with letrozole may significantly increase live birth rates controlling multiple pregnancy rates compared to CC and only human menopausal gonadotropin (hMG).[10]

- *Gonadotropins*: Gonadotropin with IUI is more successful than only gonadotropin or only IUI or CC + IUI. Gonadotropins with IUI have 10–15% chances of pregnancy as compared to 1–2% with natural cycle in idiopathic infertility. The pregnancy rates are far better when IUI is combined with gonadotropins as compared to when IUI is combined with natural cycle, CC or CC + hMG.[11]

Existing treatments, such as empirical CC and unstimulated IUI, do not offer superior birth rates compared with expectant management of unexplained infertility.[12,13] A UK randomized controlled trial (RCT) [Scottish Unexplained Infertility Trial (SUIT)] compared the effectiveness of CC and IUI with that of expectant management and concluded that neither showed superior live birth rates compared with expectant management.[14] Higher pregnancy rates are obtained when IUI is combined with gonadotropins than with antiestrogen agents.[15]

Low-dose hMG with IUI has given a higher pregnancy rate than CC with IUI and is more cost-effective. But in our experience, follicle-stimulating hormone (FSH) gives much better results in IUI cycles than HMG.

Conventional Protocol (Fig. 1)

Gonadotropins are started from Day 5 in patients with normal ovaries on baseline scan. 75 IU FSH is given daily from Day 5 to 9. If the follicle or endometrium grows, the same dose is continued; otherwise the dose is doubled for 3 days. US monitoring will help to decide whether to continue the same dose till the follicle matures or to further increase the dose to 225 IU. Gonadotropins are continued till a mature follicle and endometrium are achieved.

Step-down Protocol (Fig. 2)

If the baseline scan indicates a poor responding ovary, then we start with a higher

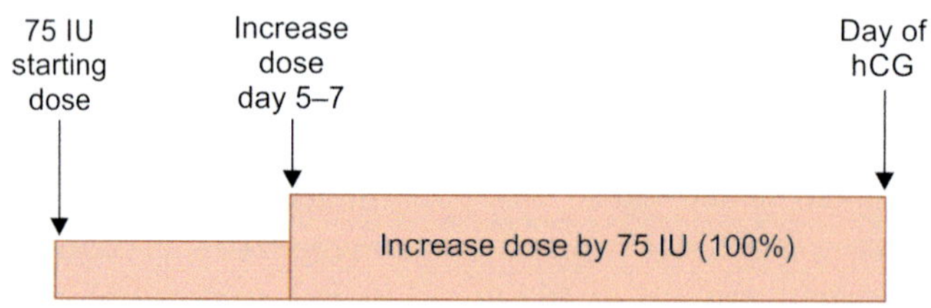

Fig. 1: Conventional protocol. (hCG: human chorionic gonadotropin)

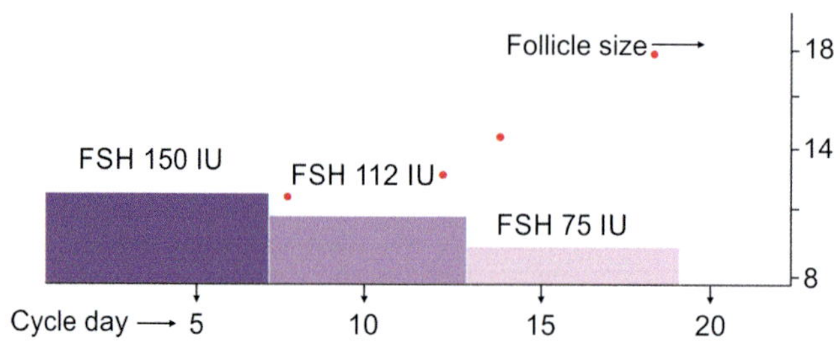

Fig. 2: Step-down protocol. (FSH: follicle-stimulating hormone)

dose for stimulation, 150–225 IU, till a follicle of 10 mm or larger appears. Then the dose is decreased to 75 IU till we get a mature follicle and receptive endometrium.

Chronic Low-dose Protocol (Fig. 3)

In polycystic ovary syndrome (PCOS) patients, stimulation is started with 37.5–75 IU and is continued up to 10–14 days before increasing the dose in spite of no follicular growth documented. This protocol is very effective in PCOS patients to decrease the incidence of ovarian hyperstimulation syndrome (OHSS) and multiple pregnancy.

The advantages of the chronic low-dose protocol are as follows[13-15] **(Fig. 4)**:

- Monofollicular development
- Multiple pregnancies can be avoided.
- Premature LH surge is avoided.
- Antagonists are not required.
- Implantation rate is improved.

A recent Cochrane review, 2007, shows that gonadotropin is the most effective drug when IUI is combined with controlled ovarian hyperstimulation (COH).[16]

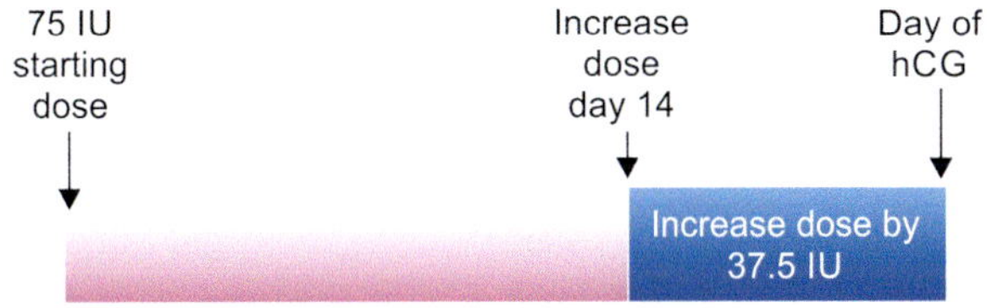

Fig. 3: Chronic low-dose protocol. (hCG: human chorionic gonadotropin)

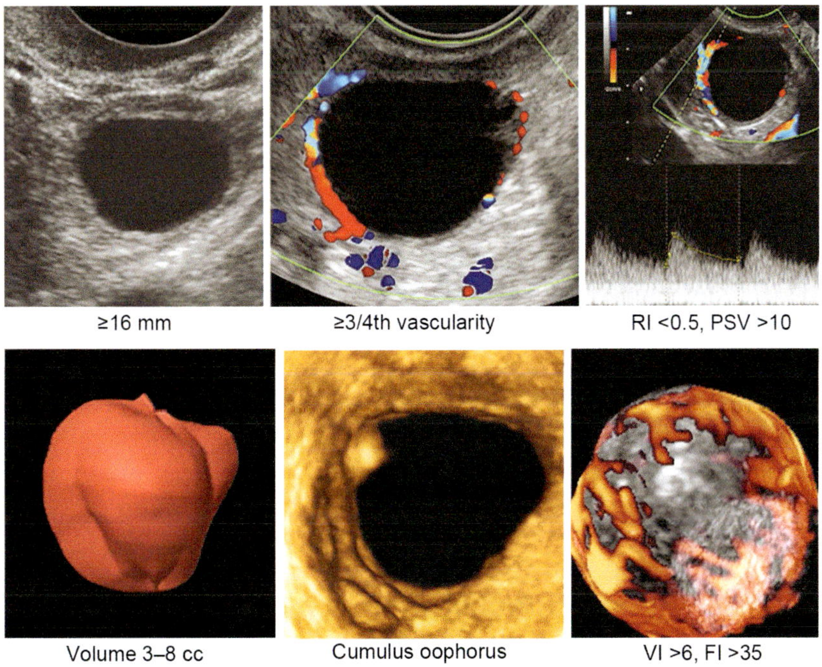

Fig. 4: Pre-hCG follicular parameters. (FI: flow index; hCG: human chorionic gonadotropin; PSV: peak systolic velocity; RI: resistance index; VI: vascularization index)

Letrozole + Gonadotropins

We have found this combination very effective in decreasing the consumption of gonadotropins and incidence of multiple pregnancy rates with equally high conception rates compared with only gonadotropins with IUI.

Letrozole is given from Day 3 to 7. From Day 7, FSH 75 IU is given daily for 5 days. Then according to the findings on US monitoring, the dose is adjusted. This is an excellent combination for poor responders.

Role of Gonadotropin-releasing Hormone Agonist and Antagonist

Gonadotropin-releasing hormone (GnRH) agonist is not used routinely in IUI protocols for downregulation. It increases the total dose of gonadotropins consumed, the incidence of OHSS, and multiple pregnancy rates. It has no advantage in IUI protocols and we never use it for IUI cycles.

Gonadotropin-releasing hormone antagonist may be used in IUI protocols. Adding GnRH antagonist in cycles with mild ovarian hyperstimulation in an IUI program routinely does not increase the live birth rate.[17] Though it is very useful in thin lean PCOS patients in whom luteinizing hormone (LH) is tonically high. Here antagonist is given when the follicle size of 14 mm is reached, till the day of trigger. It prevents premature LH surge and improves the quality of ova and embryo, which in turn gives higher pregnancy rates. But it cannot be given to all the patients of IUI.

Ultrasound Monitoring and Timing of Human Chorionic Gonadotropin

This has been discussed in the Chapter 9 of this book in detail. It is the key factor for achieving good conception rates with IUI. Good US monitoring may also give information about the hormonal milieu of the patient and hormonal assays can be omitted. Timing of hCG is the key point for the success of IUI cycles.

We decide the timing of IUI based on the following factors.[18]

Optimal Pre-hCG Follicular Parameters (Fig. 4)

- Follicular diameter of at least 16 mm and 3–7 cc volume. The optimal size of the leading follicle in ovulation induction with CC and letrozole is similar and is closely related to endometrial thickness.[19] The optimal size for the leading follicle has been suggested as 18–22 and 23–27 mm in different studies[19,20]
- Vascularity covering at least three fourths of follicular circumference
- Perifollicular resistance index (RI): 0.4–0.48
- Perifollicular peak systolic velocity (PSV) >10 cm/s
- Follicular vascularization index (VI) > 6 and flow index (FI) > 35
- Presence of cumulus oophorus

Optimal Pre-hCG Endometrial Parameters (Fig. 5)

- Endometrial thickness of at least 6 mm, preferably 8 mm
- Grade A/B endometrium
- Endometrial vascularity in zones 3–4, covering >5 mm^2 area
- Endometrial vessels RI: 0.49–0.59 and pulsatility index (PI): 1.1–2.3
- Uterine artery PI < 3.2
- Endometrial volume > 3 cc
- Endometrial FI > 40 and vascularization flow index (VFI) > 20

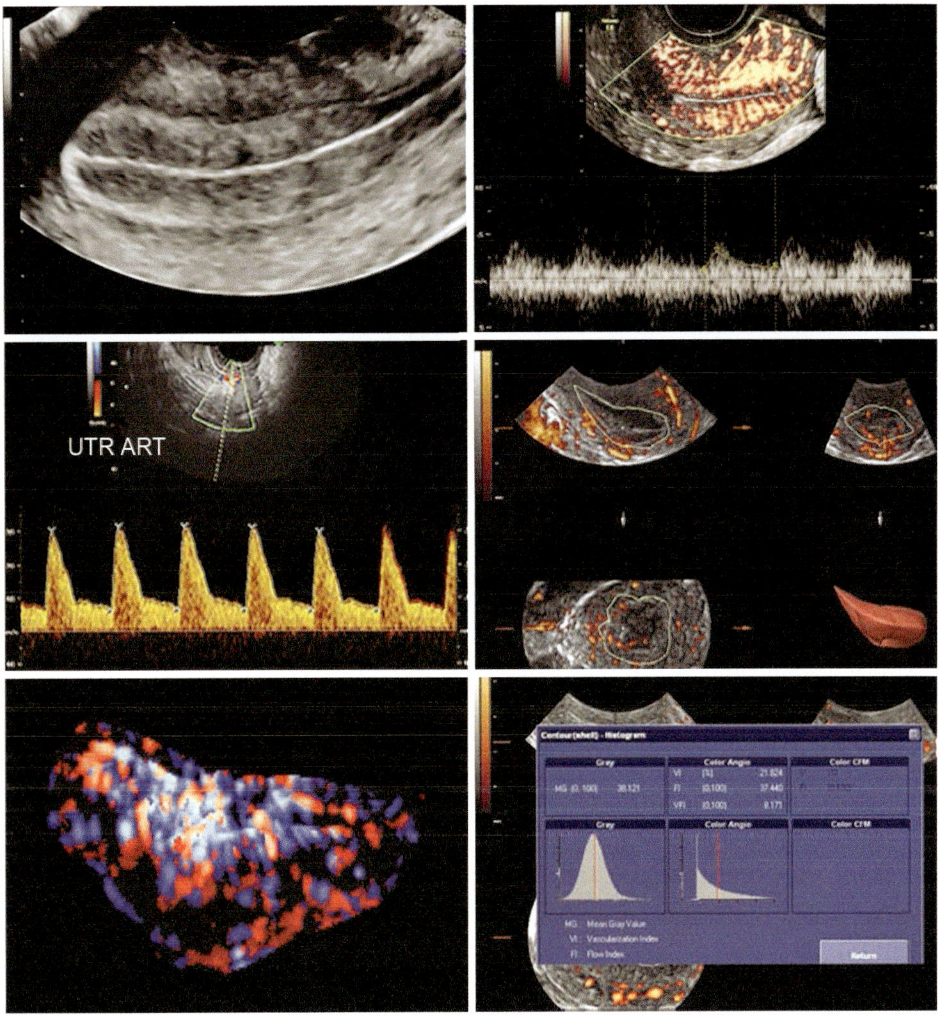

Fig. 5: Prehuman chorionic gonadotropin (hCG) endometrial parameters. (UTR ART: uterine artery)

Ovulation Trigger

- Recombinant hCG (rhCG) 250 IU is given when preovulatory follicular and endometrial parameters on US are satisfied.
- Urinary hCG (uhCG) 10,000 IU.

GnRH agonist (GnRHa): 1 mg of Leuprolide acetate. Some advocate 1.5 mg 12 hours apart in two doses and some centers use 2-mg single dose or decapeptyl 1 mg. GnRHa is given in PCOS patients when there are multiple follicles and when OHSS is anticipated. Indications of GnRHa trigger in IUI:

- In PCOS, when there is multifollicular development, GnRHa should be given as a trigger instead of hCG. IUI should be done at 36–38 hours as is done with hCG trigger. Ideally, in PCOS patients, a chronic low-dose protocol is chosen as discussed in the chapter on ovulation induction and with this, multiple follicles will not develop. But, to avoid OHSS, whenever there is multifollicular growth,

GnRHa trigger is given. With judicious luteal support, pregnancy rates are very good. We have never converted the IUI cycle to IVF.

- In patients with luteinized unruptured follicle (LUF) with hCG, GnRHa may be an effective trigger, as it also gives FSH surge, which may help in rupture of the follicle, e.g., in endometriosis.

Timing of Insemination

The life span of an ovum is about 8–10 hours, maximum. So during that time, spermatozoa should be around the ovum. A urinary LH kit is useful to decide the LH surge but we have not found it to be useful. We give trigger by deciding follicle maturity and endometrial receptivity by US and then after 36–38 hours, we do IUI in normal patients. Literature shows the following timings of insemination:

- 36–38 hours (between 32 and 38 hours)[21,22]
- 18 and 42 hours
- 24 and 48 hours
- 38 and 24 hours later if rupture is not seen on US

We have found insemination between 36 and 38 hours as excellent as it has given the highest number of pregnancies. A retrospective cohort study by Kucuk showed significantly higher cycle pregnancy rates after follicular rupture, 36–38 hours post-hCG compared with that when follicle rupture was not evident.[23]

Double Intrauterine Insemination

In the literature, it has not been quoted when to do double IUI. There are various papers which say that double IUI does not increase the pregnancy rates.[24]

The Cochrane review also suggests that double IUI adds to cost and inconvenience without improving efficacy.[25] Though double IUI may improve pregnancy rates in male factor subfertility.[25]

Physiology of Rupture of Follicle

The LH surge starts when the PSV of the follicle is 10 cm/s. It gradually increases and reaches up to 45 cm/s just before the rupture. This means that when the PSV of the follicle is higher, the follicle is not 36 hours away from rupture but is closer. This means that if hCG is given at this time, the follicle will not rupture at 36 hours but will rupture earlier and therefore IUI should be done earlier.

Our Experience on Double Intrauterine Insemination

We have done a study of 500 superovulation with IUI cycles,[26] with different stimulation protocols, namely, CC, gonadotropins, and letrozole with gonadotropins. We have found that no matter what stimulation protocol is used, if perifollicular PSV is >20 cm/s, double IUI (first one done between 12 and 14 hours after hCG and second done between 36 and 38 hours of hCG) gives significantly higher pregnancy rates as compared to single IUI done between 36 and 38 hours after hCG. This is because the higher the PSV, the earlier is the follicle likely to rupture **(Fig. 6)**. (Also refer to Chapter 9 of this book.)

Semen Preparation

It has been separately discussed in Chapter 26.

Among the factors that may affect the success of IUI:

- The most important is the age of the female. The success rate of IUI sharply decreases after 40 years of age of the female partner.[27] It has been observed that increasing male age seems to be associated with the decline in semen volume, sperm motility, and sperm morphology but not with sperm concentration.[28] This has a synergistic adverse effect when the female partner is also >35 years of age.[29] If the sperm morphology score is >4%, IUI can

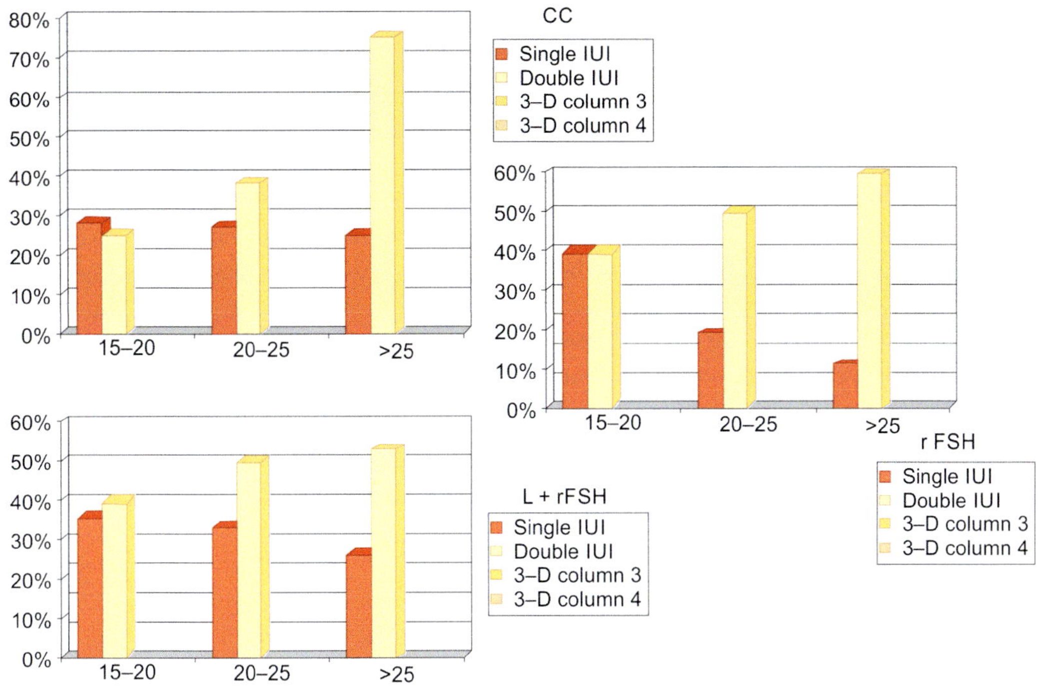

Fig. 6: Graphs showing comparative conception rates of single IUI (red columns) and double IUI (yellow columns) at different PSV values for perifollicular flow. (CC: clomiphene citrate; IUI: intrauterine insemination; rFSH: recombinant follicle-stimulating hormone)

be performed with an acceptable success rate if the insemination motile count (IMC) is >1 million.[30] The pregnancy rate per cycle is highest in the first three treatment cycles.[31] Couples with mild male subfertility, unexplained fertility, or mild endometriosis show acceptable cumulative ongoing pregnancy rates after six cycles of IUI with ovarian hyperstimulation.[32]

If time is not the issue, the couple should be offered nine treatment cycles, especially couples in which female age is <35 years.[32]

- The National Institute for Healthcare and Excellence fertility guidelines advocate up to six IUI cycles for patients of unexplained infertility, male subfertility, and moderate endometriosis.[33]
  - Single IUI is done between 36 and 38 hours.
  - Double IUI is done when perifollicular PSV is >20 cm/s.
  - Double IUI gives better results in male infertility.
  - IUI is preferred over IVF as the first line of treatment.
  - At least six cycles of IUI should be done in female ≤35 years of age.
  - Majority of the females conceive in 3 months with IUI.
  - In younger patients, up to nine cycles of IUI should be tried.

Intrauterine insemination: The important points to remember in IUI are as follows:

- Measure uterocervical length (UCL) by US at the time of baseline scan.
- IUI is done with all aseptic preparations.

- Total time from collection to insemination should be 80–120 minutes.
- There is no need to use antiseptics or saline.
- Do not touch the endometrium with an IUI cannula to avoid injury to the endometrium.
- We generally use Sims speculum and hold the anterior lip of the cervix with Alyce's forceps to straighten the cervicouterine canal. With Cusco's speculum, without using Alyce's forceps, there is often difficulty in negotiating the cannula in many cases. In our more than 12,000 IUI pregnancies, we have used Sims speculum and Alyce's forceps. When uterine contractions are seen frequently, the pregnancy rate and live birth rate increase. Myometrial contractions are necessary for achieving fertilization, as these allow the sperms to go to the fallopian tube.
- About 0.3–0.7 mL of wash sample is put inside the uterine cavity slowly.

The uterus can hold only 0.4 mL of fluid in its cavity. If it is injected in excess, it flows into the fallopian tubes or may flow out through the cervix into the vagina. We usually inject 0.5–0.7 mL of the prepared (washed) semen sample and so there is almost always some intratubal insemination. This is the reason that when the washed semen sample is being inseminated, one should be very slow and gentle. Since there is some amount of intratubal insemination almost always with intrauterine insemination, the results are similar to that of "GIFT" (i.e., gamete intrafallopian tube transfer). Therefore "GIFT" is no more practiced. As the excess amount of the prepared sample, beyond 0.4–0.5 mL, flows out of the vagina, the patient always complains of fluid dribbling out through the vagina and blames that for negative results. It is therefore essential to counsel the patient for this purpose. There is always a confusion on the part of the couple whether to keep relations before IUI or not. They should be allowed intercourse at any time during the follicular phase. Long abstinence will have dead sperms and pus cells in the semen sample. Abstinence of <2 days usually gives a higher pregnancy rate. We always ask the patient to have intercourse on the day of trigger and then the sample for IUI is collected on the day of IUI.[34]

- Allow the patient to rest for 15 minutes. About 10–15 minutes of immobilization after IUI significantly improves cumulative ongoing pregnancy rates and live birth rates.[35] Maximum six cycles of IUI should be tried. But all these six cycles should be with gonadotropins and good US monitoring.
- According to the literature, the minimum postwash sperm count required for IUI is 2 million with 4% normal spermatozoa. But in our own series, the highest pregnancy rates have been achieved when the postwash count is between 6 and 8 million.
- Advanced maternal age along with low antral follicle count (AFC) and anti-Müllerian hormone (AMH) should be offered ovum donation.
- The success rate with IUI is highest when 14% or more sperms show normal morphology, intermediate when 4–14% are normal, and very low when only <4% sperms show normal morphology.
- IUI has replaced intraperitoneal insemination, intratubal insemination, cervical cap, pentoxifylline, and estrogen therapy.

Complications

Complications are very few and very rare. If at all may occur, these are due to superovulation or incorrect semen wash.

- *Those due to superovulation are*: OHSS and multiple pregnancy.
- *Those due to incorrect semen wash are*: Infection and pain in the abdomen.

Luteal Support

Luteal support is an absolute must when superovulation is done. Protocols for luteal support may be any of the following:

- 200 mg bd, progesterone effervescent tablets
- 300–400 mg bd, micronized progesterone vaginal pessaries
- hCG 5,000 IU on Day 5 and Day 9 after IUI
- hCG 2,000 IU on Day 3-7-10 after IUI

Luteal phase support with vaginal progesterone significantly improves the live birth rates in IUI cycles with gonadotropin stimulation.[36] But it does not improve pregnancy rates in normo-ovulatory women stimulated with CC for IUI.[37]

OUR EXPERIENCES

We have so far achieved more than 12,000 pregnancies with IUI. In our experience, superovulation with recombinant FSH (rFSH) is the best. Follicular monitoring by at least color Doppler and preferably three-dimensional (3D) power Doppler is a must for precise timing of hCG. Perfect semen wash is equally important.

We have been able to achieve a success rate of 80–90% in six cycles in patients with idiopathic or dysovulatory infertility, when superovulation with rFSH or highly purified urinary FSH (uFSH-HP) is done with IUI and consistent US monitoring is done as described.

How to optimize IUI results:

- Counseling is very important as the patient should understand that IUI alone does not give pregnancy but all other factors such as stimulation to luteal phase support are equally important.
- A patient having unexplained infertility, dysovulatory infertility, and male subfertility should be offered IUI rather than IVF as the first line of treatment.
- Stimulation protocol with gonadotropins gives a higher pregnancy rate than oral ovulogens or natural cycle IUI. A chronic low-dose protocol is very useful in PCOS patients.
- FSH is better than HMG as endogenous LH is present and antagonists should be added in thin lean PCOS patients.
- US monitoring with at least color Doppler is a must to get good results of IUI.
- Ovulation trigger should be decided according to US findings, and hCG 10,000 or rhCG 250 µg gives equal results.
- Agonist trigger with judicious luteal support is given when multiple follicles develop in both ovaries.
- Double IUI is required when perifollicular PSV is >20 cm/s.
- Minimum 3–4 cycles of IUI with gonadotropins with good US monitoring should be done. The pregnancy rate increases up to six cycles. But if the age is <30 years and time is not a factor, up to nine cycles of IUI can be done. Three cycles of IUI and one IVF have the same pregnancy rate but the cost is low with IUI.
- Holding the cervix does not decrease the pregnancy rate but facilitates IUI.
- Luteal support is a must as hCG is given as a trigger.
- The gradient can be prepared for patients with male subfertility.

CARRY HOME MESSAGE

- IUI is the preferred method for dysovulatory infertility, idiopathic infertility, or male subfertility.
- Superovulation must be done by rFSH/uFSH-HP.
- Letrozole + rFSH gives excellent results.
- US monitoring by color Doppler and 3D power Doppler improves results dramatically.
- Ultrasound helps to decide the time of IUI and also whether to do single/double IUI.
- Semen preparation should be meticulous.
- Luteal support is a must in superovulation with IUI.

REFERENCES

1. Haagen EC, Nelen WLDM, Adang EM, Grol RPTM, Hermens RPMG, Kremer JAM. Guideline adherence is worth the effort: a cost-effectiveness analysis in intrauterine insemination care. Hum Reprod. 2013;28(2): 357-66.
2. Goverde AJ, McDonnell J, Vermeiden JP, Schats R, Rutten FF, Schoemaker J. Intrauterine insemination or in vitro fertilization in idiopathic subfertility and male subfertility: a randomised trial and cost-effectiveness analysis. Lancet. 2000; 355:13-8.
3. Van Ruste MME, Custers IM, Van der Veen F, van Wely M, Evers JLH, Mol BWJ. The influence of number of follicles on pregnancy rates in intrauterine insemination with ovarian stimulation: a meta-analysis. Hum Reprod Update. 2008;14:563-657.
4. Van Weert JM, Repping S, Van Voorhis BJ, Van der Veen F, Bossyut P, Mol BW. Performance of post wash total motile sperm count as a predictor of pregnancy at the time of intrauterine insemination: a meta-analysis. Fertil Steril. 2004;82(3):612-20.
5. Ghanem ME, Bakre NI, Enam MA, Al Boghdady LA, Helal AS, Elmetwally AG, et al. The effect of timing of IUI in relation to ovulation and number of inseminations on cycle pregnancy rate in common infertility etiology. Hum Reprod. 2011;26(3):576-83.
6. Ombelet W, Vandeput H, Janssen M, Cox A, Vossen C, Pollet H. Treatment of male infertility due to sperm surface antibodies: IUI or IVF? Hum Reprod. 1997;1296:165-70.
7. Hughes EG. Stimulated intra-uterine insemination is not a natural choice for the treatment of unexplained subfertility. Hum Reprod. 1998;18(5):912-4.
8. Steures P, Vander Steeg JW, Hopes PG, Bossyut PM, Habbema JD, Eijkmans MJ, et al. Effectiveness of intrauterine insemination in subfertile couples with an isolated cervical factor: A randomised clinical trial. Fertil Steril. 2007;88(6):1692-6.
9. Guzick DS, Sullivan MW, Adamson GD, Cedars MI, Falk RJ, Peterson EP, et al. Efficacy of treatment for unexplained infertility. Fertil Steril. 1998;70:207.
10. Huang S, Wang R, Rong Li, Wang H, Qiao J, Mol BW. Ovarian stimulation in infertile women treated with the use of intrauterine insemination: a cohort study from China. Fertil Steril. 2018;109(5):872-8.
11. Mahani IM, Afnan M. The pregnancy rates with intrauterine insemination (IUI) in superovulated cycles employing different protocols [Clomiphene citrate (CC), Human menopausal gonadotropin (HMG) and HMG+CC] and in Natural ovulatory cycle. J Pak Med Asso. 2004;54(10):503-5.
12. Wordsworth S, Buchanan J, Mollison J, Harrild K, Robertson L, Tay C, et al. Clomiphene citrate and intrauterine insemination as first line treatments for unexplained infertility: are they cost-effective?. Hum Reprod. 2011;26(2):369-75.
13. Verhulst SM, Cohlen BJ, Hughes E, te Velde E, Heineman MJ. Intrauterine insemination for unexplained subfertility. Cochrane Database Syst Rev. 2006;(4):CD001838.
14. Bhattacharya S, Harrild K, Mollison J, Wordsworth S, Tay C, Harrold A, et al. Clomiphene citrate or unstimulated intrauterine insemination compared with expectant management for unexplained infertility: pragmatic randomised controlled trial. BMJ. 2008;337:a716.
15. Cantineau AE, Cohlen BJ. Ovarian stimulation protocols (anti-oestrogens, gonadotropins with and without agonists/antagonists) for intrauterine insemination in women with subfertility. Cochrane Database Syst Rev. 2007;(2):CD005356.
16. Cohlen BJ, Heineman MJ. Ovarian stimulation protocols (anti-oestrogens, gonadotrophins with and without GnRH agonist/antagonist). Cochrane Database Syst Rev. 2007;(2):CD005356.

17. Cantineau AEP, Cohlen BJ, Klip H, Heineman MJ, Dutch IUI study Group Collaborators. The addition of GnRH antagonists in intrauterine insemination cycles with mild ovarian hyperstimulation does not increase live birth rates—a randomised, double-blinded, placebo-controlled trial. Hum Reprod. 2011;26(50): 1104-11.
18. Kurjak A, Chervenak FK. 3D and 3D PD assessment of Pre-HCG follicle and endometrium. Donald Sch J Ultrasound Obstetr Gynecol. 2008;2(2):35-47.
19. Palatnik A, Strawn E, Szabo A, Robb P. What is the optimal follicular size before triggering ovulation in intrauterine insemination cycles with clomiphene citrate or letrozole? An analysis of 988 cycles. Fertil Steril. 2012;97:1089-94.
20. Farhi J, Orvieto R, Gavish O, Homburg R. The association between follicular size on hCG day and pregnancy rate in clomiphene citrate treated polycystic ovary syndrome patients. Gynecol Endocrinol. 2010;26:546-8.
21. ESHRE Capri Workshop Group. Intrauterine Insemination. Hum Reprod Update. 2009; 15:265-77.
22. Ragni G, Somigliana E, Vegetti W. Timing of intrauterine insemination: where are we are? Fertil Steril. 2004;82:25-6.
23. Kucuk T. Intrauterine insemination: is the timing correct? J Assist Reprod Genet. 2008;8:427-30.
24. Bagis T, Haydardedeoglu B, Kilicdag EB, Cok T, Simsek E, Parlakgumus AH. Single versus double intrauterine insemination in multi-follicular ovarian hyperstimulation cycles: a randomised trial. Hum Reprod. 2010;25:1684-90.
25. Cantineau AE, Heineman MJ, Cohlen BJ. Single versus double intrauterine insemination in stimulated cycles for subfertile couples. Cochrane Database Syst Rev. 2003;(1):CD003854.
26. Nagori C, Panchal S. Role of double IUI in patients with high perifollicular PSV. London: 16th World Congress on Ultrasound in Obstetrics and Gynecology; 2006.
27. Broekmans FJ, Soules MR, Fauser BC. Ovarian aging: mechanisms and clinical consequences. Endocr Rev. 2009;30(5): 465-93.
28. Kidd SA, Eskenazi B, Wyrobak AJ. Effects of male age on semen quality and fertility: a review of literature. Fertil Steril. 2001;75(2): 237-48.
29. Mathieu C, Ecochard R, Bied V, Lornage J, Czyba JC. Cumulative conception rate following intrauterine artificial insemination with husband's spermatozoa: influence of husband's age. Hum Reprod. 1995;10(5): 1090-7.
30. Ombelet W, Vandeput H, Vande Putte G, Cox A, Janssen M, Jacobs P, et al. Intrauterine insemination after ovarian stimulation with clomiphene citrate: predictive potential of inseminating motile count and sperm morphology? Hum Reprod. 1997;12:1458-63.
31. Aboulghar M, Mansour R, Serour G, Abdrazek A. Controlled ovarian hyperstimulation and intrauterine insemination for treatment of unexplained infertility should be limited to a maximum of three trials. Fertil Steril. 2001;75(1):88-91.
32. Custers IM, Steures P, Hompes P, Flierman P. Intrauterine insemination: how many cycles should we perform? Hum Reprod. 2008;23(4):885-8.
33. National Institute for Health and Care Excellence. Fertility assessment and treatment of people with infertility problems. Clinical guidelines CG 11. London: NICE; 2004. [online] Available from: www.nice.org.uk/guidance/CG11 [Last accessed March, 2021].
34. Marshburu PB, Alanis M, Matthews ML, Usadi R, Papadakis MH, Kullstam S, et al. Short period of ejaculatory abstinence before intrauterine insemination is associated with higher pregnancy rate. Fertil Steril. 2010;93(1):286-9.
35. Saleh A, Tan SL, Biljan MM, Tulandi T. A randomised study of the effect of 10 minutes of bed rest after intrauterine insemination. Fertil Steril. 2000;74:509-11.
36. Erem AA, Erdem M, Atmaca S, Guler I. Impact of luteal phase support on pregnancy rates in intrauterine insemination cycles: a prospective randomised study. Fertil Steril. 2009;91:2508-13.
37. Kyrou D, Fatei HM, Tournaye H, Devroey P. Luteal phase support in normo-ovulatory women stimulated with clomiphene citrate for intrauterine insemination: need or habit? Hum Reprod. 2010;25:2501-6.

26

Chapter

Sperm Preparation in Intrauterine Insemination and In Vitro Fertilization

INTRODUCTION

After assessment of the semen sample, preparation is done. The preparation of the semen sample depends on the count, motile sperms, volume, viscosity, presence of antibodies, white blood cell (WBC), and debris.

The purpose of semen preparation is to concentrate the normal motile sperms with intact functional and genetic properties including normal morphology, with minimal deoxyribonucleic acid (DNA) damage, and intact cell membranes with functional binding properties. It makes sperms hyperactive after the removal of seminal plasma. Seminal plasma has prostaglandins, anticapacitation and antifertilization factors, dead sperms, WBC, bacteria, and germ cells.

COLLECTION OF SEMEN SAMPLE

Abstinence is not preferred before intrauterine insemination (IUI) as long abstinence may result in higher sperm volume and concentration but result in lower sperm motility and high sperm DNA fragmentation levels. Though 24 hours of abstinence is advised as abstinence shorter than that may result in poor chromatin packaging. It has been shown that IUI outcomes were optimal after 2 days of ejaculatory abstinence[1] and therefore, ≤2 days of abstinence is advised before IUI.

A semen sample is collected by the aseptic technique in a sterilized jar. Water or wet hands must not touch the semen or inner surface of the jar. Ask the patient to clean and dry parts before collection. Collection should be preferably done within the premises, but if not the case, the transport time from collection to incubator should not be >30 minutes at body temperature. Seminal plasma contains several substances that may reduce the fertilizing capacity of the sperms.[2] During transport, the semen should not be exposed to direct sunlight.

Semen is allowed to stand in the incubator at a temperature of 37°C for liquefaction for 20–30 minutes. Semen preparation should begin as soon as possible after liquefaction. Liquefaction is required for homogenous population of sperms throughout the semen sample. If liquefaction does not occur, needling through a 23 gauge needle can be done, though sperm damage is known to occur due to this.

As a rule, the liquefied sample must be examined under the microscope using Meckler chamber or Neubauer chamber for count, motility, and morphology before processing. Motility and morphologically abnormal sperms are counted as a percentage against normal sperms. The method of semen wash is decided, based on these parameters.

Split ejaculation is the collection of semen twice at a short interval. Split ejaculation collection is no longer recommended as the results are the same and spillage can occur with split ejaculation.

When antisperm antibodies are present, semen is collected directly in culture media as it decreases free antibodies and improves chances of fertilization. Similarly, semen with high viscosity is also collected in culture media.

Instruments and Equipment Required for Good Sperm Preparation

- Incubator for 37°C temperature
- Laminar airflow
- Microscope
- Centrifuge
- CO_2 incubator
- Neubauer/Makler chamber
- Semen collection jar
- *Disposables*: Double lock tubes, pipette, tips, slides, and coverslips
- Syringe
- IUI cannula

The sperm preparation laboratory should preferably be in the same setup where IUI is to be done. The laboratory should be a cool place and should not have windows and should not be in the direction of sunlight for long hours. It should preferably not be on the top floor of the building.

Composition of Sperm Preparation Media

- Earle's balance media
- Sodium pyruvate
- Synthetic serum replacement
- HEPES [4-(2-hydroxyethyl)-1-piperazineethanesulfonic acid] buffer
- Sodium bicarbonate
- Human serum albumin 1%
- Penicillin 50,000 IU/L + streptomycin 50 mg/L
- Phenol red

Proteins and buffers in media promote sperm capacitation while serum appears to be important for sperm motility. The inclusion of protein is required to prevent sperm from adhering to surfaces. Bicarbonate is required for capacitation. Media containing glucose is always better.

Selection of the method depends on:

- Motile count
- Volume of semen
- Presence of leukocytes, debris, and other cells
- Viscosity
- Whether it is for IUI, in vitro fertilization (IVF), or intracytoplasmic sperm injection (ICSI), it is important to keep in mind that a sperm preparation time of 40–80 minutes has a positive effect on pregnancy rates.[3]

SPERM PREPARATION METHODS

- Simple washing
- Swim-up
- Density gradient methods

Other methods such as migration gravity sedimentation and glass wool columns are rarely used now.

Simple Washing

Simple washing is the oldest method and is also known as simple dilution and washing technique. Only seminal plasma is removed by this technique; cellular debris, dead and nonmotile sperms, and bacteria are not removed completely as there is no swim-up. Semen is diluted with a large amount of medium (5–10 times of semen volume). It is then centrifuged at 300 g for 10 minutes with the purpose to wash it. The supernatant medium is removed and pellet is resuspended in the medium and again centrifuged at 300–500 g for 5 minutes. Again, the supernatant is removed and the pellet is resuspended in the medium appropriate for insemination and is incubated till insemination. This method is not used routinely.

Reagents for Swim-up

- *Self-prepared medium*: Earle's balanced salt solution (EBSS) + streptopenicillin [(penicillin 50,000 IU/L, streptomycin 50 mg/L + Na pyruvate + serum albumin readymade media (available from various companies)]
- Flushing medium, sperm preparation media (SPM) (MediCult, Origio)
- Cryoprep (Medline)
- G sperm (Scandinavian)
- FertiCult Flushing medium

Swim-up Methods

- Swim-up from the ejaculate
- Swim-up from pellet—different culture media have some variations

Swim-up from ejaculate: This is the ideal method as it does not require centrifugation.

- It is used only for a normal semen sample.
- It is based on the selection of the sperms based on their capability to swim-up in the media.
- Morphologically abnormal sperms and reactive oxygen species (ROS) are not filtered.
- The total yield of sperms is lower than the washing technique. It is, therefore, used for samples with a high sperm count.
- The time for which the samples are left for swim-up depends on the total sperm count, but allowing to swim-up for a long time lets more abnormal sperms to swim-up.

Method: Aliquots of liquefied semen are placed directly under medium (1 mL) in round-bottom tubes, and these tubes are placed at a 45° angle in a stand to be placed in the incubator for 30–60 minutes. The upper part of the layered medium from each test tube is collected, without disturbing the interface, and washed in 2-mL medium by centrifugating at 300–500 g for 10 minutes. Then the supernatant is removed and pellet is resuspended in the amount of medium sufficient for insemination and incubated till insemination.

Swim-up from pellet: This method is used for normal or marginally abnormal sperms, viscous samples, or samples collected in media.

Method:

- Take 2 mL of culture medium in a test tube
- Pipette 1.5 mL of semen and mix it with medium
- Centrifuge at 300–500 g for 10 minutes
- Remove supernatant
- Resuspend the pellet in another 2 mL of medium
- Centrifuge for 5 minutes at 300 g
- Remove supernatant
- Layer the pellet with 1 mL of medium
- Put it in a CO_2 incubator for swim-up for 30–60 minutes
- Gently aspirate 0.5–0.7 mL of the solution from the upper layers of the medium without disturbing the pellet.

Sperm capacitation requires the presence of bicarbonate ions. Therefore, if prepared sperms are stored before IUI, sperm buffer is recommended in a zwitterions buffered medium (such as HEPES). This will prevent premature capacitation and hyperactivated motility. If IUI is performed soon after sperm processing, the bicarbonate buffered medium can be used for the entire process.

This technique has an advantage of not using chemicals other than culture media. Most of the samples can be prepared by this method with different cultural media. But alternative methods are also described. Flushing media is most commonly used for IUI for swim-up.

Method using SPM (swim-up from ejaculate):

- Layer 1–1.5 mL of semen underneath 1–2 mL of pre-equilibrated SPM
- The tubes are kept tilted in a CO_2 incubator for 30–60 minutes.
- After swim-up, upper 0.5–1 mL is aspirated and put together.

Alternatively:

- Sample is diluted 1:3 v/v with media and is allowed to stand for 15 minutes at room temperature (+22°C).
- Centrifuge at 300 g for 10 minutes.
- Remove supernatant and resuspend in 4 mL of SPM.
- Centrifuge at 200 g for 5 minutes and remove supernatant.
- Gently overlay the pellet with 2 mL of SPM and leave in a CO_2 incubator for 120 minutes.
- Upper 0.1 mL has dead sperms and debris. Hence, this is removed.
- Then upper 0.7 mL is taken for insemination.

Variations: In nonassisted reproductive technology centers, flushing media is used rather than SPM. The difference between the two media is given in **Table 1**.

To compensate for albumin content, add 5.62 mL of human albumin solution to 125 mL of bottle of flushing media. It gives equally good results with lower costs.

Method for SPM (MediCult): Two to four test tubes with culture media are taken and in each tube, semen is put underneath the media. After 30 minutes, collect the upper portion from each tube.

TABLE 1: Difference between flushing media and sperm preparation media (SPM).

Component	*Flushing*	*SPM*
Albumin	0.1%	1.0%
pH	7–7.3	7.2–7.4
Bicarbonate	1.1	2.2

The second alternative is that we can dilute semen three times with media and after 15 minutes, centrifugation is done.

First centrifugation is at 300 g/10 min. Then resuspend in 4 mL of SPM. Then pellet is suspended with 2 mL in an incubator for 60–120 minutes.

G Sperm (Scandinavian Media):

- Take two to four tubes with 1-mL semen.
- Overlay with 2-mL media and incubate for 60 minutes.
- Aspirate 1 mL from all tubes.
- Add 5-mL media and centrifuge for 10 minutes at 300–600 g.
- Discard supernatant.
- Repeat centrifugation after adding 5-mL media with 300–600 g for 10 minutes. Resuspend in G Fert and take 0.5–0.7 mL for insemination.

Swim-up from pellet is the most widely used method as it separates motile sperms from nonmotile sperms and debris. Here, sperms are concentrated prior to swim-up and they do not have to escape seminal plasma. So it is advantageous for viscous, moderate density or moderate motility samples. It is suitable for samples collected in media or cryopreserved samples.

The disadvantage of centrifuge is production of ROS, which is harmful for fertilization.

Tips for Better Intrauterine Insemination

- Work under laminar airflow as far as possible and use a completely sterile technique.
- Gloves should not touch the inner side of the tubes as rubber is toxic for sperms.
- Work with more tubes rather than a single, large tube when the semen sample is large or the count is too high.

- Leaving for swim-up for a long time may allow the debris to swim-up. Longer time may be required for swim-up of low count or low motility samples, which means an optimum time for swim-up must be modified as per the count and motility of the sample.
- Semen processing is done within 30 minutes after collection and maximally within 1 hour.
- While loading, avoid contact of cannula with the inner side of the tube.
- The rubber of the syringe should not touch the sample which means that when the sample is loaded in the cannula with the syringe attached, there should be a small air gap between the sample column and the rubber piston.
- Air should not be injected during IUI.
- No antiseptics are applied in the vagina.
- An equal volume of pentoxifylline solution can be added before centrifugation to improve motility in oligoasthenospermia.
- *For centrifuge machine*: Different companies have different parameters of speed—the conversion formula is rpm: $\sqrt{[g/(1.118 \times r)]}$.
- Media is kept overnight in a CO_2 incubator with a loosened cap in a slanted test tube rack for equilibrium **(Fig. 1)**.
- With low count, a large amount of semen may help.
- Clean the vagina and the vulva with normal saline before wash, but it is not a must.
- Slanting test tube position during swim-up allows a larger surface and therefore a larger sperm cohort.
- Proper labeling of tubes is a must.
- A good wash sample is one which has at least 95% actively motile sperms and no debris **(Fig. 2)**.

Density Gradient Methods (Fig. 3)

This is the method that gives better recovery of sperms for IUI and IVF.

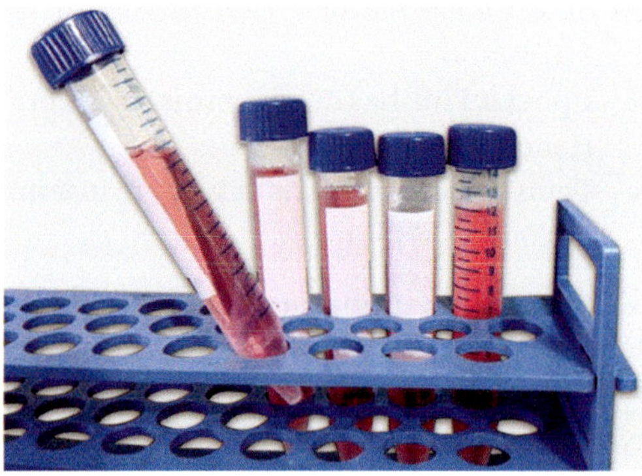

Fig. 1: Test tubes are kept in a slanting position in a rack.

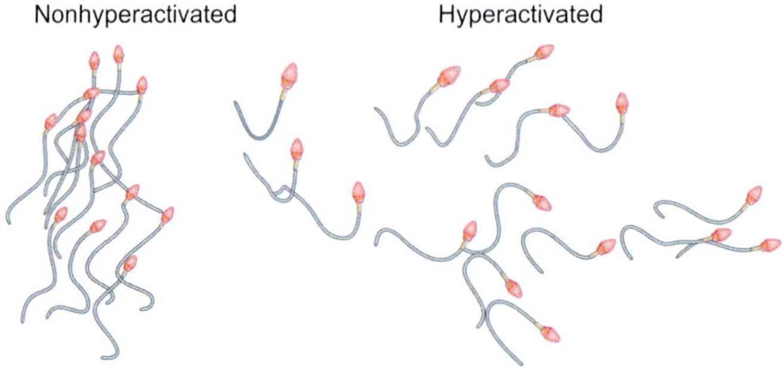

Fig. 2: Hyperactivated post semen wash sperms on the right side and nonhyperactivated sperms on the left side.

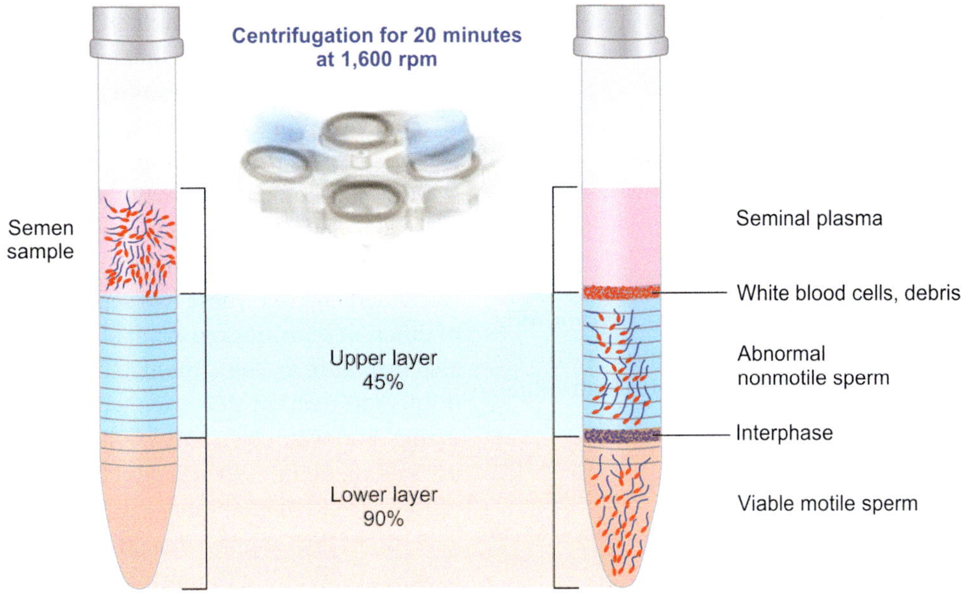

Fig. 3: Diagrammatic understanding of gradient method.

This method selects sperms according to their density and gravity (mass per unit volume) and results in cells being dispersed throughout the gradient column according to the gradient that matches their density. Normal spermatozoa have a density of 1.12 g/mL and immature abnormal sperms have a density of 1.06–1.09 g/mL. Normal sperms can be isolated in the solution with the highest concentration of gradient.

It is suitable for viscous samples as well as a sample having more debris and WBCs and low count. Dead and defective sperms and leukocytes produce ROS which causes lipid peroxidation of sperm membrane and decreases motility. These are best removed by the gradient method. Debris and immotile sperms are held in between gradient layers. Because of head density, sperms swim down and form a pellet.

Some studies have shown that the method is more useful when both the percentage of sperms with progressive motility and the proportion of sperms with good morphology are lower. But other studies say that harvest of motile sperm and normal morphology is lower with the gradient method. The same controversial results are for sperm DNA damage. Higher centrifugation for a shorter interval will give good recovery of motile sperms than when centrifugation is done at a lower speed for a longer time.

Universal Method

- From bottom to top—90% density gradient, then 45% density gradient, and then the semen sample
- Centrifuge at 1,500 rpm for 15 minutes
- Remove supernatant
- Transfer pellet to a sterile centrifuge tube (may not be required)
- Add 3–5 mL SPM and mix pellet
- Centrifuge at 1,000 rpm for 5 minutes
- Remove supernatant
- Mix pellet with 0.5–0.7 mL washing media
- Load the catheter for IUI

Gradient media available are:

- Suprasperm (MediCult)
- IxaPrep (MediCult)
- PureSperm (Nidacon)
- SpermGrad (Shivani Scientific)
- Sil-Select (Microm, UK)

Method for Suprasperm

Suprasperm is a salt solution containing a colloidal suspension of silica particles stabilized with covalently bound hydrophilic saline.

- 2 × 1 mL of semen should be used to run two gradients for each semen sample.
- Dispense 2 mL of 55% suprasperm to a test tube and dispense 2 mL of 80% medium underneath this with a pipette.
- Carefully dispense 1 mL of semen on the top of this and centrifuge at 300 g for 20 minutes.
- Remove the supernatant and resuspend the pellet in 2–3 mL of SPM and centrifuge at 200 g for 10 minutes.
- Remove supernatant, leave pellet, and repeat the wash process.
- Finally, resuspend the pellet in the desired concentration of SPM.

A final wash with a culture medium to remove the gradient solution is the drawback of this method.

Variations with Other Media

- *IxaPrep*: It has two pure, cell-separating agents: polysucrose and iodixanol with HEPES buffer. The top layer has SPM + Polysucrose. The bottom layer has SPM + Polysucrose + Iodixanol. Semen preparation is done in the same way.
- *Scandinavian method (SpermGrad)*: The bottom layer has 90% density and the upper layer has 45% and washing is done with G Fert.
- *Puresperm (gradient method)*: It has 90% and 45% solution. The first centrifugation is at 500 g for 10 minutes and the other two centrifugations are at 250 g for 5 minutes.
- *Sil-Select gradient method*: It has 80% and 40% solutions and centrifugation is done at 300–600 g for 10–20 minutes.

Gradient media are available as readymade media where two separate media of different densities are available. Media are also available as 100% media. These can be diluted to desired densities using flushing media. For example, a 45% gradient medium is to be made in a syringe of 1 mL; 0.45 mL of 100% gradient medium is taken and to that 0.55 mL of flushing medium is added. If the usage is higher, the preparation can also be made in samples of 10 mL.

Tips for a Better Yield of Sperms in the Gradient Method

- A longer centrifugation time increases the recovery of both motile and immotile sperms.
- Higher centrifugation speed increases recovery of motile sperms and low-density particles, so shorter time is required with higher speeds.
- Because of the low density, debris, round cells, and the abnormal sperms with amorphous heads and cytoplasmic droplets never reach the bottom of the tube.

The density gradient method is generally thought to be superior to other two techniques as it gives more morphologically normal sperms with grade A motility and normal DNA integrity with less chromatin and nuclear DNA anomalies in the prepared sample. It also reduces ROS and leukocyte concentration. Though in a meta-analysis by Boomsma et al. published in Cochrane review showed that there was no evidence of a difference in the effectiveness of a swim-up versus density gradient method on pregnancy rates per couple. Swim-up technique versus wash and centrifugation also showed no significant difference in pregnancy rates.[4] So no one SPM is better than the other in the present scenario though it depends on the nature of the semen sample. The recovery rate of sperms after swim-up is lower (<20%) as compared to that with the density gradient method which is >20%.[5]

For IVF: Sperm characteristics important for fertilization with standard IVF include normal morphology, normal intact acrosomes, straight line velocity (VSL), linearity (LIN) and ability to bind to zona pellucida and penetrate it and fuse with oolemma to activate ovum. Insemination of sperm in IVF is between 2,000 and 500,000 sperms/mL. Most groups inseminate 100,000 sperms/mL. Reduced exposure of oocytes to sperms improves the quality of embryo and gives high implantation rate. Oocytes are inseminated, 4–6 hours after collection. Density gradient method is more preferred for semen preparation for IVF.

For ICSI: The preferred characteristics for the sperm are same as that for IVF but morphology, motility and acrosome status are not important. Sperms for ICSI may be harvested from oil media interface after sperm containing material is placed in a drop of culture medium under oil. No difference in fertilization was observed with density gradient or swim up method. Swim up though may be an easier alternative.

Preparation from the Frozen Sample

Dealing with atypical semen samples:

- Frozen sample
- Retrograde ejaculation
- Human immunodeficiency virus (HIV)-positive sample

Frozen sample:

- Thaw the specimen 30 minutes before IUI.
- Place frozen vials in a 37° water bath for 10 minutes.
- Shake vials gently to confirm the disappearance of ice crystals.
- Then treat like a fresh sample.

Dilution is performed slowly and temperature changes should be gradual.

Retrograde ejaculation: The patient first empties his bladder. Then an alkalizer is given to the patient. After some time, he is asked to masturbate. The urine sample is collected in culture media and is centrifuged at 500 g for 8 minutes. The supernatant is removed and the pellet is washed by the gradient method.

Antiretroviral therapy must be given to reduce viral load. The sperm sample should then be tested for HIV RNA and DNA by polymerase chain reaction (PCR). Normally, cryopreservation of sample is required for complete testing. Then depending on the quantity of sperms IUI, IVF, or ICSI is done. Recently, preexposure prophylaxis (PrEP) is given to a woman while a male partner is treated. It can have spontaneous pregnancy afterward. PrEP can avoid further testing of semen samples.

Human immunodeficiency virus-positive sample: HIV viruses are found in plasma. They are not inside the sperm cell. Here, semen is prepared by the gradient method followed by swim-up. The sample can then be used for IUI.

SURGICALLY RETRIEVED PESA/MESA/TESA/TESE

- Percutaneous epididymal sperm aspiration (PESA)
- Microsurgical epididymal sperm aspiration (MESA)
- Testicular epididymal sperm aspiration (TESA)

- Testicular sperm extraction (TESE) by excisional biopsy
- Micropuncture technique (Micropuncture with nerve stimulation)

Percutaneous Epididymal Sperm Aspiration/Microsurgical Epididymal Sperm Aspiration

Fluid is aspirated from the epididymis through a fine needle (PESA) or is aspirated through a small incision on the epididymis (MESA) **(Fig. 4)**. This fluid usually contains motile and mature spermatozoa. Due to the damage to skin and microvessels, RBCs are often present in PESA/MESA samples, so heparinized (10 IU/mL) media (1:2) is used to process these sperms. The discontinuous gradient method using heparinized medium is the method of sperm wash preferred for these samples. Layer the washed pellet with heparinized media and then incubate the sample at 37°C. Motile sperms swim up into the overlayered media column and then these are loaded into ICSI dish.

Testicular Epididymal Sperm Aspiration/Testicular Epididymal Sperm Extraction

From the testis, a seminiferous tubule is aspirated from the testis into a needle (TESA) or excised from open testis biopsies (TESE) **(Fig. 4)**. The extracted tissue is minced with the help of a sharp blade and a 26 gauge needle. Chopped tissue/debris is digested in a tissue digesting buffer medium (collagenase). This digested tissue is washed in heparinized media and centrifuged at 200–250 g for 10 minutes. After centrifugation, all

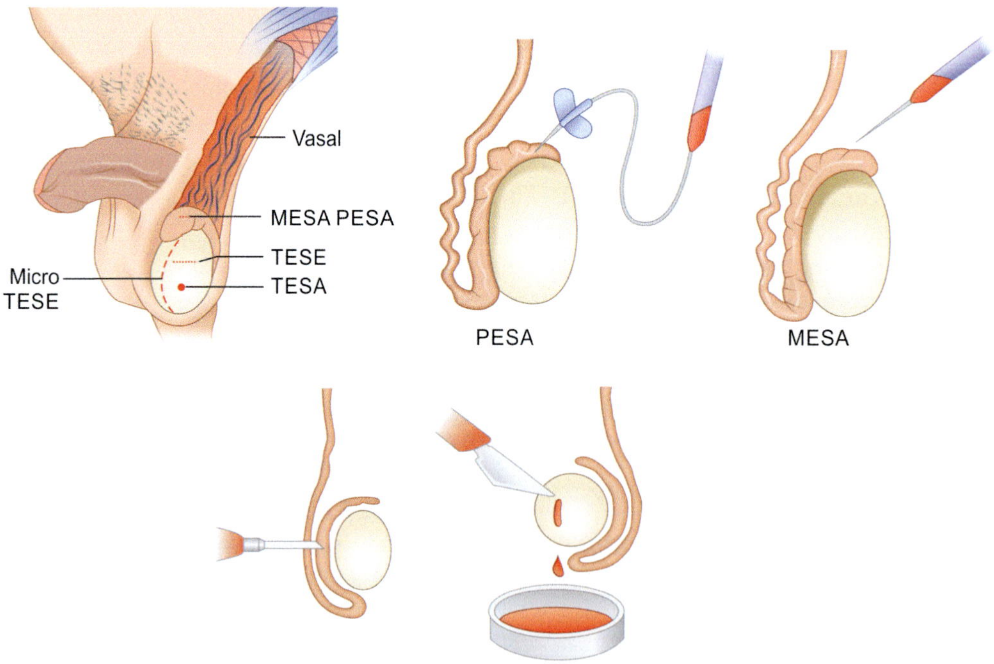

Fig. 4: Surgically retrieved sperms PESA/MESA and TESA/TESE. (MESA: microsurgical epididymal sperm aspiration; PESA: percutaneous epididymal sperm aspiration; TESA: testicular epididymal sperm aspiration)

the immotile/motile spermatozoa and debris form a pellet. Motile sperms in the pellet float in the overlaid heparinized culture media and are loaded into petri dish for ICSI.

If the pellet contains only immotile spermatozoa then:

Technique I: Pentoxifylline Treatment

The pellet is placed in the center of a petri dish, layered with 1.5–2.0 mL of pentoxifylline (POF)-supplemented media or bicarbonate media and overlayered with oil. After overnight incubation, the sperm gains motility due to the influence of pentoxifylline and swim to the edge of the media droplet. Using embryo biopsy pipette attached to the micromanipulator is used to aspirate the sperms. These are then expelled into polyvinylpyrrolidone (PVP) droplets in the ICSI dish, and ICSI is done. Spermatozoa must be washed free of any POF before being used to inseminate oocytes. Many workers use POF between 0.3 and 0.6 mmol/L which can be increased to 3.6 mmol/L, i.e., 1 mg/mL.

Technique II: Hypoosmotic Swelling Test (Figs. 5A and B)

Hypoosmotic swelling (HOS) test is based on the ability of live spermatozoa to withstand the moderate stress of a hypo-osmotic environment. This leads to swelling of live sperms. HOS assesses the osmoregulatory ability of the sperm, and therefore the functional integrity of its membranes can also be assessed. It can be used to discriminate viable from nonviable sperms even with zero or little apparent motility.

- *HOS—Research purpose*:
  - 1 mL of HOS stock solution + 100 µL washed sample
  - Incubate at 37°C for 30 minutes.
- *Modified HOS*:
  - 0.5 mL of culture medium + 0.5 mL Milli-Q Water/D.W. + 100 µL sample
  - Incubate at 37°C for 30 minutes.
  - Sperms with curved tails are only picked and put into PVP droplets to perform ICSI.
- *Other techniques*:
  - Laser pulse applied at the tail tip of immotile sperms
  - Mechanical touch technique

Advanced Sperm Selection Methods

- Selection of nonapoptotic spermatozoa—magnetic activated cell sorting (MACS; **Fig. 6**)
- Selection of motile spermatozoa—microfluidics
- Selection of motile sperm organelle morphology examination (MSOME)—intracytoplasmic morphologically selected sperm injection (IMSI)
- Sperm birefringence (polarizing microscopy)
- Hyaluronic acid sperm binding (PICSI™)—mediated sperm selection
- Surface charge sperm selection—zeta potential and electrophoretic system
- Binding with zona pellucida

Selection of Nonapoptotic Spermatozoa—Magnetic Activated Cell Sorting

Magnetic activated cell sorting separates apoptotic spermatozoa from nonapoptotic spermatozoa. (magnetic nanoparticle-based selection of live sperm without DNA fragmentation)

During apoptosis (programmed cell death), phosphatidylserine (PS) residues are translocated from the inner membrane of the spermatozoa to the outside.

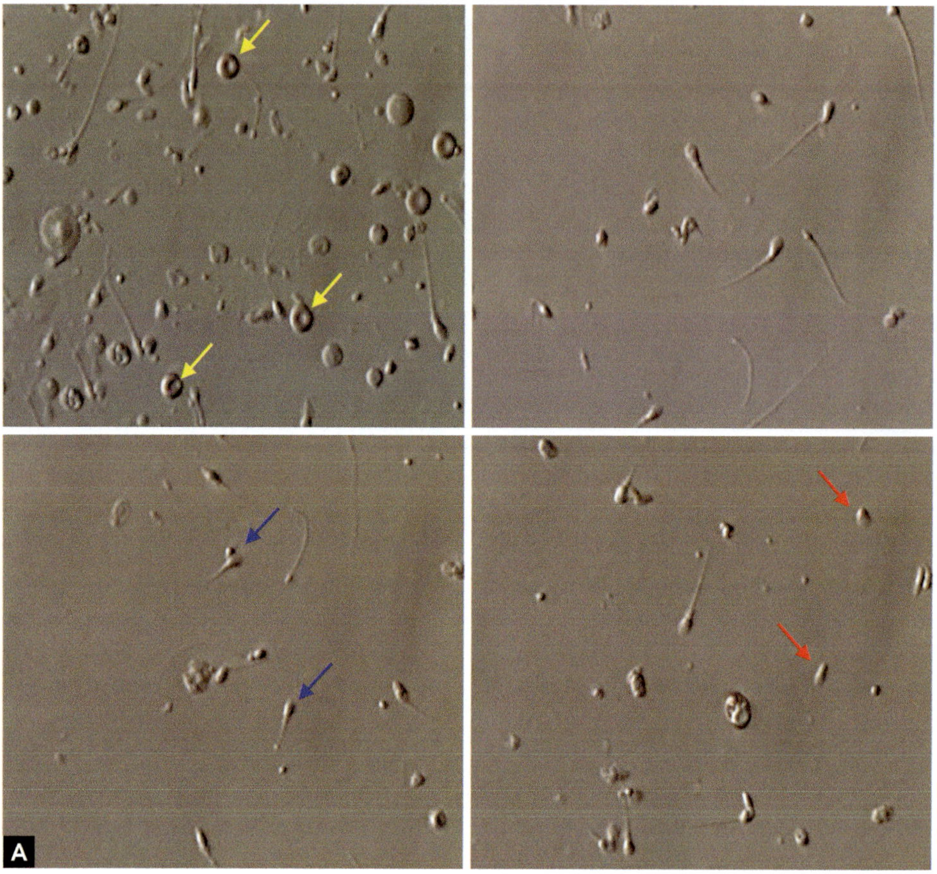

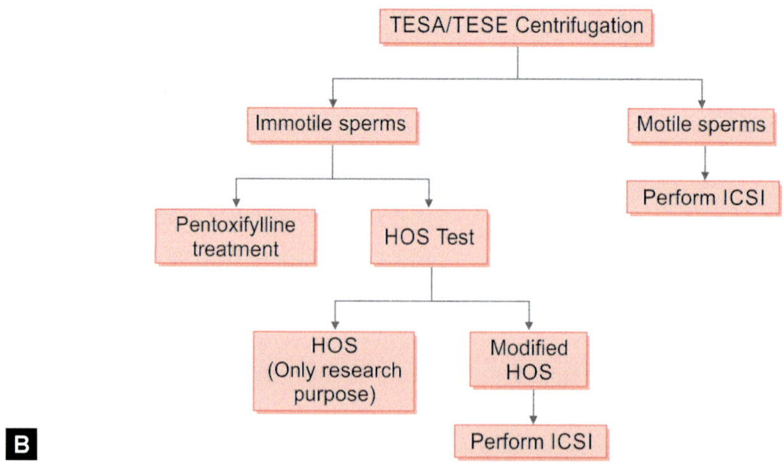

Figs. 5A and B: (A) Photomicrograph showing pattern of epididymal specimens obtained by percutaneous epididymal sperm aspiration (PESA) (*Source:* Laboratory handling of epididymal and testicular spermatozoa: What can be done to improve sperm injections outcome. J Hum Reprod Sci. 2012;5(3):233-43. doi: 10.4103/0974-1208.106333); (B) Chart for TESA/TESE. (HOS: hypoosmotic swelling; ICSI: intracytoplasmic sperm injection; TESA: testicular epididymal sperm aspiration; TESE: testicular epididymal sperm extraction)

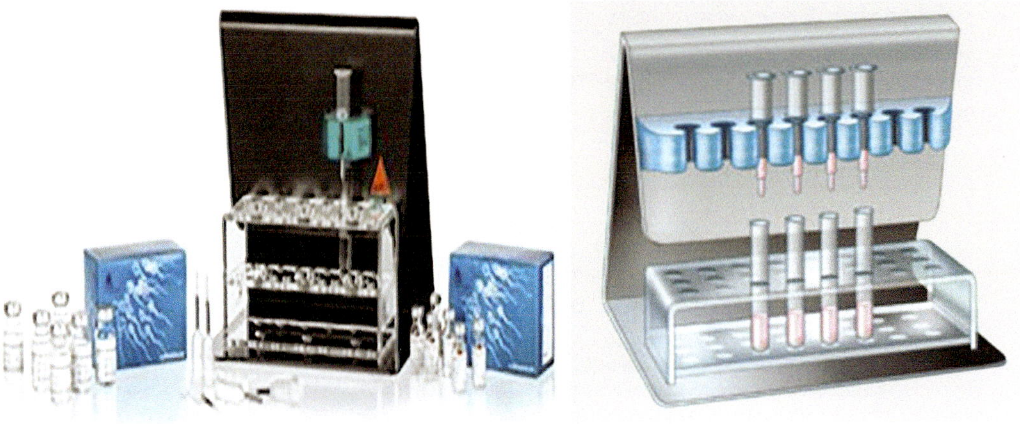

Fig. 6: Magnetic activated cell sorting.

Apoptotic cell depletion begins with magnetic labeling of apoptotic cells by the MACS assisted reproduction technology (ART) Annexin V Reagent. The labeled cells are then passed through a separation column located in a magnetic field. Unwanted cells are selectively retained in the column. Living spermatozoa are not labeled by the reagent, so they pass through the column and are collected for later use.

Instruments and reagents required for this procedure are as follows:

- Octatet magnetic collection device (maximum eight samples loading at a time)/Multistand
- Annexin V antibody beads (Magnetic)/ Microbeads
- MS column (for separation)
- Separation unit
- Annexin V reagent
- Binding buffer media
- Tubes, Pasture pipettes
- Tips and Finnpipette
- Density gradient medium
- Sperm wash medium

Method: Sperms are separated by the density gradient method/swim-up for removing leukocytes and dead spermatozoa. A 100-μL washed sperm sample is mixed with 100 μL of MACS microbeads and incubated at room temperature for 15 minutes. The mixture is loaded on top of the separation column which is placed in the magnetic field. The column is rinsed with buffer. All the unlabeled (Annexin V negative) nonapoptotic spermatozoa are passed through the column. Apoptotic fraction (Annexin V positive) is retained in the column. The column is removed from the magnetic field and Annexin V positive fraction is eluted using the Annexin V binding buffer. Viable spermatozoa without DNA fragmentation pass through the column and are collected for use in ART (IUI/IVF/ICSI/cryopreservation). Though this method is recommended for patients with advanced age, unexplained infertility, poor semen parameter, varicocele, arrested embryo development, and poor blastocyst development.

Selection of Motile Spermatozoa—Microfluidics

Microfluidic sperm sorting is a new, gentle alternative to standard sperm processing which does not require any previous processing of sperm sample or use of devices

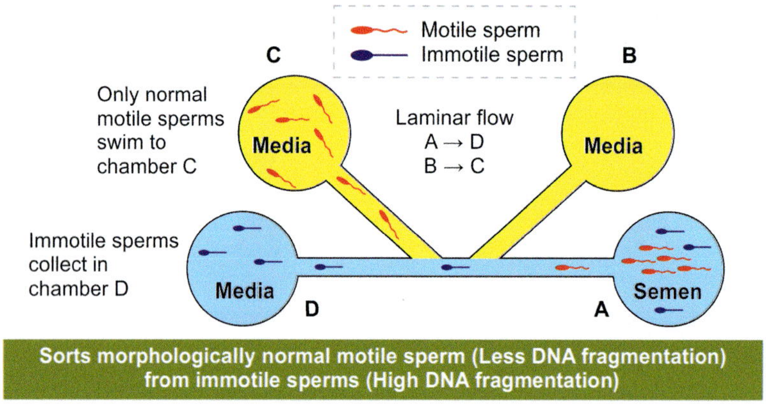

Fig. 7: Microfluidic sperm sorting "Qualis".

(e.g., centrifuge) that increase oxidative stress in sperm. Microfluidics is done in microchannels with dimensions of a few hundred micrometers. Sperm selection is done under laminar flow by gravity-driven pumps in the microchannels. Microfluidic sperm sorter selects sperm cells that have >80% improvement in DNA integrity relative to the heterogeneous population present in the raw semen, and the selection was performed for <20 minutes. There are various microfluidic devices such as microfluidic sperm sorting Qualis (MSSQ; **Fig. 7**), microfluidic sorting chip, microfluidic sperm sorting fertile device, and silicone elastomer-based microfluidic device. This procedure is recommended for recurring IUI failures, low rate of egg fertilization with ICSI in the previous cycle, recurring miscarriages, and poor-quality embryos in previous IVF cycles.

Sperm Sorting Principle "Qualis": MSSQ contains four chambers: A, B, C, and D. These four chambers are connected by two parallel channels: A–D and BC. Media is added in chambers B, C, D and laminar flow channels are allowed to form between the chambers. The sperm sample is added to chamber A. The laminar flow will help separate motile sperms from immotile sperms. The immotile sperms would passively flow in the direction of laminar flow A to D and thus collect in chamber D while the motile sperms that can swim will swim up into chamber C. After some time, only motile sperms would collect in chamber C while immotile sperms would collect in chamber D.

This method bypasses centrifugation and decreases the amount of DNA damage in the resultant sample. Separating motile sperms using the microfluidics sperm sorter and using this sample of highly motile sperms to fertilize the eggs reduce the risk of passing on sperm DNA damage or quality of the embryo.

Selection of Motile Sperm Organelle Morphology Examination—IMSI

This is based on live sperm morphology **(Fig. 8)**. Sperm evaluation at 400 magnifications for ICSI is inefficient for accurate morphological assessment of sperms. Real-time sperm evaluation is known as motile sperm organelle morphology examination. But magnification power of 6,000× can define the morphological normalcy of five sperm organelles (acrosome, postacrosomal lamina, neck, tail, and nucleus). Sperm head component correlated with sperm fertilizing capacity in vitro and pregnancy outcome performing IMSI. IMSI is a modification of ICSI, in which the injected spermatozoon is selected by the technician at high magnification using MSOME normalcy criteria. But larger trials are required to prove its efficacy.[6]

Sperm Birefringence (Polarizing Microscopy)

Another optical system is used to select live sperm for ICSI. It is based on the identification of a mature sperm nucleus that has high intrinsic birefringence due to longitudinally orientated subacrosomal protein filaments. Using polarized light microscopy, sperm birefringence can be evaluated and a mature sperm selected **(Fig. 9)**. The proportion of birefringent sperm in a sample is correlated positively with sperm concentration, motility, and viability. In addition, using this optical system, it is possible to differentiate acrosome-reacted from acrosome-intact sperm before microinjection.

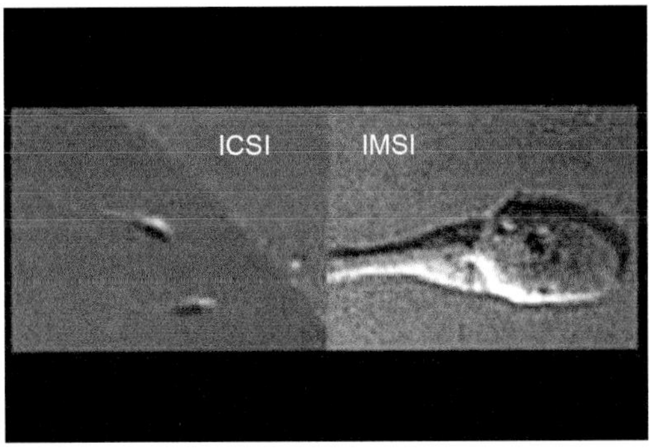

Fig. 8: Intracytoplasmic morphologically selected sperm injection.

Hyaluronic Acid Sperm Binding (PICSI™)—Mediated Sperm Selection

Hyaluronic acid–binding sites on the sperm plasma membrane indicate sperm maturity. Sperm are placed in a PICSI™ dish, which is an IVF petri dish that carries a hyaluronic acid spot. Mature sperm preferentially binds to the hyaluronan impregnated sites. Hyaluronan, a polymer, increases motility and viability of freshly ejaculated or cryopreserved thawed human spermatozoa. Add into the sperm preparation medium. Hyaluronic acid (HA) is immobilized on a solid surface [polystyrene culture dish—PICSI dish **(Fig. 10)**—enhanced with microdots of hyaluronan, where the sperm suspension is added] and the washed sperm sample allowed to interact with the HA-coated surface for 15-20 minutes. An individual sperm attached to the dish is picked up with the ICSI pipette and used for oocyte injection.[7]

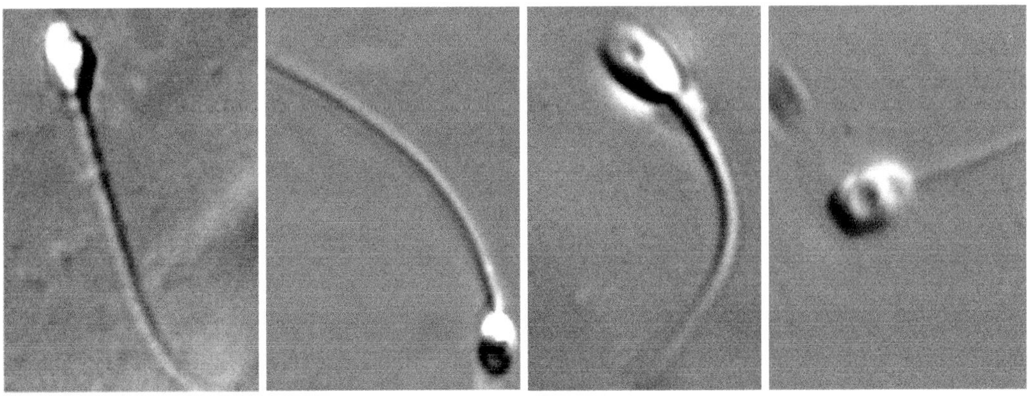

Fig. 9: Polarizing microscopy (sperm head birefringence).

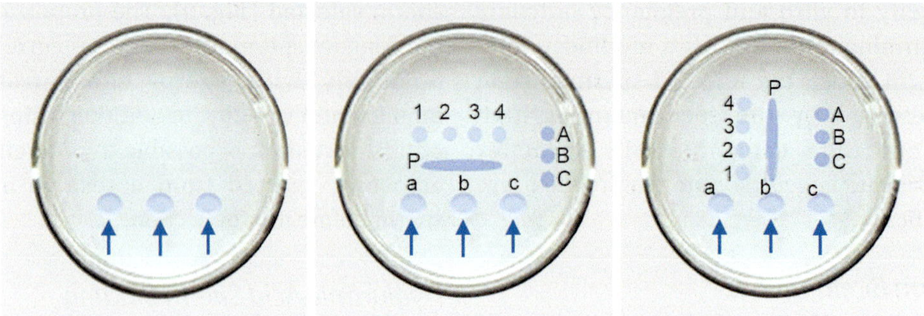

Fig. 10: PICSI™ petri dish—microdots of hyaluronan.

Surface Charge Sperm Selection

Electrophoretic sperm selection and sperm zeta potential are surface charge selection protocols utilized in both IVF and ICSI to select sperm based on the differential net electric charge on the sperm plasma membrane.

Zeta Potential Method

The zeta potential of the sperm is the electric potential between the sperm membrane and its surroundings. The zeta potential decreases with capacitation and normally differentiated sperm are charged electronegatively. A mature sperm cell has a negative zeta potential of –16 to 20 mV (differential potential between the sperm membrane and its surroundings). The zeta potential method is very simple to perform and does not require special equipment and is therefore inexpensive. Washed sperm in a serum-free medium is introduced in a conical tube placed into an electrophoretic device and a current applied. Normally, differentiated negatively charged sperm are rapidly separated and collected from an adjacent tube and nonadherent sperm fraction along with other contaminants are removed by inverting the tube. Selected adherent sperm cells are recovered by rinsing the tube with the serum-supplement medium.

Electrophoretic System

The electrophoresis-based technology uses an electric field to separate sperm cells based on size and electronegative charge. It has two outer chambers and two inner chambers (incubation and collection). The outer chambers (filled with buffer) house the platinum-coated titanium mesh electrodes. A membrane separates the outer chambers from the inner chambers allowing for the movement of small molecules, water, and ions between them. The inner chambers comprise the inoculation compartment and the collection compartment separated by a polycarbonate separation membrane. Pore size excludes leukocytes and precursor germ cells that normally contaminate semen samples. The semen specimen is loaded into the incubation chamber and allowed to equilibrate for 5 minutes before applying a current of 75 mA and variable voltage (18–21 V). The selected sperm subpopulation is recovered from the collection chamber after 5 minutes of application of the electric field.

Zona Pellucida Binding

Immature eggs from some cohorts are incubated for 2 hours with prepared sperm. Sperm that finds zona are removed and used for ICSI. Further trials are required for improvement.[8,9]

CARRY HOME MESSAGE

- For regular IUI, swim-up is a very good method and is much cheaper than the density gradient method.
- We have observed that the pregnancy rate is very high with 8–10 million post wash count.
- It is very vital that you select a method and modify it to achieve that count.
- We can have our own modification for speed of centrifugation and time of centrifugation according to the count and motility of the sample.

REFERENCES

1. Nijs M. Study of sperm parameters in assisted reproduction outcome. Maastricht, Netherlands: Datawyse Bockproducties; 2009.
2. Bjorndahl L, Mortimer D, Barratt C, Castilla JA, Menkveld R, Kvist U. Practical guide to basic laboratory andrology. Cambridge: Cambridge University Press; 2010.
3. Fauque P, Lehert P, Lamotte M, Bettahar-Lebugle K, Bailly A, Diligent C, et al. Clinical success of intrauterine insemination cycles is affected by the sperm preparation time. Fertil Steril. 2014;101(6):1618-23.e1-3.
4. Boomsma CM, Heineman MJ, Cohlen BJ, Farquhar C. Semen preparation techniques for intrauterine insemination. Cochrane Database Syst Rev. 2012;(6):CD005996.
5. Morshedi M, Duran HE, Taylor S, Oehninger S. Efficacy and pregnancy outcome of two methods of semen preparation for intrauterine insemination: a prospective randomized study. Fertil Steril. 2003;79: 1625-32.
6. Nadalini M, Tarozzi N, Distratis V, Scaravelli G, Borini A. Impact of intracytoplasmic morphologically selected sperm injection on assisted reproduction outcome. A review. Reprod Biomed Online. 2009;19(Suppl 3): 45-55.
7. Huzar G, Ozkavukcu S, Jakab A Celik-Ozenci C, Sati GL, Cayli S. Hyaluronic acid binding ability of human sperm reflects cellular maturity and fertilizing potential : selection of sperm for intracytoplasmic sperm injection. Curr Opin Obstet Gynecol. 2006;18:260-7.
8. Said TM, Land JA. Effects of advanced selection methods on sperm quality and ART outcome: a systematic review. Hum Reprod Update. 2011;17(6):719-33.
9. Paes Almeida Ferreira de Braga D, Iaconelli A Jr, Casia Savio de FR, Madaschi C, Semiao-Francisco L, Borges E Jr. Outcome of ICSI using zona pellucida bound spermatozoa and conventionally selected spermatozoa. Reprod Biomed Online. 2009;19(6):802-7.

27 Chapter

Oocyte Retrieval

INTRODUCTION

Ultrasound has proven to be a unique noninvasive modality for diagnosis and management of subfertility and also as an aid to therapeutic procedures such as oocyte retrieval and embryo transfer. For in vitro fertilization (IVF), oocytes are retrieved from the stimulated ovary. The procedure is planned about 34–35 hours after ovulation trigger, under ultrasound guidance with asepsis.

OOCYTE RETRIEVAL

Oocyte retrieval was done by laparoscopy for the first decade after the development of IVF.[1] Being highly invasive, it limited the use of the technology to very few patients. Lenz et al. first described percutaneous transabdominal or transvesical aspiration of follicles under ultrasound guidance in 1981.[2] Transvaginal ovum retrieval with transvaginal ultrasound guidance with a mechanical transvaginal sector scanner was first described by Kemeter and Feichtinger in the late 1980s.[3] This was a major breakthrough in IVF treatment and was soon universally accepted. Transvaginal oocyte retrieval is a very simple and well-accepted method with a very low complication rate. The ease of the procedure was one of the important reasons for the easy acceptability of the clinicians and the patients for the procedure.

METHOD

Preprocedure

The patient is asked to remain nil by mouth for at least 6–8 hours before the procedure. This is a requirement for anesthesia. While there is no evidence that routine antibiotics reduce the risk of infection, the administration of an intravenous bolus of antibiotics is generally recommended to women with a history of severe pelvic inflammatory disease or if an endometrioma is punctured. However, in certain units, antibiotics are routinely administered. The procedure is planned 34–35 hours after the trigger for ovulation induction is given. The trigger is planned after confirming that there are at least three follicles between 18 and 16 mm in diameter and at least three follicles in either ovary show adequate blood flows as seen on Doppler (discussed in the Chapter 9). If the ovary is low reserve and the total number of follicles larger than 14 mm are only six or less than that, it is preferred to confirm flow on Doppler in all the follicles to optimize the yield of oocytes.

Premedication and Anesthesia

It is important to provide effective anesthesia and analgesia for transvaginal oocyte retrieval as the procedure is painful. But it is also known that no technique of anesthesia, analgesia, or sedation is free from side effects, especially because anesthetic agents have been found in the follicular fluid, and these drugs may have adverse effects on oocyte fertilization and embryonic development. A prolonged period of exposure with general anesthesia (GA) can lead to lower pregnancy and delivery rates.[4]

It has been reported that due to stress, there is a 50-fold transient increase in serum prolactin levels during oocyte retrieval under GA which may affect the IVF outcome.[4]

Conscious sedation should be offered to all women undergoing the procedure as it is a safe and acceptable method of providing analgesia. Intravenous fentanyl, propofol, and midazolam are the commonly used medications. Short-acting opioids, principally fentanyl and remifentanil, do not alter IVF success rates.[5] Rosen et al. did not find the deleterious effect of N_2O on the rates of fertilization or pregnancy when used during an isoflurane-based general anesthetic technique.[6]

Though another study by Gonen et al. showed significantly lower clinical pregnancy rates in the N_2O group (14.5%) compared with the epidural group (23.7%; $p = 0.018$) or the sedation group (25.8%; $p = 0.0074$). N_2O deactivates methionine synthetase, thereby reducing the amount of thymidine available for DNA synthesis in dividing cells.[7]

Rafter and Sherry[8] in their study on 80 women found that total intravenous anesthesia (TIVA) with propofol and alfentanil is superior to inhalational anesthesia with N_2O and enflurane in view of less nausea and vomiting (64% in the inhalational group and 39% in the TIVA group), less requirement for the antiemetic medication (62% in the inhalational group and 32% in the TIVA group), and a lower probability of unplanned hospital admission (21% in the inhalational group and 5% in the TIVA group) after day-care IVF procedures.[8]

Whatever technique is used, recognized standards of practice should be adhered to and all IVF professionals should follow the safe practice of administering sedative drugs. Pharmacological exposure to the anesthetic agents should be for the least possible duration with minimal penetration to follicular fluid. Assessment of specific anesthetic drugs must be interpreted with the method of administration, dose of anesthetic agents, combination with other drugs, timing of administration, and duration of exposure. Local anesthesia is rarely used as this does not provide effective analgesia. Though paracervical block (PCB) or preovarian block (POB) has been tried. In PCB, a local anesthetic is injected into two to six sites at a depth of 3–7 mm alongside the vaginal portion of the cervix in the vaginal fornices. POB, the local anesthetic, is infiltrated in the vaginal wall under ultrasound guidance between the vaginal wall and the peritoneal surface near the ovary.[9]

Some workers have also tried spinal or epidural anesthesia, but the long recovery time and therefore longer hospitalization that is required are the disadvantages.

TECHNIQUE

All sterile precautions are taken with washing hands and wearing a sterile gown. Perfume-free washing and cleansing agents are preferred. It is best to use powder-free sterile gloves. The trolley for the procedure is prepared with all sterile precautions. The vagina can be cleaned thoroughly with normal saline. Some units use culture medium to cleanse the vagina, but this is not essential. Antiseptic agents must not be used. The ultrasound transducer is covered with a sterile plastic sleeve and then covered with a sterile condom with no spermicidal gel. Though to allow transmission of sound

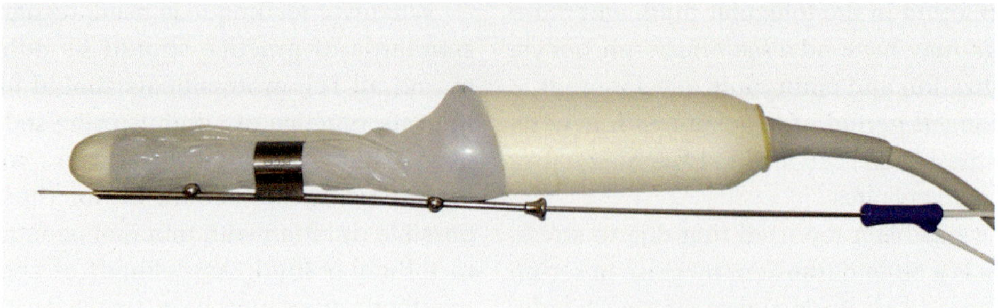

Fig. 1: Transvaginal probe prepared for ovum pick-up with biopsy guide fixed on it.

waves, ultrasound gel or saline may be used between the transducer head and the condom. When cleansing the vagina with saline, as the last step, it is douched with normal saline, which acts as a coupling agent for the ultrasound at the time of ovum pick-up. Prior to insertion into the vagina and after the procedure, the transducer should be thoroughly cleaned with the probe cleansing agents and techniques recommended by the manufacturer. It is covered by sterile sleeve and condom. The biopsy guide on the probe is fixed **(Fig. 1)**.

Place the probe in the vagina to assess the endometrial thickness, position, and accessibility of the ovaries and the number of follicles to be aspirated. Switch on the biopsy guide on the screen. The guide helps to identify the position of the needle and the path it will take when advanced through the vaginal fornix into the ovary.

The transducer is manipulated to position the follicles in the needle path (biopsy guideline) **(Fig. 2)**.

The transducer should be positioned in such a way that the ovaries are placed closest possible to the needle tip. The needle path is usually at the 2 o'clock position for puncturing the left ovary and at the 10 o'clock position for puncturing the right ovary in the vagina, lateral to the cervix. But when ovaries are fixed or positioned high up in the pelvis, the path may have to be changed. If possible, the follicle should be punctured from the side of the ovary, thus entering each follicle systematically with an aim to induce minimal damage to the ovary. As far as possible, only a single vaginal puncture with a maximum of one or two ovarian punctures should be done on each side. This approach reduces the risk of bleeding. Entering the ovary may be difficult with an ovary with a very few follicles. If ovaries are very mobile, pressure on the abdomen may be required to fix the ovaries. Find the nearest leading follicle and then the needle must be advanced.

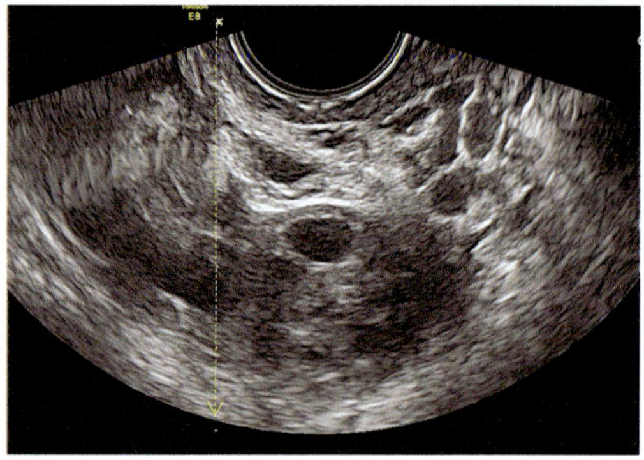

Fig. 2: Transvaginal ultrasound image with a dotted line—biopsy guideline.

Several designs of aspiration needles are available. They may have a single or double lumen to enable aspiration and flushing through different routes. The needle is usually 18–20 gauge and must have a very sharp tip to enable easy puncture of mobile ovaries, and its distal 2 cm should be roughened to enhance ultrasound visualization **(Fig. 3)**.

The needle is connected to a test tube, prewarmed at 37°C in hot blocks, by tubing, and suction is applied either from a foot-operated pump **(Fig. 4)** or manually. Before aspiration, the needle and the tubing are flushed with a flushing medium. Several media are available. One with heparin is used for this purpose. This prevents the clotting of blood in the tubing that may be aspirated along with the follicular fluid. The needle is advanced from the vagina into the ovary under vision.

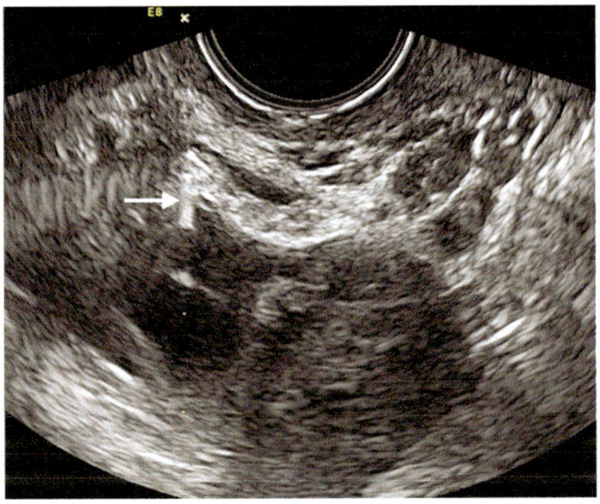

Fig. 3: Transvaginal ultrasound image with biopsy guideline and needle seen overlapping the biopsy guideline.

The needle is attached to the transvaginal ultrasound transducer through a needle guide and bracket firmly and quickly into the follicle. The negative pressure is applied at the same time when the needle punctures the follicle and should be released as soon as the follicle is completely aspirated. Pressure must not be continued while advancing to a new follicle. A negative pressure of 110–120 mm Hg is required. Always confirm that you are puncturing the follicle and not the vessel by manipulating the probe to view the follicle in the sagittal and transverse planes and if in doubt, use Doppler.

Gentle rotation of the needle helps to suck the ovum from any part of the follicle. Contents are aspirated till the follicle is empty. The next follicle is entered without withdrawing the needle out of the ovary. Keep the needle in the ovary and aspirate several follicles one after another with careful

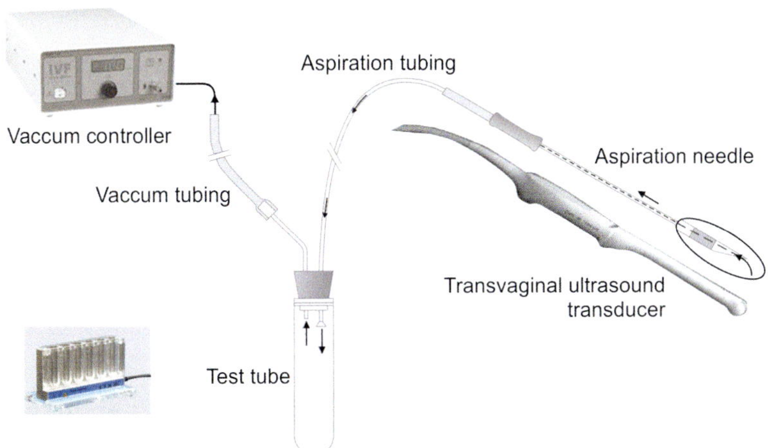

Fig. 4: Follicle aspiration equipment: An assembled follicle aspiration single-lumen needle connected to a test tube. The test tube is in turn connected to a suction pump.

Box 1: Oocyte retrieval technique.

- Light general anesthesia or conscious sedation is used
- Consider antibiotic cover
- Aseptic technique is used
- Lithotomy position of patient, and clean and drape
- Cleanse transvaginal probe and cover with sterile cover and condom with or without gel
- Set biopsy guideline on scanner and fix the biopsy guide on the probe
- Introduce the probe to image the ovary in alignment with the biopsy line
- Introduce the pick-up needle through fornix
- Apply suction as the follicle is punctured
- Aspirate all follicles one after the other and repeat the same on the other ovary
- Remove probe and check for bleeding

gentle manipulation. The order of aspiration of different follicles should be such that the needle manipulation is the least. All follicles of more than 10–12 mm size are aspirated as at times even a 10-mm diameter follicle may contain a fertilizable ovum. Aspirating all these follicles also decreases the risk of ovarian hyperstimulation syndrome (OHSS).

After aspirating all the follicles from one ovary, the probe is still in the vagina, but the needle is withdrawn and flushed with media, before reintroducing it to puncture the second ovary. After finishing the aspiration of all the follicles, remove the probe. Put the speculum and check for the bleeding from the puncture site. If required, apply pressure with a sterilized gauze for a few minutes to stop bleeding **(Box 1)**.

DIFFICULTIES AND CONTROVERSIES

Follicular flushing has been traditionally employed in the belief that it may improve the oocyte yield, although this may not improve the number of oocytes retrieved but increases the duration of retrieval and postoperative pain.[10,11] If the first aspirate does not contain an oocyte, the follicle is flushed few times until one is seen in the aspirate or the observer moves on to the next follicle. Flushing is recommended only if there are very few follicles.

Some workers do recommend twisting of the needle in the follicular lumen while aspirating. The explanation given is that it may help the ovum to be sucked into the needle from any wall of the follicle though the advantage of the same has not been proved.

Bowels in the path of the needle can be displaced by rotating and pushing movements of the probe. At times, the ovaries may not be accessible and rarely one may have to go through the uterus, but in such cases, one needs to ensure that vessels and endometrium are avoided. It is best not to puncture hydrosalpinx or endometriomas, if present, while doing oocyte retrieval. However, if a hydrosalpinx or an endometrioma is punctured inadvertently, prophylactic antibiotic should be administered. The transabdominal route may be needed rarely for oocyte retrieval, when the ovary is not approachable from the vaginal route, if it is placed high up in the pelvis, as in patients with absent uterus, or if the patient has had vaginoplasty. Though expert operators can still manage with the vaginal route.

COMPLICATIONS

Generally, very few complications are encountered during vaginal egg collections. The main risks of transvaginal oocyte recovery are pelvic infection (0.6%) and bleeding (>100 mL in 0.8% cases), which may be serious, sometimes even fatal. Appropriate preoperative vaginal preparation and minimizing the number of repeated vaginal penetrations may serve to lower the risk of infection. While there is no evidence that routine antibiotics reduce the risk of infection, the administration of an intravenous bolus of antibiotics is generally recommended to women with a history of severe pelvic inflammatory disease or if an endometrioma or hydrosalpinx is punctured. Intestinal, vascular, uterine, and tubal injuries with the aspiration needle have also been reported. Though bleeding and infections may be serious, sometimes even fatal.

Ovaries are located close to the iliac vessels, and therefore iliac vessels are vulnerable to injury during ovum pick-up in inexperienced hands. While bleeding from the major vessel is a very rare occurrence in experienced hands, care must always be taken when aspirating the follicles that are close to major vessels. Another possible site of bleeding is from the vaginal wall. This is especially common when there is congestion of the vaginal wall. This bleeding is never severe, though may be frightening for the patient. It stops by manual pressure on the bleeding site for a few minutes or by tamponing. The third possible site from where the bleeding would occur is uterine vessels. This happens when the ovary is adherent to the uterus and placed high up in the pelvis. This can be prevented by carefully managing the needle path **(Fig. 5)**.

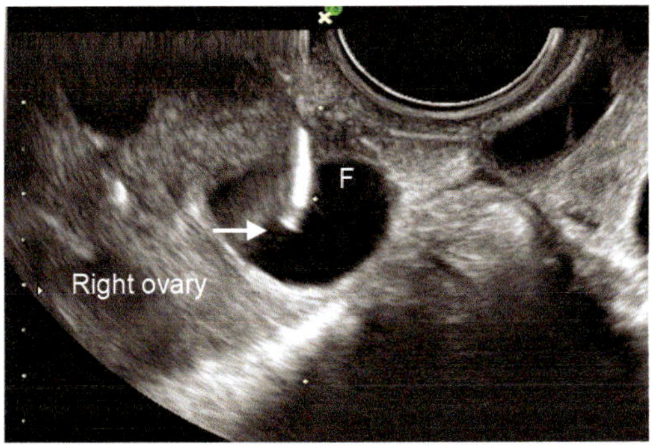

Fig. 5: Ultrasound image during vaginal egg recovery. The tip of the needle (arrow) is seen within the follicle (F).

CARRY HOME MESSAGE

- Ultrasound has proven to be reliable as a guiding tool for several procedures for managing patients with subfertility.
- Ultrasound-guided procedures are less invasive and have significantly reduced the postoperative hospital care.
- Although minimally invasive, these procedures must be done in operation theaters and all emergency drugs and gadgets must be readily available.
- Adequate asepsis, adequate anesthesia, and appropriate antibiotic cover are required.
- It is essential to master the scanning technique before trying these procedures.
- No ultrasound-guided procedure must be attempted if the ultrasound image quality is inadequate.
- Transvaginal ultrasound-guided oocyte retrieval is a very simple and well-accepted method with a very low complication rate.
- The transabdominal route may be rarely needed for oocyte retrieval, if ovaries are placed high up in the pelvis, as in patients with the absent uterus or if the patient has had vaginoplasty.

REFERENCES

1. Feichtinger W, Kemeter P. Laparoscopic ultrasonically guided follicle aspiration for in vitro fertilization. J In Vitro Fert Embryo Transf. 1984;1(4):244-9.
2. Lenz S, Lauritsen JG, Kjellow M. Collection of human oocytes for in vitro fertilization by ultrasonically guided follicular puncture. Lancet. 1981;1(8230):1163-4.
3. Kemeter P, Feichtinger W. Transvaginal oocyte retrieval using a transvaginal sector scan probe combined with an automated puncture device. Hum Reprod. 1986;1(1):21-4.
4. Hayes MF, Sacco AG, Savoy-Moore RT, Magyar DM, Endler GC, Moghissi KS. Effect of general anesthesia on fertilization and cleavage of human oocytes in vitro. Fertil Steril. 1987;48:975-81.
5. Wilhelm W, Biedler A, Hammadeh ME, Fleser R, Grüness V. Remifentanil for oocyte retrieval: a new single-agent monitored

anaesthesia care technique. Anaesthesist. 1999;48:698-704.

6. Rosen MA, Roizen MF, Eger EI 2nd, Glass RH, Martin M, Dandekar PV, et al. The effect of nitrous oxide on in vitro fertilization success rate. Anesthesiology. 1987;67:42-4.
7. Gonen O, Shulman A, Ghetler Y, Shapiro A, Judeiken R, Beyth Y, et al. The impact of different types of anesthesia on in vitro fertilization-embryo transfer treatment outcome. J Assist Reprod Genet. 1995;12:678-82.
8. Raftery S, Sherry E. Total intravenous anaesthesia with propofol and alfentanil protects against postoperative nausea and vomiting. Can J Anaesth. 1992;39:37-40.
9. Cerne A, Bergh C, Borg K, Ek I, Gejervall AL, Hillensjö T, et al. Pre-ovarian block versus paracervical block for oocyte retrieval. Hum Reprod. 2006;21:2916-21.
10. Bagtharia S, Haloob AR. Is there a benefit from routine follicular flushing for oocyte retrieval? J Obstet Gynaecol. 2005;25:374-6.
11. Kingsland CR, Taylor CT, Aziz N, Bickerton N. Is follicular flushing necessary for oocyte retrieval? A randomized trial. Hum Reprod. 1991;6:382-3.

28

Chapter

Embryo Transfer

INTRODUCTION

Embryo transfer (ET) is a critical step in determining the final outcome of IVF treatment. Though evidently simple, this procedure demands a lot of perfection and precision. It is a true blend of science and art. Optimizing the technique of ET would provide the best chance of pregnancy **(Box 1)**.

TECHNIQUE

Pretransfer ultrasound is done to check uterocervical curvature and uterocervical length. The length of the uterus is measured from the fundal end of the endometrium to the external os **(Fig. 1)**.

Asepsis is very essential. The patient lies in the lithotomy position. The vagina is cleaned with warm normal saline. Gauze soaked in normal saline is used to wipe off all the vaginal secretions. Cusco's speculum is commonly used to visualize the cervix with minimal manipulation to the cervix and uterus. Some units use Sim's speculum and Allis forceps or tenaculum to visualize the cervix and straighten the uterocervical canal to make the ET easier. However, it has been reported that this may lead to uterine contractions and may expel out the embryos and compromise the treatment outcome. But it is important to remember, on the other hand, that if the transfer is difficult, the chance of implantation may be compromised. The embryo-loaded catheter is brought to the transfer room only when everything is set. Keep the theater lights dimmed when the ET catheter is brought to the operation theater. It is also essential to maintain the room temperature at 27–29°C. Introduce the transfer catheter into the cervix, under transabdominal ultrasound guidance. If the utero-cervical canal on pretransfer ultrasound is not straight, one may electively use a stiff outer sheath or a cervical cannula

Box 1: Embryo transfer technique.

Embryo transfer can be optimized by:

- Pretransfer assessment of uterine cavity and cervical canal
- Thorough and gentle removal of cervical mucus
- Avoid touching the uterine fundus to:
  - Avoid endometrial damage
  - Avoid initiation of uterine contractions
- Confirm proper delivery of embryos inside the uterine cavity; this can be done by:
  - Confirming the location of the catheter tip
  - Visualize the easy passage of drop of media containing embryos followed by air bubble in the endometrial cavity

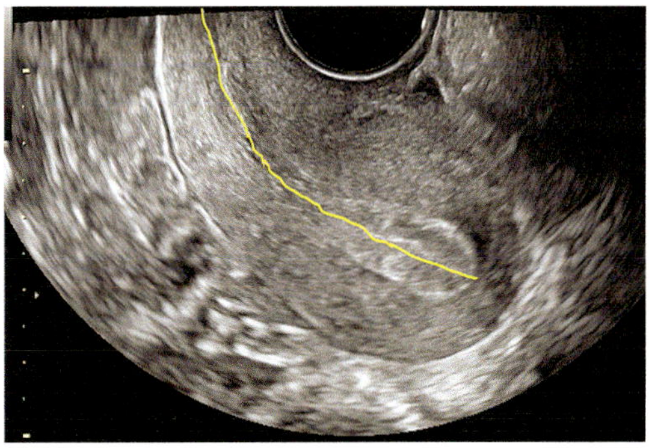

Fig. 1: Measuring the functional uterocervical length for embryo transfer.

for the introduction of the transfer catheter through it. In any case, the embryo is not retained in the catheter for more than 2 minutes. If it takes longer, the embryos are replaced back into the culture dish and reloaded later. A double-sheathed ET catheter is to be used in such cases. After introducing the outer sheath, which is firm in consistency, its position is confirmed beyond the internal os. The inner cannula is introduced through this sheath later on. The cannula tip is placed 1-1.5 cm away from the fundus of the uterus or at 5–6 cm from the external os. The transfer is done in 15–25 µm/L of the medium. Volumes of 50 µm/L or larger lead to lower pregnancy rates, as this fluid may either flow out of the uterus or may fill up the tubes. Once the cannula is introduced to the desired level in the uterus, the piston of the syringe is pushed to introduce the desired amount of fluid-containing embryos into the uterus. The ET cannula is seen as an echogenic line and can be traced from the internal os into the endometrial cavity and when the tip is placed at least 1 cm proximal to the fundal end of the endometrium. The passage of embryos with the air bubble is seen as a release of echogenic spot into the endometrial cavity and is also known as a "bullet sign" **(Figs. 2A to C)**. Then the cannula is steadily held in position for a few seconds. After that, it is gently pulled out with the piston pressed not to cause a suction action. Fluid remaining in the cannula is checked under the microscope to confirm that embryos are not remaining in the cannula. Uterine contractions, expulsion of embryos, blood or mucus on the catheter tip, bacterial contamination of catheter, and retained embryos have all been associated with difficult ETs.

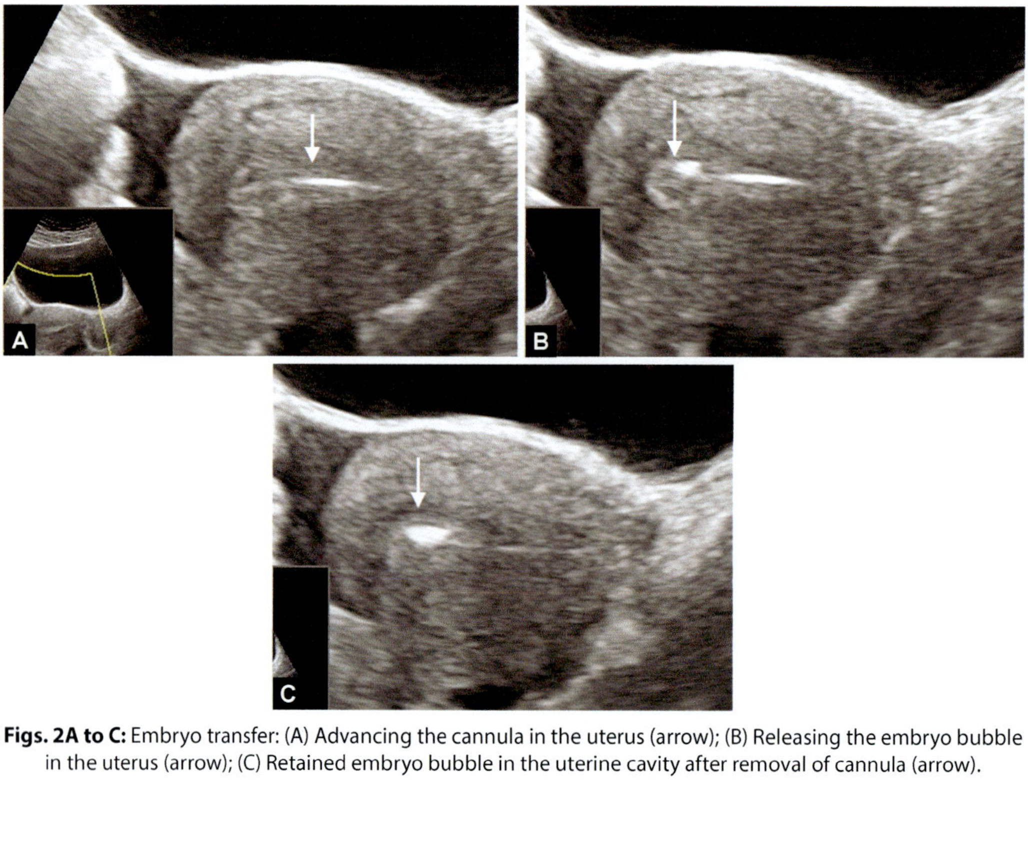

Figs. 2A to C: Embryo transfer: (A) Advancing the cannula in the uterus (arrow); (B) Releasing the embryo bubble in the uterus (arrow); (C) Retained embryo bubble in the uterine cavity after removal of cannula (arrow).

The patient may be gently shifted into the bed and allowed to rest for 20–30 minutes. Success rates are similar regardless of the time for which the patient is kept motionless.

Variables affecting implantation rates and success of ET are as follows:

- Ease of transfer and technique of transfer to avoiding uterine contractions and prevent blood or mucous on the transfer catheter
- Uterine depth and precise depth of ET in the uterine cavity
- Type of catheter used
- Catheter loading
- *Physician's experience*: Physician's perception of transfer difficulty was the most important variable.

VARIATIONS IN EMBRYO TRANSFER TECHNIQUE

Ultrasound-guided Instead of Clinical Touch Method

Ultrasound guidance in this procedure has shown advantage over clinical touch or blind ET by significantly increasing the chance of embryo implantation, ongoing pregnancy, and live birth due to the ease of transfer.[1,2] Transabdominal ultrasonographic guidance is used to determine the precise depth of embryo placement within the uterus. The tip of the catheter is placed approximately 1–1.5 cm from the uterine fundus so that the embryos are expelled gently into the mid-cavity of the uterus. Apart from the depth of the uterine cavity, the curvature of the uterine cavity, angle between the cervix and the endometrial cavity, may also be appreciated and the angle of the ET cannula may be accordingly adjusted to make the transfer easy. When the cervical canal appears curved or there is an acute angle between the cervix and the uterus, a double-sheathed catheter or a catheter with stilette is recommended. Use of stilette under ultrasound guidance to negotiate difficult cervical passage makes ET easy and less traumatic.[3]

In an exhaustive Cochrane Database Systematic Review that included 13/15 randomized controlled trials (RCTs), Brown et al.[1] reported significantly higher live birth/ongoing pregnancies per woman randomized associated with ultrasound-guided ET (452/1,376 compared with 353/1,338) for clinical touch, odds ratio (OR) 1.40, and 95% confidence interval (CI) 1.18–1.66 ($p < 0.001$) in six studies. This suggested that a population of women with a 25% chance of pregnancy using clinical touch would be increased to 32% (28–46%) using ultrasound-guided ET. Ultrasound guidance for ET is therefore recommended.

Studies have shown that no significant changes in results have been observed, whether transabdominal or transvaginal ultrasound is used for guidance.[4] However, transabdominal ultrasound is preferred as it does not interfere with the transvaginal or transcervical procedure of ET.

Ultrasound-guided ET enables the visualization of:[5]

- Guiding cannula and transfer catheter placement in relation to the endometrial surface and uterine fundus during ET
- Position and movement of a transfer-associated air bubble
- Impact of subendometrial–myometrial contractions leading to endometrial movement.

Advantages of Ultrasound-guided Embryo Transfer

- Helps placement of soft catheters
- Confirms that the catheter is beyond the internal os in cases of an elongated cervical canal.

- Allows to guide the direction of the catheter along the contour of the endometrial cavity, especially in uteri with acute curves
- Prevents damage to the endometrium and plugging of the catheter
- Full bladder that is required for transabdominal ultrasound and that straightens the uterocervical angle and helps catheter passage.
- Helps to negotiate the catheter through the difficult cervical canal
- Helps to correct position of the catheter tip for embryo deposition [point of maximum implantation potential (MIP)].

A total of eight prospective controlled trials were identified for a meta-analysis.[6] Of these studies, four were nonrandomized or quasirandomized and four were genuinely randomized. A meta-analysis demonstrated a significantly increased chance of clinical pregnancy following ultrasound-guided ET in all studies and in the genuinely randomized subgroup. The embryo implantation rate was also significantly increased following ultrasound-guided ET.[7]

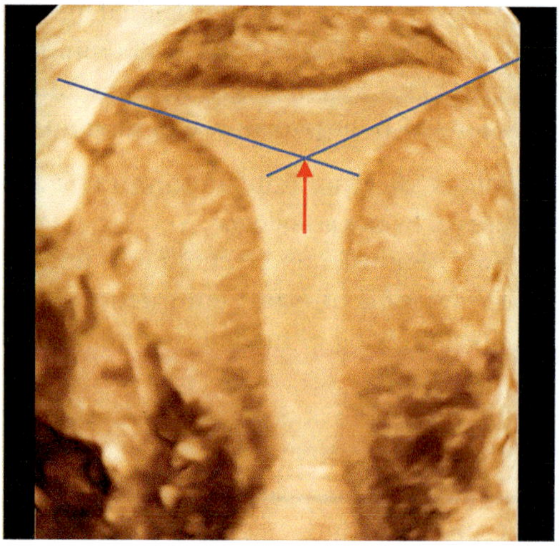

Fig. 3: Intersection of the lines drawn through the uterine cornu, indicating the point of maximum implantation potential.

Transfer at the Point of Maximum Implantation Potential

A large observational retrospective study by Gergely et al. has shown that if MIP is individually found in each patient with the help of three-dimensional (3D) ultrasound and embryos are deposited at this point, then the implantation rates can improve.[8] Point of MIP can be calculated by 3D ultrasound. On a coronal section of the uterus, two lines are drawn, one on each side parallel to the cornu. The point at which these lines intersect is the point of MIP **(Fig. 3)**.

Transvaginal ultrasound-guided ET was performed on 121 consecutive patients. The observation was made of guiding cannula and transfer catheter placement in relation to the endometrial surface and uterine fundus during ET. The position and movement of a transfer-associated air bubble and the impact of subendometrial myometrial contraction leading to the endometrial movement were observed. Results indicate that tactile assessment of ET catheter placement is unreliable in 17.4% of transfers, the outer guiding catheter inadvertently abutting the fundal endometrium. The outer guiding cannula indented the endometrium in 24.8% and the transfer catheter embedded in the endometrium in 33.1%.[9]

The use of ultrasound-guided transfer avoided tubal transfer in 7.4% of transfers. In a randomized trial, the use of transabdominal ultrasound guidance during ET improved the pregnancy rate from 33.7 to 50%.[10] In another retrospective study,[11] the pregnancy rate improved from 25 to 38% by using ultrasound during ET. However, three other prospective trials failed to show such a significant improvement.[9]

Catheter Types

Soft catheters are preferred over rigid ones as they are less likely to traumatize the cervix and endometrium and to invoke any uterine contractions. The commonly used soft catheters (Wallace) have a softer inner cannula and a stiffer outer sheath.[12] Occasionally, resistance to pass the soft inner cannula into the uterus usually at the level of internal os is encountered and in these cases, the stiffer outer sheath is advanced in the cervical canal to negotiate the resistance with the inner cannula can now be advanced into the uterine cavity.

A firmer malleable catheter with a stilette and an outer sheath is another option in difficult cases, where the catheter is advanced up to the level of the internal os. The inner stilette is then removed and the softer cannula with embryos loaded in is fed through the outer sheath to advance into the uterine cavity for transfer. The outer sheath or the malleable catheter should never be advanced beyond the internal os.

Bleeding at the time of the transfer may adversely affect the embryos. In difficult transcervical transfers, either transfer under anesthesia or a surgical transfer transfundally under ultrasound and laparoscopic guidance may be done.

Catheters with echogenic tips are better appreciated on ultrasound guidance and therefore reduce the time taken from loading the catheter to depositing the embryos in endometrial cavity. The coaxial catheter system has been preferred by some and has been claimed to be of help in difficult transfers. But in a prospective randomized study of 251 patients, no significant change was found in the implantation rate, clinical pregnancy rate, or ongoing pregnancy rate between the two catheters.[13] Another group compared soft catheters and catheters with an echogenic tip and concluded that catheters with an echogenic tip simplify the ET and also improve implantation rates.

The pump-regulated embryo-transfer (PRET) device generates a significantly smaller variance of the positioning of the embryo(s) into the uterine cavity. This resulted in an ongoing pregnancy rate of 21% in the PRET versus 17% in the manual ($p = 0.22$) transfer group; frozen-thawed ETs resulted in 17.5 versus 10.9% ($p = 0.097$), respectively.[14]

Mock Transfer

The role of mock transfers in reducing the frequency of unexpected difficult ETs has been controversial. The mock transfer is done to rehearse the transfer process so as to anticipate the difficulties and modify the selection of the catheter or speculum. Mock transfer can be done at the time of the start of ovarian stimulation or at oocytes retrieval or at the time of actual transfer. In the initial studies by Mansour et al.,[15] trial transfers have been shown to reduce the incidence of difficult transfers. However, in a study by Henne et al.,[4] it has been shown that the uterine length and position change with ovarian stimulation challenging the role of trial transfer.

Day of Embryo Transfer

The convention was to replace embryos on the second or third day post insemination, when the embryos are usually 2–8-cell stage of cleavage. With improvements in culture media and laboratory conditions, there is an increasing tendency for delaying ET till Day 5 with an aim to improve the implantation rates. Delaying ET from Day 2 or Day 3 and transfer of embryos at the blastocyst stage (Day 5/6) have shown a significant increase in live birth rate (OR: 1.35, 95% CI: 1.05–1.74) when compared with Day 2 or Day 3 transfers.[16] It is a more physiological approach, allowing synchronization of the embryo with the endometrium, and the selection of viable embryos for transfer will be more efficient.

However, the rates of embryos freezing are lower and the treatment cancellation rates are higher with blastocyst transfer. But in the selected group of couples, the practice of blastocyst transfer has the potential to favor single ET without compromising the overall success rates; however, it can significantly reduce the occurrence of multiple pregnancies. The most favored groups for blastocyst transfer are those having high numbers of eight-cell embryos on Day 3, in whom the cycle cancellation is not increased.

CARRY HOME MESSAGE

- Embryo transfer is a very important step in ART.
- Success of embryo transfer to lead to clinical pregnancy is most dependent on the ease of transfer and the time taken for the embryo to reach the female's womb from the incubator.
- Ultrasound guidance for embryo transfer has now been designated as indispensable as it facilitates the path of the cannula and allows the release of the embryos at point of maximum implantation potential.
- Aspiration of cervical mucus, mock transfer, endometrial scratching, etc., all other modifications to optimize embryo transfer procedure are yet to prove their worth.

REFERENCES

1. Brown J, Buckingham K, Abou-Setta AM, Abou-Setta AM. Ultrasound versus "clinical touch" for catheter guidance during embryo transfer in women. Cochrane Database Syst Rev. 2010;(1):CD006107.
2. Porter MB. Ultrasound in assisted reproductive technology. Semin Reprod Med. 2008;26(3):266-76.
3. Allahbadia GN, Kadam KS, Gandhi GN, Arora S, Mhatre YP, Virk S. The stilette for a Sure View. Fertil Steril. 2006;86(Suppl 3): S252.
4. Henne MB, Milki AA. Uterine position at real embryo transfer compared with mock embryo transfer. Hum Reprod. 2004;19:570-2
5. Woolcott R, Stanger J. Potentially important variables identified by transvaginal ultrasound-guided embryo transfer. Hum Reprod. 1997;12(5):963-6.
6. Buckett WM. A meta-analysis of ultrasound-guided versus clinical touch embryo transfer. Fertil Steril. 2003;80(4):1037-41.
7. Sallam HN, Sadek SS. Ultrasound-guided embryo transfer: a meta-analysis of a randomized controlled trial. Fertil Steril. 2003;80(4):1042-6.
8. Gergely RZ, De Ugarte CM, Danzer H, Surrey M, Hill D, DeCherney AH. Three-dimensional/four-dimensional ultrasound-guided embryo transfer using the maximal implantation potential point. Fertil Steril. 2005;84(2):500-3.
9. Woolcott R, Stanger J. Potentially important variables identified by transvaginal ultrasound-guided embryo transfer. Hum Reprod. 1997;12(5):963-6.
10. Coroleu B, Carreras O, Veiga A, Martell A, Martinez F, Belil I, et al. Embryo transfer under ultrasound guidance improves pregnancy rates after in-vitro fertilization. Hum Reprod. 2000;15:616-20.
11. Wood EG, Batzer FR, Go KJ, Gutmann JN, Corson SL. Ultrasound-guided soft catheter embryo transfers will improve pregnancy rates in in-vitro fertilization. Hum Reprod. 2000;15:107-12.
12. Karande V, Hazlett D, Vietzke M, Gleicher N. A prospective randomized comparison of the Wallace catheter and the Cook Echo-Tip catheter for ultrasound-guided embryo transfer. Fertil Steril. 2002;77(4):826-30.
13. Coroleu B, Barri PN, Carreras O, Belil I, Buxaderas R, Veiga A, et al. Effect of using an echogenic catheter for ultrasound-guided embryo transfer in an IVF programme: a prospective, randomized, controlled study. Hum Reprod. 2006;21(7):1809-15.
14. Caanen MR, van der Houwen LE, Schats R, Vergouw CG, de Leeuw B, Lambers MJ, et al. Embryo transfer with controlled injection speed to increase pregnancy rates: a randomized controlled trial. Gynecol Obstet Invest. 2016;81:394-404.
15. Mansour R, Aboulghar M, Serour G. Dummy embryo transfer: a technique that minimizes the problems of embryo transfer and improves the pregnancy rate in human in vitro fertilization. Fertil Steril. 1990;54:678-81.
16. Blake DA, Farquhar CM, Johnson N, Olive D. Cleavage stage versus blastocyst stage embryo transfer in assisted conception. Cochrane Database Syst Rev. 2007;(4):CD002118.

29

Chapter

3D–4D Ultrasound in Infertility

INTRODUCTION

Three-dimensional ultrasound (US) is now a well-developed technology and it has proved its superiority over the B-mode US in several applications. It is complementary to B-mode and Doppler assessment for monitoring of natural and treatment cycles in patients with infertility. For the assessment of the female, transvaginal scan is the scanning method of choice and the first-line investigation. 3D US can be used for diagnosis of polycystic ovaries, assessment of ovarian reserve [volume and antral follicle count (AFC)], ovarian follicular monitoring, endometrial receptivity assessment, and tubal patency assessment.

POLYCYSTIC OVARIES

According to the European Society of Human Reproduction and Embryology/American Society for Reproductive Medicine (ESHRE/ASRM) consensus 2018, the polycystic ovarian disease consists of various phenotypes and in majority, US showing polycystic ovaries is important.

Polycystic ovary on US according to this consensus is an ovary that is 10 cc in volume and/or has more than 20 antral follicles of 2–9 mm in diameter. But this criterion of >10 cc would fail to identify a group of ovulatory, normoandrogenic women still at risk of complications associated with polycystic ovary syndrome (PCOS), such as ovarian hyperstimulation syndrome (OHSS), failed implantation, miscarriage, and hyperinsulinemia.[1] Ovarian volume of 6.6 cc has 91% sensitivity and 91% specificity for PCOS.[2] Jonard et al. have also suggested that lowering the ovarian volume to 7 cc has allowed 67.5% sensitivity and 91.2% specificity for PCOS. The mean ovarian volume in normal ovaries was suggested as 4.5 cc in this study.[3] But, it is important to assess the correct ovarian volume and this can be done by 3D US. After the volume of the ovary is acquired by 3D US, virtual organ computer-aided analysis (VOCAL) software is used to calculate the ovarian volume. VOCAL calculates the volume of any structure by rotating it 180°. A rotating step of 6–30° can be selected. A circumference is drawn around the structure of interest at every step of rotation and at the end of 180°, the total volume is calculated by the scanner computer **(Fig. 1)**.

However, size is not the only important criterion. Histologically and biochemically, polycystic ovaries can be of normal size and a wide overlap is seen between the size of normal and polycystic ovaries. Polycystic ovarian morphology has been found to be a better discriminator than ovarian volume between polycystic ovarian syndrome and control women.[4] Among the morphological features of polycystic ovaries are the follicular number per ovary (FNPO) of more than 12 according to the old consensus and more

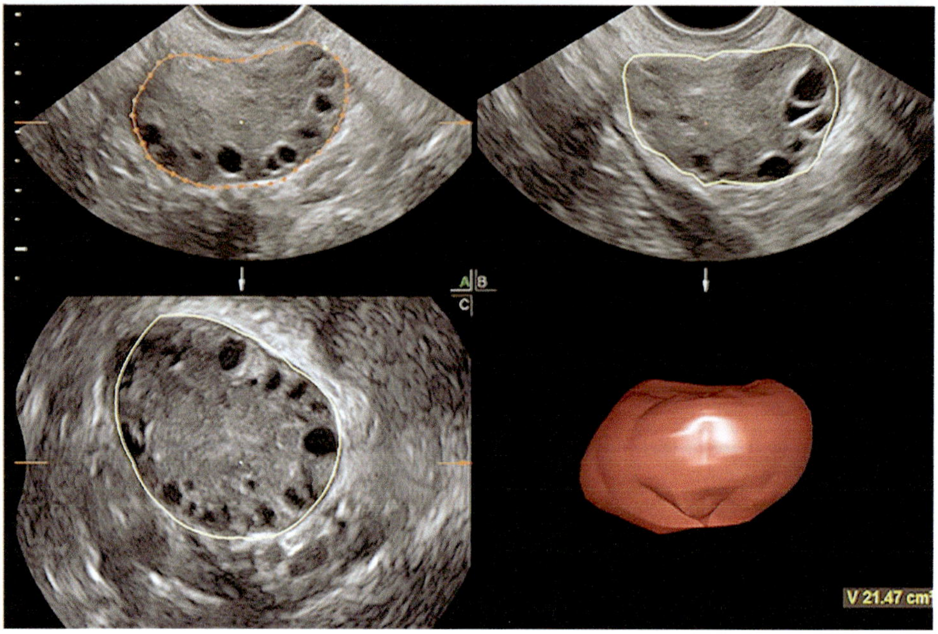

Fig. 1: Virtual organ computer-aided analysis (VOCAL) calculated volume of the ovary on 3D ultrasound-acquired volume of the ovary.

than 20 per ovary according to the 2018 consensus, the follicular arrangement that may be peripheral or generalized, and stromal abundance.

The mean FNPO of follicles 2–5 mm in size was significantly higher in polycystic ovaries than in controls, while it was similar within the 6-9-mm range. For the follicles within 2-5-mm range, a significant relationship was found between FNPO and androgens but FNPO in the range of 6–9 mm was significantly and negatively related to body mass index and fasting serum insulin level. It is believed that androgen leads to early follicular development but further progression is not normal due to hyperinsulinemia and/or other metabolic influence linked to obesity.[5] Androgen is the cause and anti-Müllerian hormone (AMH) is the result of multiple antral follicles. An average value of 26 or more follicles per ovary is a reliable threshold for detecting polycystic ovaries in women with frank manifestation of PCOS. The sensitivity and specificity for diagnosis of PCOS for FNPO (26) was 85% and 94% and for ovarian volume (10 cc) was 81% and 84%, respectively.[6]

These antral follicles that are more than 12–15 can be confidently counted only by 3D US and Sono-AVC (sonographic-based automated volume calculation) **(Fig. 2)**. Sono-AVC is based on the inversion mode and color codes the follicles, thus allowing more correct calculation of the number. More exact value of AFC was acquired when counted by 3D US. The inversion mode is the most convenient method for counting antral follicles when they are multiple.[7] Sono-AVC measured less number of follicles on AFC, though it took significantly less time to measure the size and record the number of antral follicles (132 + 56.23 seconds vs. 324.47 + 162.22 seconds).[8] Postprocessing can be used for the follicles that are missed out on automated counting. Apart from this, Sono-AVC also calculates

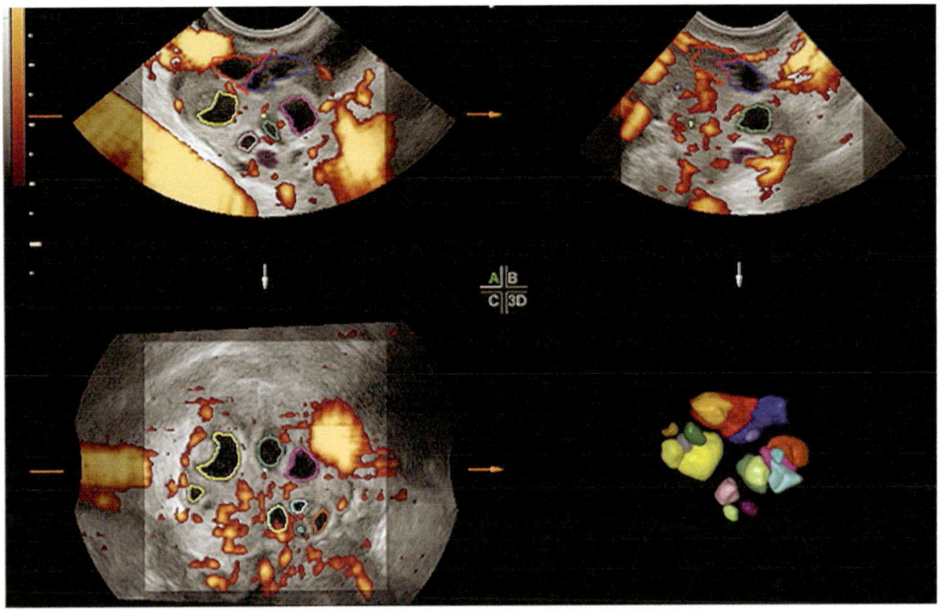

Fig. 2: 3D ultrasound-acquired volume of the ovary, with Sono-AVC showing color-coded follicles. (Sono-AVC: sonographic-based automated volume calculation)

the size of each follicle and that is important for the understanding of the variable biochemical derangement in various patients with PCOS **(Fig. 3)**. The result sheet shows *x*-, *y*-, and *z*-axis diameter, mean diameter, and volume of each follicle, respectively.

Stromal abundance is the second important feature of polycystic ovaries. The earliest description of polycystic ovaries appears to date from 1845 as "sclerocystic ovaries."[9] To identify women with a milder form of PCOS, further information, particularly about the ovarian stroma and the degree of vascularization, is required.[1] Patients having long-standing PCOS and long-standing anovulation have more dense stroma, and a cardinal feature has been shown to be the presence of a bright, highly echogenic stroma on transvaginal US.[10] Stromal hypertrophy was recognized as a frequent and specific feature in ovarian androgenic dysfunction.[11] Polycystic ovarian morphology (PCOM; stromal echogenicity) in normal women is not a morphological variant of normal ovaries but rather represents a functional entity—a silent form of PCOS.[12] Stromal abundance and echogenicity is one of the major features that discriminates polycystic ovary from multicystic ovary. This can be assessed as stromal echogenicity, stromal area, and stromal volume. Polycystic ovaries show hyperechoic[13] stroma and by ovarian area: 5.5 cm^2 (93% sensitivity and 91% specificity)—strict longitudinal ovarian section—and by stromal area: 4.6 cm^2 (91% sensitivity and 86% specificity).[14] But the most accurate assessment of stromal abundance can only be done with ovarian and stromal volume by 3D US. 3D US has the potential to address these points and improve the sensitivity and specificity of US in the diagnosis of PCOS.[15]

Both total ovarian volume and stromal volume during the early follicular phase are significantly higher in women with PCOS.[16] Stromal volume was positively correlated with

Name							Pat. ID						
Ovary:		Left					Ovary:		Right				
Total#:		26					Total#:		23				
Nr.	d(V) mm	dx mm	dy mm	dz mm	mn. d mm	V cm³	Nr.	d(V) mm	dx mm	dy mm	dz mm	mn. d mm	V cm³
	14.5	21.1	15.9	10.5	15.8	1.59		14.8	17.4	15.1	13.4	15.3	1.70
2	13.7	17.1	13.5	12.1	14.2	1.34	2	14.8	20.3	15.2	12.2	15.9	1.69
	13.5	22.2	11.5	10.8	14.8	1.28		11.7	17.8	15.1	7.0	13.3	0.84
	13.0	15.2	12.9	11.7	13.3	1.15		10.9	13.1	10.9	10.2	11.4	0.68
5	13.0	19.5	15.4	8.0	14.3	1.15	5	10.7	12.5	11.1	9.2	10.9	0.64
6	12.2	15.0	13.7	11.2	13.3	0.95	6	10.2	11.4	11.1	9.1	10.5	0.56
	9.8	13.0	10.5	7.7	10.4	0.49		10.0	13.4	9.9	8.6	10.6	0.53
8	9.5	14.3	11.4	5.8	10.5	0.45	8	10.0	14.8	11.4	7.1	11.1	0.53
9	9.5	13.5	11.5	6.4	10.5	0.45	9	9.9	15.3	9.9	7.3	10.8	0.50
10	8.8	11.8	11.3	5.4	9.5	0.35	10	9.3	14.6	12.0	6.8	11.1	0.42
11	8.7	11.0	8.3	7.8	9.1	0.34	11	8.9	13.4	8.0	7.2	9.5	0.37
12	8.6	10.2	9.2	7.5	8.9	0.33	12	8.9	12.6	8.6	7.0	9.4	0.37
13	8.5	14.2	10.5	4.9	9.9	0.32	13	8.5	13.3	9.1	5.6	9.4	0.32
14	8.1	12.7	10.5	4.7	9.3	0.28	14	7.2	10.1	7.6	5.3	7.7	0.20
15	7.9	11.5	7.6	6.4	8.5	0.26	15	7.1	11.3	6.2	5.7	7.8	0.19
16	6.9	9.9	7.2	4.9	7.3	0.17	16	6.6	9.3	7.5	4.6	7.2	0.15
17	6.3	8.1	6.4	5.3	6.6	0.13	17	6.5	8.2	7.1	5.5	6.9	0.14
18	5.8	9.1	7.2	3.3	6.6	0.10	18	5.8	8.1	6.8	4.0	6.3	0.10

Fig. 3: Result sheet of Sono-AVC showing the total number of follicles in either ovary (circles) and all three diameters, mean diameter, and volume of individual follicle marked by the relevant color in the box. (Sono-AVC: sonographic-based automated volume calculation)

serum androstenedione concentrations in patients with PCOS.[16] A statistically significant relationship was reported between ovarian volume and stromal echogenicity with serum luteinizing hormone (LH) and testosterone concentrations.[17] The ovarian volume can be calculated by VOCAL as mentioned earlier, and applying threshold volume to this can calculate the stromal volume. After the volume is calculated by VOCAL when the threshold volume is activated, a pigment appears on the VOCAL-calculated volume. Applying threshold volume on the same VOCAL-calculated volume will define stromal volume when the threshold is set to differentiate follicles from the rest of the ovarian tissues. The threshold is so adjusted that the pigmented area fills up all the follicles and only follicles. On the screen, above threshold and below threshold volumes are displayed. Below threshold is the follicular volume and above threshold is the stromal volume **(Fig. 4)**. In PCOS patients, a strong and similar correlation is seen between ovarian and stromal volumes to fasting and postprandial insulin levels.[18]

3D US not only permits improved spatial awareness and volumetric and quantitative vascular assessment, but also provides a more objective tool to examine stromal echogenicity through the assessment of the mean grayness (MG) of the ovary **(Fig. 5)**.[19] The stromal index (stromal echogenicity/total ovarian echogenicity) was significantly higher in PCOS than controls.[10]

Moreover, 3D US has clearly shown higher AFC (median 16.3 vs. 5.5 per ovary), ovarian volume (12.56 vs. 5.6 mL), stromal volume (10.79 vs. 4.69 mL), and stromal vascularization [vascularity index (VI) 3.85 vs. 2.79%, vascularity flow index (VFI) 1.27 vs. 0.85] in polycystic ovary patients.[20] Ovarian stromal flow index (FI) is higher (33.94 vs. 29.30) in hirsutism than in

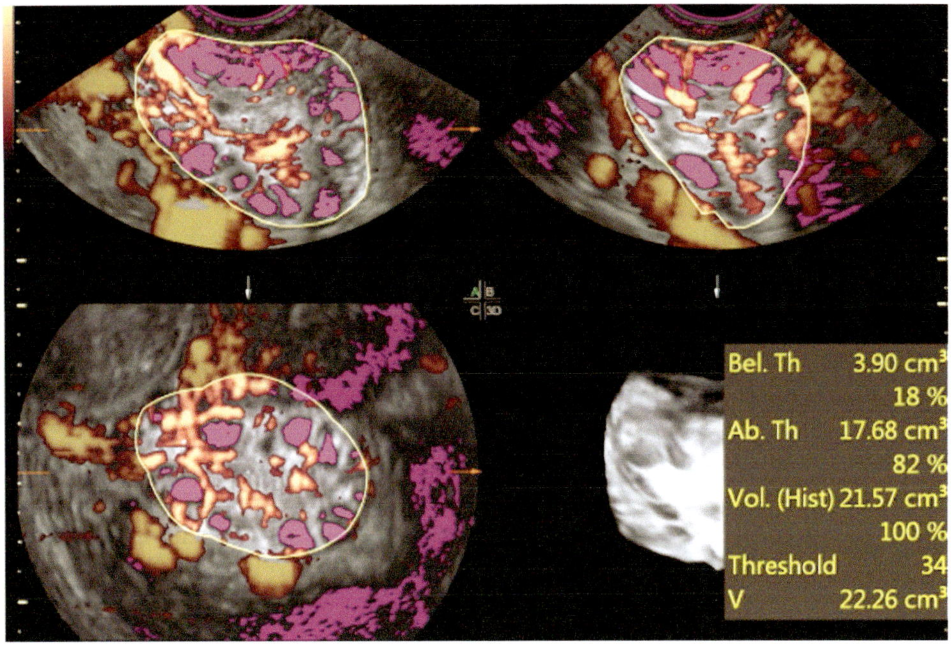

Fig. 4: 3D ultrasound acquired virtual organ computer-aided analysis (VOCAL) calculated ovarian volume with threshold volume used to calculate stromal volume of the ovary.

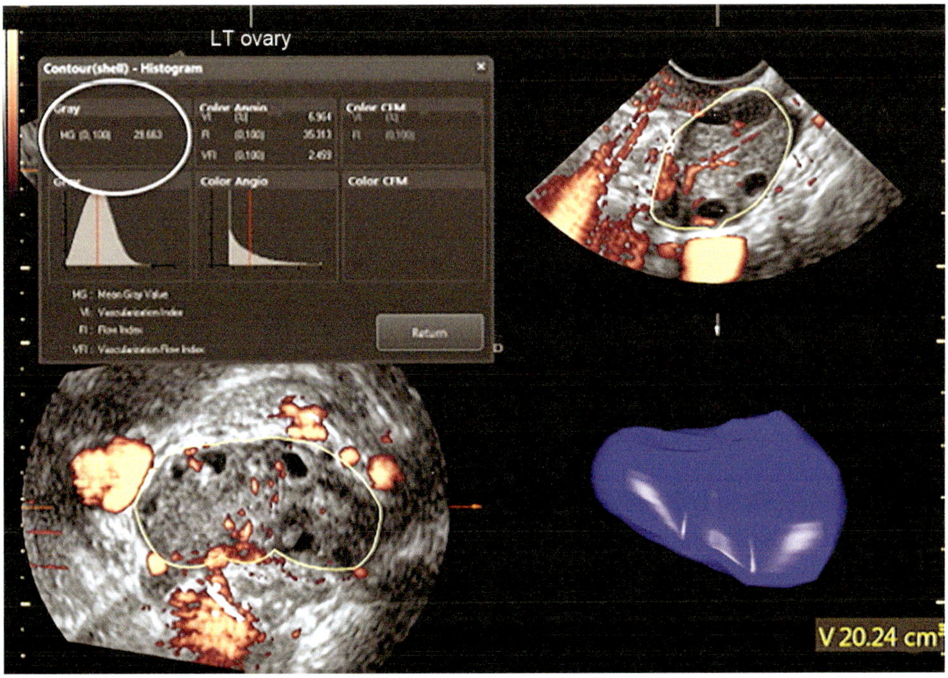

Fig. 5: 3D ultrasound-acquired VOCAL calculated ovarian volume with volume histogram, showing mean gray value of the ovary.

normoandrogenic PCOS women. But in PCOS women with obesity, the vascularity was lower than in normal weight women (VI 3.25 vs. 4.51%, VFI 1.22 vs. 1.56).[20] It is this vascularity that is responsible for hyperstimulation in the patients with PCOS.

To sum up, the morphological features of polycystic ovary that correlate the most with the biochemical derangements of PCOS, ovarian volume, stromal volume, and AFC can all be better and more precisely assessed by and correlated with by 3D US.

FOLLICULAR MONITORING

- Assessment of ovarian reserve and response
- Assessment of follicular maturity and endometrial receptivity

Assessment of Ovarian Reserve and Response

3D US is also being used to predict the ovarian response in patients on assisted reproductive techniques (ART). This volume of ovary is used to calculate ovarian volume, stromal volume, and the number of antral follicles **(Figs. 6A and B)**. Global vascular indices—VI, FI, and VFI—may be calculated from the same ovarian volume **(Fig. 7)**. VI indicates the abundance of the flow in the entire ovary, FI indicates the average intensity of the flow in the calculated volume, and VFI indicates the perfusion in the volume calculated by VOCAL software.

According to a study by Kupesic and Kurjak, the predictors of ovarian response are:[21]

- Number of antral follicles
- Stromal flow: Stromal FI
- Total ovarian stromal area
- Total ovarian volume

In that order of importance, this means that the most important predictors of ovarian response can be most precisely assessed by 3D US and 3D power Doppler.

3D US provides a new method for objective quantitative assessment of follicle count, ovarian volume, stromal volume, and blood flow in the ovary.[22] AFC, the most reliable marker for ovarian reserve, can be more exactly calculated by 3D US. The number of antral follicles when not too many can also be counted with inversion mode rendering, more precisely than eyeballing on 2D US **(Figs. 8A and B)**. Sono-AVC for

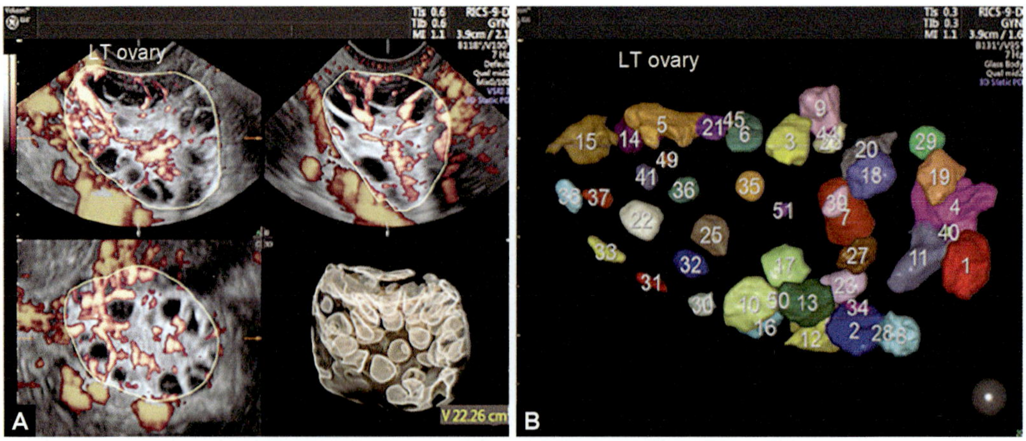

Figs. 6A and B: (A) 3D power Doppler-acquired volume of the ovary rendered in inversion mode with silhouette showing multiple antral follicles; (B) Sono-automated volume calculation with color-coded multiple follicles.

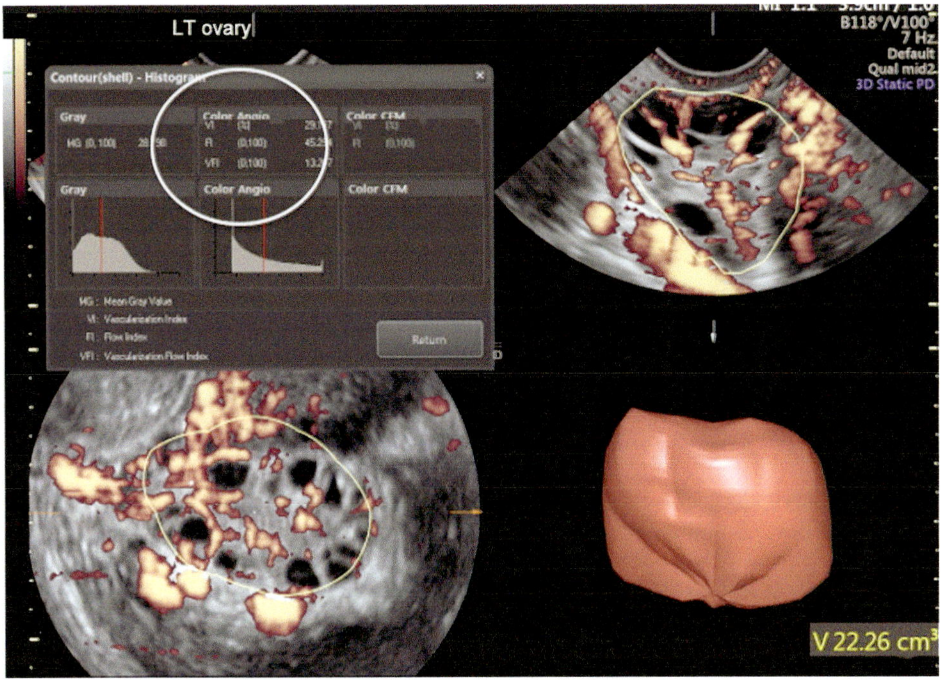

Fig. 7: 3D power Doppler-acquired volume of the ovary with volume histogram showing vascularity index (VI), flow index (FI), and vascularity flow index (VFI) values.

the assessment of the ovarian reserve can be made simpler and more precise by using Sono-AVC antral **(Fig. 8C)**. This software allows grouping the follicles into a particular size that can be designed and that helps to ignore follicles larger or smaller than the defined limit automatically. According to Rainne-Fenning and Lam, the total number of oocytes retrieved on ovum pickup is 60% of antral follicles counted on the inversion mode.[23] The advantage of the inversion mode is that it makes possible to image even very small follicles that may be missed on 2D US.

On this calculated ovarian volume with power Doppler, applying volume histogram gives values of 3D power Doppler indices, VI, FI, and VFI. Measurement of ovarian stromal flow in the early follicular phase is related to subsequent ovarian response in in vitro fertilization (IVF) treatment[24] **(Figs. 9A and B)**. 3D power Doppler with histogram can also be used to assess stromal vascularity on baseline scan. Kupesic and Kurjak have shown a correlation in the ovarian stromal FI and the number of mature oocytes retrieved in IVF cycles and pregnancy rates (stromal FI < 11: low responder; 11–14: good; >15: risk of OHSS).[21] Another group has demonstrated that VI, FI, and VFI of the ovary were significantly related to ovarian response to stimulation.[25]

These all together help to decide the stimulation protocol and also to decide any additional or supportive therapy required for a particular patient.

Pretrigger Evaluation of Follicle and Endometrium

Assessment of Follicular Maturity

A follicle that is 16–18 mm in diameter and shows perifollicular vascularity covering

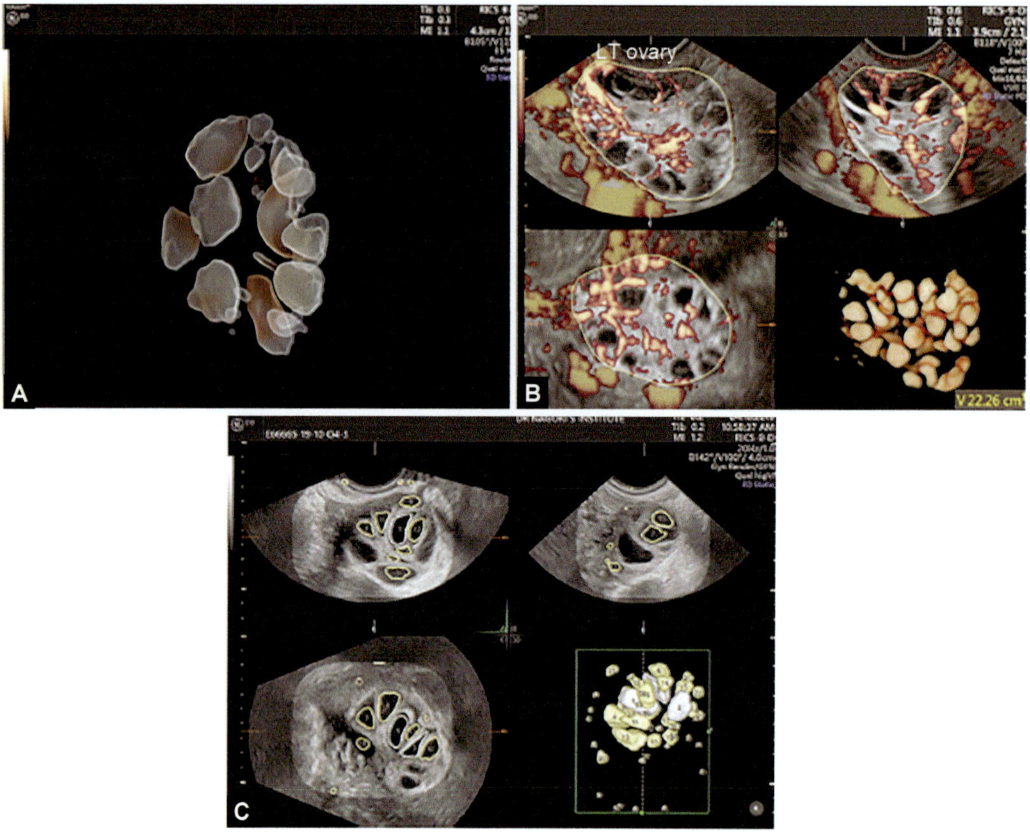

Figs. 8A to C: (A) Inversion mode HD-live with silhouette image showing antral follicles; (B) 3D power Doppler volume of ovary rendered in inversion mode to show antral follicles; (C) 3D volume of the ovary processed by Sono-AVC antral showing unicolor follicles of a defined size range.

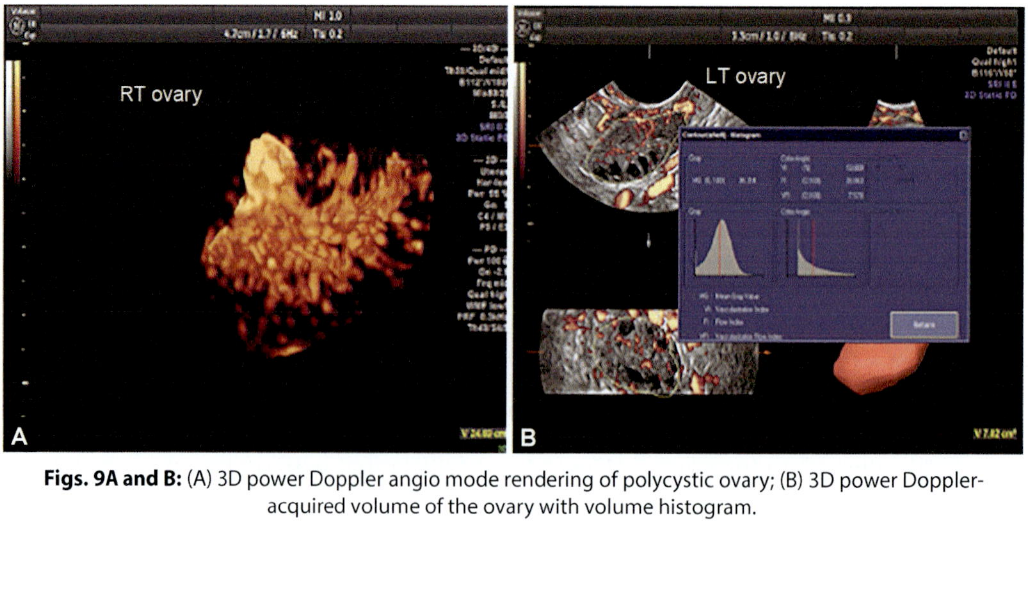

Figs. 9A and B: (A) 3D power Doppler angio mode rendering of polycystic ovary; (B) 3D power Doppler-acquired volume of the ovary with volume histogram.

three-fourths of the circumference of the follicle with resistance index (RI) of ≤0.48 and peak systolic velocity (PSV) of 10 cm/s or more is known to be functionally mature. 3D US and 3D power Doppler have been used for further assessment of these follicles.

On 3D, the follicular volume of 3–7.5 cc has been found to be optimum in our study[5] **(Fig. 10)**.[26] Follicular volumes between 3 and 7 cc are optimum for oocyte retrieval by VOCAL. The limits of agreement between the volume of the follicular aspirate and the 3D volume of the follicle were +0.96 to −0.43 with 3D and +3.47 to −2.42 with 2D volume estimation, respectively.[27]

This is because 3D US measurement is not affected by the follicular shape, as the changing contours are outlined serially to obtain the specific volume measurement. Though the follicles of <10 mm in diameter cannot be assessed accurately by 3D US because the limits of agreement are too wide for this range.

After the volume calculation, the follicle is seen plane by plane in the acquired volume by translation and rotation that is walking through the volume and rotating the volume. Using the surface smooth or light gradient mode for rendering with high threshold can show cumulus with considerable accuracy. Feichtinger et al. in their study have shown the presence of cumulus in follicles >15 mm by 3D US[28] **(Fig. 11)**. Follicles without visualization of cumulus in all three planes are not likely to contain mature oocytes.

Poehl et al.[29] also found a significant correlation between the number of detected cumuli by 3D US and the number of retrieved oocytes ($p < 0.0001$), mature oocytes ($p < 0.0001$), and fertilized oocytes ($p < 0.0001$).[29]

It has also been suggested that the follicles containing oocytes capable to produce a pregnancy have a perifollicular vascular network which is more uniform and distinctive.[30] Although it is possible to assess the follicular flow as expressed by the

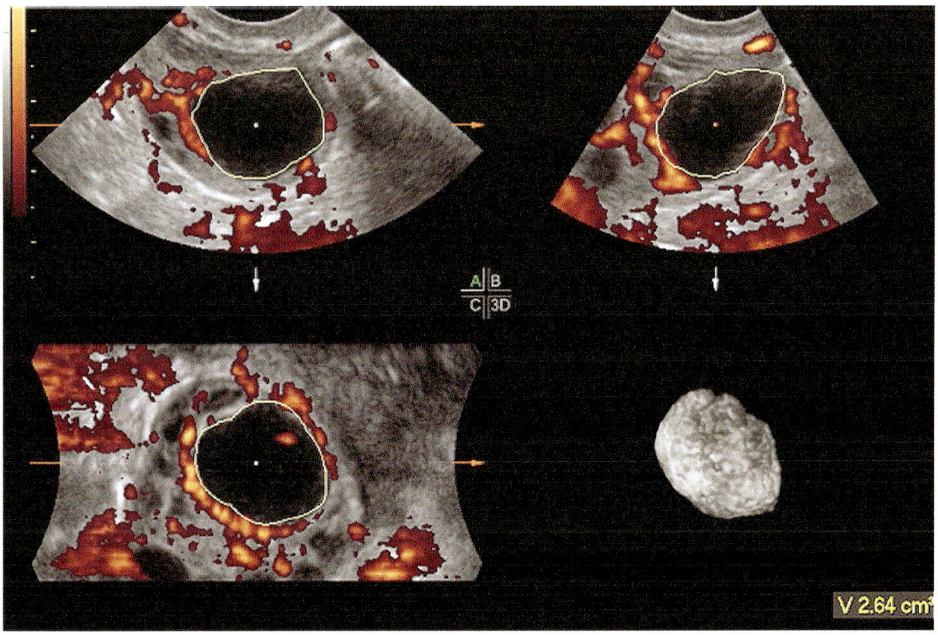

Fig. 10: 3D power Doppler volume of the follicle with VOCAL showing follicle volume calculation.

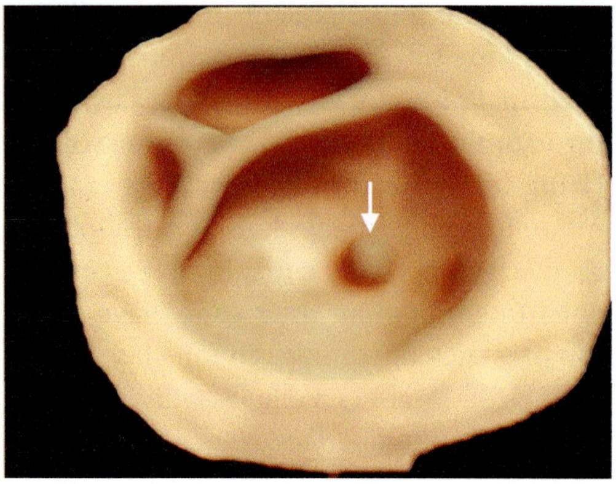

Fig. 11: Surface-rendered volume of follicle showing cumulus.

peak systolic velocity and perifollicular color map.[21] It is the 3D power Doppler, which proves the most precise information about the vascularization and follicular blood flow. 3D power Doppler gives a global assessment of the vascularity, or follicular perfusion, both qualitatively and quantitatively.

The pulse repetition frequency (PRF) settings for 3D power Doppler are fixed at 0.3 always and a 3D volume with power Doppler is taken. For the assessment of the perifollicular vascularity, the vascularity is assessed in the outside shell with the wall thickness of 2 mm, which has been found to be the most appropriate to include the perifollicular vessels **(Figs. 12A and B)**. Volume histogram of this shell will give VI, FI, and VFI values of the perifollicular vessels **(Fig. 12C)**.

We have found perifollicular VI between 6 and 20 and perifollicular FI > 35 as most optimum for fertilizable oocyte. Around 68.4% of patients conceived when VI was between 6 and 18, and 50% conceived when it was between 18 and 20. However, the pregnancy rates were <25% when VI was <6 and only 7.4% when VI was >20.[26]

This indicates that even when the follicle appeared mature according to the 2D US and color and pulse Doppler parameters, the pregnancy rates were significantly better when the follicular volume was between 3 and 7.5 cc, cumulus was present, perifollicular VI was between 6 and 20, and FI was >27.

A study by Kupesic and Kurjak shows that when the ratio of follicular volume to blood FI is between 0.4 and 0.6, the pregnancy rates are 39%; if >0.6, is the rates are 52%; and when <0.4, is the rates are only 21%.[21]

Assessment of Endometrial Receptivity

Endometrium, like follicle, is assessed by transvaginal 2D US and color Doppler. Endometrial thickness of minimum 6 mm is required on the day of trigger, but 8 mm is optimum with a multilayered morphology, preferably grade A or B[31] **(Figs. 13A and B)**.

Segmental uterine artery perfusion demonstrates a significant correlation with hormonal and histological markers of uterine receptivity, reaching the highest sensitivity for subendometrial blood flow.[32] On color Doppler the endometrium, which is mature, shows vascularity in zones 3 and 4 or in subendometrial and endometrial layers[33] **(Fig. 14)**. Zaidi et al. found that the absence of flow in the endometrial and subendometrial zones on the day of the trigger indicates total failure of implantation.[34] The vessels that reach the endometrium are the spiral arteries.

Our study[26] showed that at the endometrial volume of <2 cc, no pregnancies occurred. With endometrial volume of 2–3 cc, only 16.66% of patients conceived; between 3 and 5 cc, 47% conceived; and between 5 and 7 cc, 61.5% patients conceived.[27] Endometrial volume by 3D US volume calculation may help to correlate the cycle outcome with quantitative parameter rather than with endometrial thickness **(Fig. 15)**. For endometrial volume, the inter-CC (correlation coefficient) definition of internal

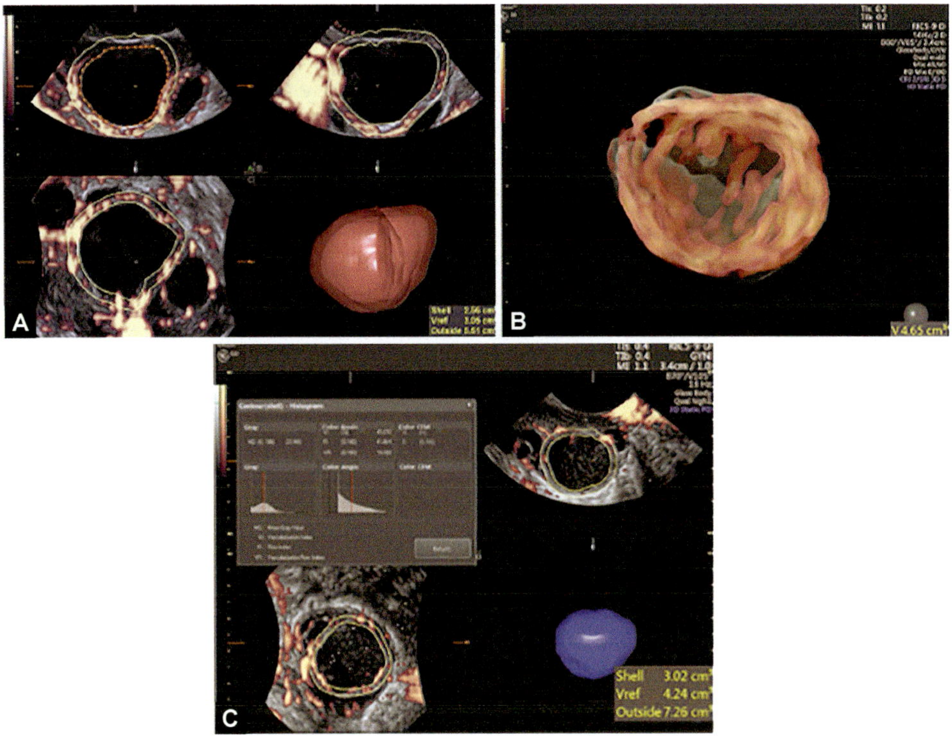

Figs. 12A to C: (A) 3D power Doppler volume of the follicle with VOCAL along with shell outside option; (B) 3D power Doppler volume of the follicle with shell outside option rendered in angio mode; (C) 3D power Doppler volume of follicle calculated with VOCAL with shell outside option. Volume histogram applied image showing VI, FI, and VFI values for the follicle. (FI: flow index; VFI: vascularity flow index; VI: vascularity index; VOCAL: virtual organ computer-aided analysis)

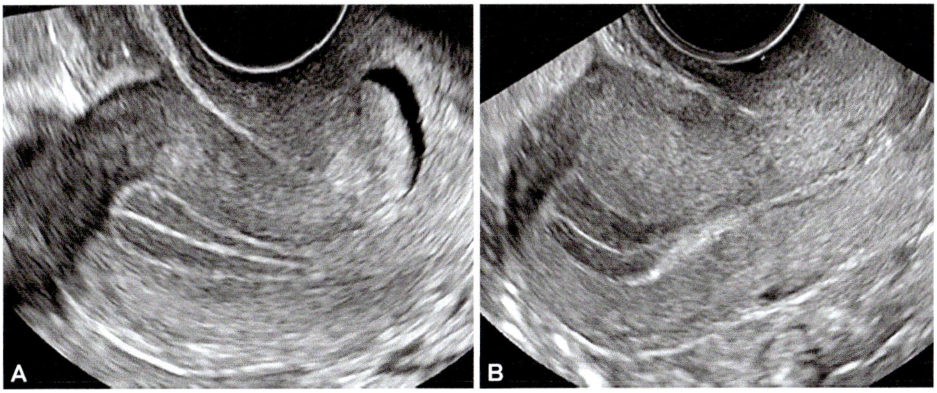

Figs. 13A and B: 2D ultrasound images of: (A) Grade A endometrium; (B) Grade B endometrium.

os (interobserver variation) was 0.82 and intra-CC (intraobserver variation) was 0.90, the chief source of error being the definition of endometrial margins.[35]

A study by Raga et al.[35] shows that pregnancy and implantation rates were significantly lower when endometrial volume < 2 mL, while no pregnancy was achieved when endometrial volume was < 1 mL. A study by Kupesic et al. also shows no pregnancy when endometrial volume was <2 mL or when it exceeded 8 mL.[36] For the same calculated volume, volume histogram is switched on and it calculates the endometrial VI, FI, and VFI **(Fig. 16)**.

A scoring system reported by Kupesic and Kurjak[21] for uterine receptivity, done on the day of embryo transfer, shows that subendometrial FI < 11 was a cut-off limit. (Subendometrial indices are calculated in the same way from the endometrial volume as we calculate the perifollicular indices from the follicular volume, i.e., by shell volume of 2-mm thickness.) No pregnancies occurred when values were 13.2 + 2.2.[37]

Contrary to this, Ng et al. documented a low endometrial VI and VFI in the pregnant group on the day of oocyte retrieval and also a nonsignificant trend of higher implantation and pregnancy rates in patients with absent subendometrial and endometrial flow.[37] Though they concluded that a number of embryos replaced and the endometrial VFI were the only two predictive factors for pregnancy. Wu et al.[38] reported that endometrial VFI was more reliable than VI and FI, and the best prediction rate was achieved by a VFI cut-off value of >0.24.

Collectively, the evidence from various studies suggests that adding 3D and 3D power Doppler for the assessment of follicular maturity and endometrial, receptivity

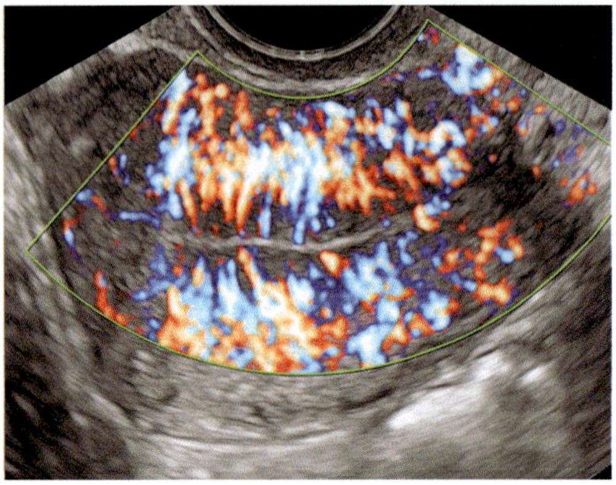

Fig. 14: HD flow Doppler image of the endometrium showing endometrial vascularity.

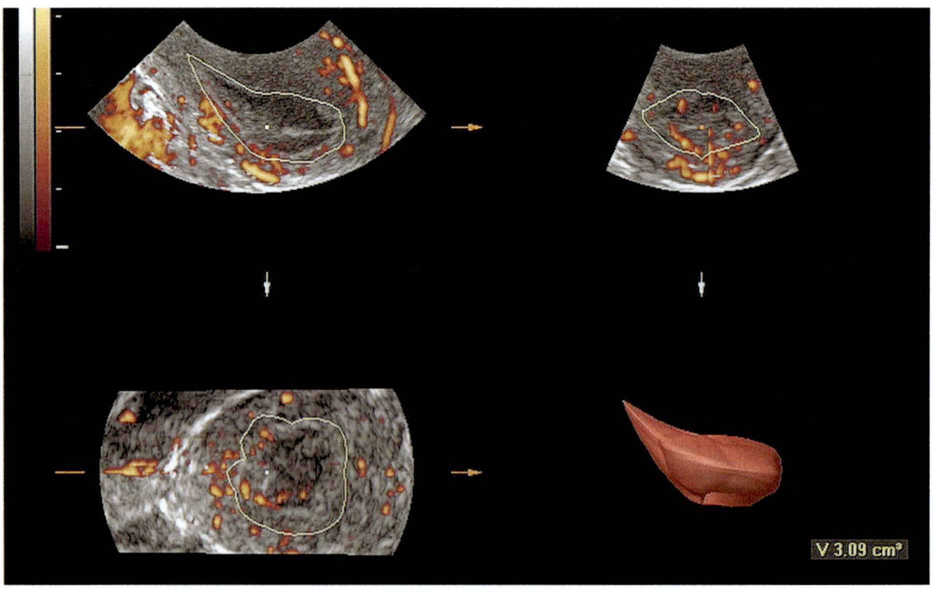

Fig. 15: 3D power Doppler-acquired volume of the endometrium, volume calculation done by VOCAL.

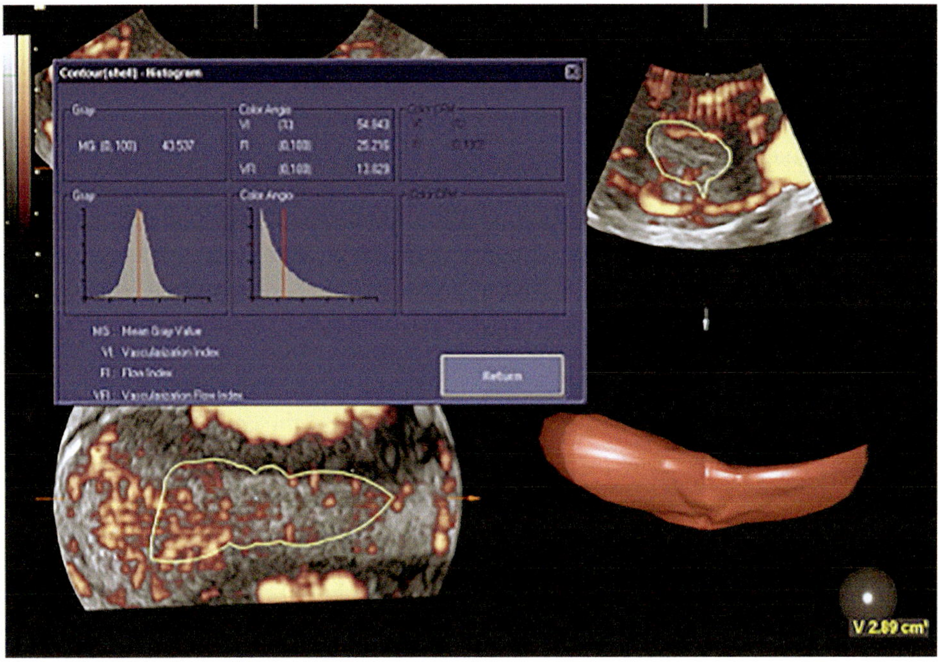

Fig. 16: 3D power Doppler-acquired volume of the endometrium, volume calculation done by VOCAL with volume histogram.

improves the outcome of the fertility treatment by assessment of global vascularity.

Spatiotemporal image correlation (STIC) commonly used for fetal cardiac evaluation can give a more real-time idea about endometrial vascularity though this is a subjective evaluation.

Tubal Patency Assessment

Tubal pathology is a cause of subfertility in 25–35% of subfertile couples. Evaluation of fallopian tubes, therefore, forms an essential part of evaluation of a subfertile female. Various nonsurgical and surgical investigative modalities have been reported to assess fallopian tubes. Nonsurgical techniques, such as hysterosalpingogram (HSG) and ultrasound-based techniques, such as saline infusion sonography (SIS) and hysterocontrast sonosalpingography (HyCoSy) are less invasive and associated with less serious risks than surgical technique such as laparoscopy and dye test (chromopertubation). Demonstration of the lumen of tubes requires visualization of the movement of fluid using highly echogenic medium.[39]

Hyperechogenic contrast medium enhances echo signals and allows detection of the flow, by both B-mode and Doppler US. HyCoSy is a safe outpatient procedure; its accuracy has been assessed in a meta-analysis, which compared the results of HyCoSy and laparoscopy and dye tests in 428 infertile women. Sensitivity was 93.3% and specificity was 89.7%.[40]

Ultrasound is also used for the assessment of tubal patency. Power Doppler with 3D US creates a good graphic presentation of fallopian tubes, when saline is injected into the uterine cavity in pulses **(Fig. 17)**.

3D HyCoSy, a recently evolved procedure, has several advantages over the routine HyCoSy. It filters out the broadband ultrasonic signals from the surrounding tissue and only the tubes are imaged that stand out being filled with microbubbles.[41] Using positive contrast, spillage of hyperechoic contrast in a completely anechoic pelvic cavity is very clear **(Fig. 18)**. Moreover, the contrast remains for a few seconds and therefore 3D acquisition can be done, making the visualization of the whole tube possible.[42]

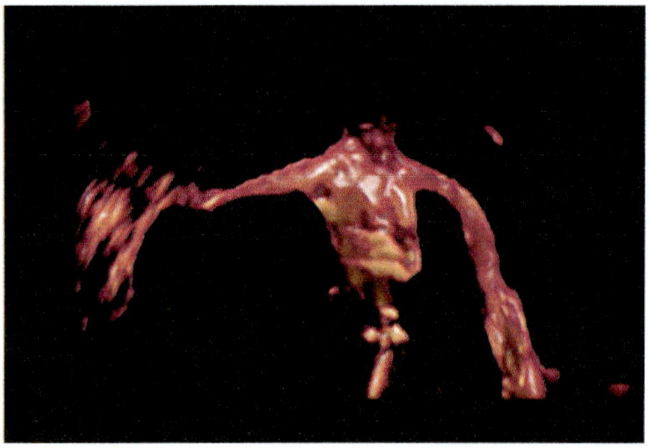

Fig. 17: 3D power Doppler acquisition of saline infusion salpingography.

A study by Exacoustos et al. has also shown that HSG and HyCoSy had the same high concordance as laparoscopy—86.7% and 86.7%, respectively.[43] 3D power Doppler was, therefore, tried to visualize the whole tube and spill. This technique has been shown to be superior to conventional HyCoSy with free spill from fallopian tubes being demonstrated in 91% of tubes using 3D power Doppler as compared to only 46% by conventional HyCoSy, and the contrast agent required was almost half for 3D power Doppler in one of these studies.[44]

There are various advantages with 3D HyCoSy techniques that allow simultaneous visualization of the uterine cavity and whole tube, short procedure time, reduced patient discomfort, requirement of less amount of contrast, and storage of the 3D volume, which allow offline review and reassessment **(Figs. 19A to D)**.

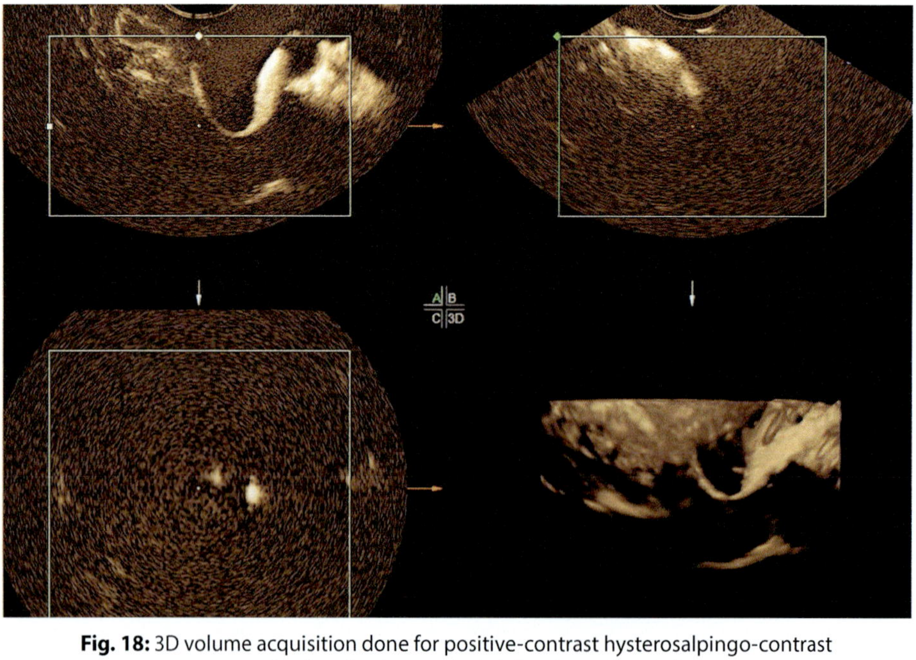

Fig. 18: 3D volume acquisition done for positive-contrast hysterosalpingo-contrast sonography showing hyperechoic tubes in sectional planes.

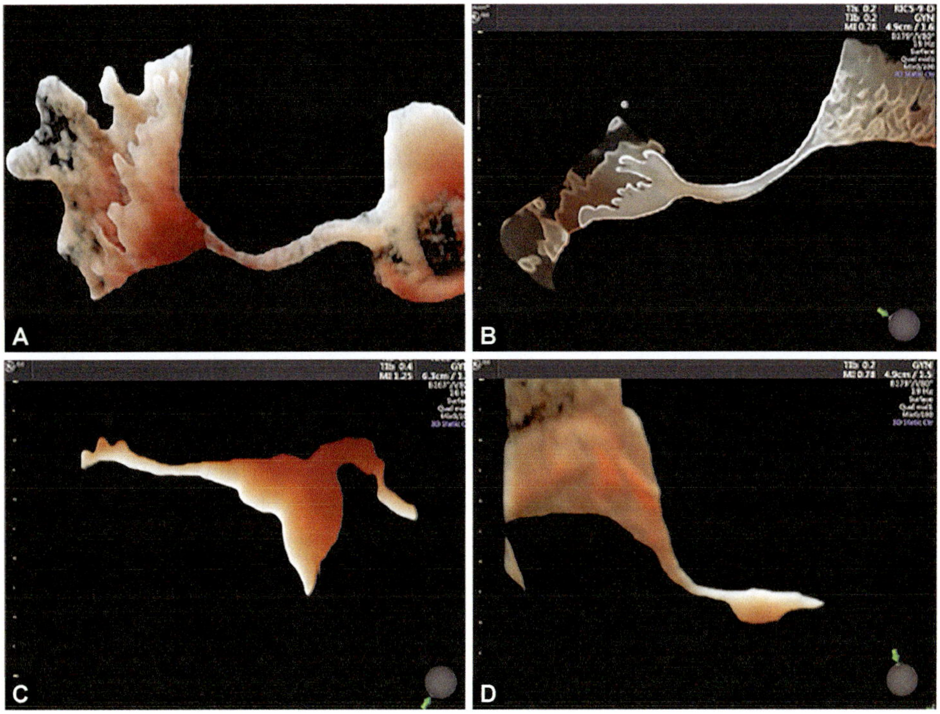

Figs. 19A to D: HD-live with silhouette rendering of 3D hysterosalpingo-contrast sonography volumes: (A) Normal right tube; (B) Normal right tube; (C) Bilateral narrow tubes, distal block on left and damaged fimbria on right; (D) Distal hydrosalpinx of left tube.

Advantages of 3D HyCoSy

- Uterine cavity and whole tube can be seen together.
- Condition of lumen and fimbriae can be studied.
- It shortens procedure time and patient discomfort.
- Less amount of contrast is required.
- Storage of volumes allows reassessment and reviews.
- Spill is better appreciated.
- It is more accurate.

Technique of 3D HyCoSy

SonoVue (Bracco) is used as the contrast agent. Patient preparation, catheter placement, and preparation of contrast media were done according to the method described earlier. Scanning is performed using a 3D US machine (e.g., Voluson E8 Expert BT 12, GE Medical Systems). A high-frequency transvaginal volume probe (6–9 MHz) is used for pelvic evaluation. Contrast mode is switched on the machine. As the contrast is slowly injected through the balloon catheter into the uterus, the transvaginal probe is so oriented that uterine cornu and ovaries are seen on the same plane. Having defined the contrast filling in the tubes, 3D is switched on and volumes are acquired for each side independently.

Rendering is done in the front back viewing direction. The surface-enhanced mode is used. Threshold is set to make the contrast path more obvious. MagiCut (electronic scalpel) is then used to cut all shadows other than the contrast path.

Then HD-live rendering mode is switched on and the direction of the light is adjusted to visualize the fimbriae and spill to its best. After the final picture is ready, both the halves are matched and put together to make a complete picture of the uterus and both tubes **(Fig. 20)**.

Hysterocontrast sonosalpingography with automated 3D-CCI (coded contrast imaging) technology retains the advantages of conventional 2D HyCoSy while overcoming the disadvantages. 2D HyCoSy is highly observer-dependent and is only accurate in the hands of experienced investigators; by obtaining a volume of the uterus and tubes, automated 3D volume acquisition permits visualization of the tubes in the coronal view and of the tubal course in 3D space and should allow less experienced operators to evaluate tubal patency status relatively easily.

Large studies have reported that 3D HyCoSy is highly accurate with 100% sensitivity, 67% specificity, 89% positive predictive value (PPV), and 100% negative predictive value (NPV) for tubal patency and concordance rate with laparoscopy of 91%.[45]

In a study by Kupesic et al., 3D HyCoSy (sensitivity, specificity, PPV, and NPV of 97.9%, 100%, 97.9%, and 100%, respectively) was found to be marginally superior to 2D HyCoSy (sensitivity, specificity, PPV, respectively) for tubal assessment.[46]

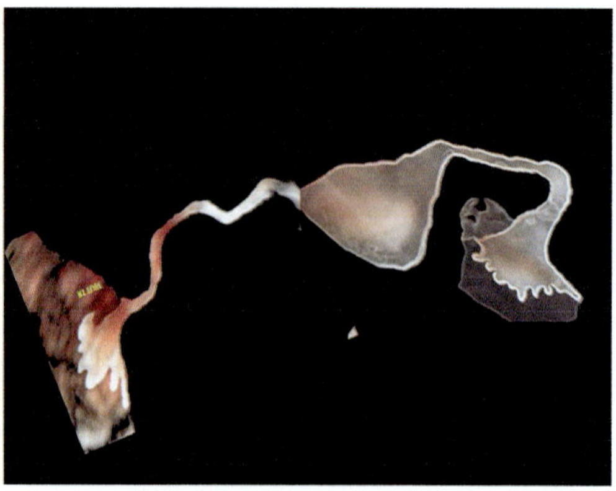

Fig. 20: Reconstructed image of 3D HyCoSy showing uterus and both normal tubes.

3D sonoVue-HyCoSy had a sensitivity of 93.5%, specificity of 86.3%, PPV and NPV of 87.8% and 92.6%, respectively, and diagnostic accuracy of 90.0%. The test-positive rates of 3D sonoVue-HyCoSy versus lap and dye were not significantly different (82/150 vs. 77/150, $p > 0.05$).[47]

Yet another study by Chan et al. has shown that the sensitivity of 3D HyCoSy for detecting tubal patency was 100% with a specificity of 67%. The PPV and NPV were 89% and 100%, respectively, and the concordance rate was 91%. The mean duration (±SD) for the 3D-HyCoSy was 13.4 ± 5.5 minutes.[44] Color-coded 3D power Doppler imaging (3D-PDI) with surface rendering allowed visualization of the flow of contrast through the entire tubal length, and free spill of contrast was clearly identified in the majority of cases. The (3D-PDI) method appeared to have advantages over the conventional HyCoSy technique, especially in terms of visualization of spill from the distal end of the tube, which was achieved twice as often with the 3D technique. The 3D-PDI technique allowed better storage of the information for re-analysis and archiving than conventional HyCoSy. The mean duration of the imaging procedure was less with 3D-PDI, but the operator time, which included postprocedure analysis of the stored information, was similar. A significantly lower volume of contrast medium (5.9 ± 0.6 mL) was used for 3D-PDI in comparison with that (11.2 ± 1.9 mL) used for conventional 2D HyCoSy.[47]

CONCLUSION

3D US can better demonstrate the uterine lesions such as polyps, endometrial synechiae, and fibroids. Better delineation of the endometrial–myometrial junction helps in the diagnosis of adenomyosis, comparable to effective by adding 3D to HyCoSy. 3D US is accurate for volume assessment for both follicle and the endometrium that are much more reliable parameters than the follicular diameter or endometrial thickness. The presence of cumulus can be confirmed by 3D US more easily than with B-mode and increases the surity of the presence of a mature ovum in the follicle. 3D power Doppler gives an idea about the global vascularity of the follicle and the endometrium. Though still larger studies are needed to establish more precise values for follicular and endometrial VI, FI, and VFI, the results are fairly promising.

CARRY HOME MESSAGE

- 3D ultrasound is a very helpful tool for assessment of antral follicle count in polycystic ovaries.
- Ovarian stromal volume and stromal vascularity are most precisely assessed by 3D ultrasound.
- Follicular volume and VI, FI and VFI values of the follicle add to the precision of assessment of follicular maturity.
- Cumulus is a surest sign for presence of ovum in follicle and is more often demonstrated by 3D than 2D ultrasound.
- Endometrial volume measured by 3D is a more precise measurement than endometrial thickness.
- 3D HyCoSy is a much more precise information about tubal lumen and fimbrial condition compared to 2D HyCoSy.

REFERENCES

1. Lam PM, Raine-Fenning N. The role of three-dimensional ultrasonography in polycystic ovary syndrome. Hum Reprod. 2006;21(9):2209-15.
2. Kupesic S, Arenas JB. Sonographic imaging in infertility. Donald School Textbook of Transvaginal Ultrasound, 1st edition. New Delhi: Jaypee Brothers Medical Publishers (P) Ltd.; 2005. pp. 357-83.
3. Jonard S, Robert Y, Dewailly D. Revisiting the ovarian value as a diagnostic criterion for polycystic ovaries. Hum Reprod. 2005; 20(10):2893-8.
4. Legro RS, Chiu P, Kunselman AR, Bentley CM, Dodson WC, Dunaif A. Polycystic ovaries are common in women with hyperandrogenic chronic anovulation but do not predict metabolic or reproductive genotype. J Clin Endocrinol Metab. 2005;90(5):2571-9.
5. Jonard S, Robert Y, Cortet-Rudelli C, Pigny P, Decanter C, Dewaillly D. Ultrasound examination of polycystic ovaries: Is it worth counting the follicles? Hum Reprod. 2003;18(3):598-603.
6. Lujan ME, Jarrett BY, Brooks ED, Reines JK, Peppin AK, Muhn N, et al. Updated ultrasound criteria for polycystic ovary syndrome: reliable thresholds for elevated follicle population and ovarian volume. Hum Reprod. 2013;28(5):1361-8.
7. Ng EH, Chan CC, Yeung WS, Ho PC. Effect of age on ovarian stromal flow measured by three-dimensional ultrasound with power Doppler in Chinese women with proven fertility. Hum Reprod. 2004;19(9):2132-7.
8. Deb S, Campbell BK, Clewes JS, Rainne-Fenning NJ. Quantitative analysis of AFC and size: a comparison of 2D and automated three-dimensional ultrasound techniques. Ultrasound Obstet Gynecol. 2010;35:354-60.
9. Dr Thatcher. Defining PCOS—a perspective: The American Infertility Association Newsletter, February 2001.
10. Buckett WM, Bouzayeb R, Watkin KL, Tulandi T, Tan SL. Ovarian stromal echogenicity in women with normal and polycystic ovaries. Hum Reprod. 1999;14(3): 618-21.
11. Falghesu A, Angioni S, Frau E, Belosi C, Apa R, Mioni R, et al. Ultrasound in polycystic ovary syndrome—the measuring of ovarian stroma and relationship with circulating androgens: results of a multicentric study. Hum Reprod. 2007;22:2501-8.
12. Franks S, Webber LJ, Goh M, Valentine A, White DM, Convay GS, et al. Ovarian morphology is a marker of heritable biochemical traits in sisters with polycystic ovaries. J Clin Endocrinol Metab. 2008;93(9): 3396-402.

13. Robert Y, Dubrulle F, Gaillandre L, Ardaens Y, Thomas-Desrousseaux P, Lemaitre L, et al. Ultrasound assessment of ovarian stroma hypertrophy in hyperandrogenism and ovulation disorders: visual analysis versus computerized quantification. Fertil Steril. 1995;64(2):307-12.
14. Dewailly D, Robert Y, Helin I, Ardaens Y, Thomas-Desrousseaux P, Lemaltre L, et al. Ovarian stromal hypertrophy in hyperandrogenic women. Clin Endocrinol (Oxf). 1994;41(5):557-62.
15. Raine-Fenning NJ, Campbell BK, Clewes JS, Kendall NR, Johnson IR. The reliability of virtual organ computer-aided analysis (VOCAL) for the semiquantification of ovarian, endometrial, and subendometrial perfusion. Ultrasound Obstet Gynecol. 2003;22(6):633-9.
16. Kyei-Mensah AA, LinTan S, Zaidi J, Jacobs HS. Relationship of ovarian stromal volume to serum androgen concentrations in patients with polycystic ovary syndrome. Hum Reprod. 1998;13(6):1437-41.
17. Pache TD, de Jong FH, Hop WC, et al. Association between ovarian changes assessed by transvaginal sonography and clinical and endocrine signs of the polycystic ovary syndrome. Feril Steril. 1993;59(3): 544-9.
18. Panchal S, Nagori CB. Assessing correlation between ovarian and stromal volumes and fasting and postprandial insulin levels in PCOS patients. Int J Infertil Fetal Med. 2014;5(1):12-4.
19. Jarvela IY, Mason HD, Sladkevicius P, Kelly S, Ojha K, Campbell S, et al. Characterization of normal and polycystic ovaries using three-dimensional power Doppler ultrasonography. J Assist Reprod Genet. 2002;19:582-90.
20. Lam PM, Johnson IR, Rainne-Fenning NJ. Three-dimensional ultrasound features of the polycystic ovary and the effect of different phenotypic expressions on these parameters. Hum Reprod. 2007;22(12):3116-23.
21. Kupesic S, Kurjak A. Predictors of IVF outcome by three-dimensional ultrasound. Hum Reprod. 2002;17(4):950-5.
22. Hackeloer BJ, Sallam HN. Ultrasound scanning of ovarian follicles. Clin Obstet Gynecol. 1983;10:603-20.
23. Rainne-Fenning NJ, Lam PM. Assessment of ovarian reserve using the inversion mode. UOG. 2006;27:104-6.
24. Zaidi J, Barber J, Kyei-Mensah A, Bekir J, Campbell S, Tan SL. Relationship of ovarian stromal blood flow at baseline ultrasound to subsequent follicular response in an in vitro fertilization program. Obstet Gynecol. 1996;88(5):779-84.
25. Merce LT, Barco MJ, Bau S, Troyano JM. Prediction of ovarian response and IVF/ ICSI outcome by three-dimensional ultrasonography and power Doppler angiography. Eur J Obstet Gynecol Reprod Biol. 2007;132(1):93-100.
26. Panchal SY, Nagori CB. Can 3D PD be a better tool for assessing the pre-HCG follicle and endometrium? A randomized study of 500 cases. Presented at 16th World Congress on Ultrasound in Obstetrics and Gynecology, 2006, London. J Ultrasound Obstet Gynecol. 2006;28(4):504.
27. Kyei-Mensah A, Zaidi J, Pittrof R, Shaker A, Campbell S, Tan SL. Transvaginal three-dimensional ultrasound: accuracy of follicular volume measurements. Fertil Steril. 1996;65(2):371-6.
28. Feichtinger W. Transvaginal three-dimensional imaging for evaluation and treatment of infertility. In: Merz E (Ed). 3D US in Obstetrics and Gynecology. Philadelphia: Lippincott Williams and Wilkins; 1998. pp. 37-43.
29. Poehl M, Hohlagschwandtner M, Doerner V, Dillinger B, Feichtinger W. Cumulus assessment by three-dimensional ultrasound for in vitro fertilization. Ultrasound Obstet Gynecol. 2000;16(3):251-3.
30. Vlaisavljevic V, Reljic M, GavricLovrec V, Zazula D, Sergent N. Measurement of perifollicular blood flow of the dominant preovulatory follicle using three-dimensional power Doppler. Ultrasound Obstet Gynecol. 2003;22(5):520-6.

31. Smith B, Porter R, Ahuja K, Craft I. Ultrasonic assessment of endometrial changes in stimulated cycles in an in vitro fertilization and embryo transfer program. J In Vitro Fertil Embryo Transf. 1984;1(4);233-8.
32. Merce LT, Barco MJ, Kupesic S, Kurjak A. 2D and 3D power Doppler ultrasound from ovulation to implantation. In: Kurjak A, Chervenak F (Eds). Textbook of Perinatal Medicine. London: Parthenon Publishing; 2005.
33. Applebaum M. The 'steel' or 'teflon' endometrium—ultrasound visualization of endometrial vascularity in IVF patients and outcome. Presented at The third World Gyneacolgy. Ultrasound Obstet Gynecol. 1993;3(Suppl 2):10.
34. Zaidi J, Campbell S, Pittrof R, Tan SL. Endometrial thickness, morphology, vascular penetration and velocimetry in predicting implantation in an in vitro fertilization program. Ultrasound Obstet Gynecol. 1995;6(3): 191-8.
35. Raga F, Bonilla-Musoles F, Casan EM, Klein O, Bonilla F. Assessment of endometrial volume by three-dimensional ultrasound prior to embryo transfer: clues to endometrial receptivity. Hum Reprod. 1999;14:2851-4.
36. Kupesic S, Bekavac I, Bjelos D, Kurjak A. Assessment of endometrial receptivity by transvaginal color Doppler and three-dimensional power Doppler ultrasonography in patients undergoing in vitro fertilization procedures. J Ultrasound Med. 2001;20: 125-34.
37. Ng EH, Chan CC, Tang OS, Yeung WS, Ho PC. The role of endometrial and subendometrial blood flows measured by three-dimensional power Doppler ultrasound in prediction of pregnancy during IVF treatment. Hum Reprod. 2006;21(1):164-70.
38. Wu HM, Chiang CH, Huang HY, Chao AS, Wang HS, Soong YK. Detection of subendometrial vascularization flow index by three-dimensional ultrasound may be useful for predicting pregnancy rate for patients undergoing in vitro fertilization-embryo transfer. Fertil Steril. 2003;79(3):507-11.
39. Jeanty P, Besnard S, Arnold A, Turner C, Crum P. Air-contrast sonohysterography as a first step assessment of tubal patency. J Ultrasound Med. 2000;19(8):519-27.
40. Holz K, Becker R, Schürmann R. Ultrasound in the investigation of tubal patency: a meta-analysis of three comparative studies of Echovist-200 including 1,007 women. Zentralbl Gynakol. 1997;119(8):366-73.
41. Exacoustos C, Zupi E, Carusotti C, Lanzi G, Marconi D, Arduini D. Hysterosalpingo-contrast sonography compared with hysterosalpingography and laparoscopic dye pertubation to evaluate tubal patency. J Am Assoc Gynecol Laparosc. 2003;10(3):367-72.
42. Balen FG, Allen CM, Gardener JE, Siddle NC, Lees WR. Three-dimensional reconstruction of ultrasound images of the uterine cavity. Br J Radiol. 1993;66(787):588-91.
43. Exacoustos C, Di Giovanni A, Szabolcs B, Romeo V, Romanini ME, Luciano D, et al. Automated three-dimensional coded contrast imaging hysterosalpingo-contrast sonography: feasibility in office tubal patency testing. Ultrasound Obstet Gynecol. 2013;41(3):328-35.
44. Chan CC, Ng EH, Tang OS, Chan KKL, Ho PC. Comparison of three-dimensional hysteron-contrast-sonography and diagnostic laparoscopy with chromopertubation in the assessment of tubal patency for the investigation of subfertility. Acta Obstet Gynecol Scand. 2005;84(9):909-13.
45. Kupesic S, Plavsic MB. 2D and 3D hysterosalpingocontrast-sonography in the assessment of uterine cavity and tubal patency. Eur J Obstet Gynecol Reprod Biol. 2007;133(1):64-9.
46. Zhou L, Zhang X, Chen X, Liao L, Pan R, Zhou N, et al. Value of three-dimensional hysterosalpingo-contrast sonography with SonoVue in the assessment of tubal patency. Ultrasound Obstet Gynecol. 2012;40(1):93-8.
47. Sladkevicius P, Ojha K, Campbell S, Nargund G. Three-dimensional power Doppler imaging in the assessment of Fallopian tube patency. Ultrasound Obstet Gynecol. 2000;16(7): 644-7.

30

Chapter

Recurrent Implantation Failure

INTRODUCTION

Despite the research in assisted reproductive technology (ART) since the last four decades, some patients do no conceive in spite of multiple embryo transfers. In the majority of cases, no identifiable cause is found; advanced maternal age, genetic abnormality of the embryo, and laboratory conditions may cause embryo loss but are not stamped as the cause of recurrent implantation failure (RIF). Apposition, adhesion, and invasion are important steps after embryo transfer.

DEFINITIONS

- It is defined as the absence of implantation after three or more transfers of a high-quality embryo.
- It is defined as the absence of implantation after transfer of >10 high-quality embryos in multiple cycles.

There is no unanimous consensus for the definitions.

CAUSES OF RECURRENT IMPLANTATION FAILURE

- *Genetics*:
  - Parental genetics
  - Embryo genetics
  - Sperm genetics
- Uterine pathologies
- Tubal pathologies
- Blastocyst culture

Genetics

Parental Genetics

In couple with translocation, i.e., reciprocal or Robertsonian translocation, are responsible for producing aneuploidy because of rearrangements during meiosis. In 15% of couples with RIF, chromosomal translocations, inversions, deletions, or mosaicism are noted.[1] So parental karyotyping should be done in patients of RIF. All the couples should be counseled for preimplantation genetic diagnosis (PGD).

Embryo Genetics

As the age of the woman advances, the aneuploidy rate increases. It is very high between the age of 38 and 45 years. With the advent of comparative genomic hybridization (CGH), it is found in the range of 58% at the age of 40 years to 100% at 47 years of age.[2] So it becomes necessary to find out aneuploidy to improve implantation rates. Biopsy and fluorescence in situ hybridization (FISH) of cleavage stage embryo are discarded because of mosaicism and self-correction capabilities of the embryo. Moreover, it has the detrimental effect of single Day 3 blastomere biopsy, and live birth rate is reported 24% as compared to 35% in control patients.[3]

Trophectoderm biopsy of blastocyst-stage embryo has improved the diagnosis of aneuploidy. Embryos are transferred in the next cycle. CGH helps to study all

24 chromosomes. But there are no authentic reports that patients of RIF are benefitted with pregenetic screening (PGS). Further studies are required to assess whether embryonic aneuploidy is responsible for RIF in absence of parental chromosomal abnormalities.[4] The negative effect of PGS in individuals with RIF was confirmed by this meta-analysis.[5]

Trophectoderm biopsy has several advantages over blastomere biopsy:

- Less mosaicism
- Multiple cells can be analyzed.
- Greater accuracy of 24 chromosome analysis
- Improves efficacy of in vitro fertilization (IVF) in older patients

In one of the studies where PGS was used in women aged 40–42 years with multiple IVF failures, PGS frozen embryo transfer showed 45% clinical pregnancy rate as compared to fresh non-PGS transfer (15.8%) or frozen non-PGS transfer which increased pregnancy rate by 19%.[6] The benefit of PGS in a young patient is less established. Biopsy and analysis do not improve implantation and increase the cost. So for young patients, it has not been found to be beneficial. Stimulation of a large number of follicles may result in poor-quality oocytes and in turn lower quality embryos. So mild stimulation is advocated by many workers to get euploid embryo. An individualized stimulation protocol is very useful and it should be so designed that 8–15 oocytes are retrieved.

There is a recent study that questions the existence of RIF due to endometrial effects. It has showed that less than 5% would fail to achieve the pregnancy with three embryos transfer. So expensive testing for endometrial cause of RIF is not required and treatment should be challenged. RIF of embryonic origin which can be minimized by transferring euploid embryo.[7]

Sperm Genetics

Regular semen analysis is a poor prediction of conception with ART. Damage of the sperm DNA is associated with poor pregnancy rate but its role in patients with RIF is uncertain.[8] Testicular sperms should be used in patients with high DNA fragmentation. DNA fragmentation in testicular sperm is 4.8% as compared to 23.6% in ejaculated sperms.[9] So many techniques have been developed to select the best sperm. These include annexin V columns, sperm hyaluronic acid-binding, confocal light absorption spectroscopy, and high magnification ICSI [intracytoplasmic morphologically selected sperm injection (IMSI)].

IMSI helps to select the sperm that are free of vacuoles considered to be normal sperms which improve implantation and pregnancy. But subsequent studies have failed to demonstrate better results than conventional ICSI.[10] So whether DNA fragmentation testing is required for patients of RIF is still not confirmed and has a doubtful role. In the same way, sperm which is tested for aneuploidy cannot be used for ICSI. So whether aneuploidy testing should be used or not remains to be established.

Uterine Pathology

All these pathologies have been discussed in detail in the chapter on recurrent pregnancy loss, but relevant points for RIF are discussed in the following text.

Fibroid

It can cause mechanical obstruction, chronic inflammation, and increased uterine contractions, which can prevent implantation. Submucous myomas should be removed. Subserous myoma does not require removal. Intramural myoma > 4–5 cm should be removed, but there is no clear evidence that its removal may improve pregnancy rates.[11]

Polyps: Pregnancy rates increase after the removal of polyps.[12]

Adhesions: Surgical corrections of adhesions improve pregnancy rate.[13]

Chronic endometritis: It is to be excluded in patients of RIF. Its incidence is as high as 30%. It is diagnosed by the presence of plasma cells in RIF. Live birth rate was 60.8% in patients in whom endometritis was treated as compared to 13.3% when it persisted after treatment.[14]

Treatment strategy:
- Patients who cultured positive for gram-negative bacteria are treated with ciprofloxacin for 10 days.
- Patients who cultured positive for gram-positive organisms are given Amoxycillin with Clavulanic acid for 8 days.
- When culture is not positive, give a single dose of ceftriaxone followed by 14 days of doxycycline and metronidazole.

Adenomyosis

Adenomyosis may be the potential cause of RIF. Ultralong GnRH agonist (GnRHa) downregulation before IVF is recommended although data are limited and further research is required.[15] Routine hysteroscopy is recommended in all the patients of RIF. Three-dimensional ultrasound of the uterus can be very effective in diagnosing abnormality of the uterus. In all patients with RIF, the myometrium and uterine cavity should be thoroughly evaluated and conditions should be diagnosed and treated. For diagnosis, hysteroscopy is a gold standard but 3D ultrasound is equally effective and saline infusion sonohysterography will be very useful.

Molecular Study of the Endometrium

The molecular study of the endometrium is done for the diagnosis in RIF. The receptivity of the endometrium is now assessed by molecular study. Dysregulation of 313 genes and 63 transcripts in the mid-secretory phase of a woman with RIF has already been documented.[16] An endometrial receptivity array has been developed by the IVI group that assesses 238 genes and is capable of identifying receptive endometrium in natural and stimulated cycles.[17] This study helps to identify the window of implantation and is better than histology. The preliminary results are good, but further confirmation is required and till then routine use is not recommended.

Tubal Pathology

Hydrosalpinx can adversely affect reproduction by various mechanisms:
- The fluid of hydrosalpinx is embryotoxic.
- Fluid may flush the embryo out.
- It can alter endometrial receptivity.

Hydrosalpinx, if evident on ultrasound, reduces the live birth rates with IVF treatment.[18] Salpingectomy restores endometrial cytokines that are useful for implantation. Specifically, Avb3 and leukemia inhibitory factor (LIF) are restored to normal levels after salpingectomy. Pregnancy rates are always better after salpingectomy.[19]

Blastocyst Culture

It is an established fact that cleavage-stage embryo development is controlled by maternal RNA transcript until 4–8-cell stage.[20] Activation of the embryonic genome begins on Day 3 of development and continues to the blastocyst stage. The implantation rate is higher with the blastocyst stage than with the cleavage-stage embryo.

Segmental media, as well as one-step media, are available according to the requirement for blastocyst development. So the rate of blastocyst formation has definitely increased. For high responders, blastocyst transfer has the advantage, But poor responders are not good candidates for prolonged culture and in these patients, Day 3 transfer or cleavage-stage transfer is preferred. Some workers recommend a sequential transfer. Day 2 and Day 5 transfers are done, but an increase in pregnancy rate is not documented by this strategy in patients with RIF.

PROCEDURES TO IMPROVE RESULTS

- Assisted hatching
- Endometrial scratching
- Co-culture
- Embryo transfer
- Miscellaneous

Assisted Hatching

Whenever zona is hard or thickened, the hatching rate is low and implantation is also poor. So cleaved embryos with thinner or reduced zona thickness have a higher implantation rate. For hatching, various processes can be used:

- Mechanical partial zona dissection
- Chemical drilling using Tyrode's solution
- Enzymatic thinning
- Laser-assisted hatching
- Piezo micromanipulation

All these techniques aid mechanical hatching as well as allow two-way exchange of nutrients and metabolites.[21] This technique should not be used routinely. It is very useful for patients elder than 38 years with thickened zona and with RIF.[22-24] There are various assisted hatching techniques, but none is established as a gold standard.

Endometrial Scratching

The principle of endometrial scratching is to induce a healing process.

It allows the release of cytokines and other growth factors that facilitate implantation. Mechanical injury to the endometrium, prior to controlled ovarian hyperstimulation, is helpful in initiating decidualization and also helps immunomodulation in the endometrium. Initial studies were promising, but subsequent workers produced contradictory reports. Few studies have reported a decrease in pregnancy rates.[25,26] Other studies suggested no benefit of endometrial scratching in unselected IVF population.[27] Endometrial scratching for women undergoing first embryo transfer does not improve the success rate.[28] But endometrial scratching was found to be useful after repeated implantation failures. There is a definite positive effect of endometrial scratching in terms of clinical pregnancy rate after three or more prior implantation failures.[29] Additional well-designed prospective randomized control trials are needed before this intervention is adopted clinically in patients with RIF.

Co-culture

For co-culture, tubal epithelium, endometrium, granulosa cells, or cumulus cells have been tried for supporting culture conditions with variable reports. Cells from animals have been tried, but there is always the risk of infection. So homologous or autologous human cells were used in the co-culture system. Tubal epithelium from the homologous source has been tried with higher pregnancy rate, implantation, and cryopreservation rate.[30] The risk of transmission of infectious agents and Creutzfeldt-Jakob disease limits the homologous technique.

Endometrial cells can be taken in the mid-luteal phase of the previous cycle of IVF. Glandular and stromal cells are separated, frozen, and used in the subsequent cycle for treatment. Embryos are put along with endometrial cells, stromal cells, Ham F10, and 15% patient's serum till the day of transfer.[31,32] It enhances embryo development. Now because of better availability of media and time-lapse microscopy, the benefit of endometrial co-culture remains to be further defined for difficult RIF patients.

Embryo Transfer

Embryo transfer should be done under ultrasound guidance. Controversy still continues as to where to place the embryos. 1, 2, and 2.8 cm caudal to the fundal end of endometrium are the options and have documented variable results. One must understand that an embryo does not remain at the place where it is placed at the time of embryo transfer. Because of the pressure that develops while placing the embryos and because of endometrial peristalsis, it may change its position. Otherwise ectopic pregnancies would not occur with IVF cycles.

Options for treatment:

- Low molecular weight heparin (LMWH)
- Intravenous immunoglobulin (IVIG)
- Intralipids
- Immunomodulators

All these drugs are given on an empirical basis to the patient of RIF. But based on the current evidence, the use of these for RIF is not recommended.

Third-party reproduction: If the problem is with embryo, genetic donation should be discussed with the patient. If the problem is with the uterus and cannot be rectified after all the treatment, surrogacy remains the only option.

Empirical use of immunomodulators such as glucocorticoids, aspirin, and LMWH, have no role in patients of RIF. Antitumor necrosis factor (anti-TNA) alpha is also not of much benefit.

Effect of GnRHa and letrozole treatment is also studied in patients of RIF. It may improve live birth rates in subsequent cycles. This improvement may be due to alteration in the endometrium receptivity or treatment of undiagnosed endometriosis.[33]

Short-term intrauterine devices (IUDs) with copper placement can improve the implantation and pregnancy rates in women with RIF. Cu IUD is kept for 2 months. It stimulates inflammatory factors in the endometrium.[34]

RIF may be managed by freeze-all policy and then a single embryo should be transferred in the next cycles. It improved the pregnancy rate in patients of RIF. In these cases, the adverse effect of controlled ovarian hyperstimulation (COH) is avoided and the pregnancy rate is better in "freeze-all" policy.[35]

CARRY HOME MESSAGE

- Parental karyotyping should be done.
- PGS has no role in young patients but in older patients it may help to rule out aneuploidy.
- Expensive testing for endometrial cause is not required.
- Aneuploidy testing or DFT is not helpful in patients with RIF.
- Chronic endometritis should be treated.
- Assisted hatching, endometrial scratching and co-cultures have controversial results.
- LHWH, IVIG, intralipids and immunomodulators are not recommended.
- Third party reproduction is the last option.

REFERENCES

1. Raziel A, Friedler S, Schachter M, Kasterstein E, Strassburger D, Ron-El R. Increased frequency of female partnet chromosomal abnormalities in patients with

high order implantation failure after in vitro fertilization. Fertil Steril. 2002;78:515-9.
2. Franasiak JM, Forman EJ, Hong KH, Werner MD, Upham KM, Treff NR, et al. The nature of aneuploidy with increasing age of the female partner: a review of 15,169 consecutive trophectoderm biopsies evaluated with comprehensive chromosomal screening. Fertil Steril. 2014;101:656-63.e651.
3. Mastenbroek S, Twisk M, van Echten-Arends J, Sikkema-Raddatz B, Korevaar JC, Verhoeve HR, et al. In vitro fertilization with preimplantation genetic screening. N Engl J Med. 2007; 357:9-17.
4. Greco E, Bono S, Ruberti A, Lobascio AM, Greco P, Biricik A, et al. Comparative genomic hybridization selection of blastocysts for repeated implantation failure treatment: a pilot study. Biomed Res Int. 2014;2014:457913.
5. Mastenbroek S, Twisk M, van der Veen F, Repping S. Preimplantation genetic screening: a systematic review and meta-analysis of RCTs. Hum Reprod Update. 2011;17:454-66.
6. Lee HL, McCulloh DH, Hodes-Wertz B, Adler A, McCaffrey C, Grifo JA. In vitro fertilization with preimplantation genetic screening improves implantation and live birth in women age 40 through 43. J Assist Reprod Genet. 2015;32:435-44.
7. Pirtea P, Ziegler DD, Tao X, Zhan Y, Ayoubi JM, Seli EM, Franasiak JM, et al. Rate of true recurrent implantation failure is low: results of three successive frozen euploid single embryo transfers. Fertil Steril. 2021;115(1): 45-53.
8. Absalan F, Ghannadi A, Kazerooni M, Parifar R, Jamalzadeh F, Amiri S. Value of sperm chromatin dispersion test in couples with unexplained recurrent abortion. J Assist Reprod Genet. 2012;29:11-4.
9. Greco E, Scarselli F, Iacobelli M, Rienzi L, Ubaldi F, Ferrero S, Franco G, et al. Efficient treatment of infertility due to sperm DNA damage by ICSI with testicular spermatozoa. Hum Reprod. 2005;20:226-30.
10. El Khattabi L, Dupont C, Sermondade N, Hugues JN, Poncelet C, Porcher R, Cedrin-Durnerin I, et al. Is intracytoplasmic morphologically selected sperm injection effective in patients with infertility related to teratozoospermia or repeated implantation failure? Fertil Steril. 2013;100:62-8.
11. Sunkara SK, Khairy M, El Toukhy T, Khalaf Y, Coomarasamy A. The effect of intramural fibroids without uterine cavity involvement on outcome of IVF treatment: a systematic review and metaanalysis. Hum Reprod. 2010;25:418-29.
12. Perez-Medina T, Bajo-Arenas J, Salazar F, Redondo T, Sanfrutos L, Alvarez P, Engels V. Endometrial polyps and their implications in the pregnancy rates of patients undergoing intrauterine insemination: a prospective randomized study. Hum Reprod. 2005; 20:1632-5.
13. Taylor E, Gomel V. The uterus and fertility. Fertil Steril. 2008;89:1-16.
14. Cicinelli E, Matteo M, Tinelli R, Lepera A, Raffaello A, Indraccolo U, et al. Prevalence of chronic endometritis in repeated unexplained implantation failure and the IVF success rate after antibiotic therapy. Hum Reprod. 2015;30:323-30.
15. Tremellen K, Russell P. Adenomyosis is a potential cause of recurrent implantation failure during IVF treatment. Aust NZ J Obstet Gynecol. 2011;51:280-3.
16. Kohler M, Achache H, Tsafrir A, Smith Y, Revel A, Reich R. Disrupted gene pattern in patients with repeated in vitro fertilization (IVF) failure. Hum Reprod. 2009;24:2541-8.
17. Diaz-Gimeno P, Maria Ruiz-Alonso, Blesa D, Bosch N, Martínez-Conejero JA, Alamá P, et al. The accuracy and reproducibility of endometrial receptivity array is superior to histology as diagnostic method for endometrial receptivity. Fertil Steril. 2013; 99:508-17.
18. Camus E, Poncelet C, Goffinet F, B Wainer B, Merlet F, Nisand I, Philippe HJ. Pregnancy rates after in vitro fertilization in cases of tubal infertility with and without hydrosalpinx: a meta-analysis of published comparative studies. Hum Reprod. 1999;14:1243-9.
19. Strandell A, Lindhard A, Waldenström U, Thorburn J, Janson PO, Hamberger L. Hydrosalpinx and IVF outcome: a prospective,

randomized multicentre trial in Scandinavia on salpingectomy prior to IVF. Hum Reprod. 1999;14:2762-9.
20. Telford NA, Watson AJ, Schultz GA. Transition from maternal to embryonic control in early mammalian development: a comparison of several species. Mol Reprod Dev. 1990;26:90-100.
21. Hershlag A, Feng HL. Effect of pre-freeze assisted hatching on post thaw survival of mouse embryos. Fertil Steril. 2005;84: 1752-4.
22. Valojerdi MR, Eftekhari-Yazdi P, Kaimian L, Ashtiani SK. Effect of laser zona pellucida opening on clinical outcome of assisted reproduction technology in patients with advanced female age, recurrent implantation failure, or frozen-thawed embryos. Fertil Steril. 2008;90:84-91.
23. Antinori S, Selman HA, Caffa B, Panci C, Dani GL, Versaci C. Zona opening of human embryos using a non-contact UV laser for assisted hatching in patients with poor prognosis of pregnancy. Hum Reprod 1996;11:2488-92.
24. Chao KH, Chen SU, Chen HF, Wu MY, Yang YS, Ho HN. Assisted hatching increases the implantation and pregnancy rate of in vitro fertilization (IVF)-embryo transfer (ET), but not that of IVF-tubal ET in patients with repeated IVF failures. Fertil Steril. 1997;67:904-8.
25. Karimzadeh MA, Ayazi RM, Tabibnejad N. Endometrial local injury improves the pregnancy rate among recurrent implantation failure patients undergoing in vitro fertilization/intracytoplasmic sperm injection: a randomized clinical trial. Aust N Z J Obstet Gynecol. 2009;49:677-80.
26. Narvekar SA, Gupta N, Shetty N, Kottur A, Srinivas, Rao KA. Does local endometrial injury in non-transfer cycle improve IVF-ET outcome in the subsequent cycle in patients with previous unsuccessful IVF? A randomized controlled pilot study. J Hum Reprod Sci. 2010;3:15-9.
27. Yeung TW, Chai J, Li RHW, Lee VCY, Ho PC[2], Ng EHY. The effect of endometrial injury on ongoing pregnancy rate in unselected subfertile women undergoing in vitro fertilization: a randomised controlled trial. Hum Reprod. 2014;29:2474-81.
28. Vitagliano A, Andrisani A, Alviggi C, Vitale SG, Valenti G, Sapia F, et al. Endometrial scratching for infertile women undergoing a first embryo transfer: a systematic review and meta-analysis of published and unpublished data from randomized controlled trials. Fertil Steril. 2019;111(4):734-45.
29. Olesen MS, Hauge B, Ohrt L, Olesen TN, Roskær J, Bæk V, et al. Therapeutic endometrial scratching and implantation after in vitro fertilization: a multicenter randomized controlled trial. Fertil Steril. 2019;112(6):1015-21.
30. Yeung WS, Lau EY, Chan ST, Ho PC. Coculture with homologous oviductal cells improved the implantation of human embryos-A prospective randomized controlled trial. J Assist Reprod Genet. 1996;13:762-7.
31. Barmat LI, Liu HC, Spandorfer SD, Xu K, Veeck L, Damario MA, et al. Human pre-embryo development on autologous endometril coculture versus conventional medium. Fertil Steril. 1998;70:1109-13.
32. Barmat LI, Liu HC, Spandorfer SD, Xu K, Veeck L, Damario MA, et al. Autologous endometrial co-culture in patients with repeated failures of implantation after in vitro fertilization-embryo transfer. J Assist Reprod Genet 1999;16:121-7.
33. Steiner N, Shrem G, Tannus S, Dahan Y, Balayla J, Volodarsky-Perel A, et al. Effect of GnRH agonist and letrozole treatment in women with recurrent implantation failure. Fertil Steril. 2019;112(1):98-104.
34. Mao X, Zhang J, Chen Q, Kuang Y, Zhang S. Short-term copper intrauterine device placement improves the implantation and pregnancy rates in women with repeated implantation failure. Fertil Steril. 2017;108(1): 55-61.
35. Magdi Y, El Damen A, Fathi AM, Abdelaziz AM, Abd-Elfatah Youssef M, Abd-Allah AAE, et al. Revisiting the management of recurrent implantation failure through freeze-all policy. Fertil Steril. 2017;108(1):72-8.

31

Chapter

Thin Endometrium

INTRODUCTION

The endometrium is the dynamic tissue that changes its thickness and morphology with estrogen, progesterone, and other autocrine and paracrine factors. It has an upper two-third layer, i.e., stratum compactum and spongiosum, and the lower one third as stratum basalis. The upper two third is the functional layer for implantation **(Fig. 1)** and the lower one-third is for regeneration of endometrium. It is the functional layer that gives thickness to the endometrium and is regenerated from the basal layer in every cycle. Normal endometrial thickness is 6–14 mm. Endometrial thickness is measured from the outer margin of the anterior hyperechoic line of the endometrium to the posterior margin of the hyperechoic line of the endometrium, perpendicular to the central line of the endometrium, at its broadest part **(Fig. 2)**.

DEFINITION OF THIN ENDOMETRIUM

There is no unanimous consensus as to how thin is thin endometrium. About 7 mm is the most accepted figure for definition by most of the workers, but some also take the cutoff as 8 mm. On the other hand, pregnancies have been documented between 5 and 15 mm thickness of the endometrium.[1] Endometrium is receptive or not can be judged by various measures:

- Hypoestrogenic endometrium is more receptive.
- Vascularity in the endometrium is more receptive.

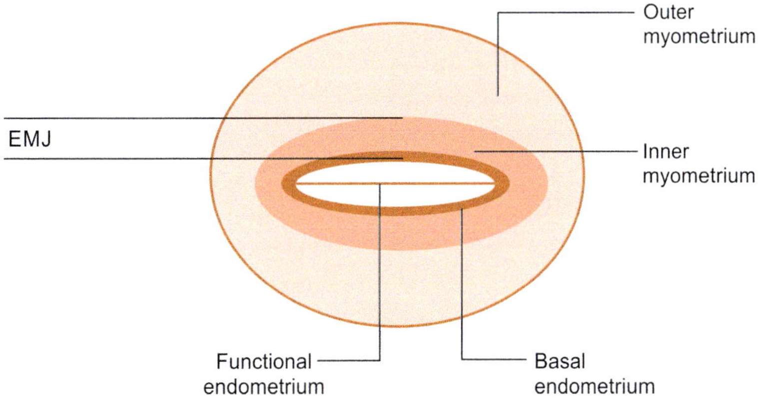

Fig. 1: Diagrammatic presentation of layers of the uterus. (EMJ: endometrial-myometrial junction)

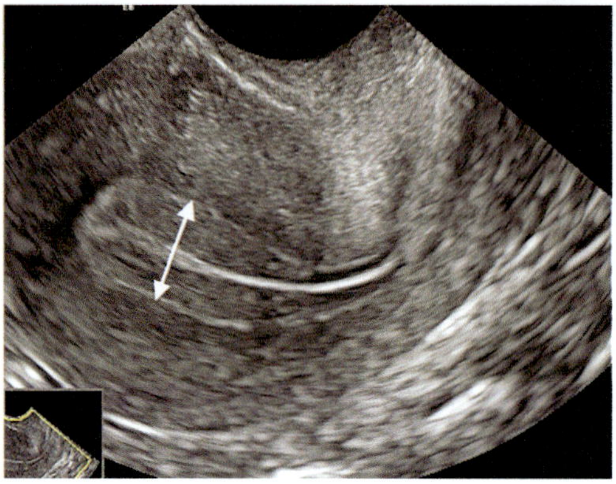

Fig. 2: Ultrasound image showing measurement of the endometrium.

- Molecular technology is considered as an excellent tool to recognize receptive endometrium.[2]

In ovarian stimulation with IUI for unexplained infertility, endometrial thickness is not significantly associated with live birth rate when adjusted to ovarian stimulation treatment type. Appreciable live birth rate is seen in all endometrial thickness groups, even in those with endometrial thickness of ≤ 5 mm. This suggests that ovarian stimulation with IUI cycles should not be canceled for thin endometrium.[3]

Clinical pregnancy rate and live birth rates decrease with each millimeter of endometrial thickness below 8 mm in fresh IVF cycles and below 7 mm for frozen embryo transfer cycles. Nevertheless viable pregnancy rates remain reasonably acceptable in patients with an endometrial thickness between 4 and 6 mm.[4]

CAUSES OF THIN ENDOMETRIUM

- Surgical
- Radiotherapy
- Infections
- Congenital Müllerian abnormalities
- Other causes
- Idiopathic

Surgical

- *Dilatation and curettage*: 90% of cases of intrauterine adhesions and thin endometrium is due to cervical dilatation and postabortal curettage.[5] Adhesions interfere with implantation and sperm migration. Isthmus and cornual are the common locations. When severe adhesions occur, it is called "Asherman's syndrome." Intrauterine adhesions or synechiae are diagnosed on 2D ultrasound by persistently thin endometrium even in preovulatory and secretory phases of the menstrual cycle **(Fig. 3A)**. On 3D ultrasound, especially with sonohysterography, it is better diagnosed as echogenic strands between the endometrial layers **(Fig. 3B)**.
- *Intrauterine surgeries*: The most common cause is hysteroscopic resection of multiple fibroids, particularly when a resectoscope is used. The incidence is as high as 30–45%.[6] Bipolar resectoscope causes lesser adhesions as much as 7–8%. After hysteroscopic metroplasty, hormone replacement of intrauterine contraceptive device (IUCD) insertion is not required. The second most common cause is septoplasty 86% and they did not find adhesions after polypectomy. So assisted reproductive technology (ART) is not recommended for 3 months after all these procedures or adhesiolysis.[7] But polypectomy does not affect the line of treatment.[8]
- *Strassman operation*: Unification of the uterus has been advocated in the bicornuate uterus. But now it has become obsolete. Strassman operation is also not performed commonly these days unless there is a history of premature deliveries with a complete bicornuate uterus. Because of progesterone, cervical

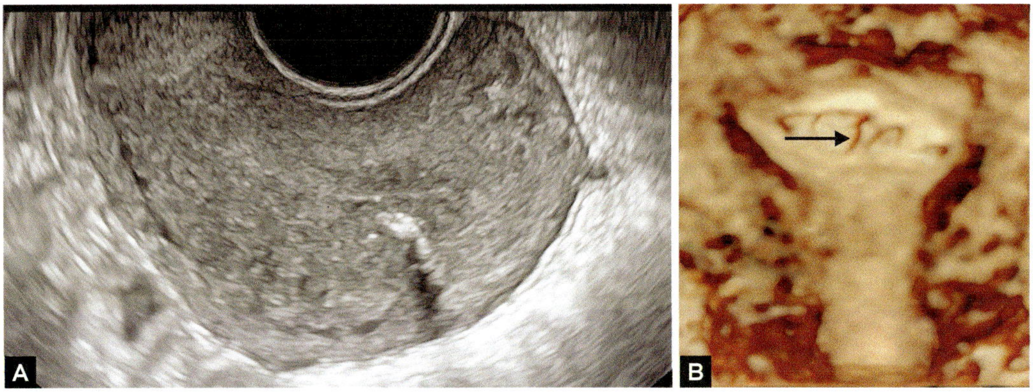

Figs. 3A and B: (A) B-mode image of thin endometrium; (B) Sonohysterography with 3D of the same uterus showing synechiae.

encerclage and good neonatal care, such operations are rarely performed and so now it is a rare cause for intrauterine adhesions and thin endometrium.

Radiotherapy

Radiotherapy can damage the endometrium and it can become atrophic and nonresponsive to hormonal therapy. Radiation-induced uterine damage is age and dose-dependent. The growing uterus is more vulnerable. Older patients show a better response to hormonal therapy. Miscarriage rates and preterm deliveries are very high.

Infections

Chronic endometritis is a very common cause of thin endometrium. It hampers the uterine receptivity. It also changes the endometrial peristaltic wave pattern which causes infertility.[9] Chronic endometritis is difficult to diagnose. The patient may have dysfunctional uterine bleeding, pelvic pain, and dyspareunia. Hysteroscopy may reveal micropolyps, adhesions, focal hyperemia, and edema with diagnostic accuracy (93%).[10]

Tuberculosis is very common in our country and can be strongly suspected on ultrasound. Though most ultrasound features are not specific to tuberculosis, persistently thin endometrium with endometrial, sub-endometrial, and myometrial calcifications **(Fig. 4A)**, contracted narrow endometrial cavity **(Fig. 4B)**, or synechiae **(Fig. 4C)** are the signs that raise the suspicion of tuberculosis. Tuberculous endometritis may also present as fluid in the endometrial cavity in the mid proliferative phase with hyperechoic endometrial lining **(Fig. 4D)** or micropolyposis **(Fig. 4E)**. One of the most specific signs is vertical orientation of the interstitial part of the tube **(Fig. 4F)**.

In patients with recurrent implantation failure, chronic endometritis is the frequent cause. The cure rate is very high after antibiotics. So diagnosis by hysteroscopy and treatment with antibiotics improve the implantation rate.[11] Doxycycline 100 mg bd for 10–14 days is recommended. Azithromycin is also a good option for endometritis.

Congenital Müllerian Abnormalities

Müllerian abnormalities are associated with poor reproductive outcomes. It may have abnormal karyotype in 87% of cases. The implantation failure and thin endometrium

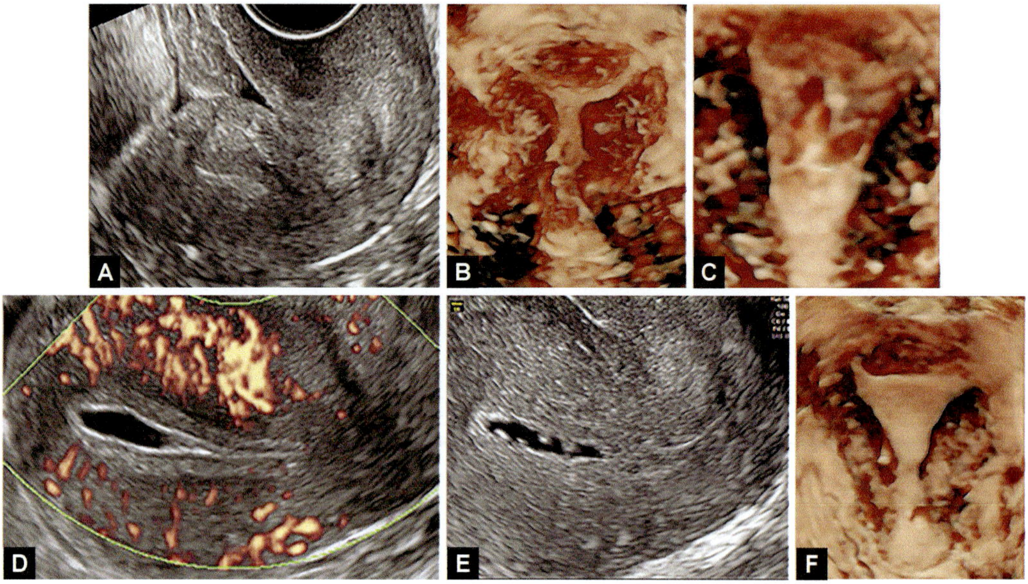

Figs. 4A to F: (A) Micropolyposis; (B) Fluid in endometrial cavity with hyperechoic margins; (C) Thin endometrium; (D) Contracted endometrial cavity; (E) Vertical orientation of the interstitial part of the tube; (F) Synechiae.

are poorly understood. There may be alteration in *HOXA* genes.

Other Causes

- *Estrogen deficiency*: In patients with hypogonadotropic hypogonadism, there is a low estrogen level. So the endometrium is thin. By stimulating with human menopausal gonadotropin (HMG), follicles develop, estrogen level rises, and endometrium can grow to more thickness.
- *Clomiphene citrate*: Repeated cycles of clomiphene for ovulation induction cause accumulations of Zuclomiphene which causes thinning of the endometrium as estrogen receptors are occupied and estrogen cannot show its effect on the endometrium.
- *Oral contraceptive (OC) pills*: Long-term use of OC pills can cause thinning of endometrium, but it is regained after stopping the drug.
- *Long-term use of progesterone*: It compacts the endometrium and decreases the thickness but the effect is reversible.

MANAGEMENT

Drugs

- Low-dose aspirin
- Sildenafil
- Tocopherol
- Pentoxifylline
- Nitroglycerine
- L-arginine
- Gonadotropin-releasing hormone agonist (GnRHa)
- Estrogen
- Tamoxifen
- Human chorionic gonadotropin (hCG)
- Ovulation induction

Procedures

- Endometrial scratching
- Granulocyte colony-stimulating factor (G-CSF)

- Platelet-rich plasma (PRP)
- Stem cell therapy

DRUGS

- *Low-dose aspirin*: Low-dose aspirin improves endometrial thickness and implantation by improving uterine endometrial blood flow and by reducing uterine artery resistance [pulsatility index (PI)]. It reduces subendometrial contractility and minimizes inflammation. The recommended dose is 75–150 mg/day.
  It is widely used in in vitro fertilization (IVF) cycles, but no beneficial effect on implantation has been documented. Weckstein et al. found improved pregnancy rates without increasing endometrial thickness due to improvement in the blood flow.[12] A Cochrane review in 2010 found no benefit in endometrial preparation with Aspirin.[13] A recent meta-analysis in 2017 by Wang et al. did not find any difference in the implantation rate in with aspirin and without aspirin groups.[14] So the current evidence to support the beneficial effect of aspirin in patients with thin endometrium is lacking and is controversial.
- *Sildenafil*: It has a vasodilator effect. It relaxes the smooth muscles of the blood vessels and increases the blood flow to the endometrium and is also claimed to increase the endometrial thickness and receptivity. The dose is 25 mg 6 hourly vaginally up to the day of trigger or embryo transfer.[15] However, a Cochrane review 2014 found insufficient evidence for Sildenafil to improve the thickness of the endometrium and live birth rate.[16] The clinical benefit of sildenafil in women with a recurrent thin endometrium is lacking, and only a few studies with a small group of patients are available.
- *Tocopherol (Vitamin E)*: It is a vasodilator as well as an antioxidant. Generally, it is used with pentoxifylline in radiation fibrosis. A significant increase in uterine diastolic blood flow and endometrial thickness was observed with 1,000 IU of vitamin E and 800 mg of pentoxifylline daily for 9 months. An increase in the endometrial thickness was also found in refractory thin endometrium in patients with premature ovarian failure.[17] But except for radiation fibrosis, other studies are lacking for vitamin E and pentoxifylline combination to improve endometrial thickness in regular practice.
- *Pentoxifylline*: It has a vasodilating effect and reduces blood viscosity along with vitamin E. It can be used in radiation fibrosis.[18]
- *Nitroglycerine*: It releases nitric oxide (NO) and has a vasodilator effect. There is no specific publication on it. Ohl et al. used a nitroglycerine patch on the day before embryo transfer in recurrent implantation failure patients.[19] But no positive effect was documented. There is no current evidence to use a nitroglycerine patch in women with thin endometrium.
- *L-arginine*: It is a precursor of nitric oxide. It acts as a vasodilator and also activates the immune system and inflammatory process. Takasaki et al. gave 6 mg/day of L-arginine in patients with thin endometrium. They observed an endometrial thickness of >8 mm in 67%.[20] But other evidences are not available. It is also used in radiation fibrosis by some workers.
- *GnRHa*: The patient is given luteal support by triptorelin 0.1 mg on the day of oocyte retrieval, day of embryo transfer,

and 3 days later.[21] Qublan et al. found significant improvement in implantation and pregnancy rates. However, no other studies have validated these findings.

- *Estrogen*: The dose of estrogen to prepare endometrium is 68 mg and can be increased up to 16 mg. The minimum duration of exposure required for estrogen stimulation is 12 days and the maximum is 28 days. Estrogen, when given for a longer duration, has shown poor results. Endogenous estrogen is not required when exogenous estrogen is given. In all frozen embryo transfer (FET) cycles, it is continued up to 9 weeks of pregnancy. Estrogen can also be administered vaginally but should not be used vaginally with progesterone. Twice-a-week injection of 4 mg can be given when other routes fail.
  Estrogen helps endometrial preparation by causing spiral artery contraction and reduced oxygen tension in the functional layer, which in turn facilitates embryo implantation.[22] Though the step-up protocol of estrogen is popular, recent studies suggest that this is not required. estrogen can be started as a 6–8 mg dose, maximum up to 16 mg per day from day 1. Though only 2 mg can block follicular development and so downregulation from the luteal phase is not required.
- *Tamoxifen*: In patients having thin endometrium, tamoxifen can increase the thickness. For FET cycles, Chen et al. reported tamoxifen 20 mg for 5 days and if the patient did not respond, an extended regimen can be tried.[23] Tamoxifen can also be used in patients having thin endometrium because of clomiphene citrate.
- *hCG in proliferative phase*: It is produced by endometrial epithelial cells in the secretory phase.[24] hCG has a local paracrine role in differentiating endometrial receptivity by regulating different cytokines and growth factors.[25] Intrauterine injection of 500 IU of hCG increases leukemia inhibitor factor (LIF) and vascular endothelial growth factor (VEGF).
  Papanikolaou et al. introduced 150 IU of hCG daily subcutaneously for 7 days from Day 8 of the cycle for those who did not respond to 17-β-estradiol 8 mg/day. They found an increase in endometrial thickness and clinical outcome. hCG was stopped when progesterone was started.[26] If the dose is increased or is given to the patients with normal endometrium, it can have a deleterious effect on endometrial receptivity.

PROCEDURES

Endometrial Scratching

Endometrial scratching causes an inflammatory reaction and this injury to the endometrium may increase the chances of implantation.[27] Injury leads to favorable changes in cytokines, natural killer (NK) cells, and macrophages to improve the implantation rate.

A recent Cochrane review suggests a favorable outcome with endometrial scratching.[28] Scratching causes the growth of the endometrium and increases endometrial thickness. It is useful in cases with recurrent implantation failure also. Xu et al. in 2015 documented that a combination of G-CSF and endometrial scratching gives a favorable pregnancy rate.[29] Though more studies are required to prove its role in patients with thin endometrium. A recent study by Mackens et al. in 2020 has documented that intentional endometrial injury in the follicular phase of ovarian stimulation warrants further attention in future research as it may be harmful.[30]

According to SCRaTCH trial, the results suggest that a possible effect of scratching may be smaller than anticipated and may apply to only specific groups of women. At present scratching should not be applied outside of clinical trials.[31]

Granulocyte Colony-stimulating Factor

It is produced in various tissues in the body including vascular endothelium. It acts as a growth factor and cytokine. It causes proliferation and differentiation of the endometrium as it causes endometrial stromal cell decidualization. G-CSF may stimulate endometrial stem cells or mobilize bone marrow cells promoting the growth of the endometrium. G-CSF modulates gene expression of endometrial vascular remodeling, immune regulation, and cell adhesions.[32] The first successful experience was described by Gleicher et al., which resulted in four pregnancies after increasing the endometrial thickness.[33] Patients were treated with intrauterine perfusion of 30 IU of G-CSF (300 μg/mL), approximately 6–12 hours prior to hCG injection. If during egg retrieval, endometrial thickness is <7 mm, the dose was repeated. The thickness was 9.3 ± 2.1 mm versus 6.4 ± 1.4 mm. But a randomized controlled trial (RCT) was lacking and there was no control group for comparison. Eftekhar et al. documented improved endometrial receptivity in FET cycles when the endometrial thickness was <7 mm.[34] However, Barad et al. who are pioneers of this concept were unable to demonstrate any effect of G-CSF on endometrial growth or pregnancy rate.[35]

So, even though nonrandomized studies have given good results, the published RCT failed to show any beneficial effect so more trials are required to prove its efficacy. The present evidence is not supportive. G-CSF does not improve pregnancy outcome when the endometrial thickness is normal.[36]

Autologous Platelet-rich Plasma

Platelet-rich plasma releases cytokines and growth factors such as VEGF, transforming growth factor beta 1 (TGFβ1), and epidermal growth factor (EGF). It was introduced after 10 days of estradiol valerate 12 mg in patients where endometrial thickness was <7 mm. In all five patients, endometrial thickness increased and resulted in conception after embryo transfer.[37] Shahrzad et al. did the pilot study in 2017. PRP was introduced on day 11–12 and repeated on Day 13–14. Endometrial thickness increased >7 mm after the second PRP in all patients and got 5 pregnancies in 10 patients. So growth factors and cytokines from PRP may improve endometrial receptivity.[38] As PRP is autologous, there is no risk of transmission of infectious diseases and immunological reactions.

Platelet-rich plasma infusion is done 48 hours before embryo transfer. 8 mL of venous blood is drawn and centrifuged at 1,500 g for 10 minutes.

- Collect blood
- Spin at 200 g for 15 minutes
- Then spin at 600 g for 6 minutes. The repeated reversal of the tube allows PRP at the concentration required.
- 0.5–6.8 mL obtained is infused with intrauterine insemination (IUI) cannula.
- After 48 hours assess endometrium, otherwise introduce a second dose.

Still, the evidence is limited. Further studies are required for thin endometrium. According to Urman et al., caution is required prior to using PRP on a wide scale and await the results of a well-designed study.[39]

Stem Cells

The first case of endometrial regeneration by stem cells followed by conception was published by us in 2011.[40] Autologous bone marrow cells obtained from the iliac crest were infused on Day 2 after curettage into the uterus with Asherman's syndrome and thin endometrium that was unresponsive to estrogen grew after cyclical hormonal therapy. Aspiration was done using a bone marrow biopsy needle and a 10-mL syringe prewashed with heparin. A total of 45 mL of bone marrow was aspirated. The collection was done in citrate-phosphate dextrose anticoagulant (CPDA) medium using 1 mL of medium for 7 mL of bone marrow. It was sent to a dedicated stem cell laboratory working as per the clinical Good Manufacturing Practice/Good Tissue Practice (GMP/GTP) standard and having a working area with laminar airflow to class 100.

Bone marrow was centrifuged using a histopaque density gradient at 1,000 rpm for 10 minutes and 102 million mononuclear cells were separated. These cells were then treated by the column separation technique, and customized cocktail of CD9, CD90, and CD133 antibodies was used for immunomagnetic isolation of endometrial angiogenic stem cells. The markers used for endometrial angiogenic stem cells were CD9, CD44, and CD90. Gene expression study for CD9, CD44, and CD90 using the reverse transcription-polymerase chain reaction (RT-PCR) technique was done for differentiated cells. A total of 39 million marker positive endometrial angiogenic cells were supplied in 0.7 mL of phosphate buffer saline (PBS) with 2% autologous (patient's own) heat-inactivated serum for transplantation on the next day.[41-45]

Curettage was done under anesthesia. With the patient in lithotomy position and Sim's speculum in place, an anterior retractor was used to retract the anterior vaginal wall and vulsellum was used to hold the anterior lip of cervix. An embryo transfer cannula (Frydman® Classic Catheter 4,5, Laboratoire C.C.D., France) attached with 1-mL syringe and filled with 0.7-mL stem cell suspension was advanced through cervix up to the fundal end of the endometrium under transabdominal ultrasound guidance. With the tip of the catheter being 0.5 cm distal to the fundus, the piston was very slowly advanced to allow a slow steady flow of cell suspension in the uterine cavity. After instilling 0.3 mL of stem cell suspension at the fundus, injection was continued when cannula was gradually withdrawn out, till the tip reached the mid cavity of the uterus. It was very gently and slowly withdrawn from the internal os and then the external os, continuously maintaining pressure on the piston to prevent any backflow.

This is followed by cyclical estrogen and progesterone therapy for 3–4 months, with Aspirin 75 mg daily. This resulted into 7 mm + endometrium with vascularity reaching the inner zones of the endometrium as confirmed by Doppler studies. Embryo transfer was done after that and it resulted in conception.

Three main sources of endometrial cell reconstruction have been proposed:

1. Clonogenic cells in the endometrium
2. Epithelial progenitor cells and mesenchymal stromal stem cells from bone marrow
3. Human embryonic stem cells

These are pluripotent stem cells and are not obtained from the fibroblasts of a female with Asherman's syndrome.

Subendometrial autologous stem cell transplantation of mononuclear stem cells from the iliac crest also increases endometrial thickness in patients with Asherman's syndrome. Exogenous estrogen therapy is given.

This gives good results and resumption of menstruation is also observed.[46]

Santamaria et al. also did autologous stem cell therapy with CD133+ bone marrow-derived stem cells and has claimed good results.[47] According to them, some women are prone to Asherman's syndrome and these should be identified. In another study, somatic cell nuclear transfer derived hPSC (human pluripotent stem cells) 5 MPCs (mesenchymal progenitor cells) could be an advanced therapeutic strategy for specific diseases in the field of regenerative medicine.[48]

CARRY HOME MESSAGE

- 7 mm is the cutoff for endometrial thickness.
- Vascularity is more important than only thickness.
- Obstetric D&C is the most common cause for thin endometrium.
- Hysteroscopic surgery for fibroids and septum can cause intrauterine adhesions.
- Endometritis is treatable and a good outcome is achievable.
- There is insufficient evidence for low-dose aspirin, sildenafil.
- Vitamin E and pentoxifylline are useful in radiation fibrosis.
- Extended estrogen therapy is useful.
- Subcutaneous hCG for 7–8 days is under trial.
- L-arginine 6 mg/day requires more evidence.
- Endometrial scratching has mixed opinions.
- G-CSF for improving receptivity requires double-blind studies.
- PRP is safe and larger studies are required.
- Stem cell is the future.

REFERENCES

1. Cai QF, Wan F, Huang R, Zhang HW. Factors predicting the cumulative outcome of IVF/ICSI treatment: a multivariable analysis of 2450 patients. Hum Reprod. 2011;26:2532-40.
2. Cruz F, Bellver J. Live birth after embryo transfer in an unresponsive thin endometrium. Gynecol Endocrinol. 2014;30: 481-4.
3. Quaas AM, Gavrizi SZ, Peck JD, Diamond MP, Legro RS, Robinson RD, et al. Endometrial thickness after ovarian stimulation with gonadotropin, clomiphene or letrozole for unexplained infertility, and association with treatment outcomes. Fertil Steril. 2021; 115(1): 213-20.
4. Liu KE, Hartman M, Hartman A, Luo ZC, Mahutte N. The impact of a thin endometrial lining on fresh and frozen thaw IVF outcomes: an analysis of over 40,000 embryo transfers. Hum Reprod. 2018;33(10):1883-8.
5. Schiper E, Valle RF, Nezhat C. Intrauterine adhesions: hysteroscopic evaluation and treatment, prevention and management, 3rd Edition. Society of Laparoscopic Surgeons. pp. 1-3.
6. Taskin O, Sadik S, Onoglu A, Gokdeniz R, Erturan E, Burak K, et al. Role of endometrial suppression on the frequency of intrauterine adhesions after surgery resectoscope. J Am Assoc Gynecol Laparosc. 2000;7:351-4.
7. Young SL. Oestrogen and progesterone action on endometrium: a translational approach to understanding endometrial receptivity. Reprod Biomed Online. 2013;27: 497-505.
8. Pereira N, Amrane S, Estes JL, Lekovich JP, Elias RT, Chung PH, et al. Does the time interval between hysteroscopic polypectomy and start of in vitro fertilization affect outcomes? Fertil Steril. 2016;105:539-44.
9. Pinto V, Matteo M, Tinelli R, Mitola P, De Ziegler D, Cicinelli E. Altered uterine contractility in women with chronic endometritis. Fertil Steril. 2015;103:1049-52.
10. Cicinelli E, Matteo M, Tinelli R, Lepera A, Alfonso R, Idraccolo U, et al. Prevalence of chronic endometritis in repeated unexplained implantation failure and the IVF success after antibiotic therapy. Hum Reprod. 2015;30:323-33.
11. Zolghadri J, Momtahan M, Aminian K, Ghaffarpasand F, Tavana Z. The value of hysteroscopy in diagnosis of chronic endometritis in patients with unexplained recurrent spontaneous abortion. Eur J Obstet Gynecol Reprod Biol. 2011;155:217-20.
12. Weckstein LN, Jacobson A, Galen D, Hampton K, Hammel J. Low dose aspirin for oocyte donation recipients with a thin

endometrium: prospective, randomized study. Fertil Steril. 1997;68:927-30.
13. Glujovsky D, Pesce R, Fiszbajn G, Sueldo C, Hart RJ, Ciapponi A. Endometrial preparation for women undergoing embryo transfer with frozen embryos or embryos derived from donor oocytes. Cochrane Database Syst Rev. 2010;20(1):CD006359.
14. Wang H, Huang X, Li X, Lv F, He X, Pan Y, et al. Efficacy evaluation if low dose aspirin in IVF/ICSI patients evidence from 13 RCTs: a systematic review and meta-analysis. Medicine. 2017;96:e7720.
15. Sher G, Fisch J. Vaginal Sildenafil (Viagra): a preliminary report of a novel method to improve uterine artery blood flow and endometrial development in patients undergoing IVF. Hum Reprod. 2000;15:806-9.
16. Gutarra-Vilchez RB, Urrutia G, Glujovsky D, Coscia A, Bonfill Cosp X. Vasodilators for women undergoing fertility treatment. Cochrane Database Syst Rev. 2014;10: CD010001.
17. Letur-Konirsch H, Guis F, Delanian S. Uterine restoration by radiation sequelae regression with combined pentoxifylline-tocoferol: a phase II study. Fertil Steril. 2002;77:1219-26.
18. Chiao TB, Lee AJ. Role of pentoxifylline and vitamin E in attenuation of radiation induced fibrosis. Ann Pharmacother. 2005;39:516-22.
19. Ohl J, Lefebvre-Maunoury C, Wittemer C, Nisand G, Laurent MC, Hoffman P. Nitric oxide donors for patients undergoing IVF. A prospective, double blind, randomized, placebo controlled trial. Hum Reprod. 2002;17:2615-20.
20. Takasaki A, Tamura H, Miwa I, Taketani T, Shimamura K, Sugino N. Endometrial growth and uterine blood flow: a pilot study for improving endometrial thickness in the patients with a thin endometrium. Fertil Steril. 2010;93(6):1851-8.
21. Qublan H, Amarin Z, Al-Qudah M, Diab F, Nawasreh M, Malkawi S, et al. Luteal phase support with GnRHa improves implantation and pregnancy rates in IVF cycles with endometrium of ≤7mm on day of egg retrieval. Hum Fertil (Camb). 2008;11:43-7.
22. Casper RF. It's time to pay attention to the endometrium. Fertil Steril. 2011;96:519-21.
23. Chen X, Chen SL. Successful pregnancy in recurrent thin endometrium with new uses for an old drug. J IVF Reprod Med Genet. 2013;1:2.
24. Paiva P, Hannan NJ, Hincks C, Meehan KL, Pruysers E, Dimitriadis E, et al. Human chorionic gonadotropin regulates FGF2 and other cytokines produced by human endometrial epithelial cells, providing a mechanism for enhancing endometrial receptivity. Hum Reprod. 2011;26:153-62.
25. Licth P, Flur H, Neuwinger J, Wallwiener D, Wildt L. Is human chorionic gonadotropin directly involved in the regulation of human implantation? Mol Cell Endocrinol. 2007;269:85-92.
26. Papanikolaou EG, Kyrou D, Zervakakou G, Paggou E, Humaidan P. Follicular hCG endometrial priming for IVF patients experiencing resisting thin endometrium. A proof of concept study. J Assist Reprod Genet. 2013;30:1341-5.
27. Barasch A, Dekel N, Fieldust S, Segal I, Schechtman E, Granot I. Local injury to the endometrium doubles the incidence of successful pregnancies in patients undergoing in vitro fertilization. Fetil Steril. 2003;79:1317-22.
28. Nastri CO, Lensen SF, Gibreel A, Rainne-Fenning N, Ferriani RA, Bhattacharya S, et al. Endometrial injury in women undergoing assisted reproductive techniques. Cochrane Database Syst Rev. 2015;22(3):CD009517.
29. Xu B, Zhang Q, Hao J, Xu D, Li Y. Two protocols to treat thin endometrium with granulocyte colony stimulating factor during frozen embryo transfer cycles. Reprod Biomed Online. 2015;30(4):349-58.
30. Mackens S, Racca A, Van De Velde H, Drakopoulos P, Tournaye H, Stoop D, et al. Follicular phase endometrial scratching: a truncated randomized controlled trial. Hum Reprod. 2020;35(5):1090-8.
31. van Hoogenhuijze NE, Mol F, Laven JSE, Groenewoud ER, Traas MAF, Janssen CAH, Teklenburg G, et al. Endometrial scratching

in women with one failed IVF/ICSI cycle-outcomes of a randomised controlled trial (SCRatch). Hum Reprod. 2021;36(1):87-98.

32. Rahmati M, Petitbarat M, Dubanchet S, Bensussan A, Chaouat G, Ledee N. Granulocyte-colony stimulating factor related pathways tested on an endometrial ex-vivo model. PLoS One. 2014;9(9):e102286.
33. Gleicher N, Vidali A, Barad DH. Successful treatment of unresponsive thin endometrium. Fertil Steril. 2011;95:2123.e13-7.
34. Eftekhar M, Sayadi M, Arabjahvani F. Transvaginal perfusion of G-CSF for infertile women with thin endometrium in frozen ET program: a non-randomized clinical trial. Iran J Reprod Med. 2014;12:661-6.
35. Barad DH, Yu Y, Kushnir VA, Shohat-Tal A, Lazzaroni E, Lee HJ, et al. A randomized clinical trial of endometrial perfusion with granulocyte-colony stimulating factor in in vitro fertilization cycles: impact on endometrial thickness and clinical pregnancy rates. Fertil Steril. 2014;101:710-5.
36. Eftekhar M, Hosseinisadat R, Baradaran R, Naghshineh E. Effect of granulocyte-colony stimulating factor (G-CSF) on IVF outcomes in infertile women: a RCT. Int J Reprod Biomed. 2016;14(5):341-6.
37. Chang Y, Li J, Chen Y, Wei L, Yang X, Liang X. Autologous platelet rich plasma promotes endometrial growth and improves pregnancy outcome during in vitro fertilization. Int J Clin Exp Med. 2015;8:1286-90.
38. Shahrzad Z, Saghar S, Nasrin S, Leila N. Treatment of thin endometrium with autologous platelets rich plasma: a pilot study. JBRA Assist Reprod. 2017;21(1):54-6.
39. Urman B, Boza A, Balaban B. Platelet rich plasma another add-on treatment getting out of hand? How can clinicians preserve the best interest of their patients? Hum Reprod. 2019;34(11):2099-103.
40. Nagori CB, Panchal S, Patel H. Endometrial regeneration using autologous adult stem cells followed by conception by in vitro fertilization in a patient of severe Asherman's syndrome. J Hum Reprod Sci. 2011;4(1):43-8.
41. Yin AH, Miraglia S, Zanjani ED, Almeida-Porada G, Ogawa M, Leary AG, et al. AC133, a novel marker for human hematopoietic stem and progenitor cells. Blood. 1997;90:5002-12.
42. Miraglia S, Godfrey W, Yin AH, Atkins K, Warnke R, Holden JT, et al. A novel five-transmembrane hematopoietic stem cell antigen: isolation, characterization, and molecular cloning. Blood. 1997;90:5013-21.
43. Uchida N, Buck DW, He D, Reitsma MJ, Masek M, Phan TV, et al. Direct isolation of human central nervous system stem cells. Proc Natl Acad Sci USA. 2000;97:14720-5.
44. Cummings BJ, Uchida N, Tamaki SJ, Salazar DL, Hooshmand M, Summers R, et al. Human neural stem cells differentiate and promote locomotor recovery in spinal cord-injured mice. Proc Natl Acad Sci USA. 2005;102:14069-74.
45. Bussolati B, Bruno S, Grange C, Buttiglieri S, Deregibus MC, Cantino D, et al. Isolation of renal progenitor cells from adult human kidney. Am J Pathol. 2005;166:545-55.
46. Singh N, Mohanty S, Seth T, Shankar M, Bhaskaran S, Dharmendra S. Autologous stem cell transplantation in refractory Asherman's syndrome: a novel cell based therapy. J Hum Reprod Sci. 2014;7:93-8.
47. Santamaria X, Cabanillas S, Cervello I, Arbona C, Raga F, Ferro J, et al. Autologous stem cell therapy with CD133+ bone marrow-derived stem cells for refractory Asherman's syndrome and endometrial atrophy: a pilot cohort study. Hum Reprod. 2016;31(5):1087-96.
48. Jun SM, Park M, Lee JY, Jung S, Lee JE, Shim SH, et al. Single cell-derived clonally expanded mesenchymal progenitor cell from somatic cell nuclear transfer derived pluripotent stem cells ameliorate the endometrial function in the uterus of a murine model with Asherman's syndrome. Cell Prolif. 2019;52(3):e12597.

32 Chapter

Recurrent Pregnancy Loss

INTRODUCTION

Recurrent pregnancy loss (RPL) is a social stigma and the couple has tremendous stress, frustration, and uncertainty regarding future reproductive outcomes. According to the Royal College of Obstetricians and Gynaecologists (RCOG) and European Society of Human Reproduction and Embryology (ESHRE) guidelines, RPL is defined as three or more consecutive pregnancy losses. But according to the American College of Obstetricians and Gynecologists (ACOG), RPL is two or more pregnancy losses. This does not include loss of biochemical pregnancy. About 80% of these losses occur in the first 12 weeks of pregnancy, but only 20% of pregnancy losses in RPL occur after the cardiac activity has been established. The incidence of RPL is 1–2% in the fertile population.

Detailed history must be taken which in the majority of cases gives a clue to the diagnosis. A correct diagnosis is the basis for successful treatment. Though 50% of cases of RPL will not have a clearly defined etiology.[1] Counseling plays a very important role in treating these couples. Bed rest does not help in improving the reproductive outcome. The patient should be allowed to do her regular work and exercise program.

CAUSES

- Anatomical
- Autoimmune
- Thrombophilia
- Genetic
- Alloimmunity
- Infections
- Environmental
- Endometriosis
- Psychological
- Endocrinal
- Male factor

ANATOMICAL CAUSES

The incidence is 1–4% and in RPL 15–25%.

Congenital Causes

These are also called Müllerian duct abnormalities and are a result of:

- Failure of one or more Müllerian duct to develop
- Failure of the ducts to canalize
- Failure to fuse or abnormal fusion of Müllerian ducts
- Failure of resorption of midline uterine septum

These were earlier classified by the American Fertility Society (AFS) in 2003,[2] as unicornuate, bicornuate, didelphys, septate, and arcuate uterus. But in 2013, a new classification—ESHRE/ESGE (European Society of Human Reproduction and Embryology/European Society of Gynaecological Endoscopy)[3] was published and was claimed to be more practical and treatment-oriented; hence, since then, the new classification is used **(Table 1 and Fig. 1A)**.

TABLE 1: ESHRE/ESGE classification of female genital tract anomalies.

ESHRE/ESGE Classification Female Genital Tract Anomalies				
Uterine anomaly			*Cervical/Vaginal anomaly*	
	Main class	*Subclass*	*Coexistent class*	
U0	Normal uterus		C0	Normal cervix
U1	Dysmorphic uterus	a. T-shaped b. Infantilis c. Others	C1	Septate cervix
U2	Septate uterus	a. Partial b. Complete	C2	Double "'normal" cervix
U3	Bicorporeal uterus	a. Partial b. Complete c. Bicorporeal septate	C3	Unilateral cervical aplasia
U4	Hemiuterus	a. With rudimentary cavity (communicating or not horn) b. Without rudimentary cavity (horn without cavity/no horn)	C4	Cervical aplasia
U5	Aplastic	a. With rudimentary cavity (bi- or unilateral horn) b. Without rudimentary cavity (bi- or unilateral uterine remnants/aplasia)	V0	Normal vagina
U6	Unclassified malformations		V1	Longitudinal non-obstructing vaginal septum
			V2	Longitudinal obstructing vaginal septum
			V3	Transverse vaginal septum and/or imperforate hymen
			V4	Vaginal aplasia
U			***C***	***V***

(ESGE: European Society for Gynaecological Endoscopy; ESHRE: European Society of Human Reproduction and Embryology)[3]

According to this classification, Müllerian duct abnormalities are divided into seven classes and cervical and vaginal shape is also divided into classes.

Investigations to Diagnose these Abnormalities

- *Ultrasonography*: Three-dimensional (3D) ultrasound (US) has a major role to play in the diagnosis of uterine anomaly. It is known as virtual hysteroscopy. The sensitivity and specificity of volume US for detection of congenital uterine abnormality are almost 100% and therefore are considered to be a gold standard for diagnosis of these abnormalities **(Figs. 1B to D)**.
- *Hysterosalpingogram (HSG)*: It has a very limited role for differential diagnosis of congenital uterine abnormalities such as bicornuate, septate, and arcuate uterus.
- *Saline infusion sonohysterography (SHG)*: SHG along with 3D is also useful.

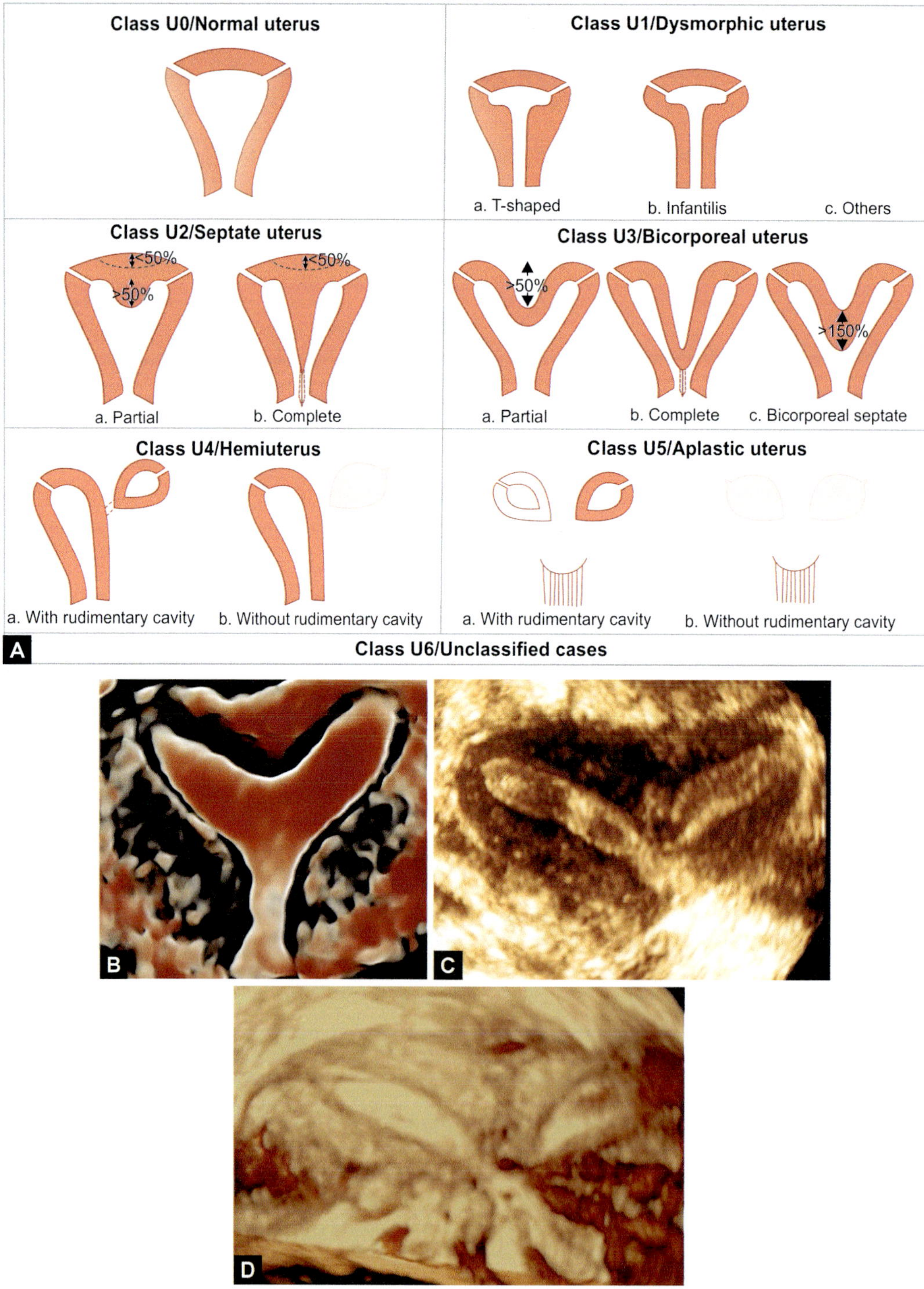

Figs. 1A to D: (A) Diagrammatic explanation of the ESHRE-ESGE classification of Müllerian duct abnormalities; (B to D) Different duplication abnormalities as demonstrated on 3D ultrasound.[3] (ESGE: European Society for Gynecological Endoscopy; ESHRE: European Society of Human Reproduction and Embryology)

- *Magnetic resonance imaging (MRI)*: This is not required most of the times as 3D US is sufficient. Moreover, it is much more inconvenient and expensive for the patient. It is used only when the uterus is poorly visualized on ultrasound.
- *Diagnostic laparoscopy and hysteroscopy*: They have the same diagnostic accuracy as achieved by volume US, but are highly invasive and so are not preferred over the 3D US. These procedures are used only for operative corrections of these abnormalities.
- *Intravenous pyelography (IVP)*: This is done to rule out renal abnormalities which are common to Müllerian abnormalities.

Classification of Müllerian Duct Abnormalities

- *Class U0*: Normal uterus
- *Class U1*: Dysmorphic uterus

Dysmorphic uterus is divided into two subclasses: (1) T-shaped uterus and (2) uterus infantalis. The latter was earlier named as the hypoplastic uterus.

Ultrasound findings: The US findings of class U1 are described in **Table 2**.

Clinical significance of diethylstilboestrol (DES) exposed (T-shaped) uterus is rapidly decreasing as the population of women exposed to DES now has crossed the active reproductive age. This is so because DES was used from 1948 to 1971. Since then, it is banned and the women who might have taken it in 1971 also now must be 50 years old. But correct identification of T-shaped uterus is still important because the narrow uterine cavity is often diagnosed as T-shaped uterus. This may be Koch's affected uterus. In these cases, delivery at term is extremely rare. About 50% abort by the end of the second trimester.

TABLE 2: Ultrasound findings of T-shaped uterus and uterus infantalis.

T-shaped uterus (class U1a) **(Fig. 2A)**	*Uterus infantalis (class U1b)* **(Fig. 2B)**
• Narrow cavity • Normal uterocervical ratio • Thick lateral wall	• Narrow cavity • Reverse uterocervical ratio • Normal walls

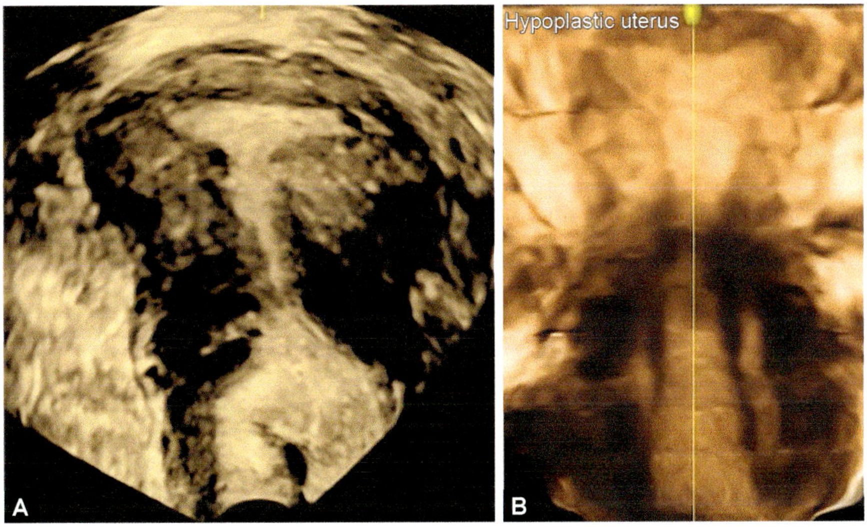

Figs. 2A and B: (A) T-shaped uterus; (B) Hypoplastic uterus on 3D ultrasound.

Hysteroscopic metroplasty followed by cervical encerclage during pregnancy can be very useful. The hypoplastic uterus does not require any specific treatment except cyclical hormone therapy.

Data about uterine enlargement with metroplasty for dysmorphic uterus in cases with RPL is controversial. International guidelines do not recommend this.[4]

- *Class U2*: Septate uterus.

  This class is subclassified into:
  - Partial septum **(Fig. 3A)**
  - Complete septum **(Fig. 3B)**

  With normal outer fundal contour, there is a septum dividing the endometrial cavity. The indentation of the endometrial fundus should be >50% of the total myometrial wall thickness. If this septum reaches the internal os, it is complete septum and short of that is partial septum.

  This is the most common uterine anomaly amongst the patients presenting with RPL. The causes postulated for abortion in the septate uterus are as follows:
  - The septum has less connective tissue resulting in poor decidualization and placentation.
  - Increased muscle mass in the septum causes local uncoordinated myometrial contractility.
  - High-resistance vascularity in the septum leads to poor blood supply to the endometrium overlying the septum.
  - When there is a high septal length to uterine cavity ratio, the chances of abortion are higher.[5]
  - Cervical incompetence

Management of septate uterus:
- Operative hysteroscopy for septum resection has a good outcome but there is no definite data to justify its widespread use.[6,7]
- No pre- or postsurgical treatment is required if surgery is planned.
- Surgery should be deferred before pregnancy loss.[6,7]
- Risk of uterine rupture is increased in subsequent pregnancy after surgery.[8]
- Cervical encerclage is beneficial along with progesterone.
- ASRM and French guidelines recommend septum resection in cases with RPL, while RCOG concludes that there is insufficient

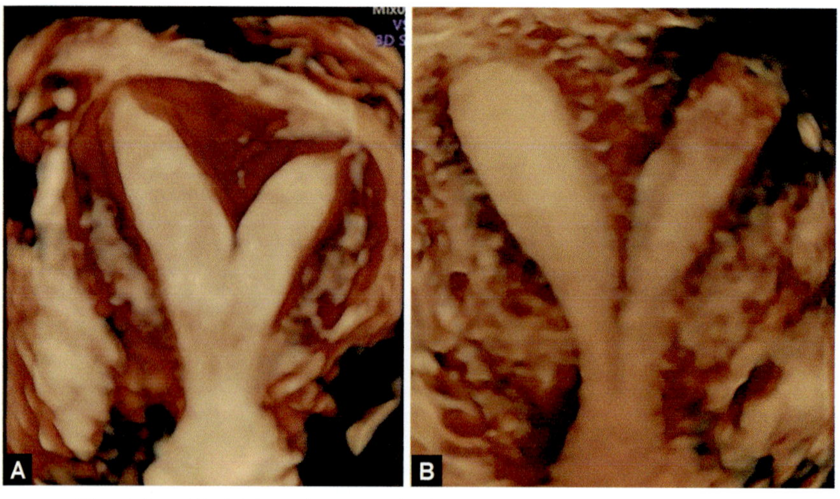

Figs. 3A and B: (A) Partial septum; (B) Complete septum on 3D ultrasound.

evidence for surgical correction of uterine septum.

- *Class U3*: Bicorporeal uterus with two corpora (body).

  This class is further subclassified into:
  - Partial bicorporeal **(Fig. 4A)**
  - Complete bicorporeal **(Fig. 4B)**
  - Bicorporeal septate **(Fig. 4C)**

Uteri are placed in this class when the uterine outer contour shows indentation, >50% of the myometrial wall thickness along with the division of the endometrial cavity also. When this indentation divides the corpus of the uterus till internal os, it is complete bicorporeal and if it is short of that it is partial bicorporeal. But if in spite of indentation of the fundus, the thickness of the dividing wall between the two endometrial cavities is 1.5 times the myometrial wall thickness, it is named as bicorporeal septate uterus. The anomalies included in this class were earlier named as bicornuate uterus and uterus didelphys. If a complete bicorporeal uterus also has a double cervix, it is uterus didelphys according to the AFS classification.

For bicorporeal uterus, pregnancy prognosis is the best (64%) amongst all congenital uterine abnormalities. Unification of uterus is rarely required. Particularly in this era of good neonatal care, late-trimester babies can be well managed in neonatal intensive care units. Cervical incompetence is present in up to 40% of patients. Cervical encerclage is the primary line of treatment and the results are parallel to metroplasty (Strassman's operation). The abortion rate quoted in literature for bicorporeal uterus is 20–40%.

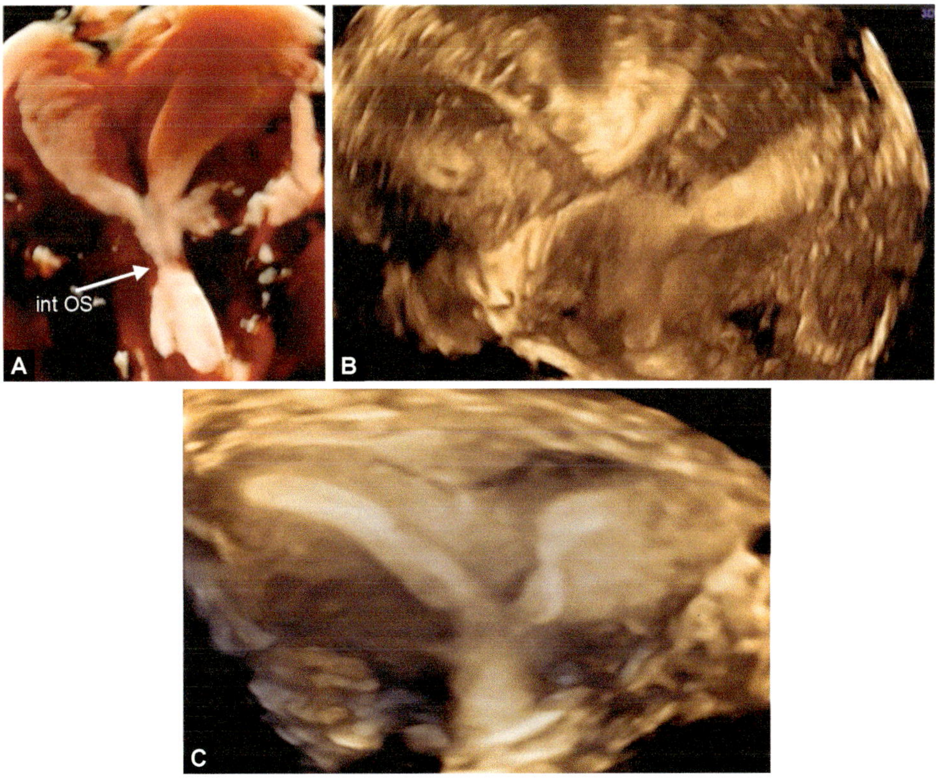

Figs. 4A to C: (A) Partial bicorporeal; (B) Complete bicorporeal; (C) Bicorporeal septate uterus on 3D ultrasound.

Arcuate uterus ***(Figs. 5A and B)***: Uterus is called arcuate when indentation in the endometrial cavity is <50% of the myometrial wall thickness with normal fundal contour. This is no more considered an abnormal shape. Evidently, it does not require any treatment.

- *Class U4*: Hemi uterus (unicornuate uterus) **(Figs. 6A and B)**:

Its subclasses are: (1) With rudimentary horn and (2) without rudimentary horn.

Unicornuate uterus is seen in 6–20% of all congenital uterine malformations. About 90% of patients having hemi uterus have rudimentary horn but it may be communicating or noncommunicating with the well-formed cornu. The rudimentary horn should be removed in case of hematometra, ectopic pregnancy, or severe dysmenorrhea. In 40% of cases, these are associated with renal anomalies.

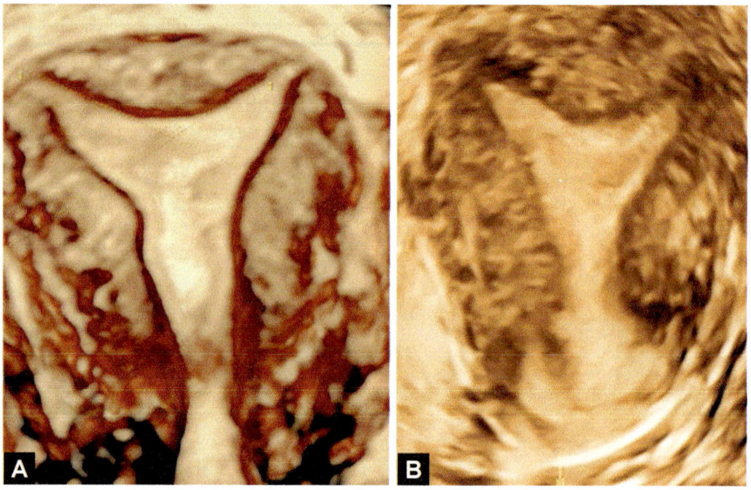

Figs. 5A and B: Arcuate uterus on 3D ultrasound.

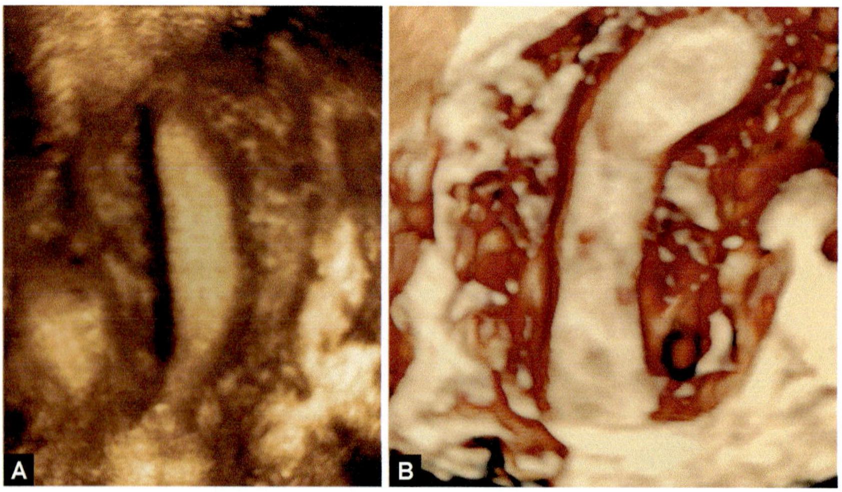

Figs. 6A and B: Unicornuate uterus.

It has the worst outcome amongst all congenital uterine malformations.[2] Fetal loss can be up to 40–45% before completion of the second trimester. Preterm deliveries are extremely common. Abortions are due to abnormal vasculature, decreased muscle mass, and reduced space. Prophylactic cervical encerclage is extremely useful. Vaginal micronized progesterone is useful to prevent uterine contractions.

Acquired Causes (Figs. 7A to C)

- Myomas
- Polyps
- Intrauterine adhesions
- Cervical incompetence
- Chronic endometritis

Myoma (Fibroid)

The myomas that are considered to affect pregnancy prognosis are:

- Submucous myomas >2 cm in size. ESHRE guidelines surprisingly concludes that there is insufficient evidence supporting the hysteroscopic removal of submucous fibroid in RPL.[4]
- Intramural myomas >4 cm—disturb endometrial vascularity. Surgery for myoma of >4 cm diameter also remains controversial according to certain workers. Though they agree that presence of multiple fibroids is a significant predictor one or more pregnancy loss.
- Though any myoma touching the endometrium can cause abortion because of interference with vascular supply and distortion of endometrial cavity.
- Myomas are more commonly associated with mid-trimester losses, and resecting the fibroids that distort the endometrial cavity can double the live birth rate in subsequent pregnancies.[9]

Myomas adversely affect pregnancy development because of altered uterine contractility, disturbances in endometrial cytokine expression, abnormal vascularization and chronic endometrial inflammation. Mechanical stretching of the endometrium leads to difference in the gene-expression and HOXA 10 levels are reduced. But receptivity related gene-expression is not affected and ART success rate is not altered.[10]

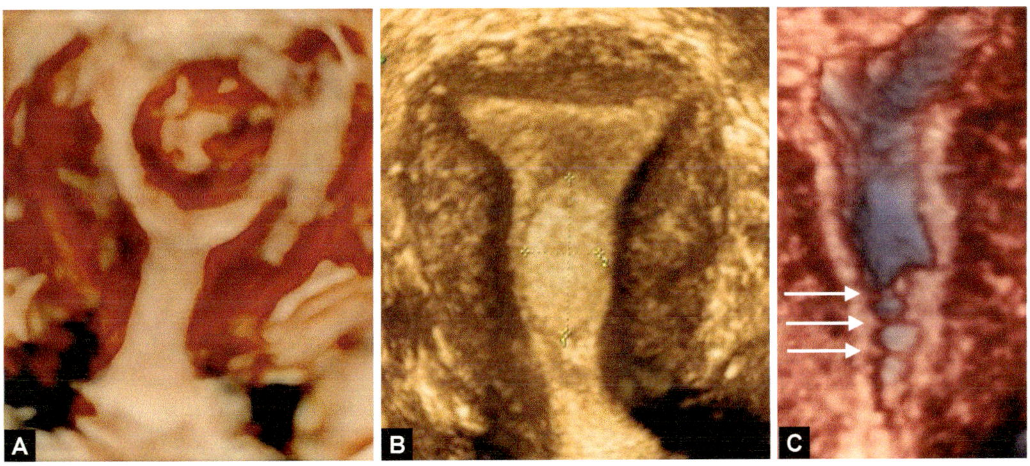

Figs. 7A to C: (A) Endometrial fibroid on 3D ultrasound; (B) Endometrial polyp; (C) Intrauterine adhesions on 3D ultrasound.

Myomectomy should be done by endoscopy. Laparoscopy-assisted myomectomy (LAM) is very popular. Myomectomy is preferred over uterine artery embolization if fertility is to be preserved because embolization can cause transient ovarian failure, endometrial atrophy, and amenorrhea. MRI-guided focused high-frequency ultrasound (HIFU) ablation has been proved by the United States Food and Drug Administration (US FDA) as an effective treatment option.

Polyps

Polyp is usually not a cause of RPL. But when RPL is present and no other cause than polyp is found, the polyp should be removed. Chronic inflammation and polyp may act as foreign body and therefore lead to abortion. If polypectomy is done with resectoscope, the recurrence rate is very low, and if done with polyp forceps, the recurrence rate is approximately 17%. Bipolar forceps can also be used.

In up to 27% of cases of spontaneous abortion, spontaneous resolution of polyp is documented. Polyp affects fertility by mechanical interference and at molecular level by increasing glycodelin aromatase and inflammation markers. There is insufficient data to recommend its surgical removal for recurrent pregnancy loss.

Intrauterine Adhesions

These are expected to be more common among patients with RPL. About 21% of patients had intrauterine adhesions who otherwise had no cause for three abortions.[11] Hysteroscopic surgery may be beneficial.

ESHRE and ASRM guidelines conclude that there is insufficient evidence of a benefit by surgical removal of intrauterine adhesions in women with RPL. However, removal of mild-to-moderate adhesions have positive impact on subsequent fertility.

Cervical Incompetence

Congenital cervical incompetence is more common as compared to iatrogenic as surgeries on the cervix such as Manchester's operation and cone biopsy of the cervix, are now rarely done.

History of ruptured membranes without pain and setting in of labor is the most common presentation. Easy passage of No. 8 Hegar's dilator is diagnostic of cervical incompetence. But now US has replaced Hegar's test as well as HSG.

Chronic endometritis: Low grade persistent inflammation of the endometrial lining is chronic endometritis due to altered endometrial microbiota. It may be asymptomatic or with mild symptoms such as abnormal uterine bleeding, pelvic discomfort and leukorrhea. Diagnosis can be done by hysteroscopy by presence of focal or diffuse hyperemia and presence of micropolyps.[12]

Histopathology is the Gold standard. Presence of plasma cells in endometrial stroma by immunohistochemical staining with CD138 is simple and a reliable test. Chronic endometritis can cause infertility, implantation failure and RPL.[13]

Ongoing pregnancy rates can be improved by antibiotics. Chronic endometritis causes cellular and biochemical alterations, disturbing endometrial receptivity. Antibiotics are useful in improving live birth rate.[14]

Ultrasound findings:

- Cervical length < 3 cm **(Fig. 8A)**
- Funneling of internal os **(Fig. 8B)**
- Internal os diameter >1.5 cm in the first trimester and >2 cm in the second trimester
- Bulging membranes into the cervical canal through internal os
- Thinning of the anterior part of lower segment

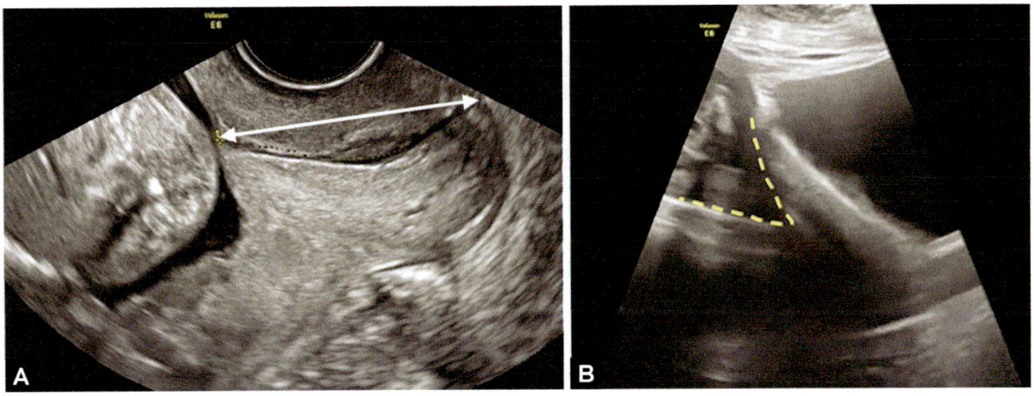

Figs. 8A and B: (A) Measurement of cervical length in pregnancy on transvaginal scan; (B) Dashed yellow line showing funneling of cervix.

- *Cervical index*: Funnel length + 1/Endo-cervical length. If the value is >0.52, it increases the chances of preterm labor.
- *Elastography*: This is a new modality assessing the elasticity or firmness of tissues. Soft cervix on elastography increases the risk of the opening of cervical canal with increasing fetal weight.

Dr Shirodkar (India) was the first person to suggest surgery for cervical incompetence in 1955. He recommended fascia lata for os tightening but now Merceline tape is used in its place. This is technically difficult; majority of the surgeons use McDonald's operation, in which silk is tied at the lower level without opening the vaginal wall. There are more than 10 different surgeries suggested but are not used routinely.

ANTIPHOSPHOLIPID SYNDROME

Definition: It is a triad of:

- Arterial/venous thrombosis
- RPL
- Thrombocytopenia with elevated levels of antiphospholipid (APL) antibodies, i.e., lupus antigen (LA) and/or anticardiolipin antibody (ACA)

This syndrome is systemic and affects all tissues and organs of the body.

Etiology

- There is no single specific cause for antiphospholipid syndrome (APS) but the combination of environmental, hormonal, and genetic factors is proposed and has genetic susceptibility.
- APL antibodies bind with β2 glycoprotein I (β2GPI) antigen, i.e., cofactor. This complex has an affinity for membrane phospholipids.
- Skin infections, human immunodeficiency virus (HIV), cytomegalovirus (CMV), TORCH (Toxoplasmosis, Other agents, Rubella, Cytomegalovirus, and Herpes simplex), pneumonia, hepatitis C, urinary tract infection (UTI), and *Helicobacter pylori (H. pylori)* are associated with APS. Molecular mimicry between β2GPI and bacterial and viral epitopes is the principal mechanism that links infection to APS.
- In false-positive tests for syphilis, only APL antibody is raised but in APS, β2GPI is recognized by raised antibody titer.

- There is no single specific cause for APS, but a combination of environmental, hormonal, and genetic factors is proposed.

Mechanism of Reproductive Failure in Antiphospholipid Syndrome

- *Thrombosis*:
  - Altered activity of platelets, fibrinolysis, coagulation cascade, and tissue factor
  - Complement activation has been recently proved.
  - APL inhibits arachidonic acid release and so prostaglandin I2 (PGI2) production is reduced.
  - Thromboxane A2 (TXA2)/PGI2 ratio is changed because of activation of platelets.
  - Systemic thromboembolism is the principal manifestation and placental vessel thrombosis may also occur.
- *Anticytokine effect*: Anti-inflammation cytokine interleukin 3 (IL3) is decreased and leads to fetal loss. Aspirin and ciprofloxacin can revert this.
- *Induction of placental apoptosis*: APL affects adhesion molecules between elements of syncytiotrophoblast and damages the trophoblasts. This effect is unrelated to thrombosis. So there is a role of steroid in early pregnancy loss. Cell adhesion molecule 1 (CAM1) and vascular cell adhesion molecule 1 (VCAM1) levels are increased and there is no protection to trophoblast.
- APL decreases human chorionic gonadotropin (hCG) production, and therefore supplementation of hCG is useful.
- Production of autoantibodies and so there is a role of immunoglobulins and steroids.
  - Autoantibodies to proteins C and S
  - Autoantibodies to plasmin and plasminogen
  - Autoantibodies to annexin V, which otherwise protects phospholipids
- APL antibodies can be directly toxic to the fetus.
- APL can reduce vascular endothelial growth factor (VEGF) which is corrected by heparin.

Diagnosis

Detection of Antiphospholipid (APL)

- *Not prolonging clotting*: Anticardiolipin (aCL), antiphosphatidylethanolamine (aPE), antiphosphatidylserine (aPS), antiphosphatidylcholine (aPC), antiphosphatidylglycerol (aPG),antiphosphatidylinositol (aPI) antiphosphatidic acid (aPA), and aβ2GPI
  - 1 APL unit = 1 μg/mL phospholipid-binding capacity
  - Antibody may be immunoglobulin G (IgG), IgM, IgA and called G phospholipids (GPL), M phospholipids (MPL), or APL.
- *Prolonging clotting assays*: Lupus anticoagulant (LA).

  These include:
  - Activated partial thromboplastin time (APTT)
  - Diluted Russel Viper Venom test (dRVVT)
  - Kaolin clotting time (KCT)

Diagnosis of Antiphospholipid Syndrome

For diagnosis of APS, at least one laboratory and one clinical criterion should be present.

Laboratory features:
- LA
- ACA

Laboratory results must be assessed twice at least 6 weeks apart.

Clinical features:

- Arterial, venous, or small vessel thrombosis
- *Pregnancy complications*:
  - Three abortions before 10 weeks, or
  - One abortion after 10 weeks or positron emission tomography (PET), or
  - Fetal growth restriction (FGR) with pregnancy at <34 weeks because of thrombosis, pregnancy-induced hypertension (PIH), pregnancy complications, and endometriosis.

Early losses are due to noninvading blood vessels and direct action on the trophoblast.

Types

Lupus anticoagulant and ACA independently increase the pregnancy loss. In reproductive autoimmune failure syndrome (RAFS), full APL panel should be measured. This includes LA, ACL, aPE, aPS, aPC, aPG, aPI, aPA, and aβ2GPI.

aPS and aPE are responsible for early loss as these affect trophoblastic functions. Here in isotype, high IgM may be due to infection and drugs. High IgG > 40 GPL is diagnostic and the patient will benefit from drug prophylaxis. Levels lower than 40 GPL have doubtful significance. Both IgM and IgG should be measured. The APL panel other than ACA has a controversial role and in clinical practice, only ACA is done.

Time of Testing

- The test should be performed during pregnancy or close to pregnancy loss.
- Increased titers of aPL must be present in serum in two measurements at the interval of 6 weeks.
- Occasionally, aCL may be high outside.
- β2 glycoproteins, aPS, and Annexin do not provide additional information and are not done routinely. But few centers include β2GPI for APL-related abortions.
- Antinuclear antibody (ANA) and antithyroid antibody (ATA) assays are not required in RPL because there is no logic or proven treatment and they have uncertain relevance.
- LA is more responsible for an adverse outcome than aCL.
- ACL is for late complications.

Treatment

- Aspirin 75 mg
- Heparin 20,000 IU
- Warfarin
- Hydroxychloroquine
- Prednisolone 40–60 mg
- Immunoglobulins
- Plasma exchange

Aspirin

Aspirin affects embryo implantation and placental development by modulating balance of thromboxane, prostaglandin, and IL3 production. Aspirin in a dose of 75 mg daily should be started as soon as the pregnancy is confirmed. Majority of papers believe that it is very useful, but several papers indicate that it has no role.[15,16] Low-dose aspirin is recommended by the ACOG Practice Committee Recommendations 2010. It is to be stopped 7 days before labor or surgery.

Heparin

Low molecular weight heparin (LMWH) is extremely useful and a standard treatment for APS. It should be started on confirmation of intrauterine pregnancy and it improves live birth rate by 80%. The dose of LMW heparin in RPL without a history of thrombosis is 1 mg/kg/day but when thrombosis is present the dose is doubled to 1 mg/kg/bd. This same dose is given when there is a history of previous loss after 10 weeks. For APS with early pregnancy losses (three or more), lower doses of 1 mg/kg/day are used. Heparin is stopped 12 hours before labor or surgery. A combination of heparin and aspirin gives better pregnancy rates than one of them alone.[17]

Although generally LMWH has no side effects, occasionally it may cause hemorrhage, osteopenia, and thrombocytopenia. LMWH does not cause overlap between anticoagulant and antithrombotic effects and so there is no bleeding and therefore there is a little need of monitoring. LMWH does not prolong partial thromboplastin time (PTT) and so is monitored by Factor Xa.

Mechanism of action of heparin:

- It has an anticoagulant effect.
- It binds directly to APL.
- Heparin inhibits complement activation.
- It has an antithrombotic effect.

Warfarin

Warfarin is to be avoided in the first trimester of pregnancy due to its teratogenic effect. But it can be used instead of heparin after the first trimester. It is cheaper than heparin, and complications of heparin such as osteopenia can be avoided. At the end of the third trimester, the patient should be shifted to heparin again.

Hydroxychloroquine

Hydroxychloroquine restores annexin A5 expression and has an antithrombotic effect. It can be used as an adjuvant therapy or for those patients who are resistant to heparin and aspirin combination. It is safe to use during pregnancy.

Glucocorticoids

- Glucocorticoid is very useful in patients having APS secondary to systemic lupus erythematosus (SLE).
- It has been found to be very useful in early pregnancy loss but should be stopped after 10 weeks.
- It also prevents complement activation which is proinflammatory and procoagulant.
- Corticosteroids correct defective decidualization that has occurred because of an increase in uterine natural killer (uNK) cell density. It reduces uNK cells and causes angiogenesis.[18]
- Corticosteroids are useful when ANA is present.

Intravenous Immunoglobulin

Intravenous immunoglobulin improves thrombogenicity in experimental APS. However, clinical trials have found that it is not more effective in preventing pregnancy loss than heparin with aspirin. Intravenous immunoglobulin (IVIG) is found to be more effective in late pregnancy complications such as PIH or intrauterine growth restriction (IUGR). Now it seems that IVIG may have a place as a second line of treatment in patients who are refractory to heparin or who suffer from late obstetric complication. But heparin and aspirin are to be continued. The dose of IVIG is 400–1,000 mg/kg daily for 5 days every month. Cost is prohibitive and it does not decrease the pregnancy loss better than heparin with aspirin.

Plasma Exchange

Plasma exchange can be used for patients refractory to heparin and aspirin treatment. It is given as one to four sessions in a week, throughout pregnancy.[19] But additional studies are warranted.

THROMBOPHILIA

In a nonpregnant state in a hemostatic pathway, there is equilibrium between:

- *Procoagulant factors*: Factors V, VII, VIII, and fibrinogen
- *Anticoagulant factors*: Protein C, Protein S, and antithrombin III
- *Fibrinolytic factors*: High PAI (plasminogen activator inhibitor) 1 and 2 genes

These are all shifted in favor of a procoagulant state during pregnancy.

Hereditary/congenital thrombophilia can be classified as follows:

- Antithrombin III deficiency
- Protein C deficiency
- Protein S deficiency

These are less common but more thrombogenic and there are others which are more common but weak thrombogenic factors. These are endogenous inhibitors of coagulation.

- *Factor V Leiden (FVL)*: Mutations/APCR (Northern Europe) (G1691A) are common but are rare in Asians and Africans.
- *Prothrombin G (20210A) mutations (Southern Europe)*:
  Methylenetetrahydrofolate reductase (MTHFR) (C677T): There is an increased level of the procoagulant factor. The risk is higher when it causes two mutations, A1298C and C6777T locus, in MTHFR.[20]
  - *Antithrombin III deficiency*: It is an inhibitor of thrombin and prevents the conversion of fibrinogen to fibrin. Antithrombin III has a thrombin-binding site and a heparin-binding site. The latter of the two has 100-fold higher antithrombin activity. As a large number of mutations are seen in the antithrombin III gene, its deficiency can be assessed by functional clot-based assays like thromboelastography.

What is Thromboelastography?

Hemostasis is a dynamic process of interaction between prothrombotic and antithrombotic cellular and plasma components. Measurement of any single factor is therefore not useful, but the net result of the process must be studied. Elastography assesses the whole process and decides if it is a hypo- or hypercoagulation state and so gives dynamic information.

- *Protein C deficiency*: Protein C is activated by thrombin to exert an anticoagulant effect. It inactivates factors Va and VIII. Protein C deficiency also can be diagnosed by a clot-based assay.
- *Protein S deficiency*: Protein S is a co-factor for Protein C and is Vitamin K dependent. It inactivates factors V and VII and requires a clot-based assay for diagnosis.
- *FVL mutations*: Substitution of glutamine from arginine at amino acid 506 in factor V protein abolishes the cleavage site for activated protein C, and so factor V is resistant to activated protein C. It is seen in 10–15% of people of Northern European origin. It is a single-point mutation. It has a weak thrombogenic potential but if it is a heterogeneous mutation, it is 3–8-fold more thrombogenic, and if homogeneous mutation it is 80-fold more thrombogenic.
- *Hereditary factor XIII deficiency*: Autosomal recessive trait. Its concentration decreases to 50% in normal pregnancy and only 0.5–2% is required for normal hemostasis. This is important for implantation and attachment of the placenta to uterus. Its deficiency affects fibrin-fibronectin cross-linking adversely. Recombinant factor XIII is available with a half-life of 10–12 days and is to be given in a dose of 20 IU/kg, once in every 4 weeks.

- *Fibrinogen deficiency*: This may present as afibrinogenemia, hypofibrinogenemia, or dysfibrinogenemia. The normal fibrinogen level to maintain pregnancy is 60 mg/100 mL. Its half-life is 4 days and its infusion in case of deficiency is given twice a week. It may lead to catastrophic thrombosis and therefore heparin is advocated.

Acquired Thrombophilia

Hyperhomocysteinemia

Homocysteine is an intermediate by-product formed during the metabolism of methionine. It generates H_2O_2 through its effect on endothelium and impairs endothelial cell thrombomodulin. Its modest elevation is described in association with inherited polymorphism of MTHFR with Vitamin B_{12} and folic acid deficiency. C to T mutations at nucleotide 677 in gene coding of MTHFR enzyme leaves only 30% of functionally active enzyme. This results in increased homocysteine levels and increases thrombogenicity by 2–3-fold.

Currently, identified thrombophilia is less common in African and Asian population. A meta-analysis from 31 studies found that thrombophilias are commonly associated with second- and third-trimester losses. Evidence says that thrombophilia predispose to a high risk of both early and late pregnancy loss. But reproductive performance is normal with thrombophilia in some patients. It is not possible to establish as to which patient with RPL has an increased risk with thrombophilia.

Pathophysiology of Pregnancy Loss in Thrombophilia

- Thrombosis in placental vessels in the second and third trimesters causes fetal loss.
- Placental contact of the spiral artery and placental intervillous space starts developing only after 8 weeks and therefore pregnancy loss before 10 weeks may not be related to hemostasis. Early pregnancy loss in patients with thrombophilia therefore cannot be explained.
- Fetal thrombophilia can cause thrombosis in fetal vessels. Paternal thrombophilia can also cause fetal vessel thrombosis when the fetus is homozygous or there is a combined maternal and paternal defect. Genetic mutation, therefore, increases the risk of pregnancy loss in subsequent pregnancies.
- Only a minority of patients with thrombophilia experience RPL. It is a combination of genetic and acquired risk factors usually.
- Though several studies have found no correlation of thrombophilia with pregnancy loss. It causes venous thrombosis and not arterial.
- FVL deficiency is usually responsible for third-trimester loss.
- Prothrombin 20210A mutation may lead to late trimester but nonrecurrent fetal loss.
- Protein S deficiency also causes late trimester fetal loss.
- MTHFR, Protein C, and antithrombin III deficiency are not associated with fetal loss.

It has been shown in a meta-analysis by Rey et al.[21] that:

- Thrombophilia increases fetal loss.
- However, not all thrombophilias are associated with fetal loss.
- First-trimester losses are associated with FVL, protein C deficiency, and prothrombin mutation. These are not recommended in patients of RPL.

- Late trimester losses are associated with FVL deficiency and prothrombin mutation.

Thrombophilia: To Conclude

- Thrombophilia increases the risk of pregnancy loss by 3–8-fold.
- Screening for thrombophilia is done in patients with three or more first-trimester losses after 8 weeks or in patients with two or more second-trimester losses or with past history or family history of RPL.
- Patients with unexplained stillbirth must also be screened.
- The patient should be counseled for the clinical uncertainty of the results and should be referred to a hematologist.
- For inherited thrombophilias, there is little evidence that treatment affects outcome of RPL and therefore, screening should be limited to patients who have personal or strong family history of venous thrombosis.[22]
- At present heparin or aspirin is recommended only for acquired thrombophilia, i.e., antiphospholipid syndrome.

Treatment

- *Prophylactic LMWH*: It is safe and has minimal risk of allergic reaction. It has high bioavailability and a long half-life with a predictable therapeutic response. It is given in a dose of 40 mg daily. Rarely, it may cause thrombocytopenia or osteoporosis. But it is not useful in unexplained RPL.

  Low molecular weight heparin therapy should be monitored by:
  - Baseline assessment of platelets, repeated after 1 week and repeated every month during therapy
  - Antifactor Xa levels are assessed for assessment of the drug response. But the results are not very consistent and so are less suitable to follow.
  - Tissue factor pathway inhibitor (TFPI) can also be used for monitoring LMWH therapy.
  - If the patient requires a regional anesthesia, the dose of LMWH is omitted for a day to prevent spinal hematoma.
- Aspirin is still an optional treatment. It is given in a dose of 100 g/day. But the majority of trials did not show a significant effect in unexplained RPL.
- Progesterone produces IL-4 cytotoxins and therefore Th2 response.
- hCG helps in cytokine production of the endometrium [tumor necrosis factor-alpha (TNF-α) and IL-4].

But heparin is preferred in patients with pregnancy loss after 10 weeks. Most of the times, both heparin and aspirin are combined. Heparin also has an anti-inflammatory effect. Its anti-inflammatory effect is by increasing serum TNF-α binding protein. Heparin inhibits TNF-α production. It has a direct effect on the trophoblast and increases hCG production.

More research is required to find out why only few women get pregnancy loss. There are some other factors that play a role in coagulation such as protein Z and vitamin K. These factors need further study. There are some more mutations that have been found to be responsible such as thrombomodulation gene, plasminogen activation gene, and factor V Cambridge mutation. These mutations also need further research to know their exact role.

GENETIC CAUSES

Genetic factors are common causes of sporadic abortions (50–80%) while single-gene defects are a common cause of birth defects. A Japanese study has shown that abnormal karyotype is the most common cause of recurrent miscarriage and only in 24.5% of patients with RPL, the cause was unexplained. In 41.1%, the cause is abnormal embryonic karyotype.[23] Comparative genomic hybridization (CGH) microassays [or multiplex fluorescence in situ hybridization (M-FISH)] also may show anomalies in abortus not found in karyotype.

Chromosomal abnormalities may be autosomal trisomy, double trisomy, polyploidy, tetraploidy, monosomy X, and sex chromosomal polysomy.

The question is: Does recurrent aneuploidy exist? Recurrent aneuploidy can be seen in certain families. So if the first abortus is abnormal, the chances of abnormal abortus is increased. Maternal age plays a major role. The higher the age, recurrent aneuploidy may be more possible. Structural chromosomal derangements include translocations and inversions which play a major role in repeated losses.

Balanced translocation is higher in females. There may be a history of stillborn or abnormal live born. There are two types of translocations: (1) Robertsonian and (2) reciprocal. In a couple having balanced translocation with RPL, preimplantation genetic diagnosis (PGD) should be offered. Other rare causes may be mendelian and polygenic or multifactorial etiology. There may be uniparental disomy (UPD) where the sole contribution is from a single parent.

It has been shown in a very interesting study that the cumulative chance of a healthy child is the same for carrier couples as for noncarrier couples, and therefore selective karyotyping is advised instead of offering karyotyping to all couples with RPL.[24] It is recommended only in unbalanced chromosomal abnormalities detected in fetal karyotype (RCOG). Parental karyotyping does not provide a diagnosis or prognosis for future outcome and treatment.

Place of Fetal Karyotyping in Recurrent Pregnancy Loss

- *In favor*:
  - Karyotyping of the abortus allows the patient to be given prognostic information regarding the subsequent outcome.
  - Aneuploidy report can save further investigations and treatment. It assures to have a better chance of normal embryo.
  - If repeated abnormal karyotype abortuses are found, PGD is offered.
- *Against*:
  - About 60–70% of women with unexplained RPL will have a successful next pregnancy.
  - As the number of miscarriages increases, the possibility of chromosomal abnormality decreases.
  - Current laboratory techniques are obstacles in making the diagnosis because of contamination and growth of maternal cells; cytogenic analysis is expensive. Histological features are not useful.
  - About >86% of chromosomally abnormal abortuses have numerical abnormality which occurs randomly and incidentally.
  - ACOG, RCOG, Royal College of Pathologists (RCPath), and international workshop (Denmark' 2002) do not advise karyotyping of abortus as a routine procedure.

Role of Preimplantation Genetic Diagnosis

- It is very expensive as the patient has to take in vitro fertilization (IVF)/

intracytoplasmic sperm injection (ICSI) cycles only.

- PGD does not perform better than expectant management.
- Even in couples who are carriers of structural chromosomal rearrangements, PGD does not improve pregnancy rates as compared to expectant management. So routine use of preimplantation genetic screening (PGS) and PGD is not justified in RPL.

ALLOIMMUNITY

Normal pregnancy requires maternal immunological recognition and response to paternally derived antigens on embryonic tissue, and abnormality in this response may lead to RPL. Large proportions of unexplained RPL (80%) may be due to immunological causes. In alloimmune abortions, the maternal immune system reacts against the embryo and damages trophoblasts through allogenic rejection-type reactions.

Apart from ANA and ATA, there is increase in CD19+ and CD5+ cells which produce antibodies against estradiol (E2), progesterone, hCG, and neurotransmitters such as endorphins and serotonin. These cause insufficient decidualization and decreased blood supply to endometrium. The genetic background of human leukocyte antigen (HLA)-DQAI*0505 sharing is found in patients with RPL. Th2 type reaction favors implantation while Th1 type causes the reaction. Progesterone from corpus luteum favors Th2 response. Increased NK cell activity favors abortion.

Immune Response in Normal Pregnancy

There is an immunological paradox of pregnancy because the embryo is not rejected even though it has genes inherited from the father. This is because facilitation reaction prevails over the rejection reaction.

This is because of:

- *Th2 type immune response instead of Th1 type response*: Th2 type cytokines (IL-4, IL-5, IL-10) predominate over Th1 type cytokines [IL2 and interferon-γ (IFN-γ)] and prevent antitrophoblast cytotoxic reaction. Granulocyte/macrophage colony stimulating factor (GM-CSF), IL-3, and transforming growth factor-beta (TGF-β) also favor implantation. Progesterone influences Th2 type response by inducing production of IL-4 by γδ T-lymphocytes.
- *Role of NK cells in monitoring pregnancy*: uNK cells are characteristically CD56 antigen. Peripheral NK (pNK) cells have CD16 and CD3 antigens. uNK cells participate in an alternative defense system against microbiological and malignant invasion called innate immune system. These are increased in luteal phase and may be due to progesterone. But they do not express progesterone receptors. Percentage of uterine NK cells dramatically increase to reach 70–80% of total leukocytes. Macrophages are 30% while T-cells decrease to 10% in response to estradiol and progesterone signals. Uterine NK cells are absent before menarche and after menopause. They have prolactin and estrogen receptors. uNK cells help decidualization of endometrial stroma and control trophoblast invasion. uNK cells become active and play a major role for the production of INF-γ and Th2 type reactions. The function of uNK cells is to regulate endometrial angiogenesis important for implantation.[25] It helps in placental augmentation and local immunosuppression and immunomodulation. uNK cells cause production

of an array of cytokines such as TNF-α, INF-α, leukemia inhibitory factor (LIF), and GM-CSF.

Direct antigen–receptor interactions between uNK cells and extravillous trophoblast occur[26] and polymorphism of uNK cell receptor and trophoblast antigen have been associated with RPL.[27] Defective decidualization correlates with high uNK cell density > 5% and a lack of 11-β-hydroxysteroid dehydrogenase type 1 in stromal cells.[28] 11-β-hydroxysteroid dehydrogenase type 1 activates cortisol; hence, the administration of glucocorticoid prednisolone may overcome this deficit and also reduce endometrial uNK cell density and production of angiogenic cytokines to help endometrial angiogenesis.[25] There is interaction with HLA-G molecule which is in placenta only. NK cells of conventional CD3–, CD56+, and CD16+ types are increased in abortion. They are also increased in blood. uNK cells do not express classical HLA antigens—HLA-C, HLA-G, and HLA-E. Placentation is regulated by interaction between maternal KIRs (killer cell immunoglobulin-like receptors) expressed by uterine NK cells and fetal HLA-C molecules expressed by EVT (extravillous trophoblast) cells. So at present, KIR and HLA-C are useful investigations.

To summarize, the role of uNK cells:

- These are hostile to invading trophoblast.
- These may facilitate abnormal blastocysts.
- More uNK cells mean a poor pregnancy outcome.

Diagnostic Tests

- Antipaternal lymphocytic antibodies
- Maternal blocking antibody
- HLA sharing
- Maternal immune suppression
- Mixed lymphocyte culture reactivity
- Peripheral blood NK cells

But these tests have no clinical utility.

The prognostic value of measuring pNK or uNK cell parameters in women with RPL remains uncertain as a predictive test for screening women who may benefit from immunotherapy.[29]

Treatment

- Active immunization of a woman using paternal or third-party lymphocytes. Cochrane review 2006 does not support this therapy. This therapy has only marginal benefits. According to the American Society for Reproductive Medicine (ASRM), it has a higher rate of side effects.
- Passive immunization by IVIG. It is very useful in increasing NK cells in peripheral blood. IVIG shifts to Th2 type response.
- IVIG appears to include CD200-dependent activity that results in suppression of NK cells. The dose is 0.5 g/kg at 5 weeks, followed by 0.35 g/kg every 3 weeks till 24 weeks. This treatment is very useful in very early abortions when NK cells are raised as it decreases NK cells and enhances CD8+ cell activity. Cochrane review does not support this therapy. Cytokines such as GM-CSF and TGF-β are the future. IVIG therapy requires documentation of immunological cause and absence of nonimmunogenic risk factors. It is more useful in patients who have not responded to aspirin, prednisolone, and heparin. The treatment should be started prior to conception or the previous day of embryo transfer.

Though several trials and meta-analyses concluded that IVIG is ineffective for primary RPL.[30]

How does IVIG act?

- It decreases the killing action of NK cells.
- It increases the activity of suppressor T-cells.
- It suppresses B-cell production of autoantibodies.
- It has antibodies to idiopathic antibodies.
- It binds with the Fc component of IgG.
- It decreases Th1 cytokine activity.

- Preconceptional prednisolone or intra-uterine prednisolone 20 mg/day from day 1–2 of the cycle for 4 weeks, prior to embryo transfer, has been recommended.
- High proportion of women with RPL have vitamin D deficiency and this has immunological implications in RPL. Vitamin D is associated with B and NK cell immunity and Th1/Th2 balance. Women with low vitamin D have a tendency to develop APA and other autoantibodies related to autoimmune disorders and poor reproductive outcome.[31]
- Cytokines GM-CSF and TGF-β are likely to replace parental leukocytes and IVIG.
- Intralipid administration intravenously enhances implantation and maintenance of pregnancy. It is 20% fat emulsion. It decreases NK cell cytotoxicity. Pregnancy rates were the same with intralipid when compared with IVIG.[30] But there are no published results for RPL.
- Progesterone and hCG favor Th2 > Th1.

Points against parental lymphocyte immunization:

- A meta-analysis of trials on paternal leukocytes immunization concluded that it had no beneficial effect.[32]
- Increased sharing of HLA class I alleles between partners has been refuted in a recent meta-analysis.[33]
- Hypothesis of blocking antibodies is not validated.
- Miscarriage occurs despite blocking antibody.
- A patient without blocking antibody has successful pregnancy.

Points against IVIG:

- The relation between peripheral blood NK cells and reproduction failure is most controversial.
- It is unclear regarding the number of NK cells which is abnormal.
- Rise in NK cells is mostly transient and not chronic.
- The beneficial effect is not observed and it is difficult to define who will be benefitted with IVIG.

Granulocyte Colony Stimulating Factor as Immunomodulator

- Both GM-CSF and granulocyte colony stimulating factor (G-CSF) stimulate bone marrow to produce granulocytes and stem cells released into blood stream. Receptors are found on the trophoblast and decidua and human placenta.
- In follicular fluid, it helps in improving oocyte competence and implantation potential of the embryo.
- It is useful in idiopathic RPL.
- Dose is 1 μg/kg from the sixth day of ovulation to menstruation, or 9 weeks of gestation gives a live birth rate of 82.8% compared to 48%.[34]

INFECTIONS AND RECURRENT PREGNANCY LOSS

The role of infection in RPL is unclear. Various infections quoted in the literature are:

- Tuberculous
- Listerioses
- TORCH
- Chlamydia
- Syphilis

- Bacterial vaginosis
- Mycoplasmas

  Infections are not the cause of RPL.

  Investigations of TORCH and other organisms should be abandoned (RCOG Guidelines, 2011).

ENVIRONMENTAL FACTORS

- Smoking
- Alcohol
- Heavy coffee
- Anesthetic gases
- Heavy metals
- Herbicide
- Radiation
- Electromagnetic field
- Wilson's disease
- Chemicals
- *Obesity*: Obesity in pregnancy is defined as a body mass index (BMI) of 30 kg/m^2 or more at the first antenatal visit. The risk of early miscarriage is more with obese patients rather than with BMI < 30 kg/m^2. The reason for abortion is either poor endometrial development or poor oocyte quality. There is increased production of inflammatory and prothrombotic agents. Plasminogen activator inhibitory type I is increased in obese mothers which is associated with an increased risk of miscarriage.

The role of these factors in causing RPL is not proved; these factors may have a supporting role for pregnancy loss. Change in lifestyle may also be recommended in patients with RPL.

Serum ferritin level is inversely related to number of previous pregnancy losses in patients of RPL. So women with low ferritin level may benefit from iron therapy and iron status should be evaluated in patients of RPL.[35]

ENDOMETRIOSIS

Milder cases of endometriosis have the highest risk for causing pregnancy loss as these are functionally more active. Spontaneous abortion rate decreases after treatment. But sufficient data is not yet available for considering it as a cause of RPL. It causes progesterone resistance by changing the expression of estrogen receptors and so does not respond to progesterone therapy.

Endometriosis have more effect on spontaneous pregnancy than pregnancy with ART. In spontaneous pregnancy, it affects oocyte quality by pelvic toxic factors during temporary exposure while passing through the tube. It increases the risk of aneuploidy. In endometriosis because of progesterone resistance there is inflammation-mediated histological changes. There is estrogen receptor dominance in secretory phase. It is the root cause of impaired implantation because of altered endometrial receptivity. Aromatase is over expressed and increases E2 level which inihibits beta3 integrins which is for implantation.

Endometriosis can act through:

- *Local factors*:
  - Alteration in meiotic spindle
  - Endometrial stromal cell proliferation
  - High macrophage cytotoxicity
  - High cytokine
  - Low NK cell activity
- *Systemic factors*:
  - Raised immunoglobulin production
  - More T1 helper cells
  - Embryotoxicity
  - Suppression of NK cells
  - Low cell immunity
  - Abnormal autoimmune function

Current recommendations are to offer freeze all and deferred embryo transfer strategy in endometriosis. (Bishop et al. observed no difference in pregnancy outcome in cases of FET of euploid blastocysts in patients with endometriosis with their counter part undergoing ART for male factor.[36]

Adenomyosis alters the normal response to progesterone because of cellular and biochemical alteration because of inflammatory process. It is like endometriosis. It affects uterine contractions and endometrial peristalsis. GnRHa can reduce junctional zone thickness but future pregnancy outcomes is not validated.

PSYCHOLOGICAL CAUSES

Role of stress:

- Stress-related hormones have an endocrine role and affect placental hormones.
- They have autocrine and paracrine roles.
- Hypothalamo-pituitary-ovarian axis reacts to anxiety and depression.
- Secretion of catecholamines plays a vital role in steroidogenesis.
- Peripheral NK cells are increased.

Patient's perspective:

- The need for children is more intense than to live.
- Because of depression and anxiety, it disturbs personal relation, sexual life, and quality of life.
- There is fear of the next pregnancy which aggravates all symptoms.

Role of tender loving care (TLC):

- Limbic system is the seat of emotional activity.
- There is a link between the limbic system and the immune system.
- The immune system prevents implantation.
- TLC creates lifelong bond and helps in preventing pregnancy loss.
- Narrating the fact that the risk of recurrent miscarriage is 25–30% after three miscarriages means that 75% deliver normally even without treatment, and the chances of a successful full-term pregnancy after three abortions being 55–60% give considerable mental relief and psychological support to the patient. Psychological support definitely increases live birth rates. Psychological support can be added by meeting other patients of RPL, recommending activities that reduce anxiety, teaching relaxation methods, and counseling.

"ESHRE special interest group concluded that the only interventions that do not require more randomized controlled trials are TLC and health advice."[37]

ENDOCRINE CAUSES

- Hypohyperthyroidism
- Diabetes mellitus
- Luteal phase defect (LPD)
- Hyperprolactinemia
- Polycystic ovarian syndrome (PCOS)

Thyroid

There is no direct evidence that subclinical hypo- or hyperthyroidism causes RPL.[38] Antithyroid antibodies may be high due to autoimmune causes. Though it has been shown that a transient impairment of thyroid function in early pregnancy may cause inadequate adaptation to the increased thyroid requirement and may be implicated in RPL.[39]

Recently, the upper limit of thyroid-stimulating hormone (TSH) that has been revised is 2.5 IU/L for subclinical hypothyroidism. Clinical practice guidelines by the American Association of Clinical Endocrinologist and Antithyroid Association state that antithyroid peroxidase (TPO) and antithyroglobulin (TG) measurements should be considered during the evaluation of RPL. They suggest that in patients of normal TSH with the presence of anti-TPO, L-thyroxine should be given if there is a history of miscarriage. But in few studies, there is no statistical difference in RPL. Hyperthyroidism is not correlated with infertility and RPL. However, the affected mother has an increased rate of miscarriage. But it is not confirmed that it causes RPL.

Diabetes Mellitus

- High glycated hemoglobin (HbA1c) in the first trimester can cause abortion or malformation.
- In the uncontrolled group, pregnancy loss is high and it can cause infertility.
- HbA1c assessment should be done for patients with RPL (ASRM guidelines).
- It is recommended to maintain at <7.5.
- Approximately 5–14% of patients with a diagnosis of type 2 diabetes mellitus have diabetes associated auto-antibodies. So screening of these antibodies in RPL is a new horizon in RPL.

Luteal Phase Defect

It has been shown that increased uterine artery resistance may be a contributing factor to some causes of RPL.[40,41] Here we shall discuss LPD in relation to RPL only. Literature quotes incidence of LPD between 23% and 60%.

- Transvaginal sonography (TVS) with Doppler can give information regarding impaired uterine perfusion and this can be used as a screening test in RPL.
- High pulsatility index (PI) is related to low estradiol (E2) and progesterone (P).
- Mid luteal phase Doppler is informative and important.
- Low-dose aspirin and omega 3 fatty acids are effective in improving uterine artery blood flow velocity in women with recurrent miscarriage due to abnormal uterine perfusion.[42]

Role of Progesterone Supplementation in Recurrent Pregnancy Loss

- It creates the environment for implantation.
- It corrects abnormal progesterone secretion.
- It acts on the immune system and causes cytokine synthesis and function of NK cells.
- Th2 dominance (IL-10) response is created by progesterone and progesterone decrease in Th1 cytokines (IL-2, IFN-γ).
- Periconceptional progesterone is more effective if administered during the luteal phase before confirmation of pregnancy in patients of RPL. This may be because of the immunomodulatory effect of progesterone.[43]

Progesterone Supplementation

Progesterone-induced blocking factor (PIBF) expression was less in patients who aborted than the healthy pregnant women. For donor oocyte programs also, progesterone is given for 8 weeks.

As the diagnosis of LPD is very difficult to establish, progesterone should be given in suspected cases or on an empirical basis. The argument in favor of empirical therapy is that it prevents a 33% miscarriage rate when it is given to 100% of patients. Follicular-maturing drugs may not correct the luteal phase, but progesterone supplementation reduced the miscarriage rate from 28 to 6%.[44,45] Progesterone is started after ovulation which is the preconceptional stage.

Whenever serum progesterone is <8 ng/mL, progesterone supplementation will salvage 60% of pregnancies.[46] So with lower serum progesterone pregnancy, wastage is high. A recent Cochrane review evaluating 15 trials concluded that there was a benefit to the routine administration of progesterone to all the women with a history of RPL.[47] Therefore, it is very convincing that it is better to give benign treatment that is later found not effective rather than not to treat her.

My personal opinion is to give progesterone to all patients of RPL, particularly when ovulation-inducing drugs are used, or in patients of RPL when loss occurs very early in pregnancy.

Human Chorionic Gonadotropin Supplementation

Patients with LPD are more likely to have early pregnancy losses before the appearance of fetal cardiac activity. hCG supplementation is particularly useful in patients with oligomenorrhea.[48,49] Majority of these women have PCOS. LPD is common in PCOS patients and so hCG supplementation is justified. If we stick to early pregnancy loss and oligomenorrhea, 30% of patients with RPL are in this group and hCG supplementation gives favorable results in 85% of these patients.[50]

I have been using hCG for LPD since the last 30 years and a combination of progesterone and hCG since the last 18 years as progesterone was introduced in India only 18 years back.

Hyperprolactinemia and Pregnancy Loss

A high prolactin level interferes with corpus luteum function. A high prolactin level in the follicular phase interferes with progesterone secretion in the luteal phase. Patients with hyperprolactinemia, treated with bromocriptine, have better chances of a successful pregnancy. Therefore, the normal level of prolactin may play an important role in the growth and implantation of the early embryo. But its role in RPL requires further studies.

Polycystic Ovarian Syndrome

Pregnancy loss in RPL is because of high LH, which in turn causes high androgen and high insulin levels. These are detrimental to ova and embryo and lead to a poor implantation rate and a high early miscarriage rate. Ovarian drilling is very useful in reducing pregnancy loss as it decreases LH levels. An antagonist can be used in thin, lean PCOS to prevent early pregnancy loss or infertility. The role of metformin is debatable at present. Majority of the studies have shown that metformin has no role in ovulation induction or to prevent pregnancy loss. Metformin actually should be stopped during pregnancy as it crosses the placenta. It does not decrease early pregnancy loss.

MALE FACTOR

Significant DNA fragmentation, abnormal sperm morphology, and decreased scores of sperm function tests are found in the male partners of patients with RPL. Sperms do not have the power of endogenous DNA repair. Damaged DNA is a major source of embryonic mortality. Spermatozoa is vulnerable to reactive oxygen species (ROS) as it has less cytoplasm and so limited supply of antioxidants. Also, plasma membrane is rich in unsaturated fatty acids and so it is vulnerable to oxidative stress.

There are two tests that are required:

1. *DNA fragmentation index (DFI)*: The men may have normal sperm morphology

in spite of damaged DNA. This causes alteration in sperm quality, function, implantation, and early embryonic development. But damaged DNA does not prevent zygote formation. Sperm DNA fragmentation decreases after varicocele repair. Defects in DNA methylation, genetic mutations and epigenetic mutations in sperm increases susceptibility to RPL.[51]

Sperm with high DNA fragmentations are treated by ICSI and it may compensate for lower pregnancy rate. Sperm sorting helps in selecting optimal sperm function is useful in patients of RPL. It is done by: (i) microfluidics, (ii) magnetic-activated cell sorting (MACS), and (iii) fluorescence-activated cell sorting. (FACS). Sperm selection technique like IMSI (intracytoplasmic morphologically selected sperm) and hyaluronidase binding assay (HA) with ICSI has not shown promising results. All other sperm selection techniques including MACS and zeta sperm selection has no impact on pregnancy, miscarriage or live birth.

2. *FISH for evaluating sperm aneuploidy*: There is no association between sperm DNA fragmentation and sperm aneuploidy. Sperm aneuploidy increases with chemotherapy agents and environmental pollutants. The incidence of aneuploidy increases with surgically removed sperms from testis.[52] About 40% of men with RPL have sperm aneuploidy. In these patients, IVF with PGS is recommended. Count less than 10 million have a higher aneuploidy rate. But despite 50 years of innovation and progress, we are no closer to understanding the mechanisms of the contribution of male factor to pregnancy loss. So routine testing of DFI and FISH is not recommended according to the practice committee of ASRM 2012.

LIST OF INVESTIGATIONS FOR RECURRENT PREGNANCY LOSS

The RCOG protocol, ASRM protocol, and ESHRE protocol differ in asking for certain investigations or treatment of RPL.

- *Anatomical*: 3D of the uterus—3D ultrasound
- *APS*:
  - Lupus anticoagulant
  - APTT
  - dRVVT
  - KCT
  - ACA ANA β_2 glycoprotein
  - APL antibodies
- *Genetic (karyotyping)*:
  - Male
  - Female
  - Fetus
- *Endocrine*:
  - Baseline scan day 2–3
  - Midluteal scan, mid-luteal progesterone
  - Triiodothyronine (T3), thyroxine (T4), TSH
  - Blood sugar
  - Insulin resistance, Hb1c
  - Prolactin
  - Minor preoperative profile
- *Alloimmunity*:
  - Anti-HLA antibody
  - NK cell activity
  - HLA sharing
  - Homocysteine
- *Thrombophilia*:
  - Protein C
  - Protein S
  - Antithrombin
  - FVL
  - Factor I L

CARRY HOME MESSAGE

- *Anatomical*:
  - *Congenital*:
    - Expectant management
    - Cervical encerclage
    - Septum resection
  - *Acquired*:
    - Removal of fibroid (intramural >4 cm, sub-endometrial >2 cm) or polyps
    - Cervical encerclage
- *Antiphospholipid syndrome*:
  - Aspirin 75 mg/day
  - LMWH 60 mg/day
  - Prednisolone 10 mg qds in selected patients
  - hCG 5,000 IU twice a week
  - IVIG 0.35 g/kg every 3 weeks (in resistant patients)
- *Genetic causes*:
  - Fetal karyotyping is not required
  - Parental karyotyping in cases of affected fetus
  - Chorion biopsy or PGD for translocations
- *Alloimmunity*:
  - Micronized vaginal progesterone 400 mg TDS
  - Parenteral or third-party lymphocytes are not recommended because of only marginal benefit.
  - hCG 5,000 IU twice a week
  - IVIG 0.5 g/kg followed by 0.35 g/kg every 3 weeks in very early losses
- *Infections*: They are not a cause of RPL.
- *Environmental*: They are not a cause of RPL.
- *Endometriosis*: They are not a cause of RPL.
- *Psychological*:
  - TLC
  - Health advice
- *Endocrine*:
  - *LPD*:
    - Micronized vaginal progesterone
    - hCG 5,000 IU twice a week
  - *PCOS*:
    - Ovarian drilling
    - Antagonist and/or chronic low-dose FSH stimulation protocol
    - Micronized vaginal progesterone
    - hCG 5,000 IU twice a week
- *Hereditary—Thrombophilia*: LMWH 40–80 mg/day

REFERENCES

1. The Practice Committee of American Society of Reproductive Medicine. Evaluation and treatment of recurrent pregnancy loss: a committee opinion. Fertil Steril. 2012;98:1103-11.
2. The American Fertility Society classification of adnexal adhesions, distal tubal occlusion secondary to tubal ligation, tubal pregnancies, Müllerian anomalies and intrauterine adhesions. Fertil Steril. 1998;49:944-55.
3. Grimbizis GF, Gordts S, Di Spiezio Sardo A, Brucker S, De Angelis C, Gergolet M, et al. The ESHRE/ESGE consensus on the classification of female genital tract congenital anomalies. Human Reprod. 2013;28(8):2032-44.
4. ESHRE Guideline Group on RPL; Atik RB, Chrstisnsen OB, Elson J, Kolte AM, Lewis S, et al. ESHRE guideline: recurrent pregnancy loss. Hum Reprod Open. 2018;2018(2):hoy004.
5. Salim R, Regan L, Woelfer B, Backos M, Jurkovic D. A comparative study of the morphology of congenital uterine anomalies in women with and without a history recurrent first trimester miscarriage. Hum Reprod. 2003;18:162-6.
6. Homer HA, Li TC, Cooke ID. The septate uterus: a review of management and reproductive outcome. Fertil Steril. 2000;73:1-14.
7. Heinonen PK. Complete septate uterus with longitudinal vaginal septum. Fertil Steril. 2006;85:700-5.
8. Sentilhes L, Sergent F, Roman H, Verspyck E, Marpeau L. Late complications of operative hysteroscopy: predicting patients at risk of uterine rupture during subsequent pregnancy. Eur J Obstet Gynecol Reprod Biol. 2005;120:134-8.
9. Saravelos SH, Yan J, Hassan R, Tin-Chiu Li. The prevalence and impact of fibroids and their treatment on the outcome of pregnancy in women with recurrent miscarriage. Hum Reprod. 2011;26(12):3274-9.
10. Horcajadas JA, Goryri E, Higon MA, Martinez-Conejero JA, Gambadauro P, Garcia G, et al. Endometrial receptivity and implantation are not affected by the presence of uterine intramural lieomyomas: a clinical and functional genomics analysis. J Clin Endocrinol Metab. 2008;93:3490-8.

11. Ventolini G, Zhang M, Gruber J. Hysteroscopy in the evaluation of patients with recurrent pregnancy loss: a cohort study in a primary care population. Surg Endosc. 2004;18:1782-4.
12. Moreno I, Cicinelli E, Garcia-Grau I, Gonzalez-Monfort M, Bau D, Vilella F, et al. The diagnosis of chronic endometritis in infertile asymptomatic women: a comparative study of histology, microbial cultures, hysteroscopy, and molecular microbiology. Am J Obstet Gynecol. 2018; 218 (6):602.e1-602.e16.
13. Kimura F, Takebayashi A, Ishida M, Nakamura A, Kitazawa J, Morimune A, et al. Review: chronic endometritis and its effect on reproduction. J Obstet Gynaecol Res. 2019;45(5):951-60.
14. McQueen DB, Perfetto CO, Hazard FK, Lathi RB. Pregnancy outcomes in women with chronic endometritis and recurrent pregnancy loss. Fertil Steril. 2015;104: 927-31.
15. Pattison NS, Chamley LW, Birdsal M, Zanderigo AM, Liddell HS, McDougall J. Does aspirin have a role in improving pregnancy outcome for women with the antiphospholipid syndrome? A randomised controlled trial. Am J Obstet Gynecol. 2000;183:1008-12.
16. Cowchock S, Reece EA. Do low risk pregnant women with antiphospholipid antibodies need to be treated? Organising Group of the Antiphospholipid Treatment Trial. Am J Obstet Gynecol. 1997;176:1099-100.
17. Kutteh WH. Antiphospholipid antibody-associated recurrent pregnancy loss: treatment with heparin and low dose aspirin is superior to low dose aspirin alone. Am J Obstet Gynecol. 1996;174:1584-9.
18. Triolo G, Ferrante A, Ciccia F, Accardo-Palumbo A, Perino A, Castelli A. Randomized study of subcutaneous low molecular weight heparin plus aspirin versus intravenous immunoglobulin in the treatment of recurrent fetal loss associated with antiphospholipid antibodies. Arthritis Rheum. 2003;48:728-31.
19. Frampton G, Cameron JS, Thom M, Jones S, Raftery M. Successful removal of antiphospholipid antibody during pregnancy using plasma exchange and low dose prednisolone. Lancet. 1987;2:1023-4.
20. Yajuan X, Ban Y, Ran L, Yu Y, Zhai S, Sun Z, et al. Relationship between unexplained recurrent pregnancy loss and 5,10-methylenetetrahydrofolate reductase) polymorphisms. Fertil Steril. 2019;111(3):597-603.
21. Rey E, Kahn SR, David M, Shrier I. Thrombophillic defect and fetal loss: a meta-analysis. Lancet. 2003;361:901-8.
22. American college of Obstetricians and Gynecologists' Committee on Practice Bulletins-Obstetrics. ACOG Practice Bulletin No. 197: Inherited Thrombophilias in Pregnancy. Obstet Gynecol. 2018; 132(1):e18-34.
23. Sugira-Ogasawara M, Ozaki Y, Katano K, Suzumori N, Kitaori T, Mizutani E. Abnormal embryonic karyotype is the most frequent cause of recurrent miscarriage. Hum Reprod. 2012;27(8):2297-303.
24. van den Boogaard E, Hermens RPMG, Verhoeve HR, Kremer JAM, van der Veen F, Knegt AC, et al. Selective karyotyping in recurrent miscarriage: are recommended guidelines adopted in daily clinical practice? Hum Reprod. 2011;26(8):1965-70.
25. Quenby S, Nik H, Innes B, Lash G, Turner M, Drury J, et al. Uterine natural killer cells and angiogenesis in recurrent reproductive failure. Hum Reprod. 2009;24:45-54.
26. Moffett-King A. Natural killer cells and pregnancy. Nat Rev Immunol. 2002;2;656-63.
27. Hiby SE, Regan L, Lo W, Farrel L, Carrington M, Moffett A. Association of maternal killer-cell immunoglobulin-like receptors and parental HLA-C genotypes with recurrent miscarriage. Hum Reprod. 2008;23:972-6.
28. Kuroda K, Venkatakrishnan R, Salker MS, Lucas ES, Shaheen F, Kuroda M, et al. Induction of 11-β-hydroxyl steroid dehydrogenase type 1 and activation of distinct mineralocorticoid receptor and glucocorticoid receptor-dependent gene networks in decidualizing human endometrial stromal cells. Mol Endocrinol 2012;27:192-202.

29. Tang AW, Alfirevic Z, Quenby S. Natural killer cells and pregnancy outcomes in women with recurrent miscarriage and infertility: a systematic review. Hum Reprod. 2011;26(8):1971-80.
30. Ata B, Tan SL, Shehata F, Holzer H, Buckett W. A systematic review of intravenous immunoglobulin for treatment of unexplained recurrent miscarriage. Fertil Steril. 2011;95: 1080-5.
31. Ota K, Dambaeva S, Ae-Ra Han, Beaman K, Gilman-Sachs A, Kwak-Kim J. Vitamin D deficiency may be a risk factor for recurrent pregnancy loss by increasing cellular immunity and autoimmunity. Hum Reprod. 2014;29(2):208-19.
32. Porter TF, LaCoursiere Y, Scott JR. Immunotherapy for recurrent miscarriage. Cochrane Database Syst Rev. 2014;2014(10): CD000112.
33. Beydoun H, Saftlas AF. Association of human leukocyte antigen sharing with recurrent spontaneous abortions. Tissue Antigens. 2005;65:123-35.
34. Scarpellini F, Sbracia M. Use of granulocyte colony-stimulating factor for the treatment of unexplained recurrent miscarriage: a randomised controlled trial. Hum Reprod. 2009;24:2703-8.
35. Georgsen M, Krog MC, Korsholm AS, Hvidman HW, Kolte AM, Rigas AS, et al. Serum ferritin level is inversely related to number of previous pregnancy losses in patients of RPL. Fertil Steril. 2021;115(2): 389-95.
36. Bishop LA, Gunn J, Jahandideh S, Devine K, Decherney AH, Hill MJ. Endometriosis does not impact live-birth rates in frozen embryo transfers of euploid blastocysts. Fertil Steril. 2021;115:416-22.
37. Jaunianx E, Farquarson RG, Christiansen OB, Exalto N. Evidence-based guidelines for investigation and medical treatment of recurrent miscarriage. Hum Reprod. 2006;21:2216-22.
38. Bernardi LA, Cohen RN, Stephenson MD. Impact of subclinical hypothyroidism in women with recurrent early pregnancy loss. Fertil Steril. 2013;100(5):1326-31.
39. Lago AD, Vaquero E, Pasqualetti P, Lazzarin N, Carolis CD, Perricone R, et al. Prediction of early pregnancy maternal thyroid impairment in women affected with unexplained recurrent miscarriage. Hum Reprod. 2011;26(6):1324-30.
40. Lazzarin N, Vaquero E, Exacoustos C, Romanini E, Amadio A, Arduini D. Mid-luteal phase Doppler assessment of uterine artery blood flow in nonpregnant women having a history of recurrent spontaneous abortions: correlation to different etiologies. Fertil Steril. 2007;87;1383-7.
41. Habara T, Nakatsuka M, Konishi H, Asagiri K, Noguchi S, Kudo T. Elevate blood flow resistance in uterine arteries of women with unexplained recurrent pregnancy loss. Hum Reprod. 2002;17(1):190-4.
42. Lazzarin N, Vaquero E, Exacoustos C, Bertonotti E, Romanini ME, Arduini D. Low-dose aspirin and omega 3 fatty acids improve uterine artery blood flow velocity in women with recurrent miscarriage due to impaired uterine perfusion. Fertil Steril. 2009;92(1):296-300.
43. Stephenson MD, McQueen Dana, Winter M, Bertonotti E, Romanini ME, Arduini D. Luteal phase vaginal micronized progesterone improves pregnancy success in women with recurrent pregnancy loss. Fertil Steril. 2017;107:84-94.
44. Check JH, Nowroozi K, Wu CH, Adelson HG, Lauer C. Ovulation inducing drugs versus progesterone therapy for infertility in patients with luteal phase defects. Int J Fertil. 1988;33:252-6.
45. Check JH, Chase JS, Wu CH, Adelson HG, Teichman M, Rankin A. The efficacy of progesterone in achieving successful pregnancy: I. Prophylactic use during luteal phase in anovulatory women. Int J Fertil. 1987;32:15-8.
46. Choe JK, Check JH, Nowroozi K, Benveniste R, Barnea ER. Serum progesterone and 17-hydroxyprogesterone in the diagnosis of ectopic pregnancies and the value of progesterone replacement in intrauterine pregnancies when serum progesterone levels are low. Gynecol Obstet Invest. 1992;34:133-8.

47. Haas DM, Ramsey PS. Progestogen for preventing miscarriage. Cochrane Database Syst Rev. 2008;(4):CD003511.
48. Quenby S, Farquharson RG. Human chorionic gonadotrophin supplementation in recurring pregnancy loss: a controlled trial. Fertil Steril. 1994;62:708-10.
49. Scott JR, Pattison N. Human chorionic gonadotrophin for recurrent miscarriage. Cochrane Database Syst Rev. 2000;(2): CD000101.
50. EI-Zibdeh MY. Dydrogesterone in the reduction of recurrent spontaneous abortion. J Steroid Biochem Mol Biol. 2005;97:431-4.
51. Khambata K, Raut S, Deshpande S, Mohan S, Sonawane S, Goankar R, et al. DNA methylation defects in spermatozoa of male partners from couples experiencing recurrent pregnancy loss. Hum Reprod 2021, 36(1):48-60.
52. Martin RH. Mechanisms of nondisjunction in human spermatogenesis. Cytogenet Genome Res. 2005;111:245-9.

33 Chapter

What Should a Gynecologist Know about Embryology?

INTRODUCTION

The basic knowledge of embryology is essential for every gynecologist. This helps the clinician to correlate the quality of ova, oocytes retrieved, fertilization rate, and blastocyst rate with the drugs used for ovulation induction. Pre-IVF (in vitro fertilization) and post-IVF counseling can be based on this, which helps to build a stronger confidence of the patient in the clinician.

It is unfortunate that when the embryologist is busy handling the gametes and embryos, clinicians are busy in oocyte retrieval, patient counseling, and patient consultation and therefore can rarely take an active part in the laboratory.

We will discuss certain basic facts and procedures about the processing of the gametes and embryos in the laboratory.

CHECKLIST WHEN PREPARING FOR OOCYTE RETRIEVAL

- Inform the embryologist, anesthetist, and the supporting staff about the time of trigger and the time for oocyte retrieval.
- The whole laboratory, instruments, tabletops, laminar airflow, intracytoplasmic sperm injection (ICSI) machine should all be cleaned and disinfected preferably 36–48 hours before the oocyte retrieval. It is essential to use oocyte and embryo-safe reagents.
- All the equipment, including the suction pump in the oocyte retrieval operation room, must be checked on the day of trigger.
- The embryologist must be informed about the number of oocyte retrievals and the total expected number of ova. With hi-tech ultrasound scanners, the number of ova likely to be retrieved can be precisely predicted. This is important for the embryologist to calculate the amount of media and disposables required. This is essential because the media needs to be placed in a CO_2 incubator, 8–10 hours/overnight prior to oocyte retrieval. The CO_2 incubator is set at 37°C and 5–6% of CO_2.
- Disposables are all labeled before the procedures start.
- Laminar airflow and high-efficiency particulate air (HEPA) filters should be started at least 20 minutes before oocyte retrieval for clean air.
- The patient should be referred to the physician and anesthetist to confirm fitness for anesthesia and procedure.

OOCYTE RETRIEVAL

- Quick and efficient handling of the oocytes is very important for success.
- The procedure is planned 34–35 hours after the trigger. It is usually done under short general anesthesia but can be done under sedation or local anesthesia.
- The test tubes for oocyte retrieval in the operation theater (OT) should be heated

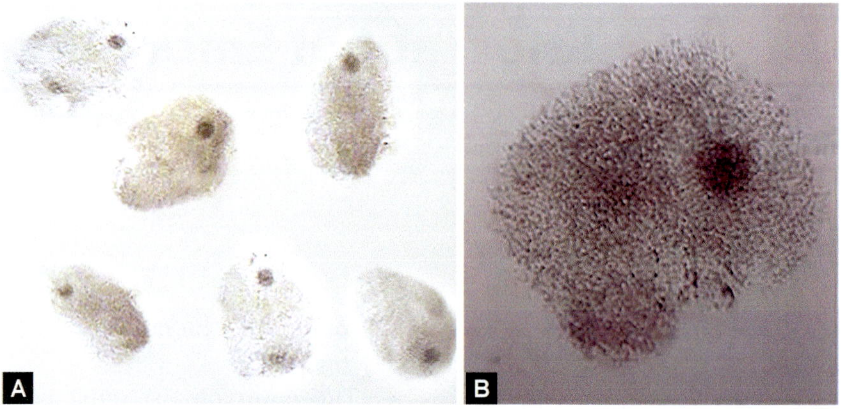

Figs. 1A and B: (A) Oocyte cumulus (OC) complexes in the Petri dish; (B) OC complex aspirated by a pipette and placed into the central well organ culture Petri dish in flushing (HEPES buffer) media.

at 37°C in the warmer block. The number of test tubes required must also be calculated as a maximum of 2–3 oocytes should be collected in a single test tube **(Fig. 1A)**.

- Test tubes are transferred to the laboratory from the OT via a bypass window.
- As soon as the embryologist receives the test tube, the contents are poured into the Petri dish, under the stereo zoom microscope mounted on warm (37°C) stage, the oocyte cumulus complexes are looked for. These are aspirated by a pipette and placed into the central well organ culture Petri dish in flushing (HEPES buffer) media. Not more than three complexes are lodged in one Petri dish. The entire process is done under laminar airflow **(Fig. 1B)**.
- These Petri dishes are shifted to the CO_2 incubator. The time from oocyte retrieval to the incubator should be the shortest possible. Exposure of oocytes to light should also be the shortest possible.

Normal Oocyte Morphology (Fig. 2)

A normal oocyte is round in shape with uniform zona pellucida. The cytoplasm is homogeneous and transparent. A polar body is seen.

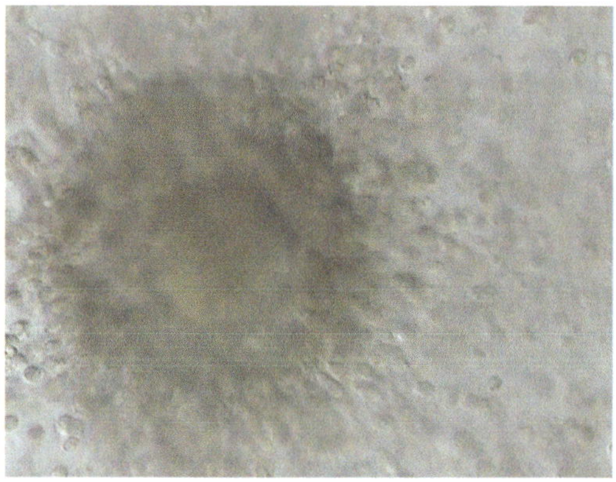

Fig. 2: Normal oocyte.

Oocytes are graded depending on nuclear maturity corona cells and cumulus structure into immature, intermediate, mature, and postmature.

- *Immature oocytes*: Germinal vesicle (GV), tightly packed corona cells, and scanty cumulus **(Fig. 3A)**
- *Intermediate oocytes*: Metaphase I (MI)—tightly packed corona cells and cumulus cells **(Fig. 3B)**
- *Metaphase II (MII) oocyte* ***(Fig. 4)***: MII oocyte is considered a mature oocyte, but it can have morphological abnormalities.

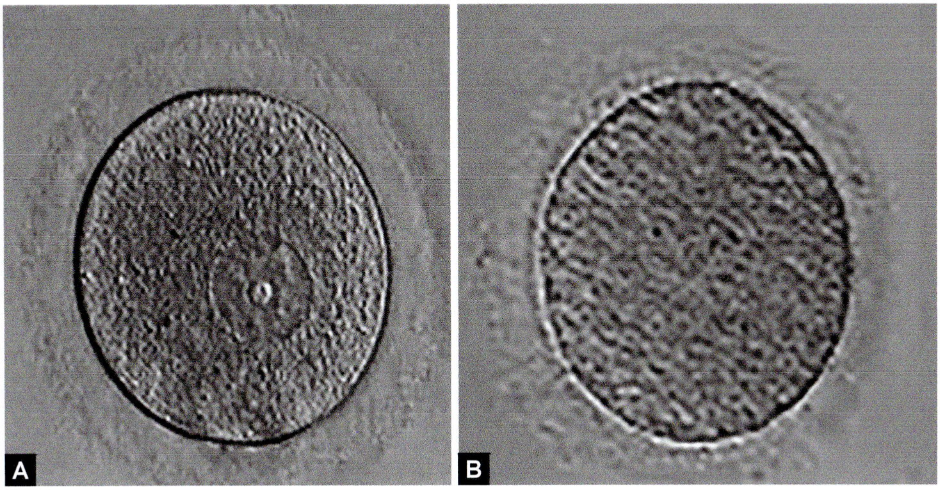

Fig. 3A and B: (A) Immature oocyte; (B) Intermediate oocyte.

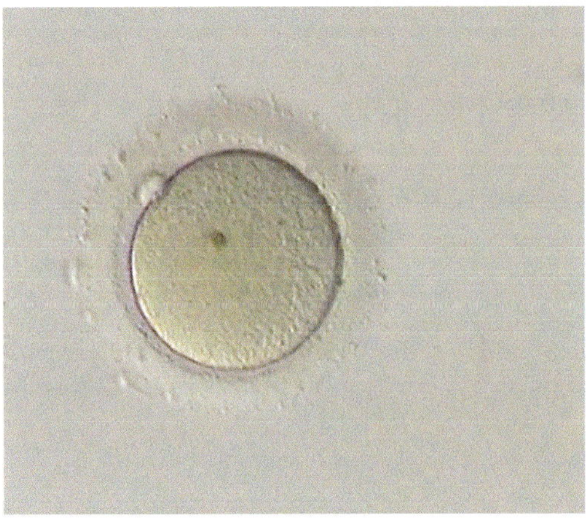

Fig. 4: Metaphase II oocyte.

There is a sunburst appearance of corona cells and fully expanded abundant cumulus cells.

- *Extracytoplasmic abnormality* ***(Figs. 5A to F)***: It may have an abnormal shape and altered zona pellucida. Perivitelline space may be large or with granulation. The polar body may be abnormal.
- *Cytoplasmic abnormalities*:
  - Dark granulation with dark color cytoplasm
  - Excessive whole or centrally located granulation
  - Refractile bodies, vacuoles in the ooplasm
- *Postmature oocytes*: MII, dark oocyte cumulus complex (OCC), gelatinous or mucified cumulus cells, and corona cells have begun to degenerate.

SPERM PREPARATION

This has been discussed in detail in the Chapter 26: Sperm Preparation in Intrauterine Insemination and In Vitro Fertilization. Here, the gradient wash is done. Gradient wash is done for sperm preparation. It is safe to always keep one frozen sample in spare to be utilized in case the male partner is not able to produce the sample on the day of oocyte retrieval. Sperm retrieval from epididymis or testis is done prior to pickup or even in any of the previous days and can be frozen.

INSEMINATION OF OOCYTES

Oocytes can be inseminated by conventional IVF or ICSI. The insemination/injection time should be decided based on the number

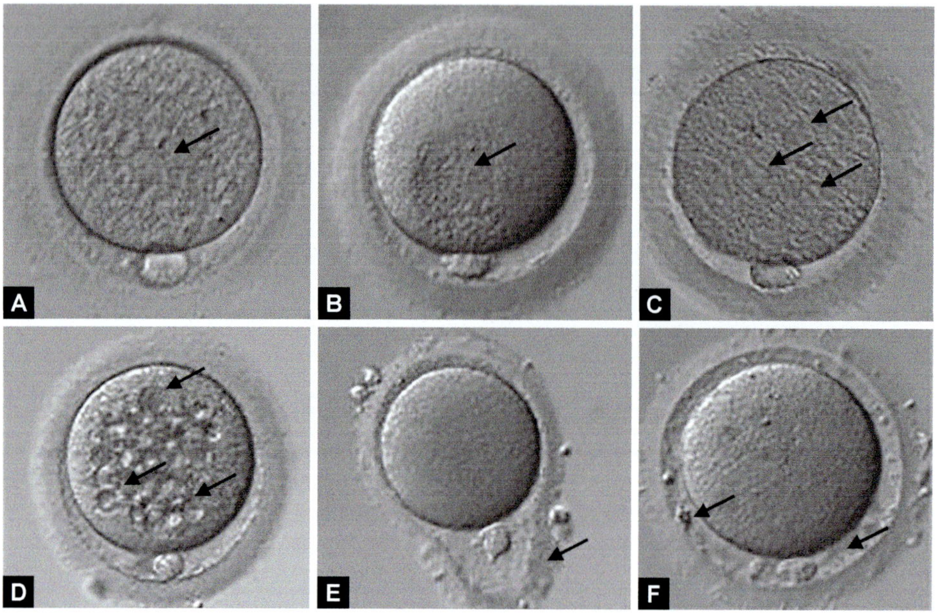

Figs. 5A to F: (A and B) Oocytes with granulation; (C and D) Oocytes with vacuoles; (E and F) Oocytes with large perivitelline space.

of hours that have elapsed from ovulation trigger and/or oocyte retrieval. Also, one must keep in mind that fertilization needs to be checked 16–18 hours after insemination and so the timing of insemination should also be adjusted considering that.

CONVENTIONAL IVF (FIG. 6)

For conventional IVF, motile sperm concentration between 0.1 and 0.5 million/mL or 25,000 sperms per oocyte are required for insemination. Co-incubation of cumulus oocyte complexes and sperm is usually performed overnight or for minimum 6 hours and maximum 18 hours. Then check for fertilization.

INTRACYTOPLASMIC SPERM INJECTION

Oocytes are checked for maturity and staging is done. Only MII oocytes are used for ICSI.

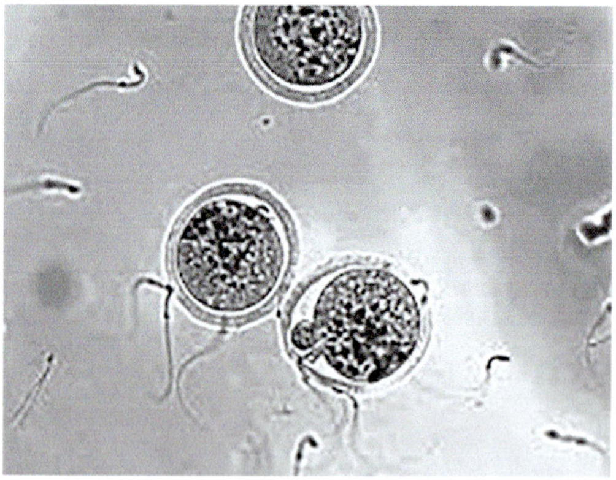

Fig. 6: Oocytes with sperms around the Petri dish for conventional in vitro fertilization.

Before ICSI, cumulus cells are removed **(Fig. 7)**. During this process, exposure of oocytes to light and hyaluronidase is minimized. It ideally should be <30 seconds.

Do's and Don'ts of ICSI

- Only MII oocytes are used.
- Do not use giant oocytes.

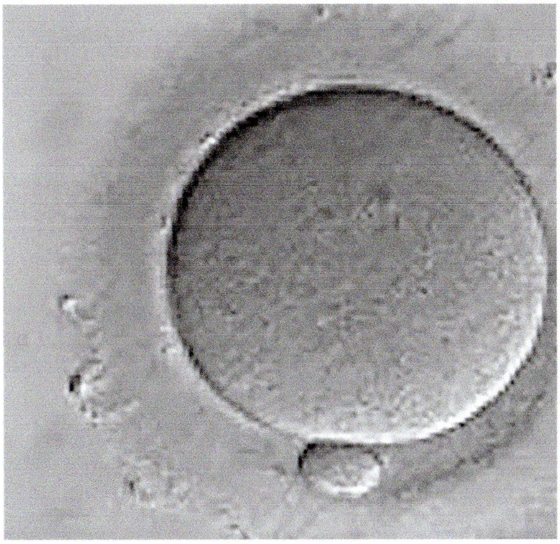

Fig. 7: Denuded metaphase II oocyte.

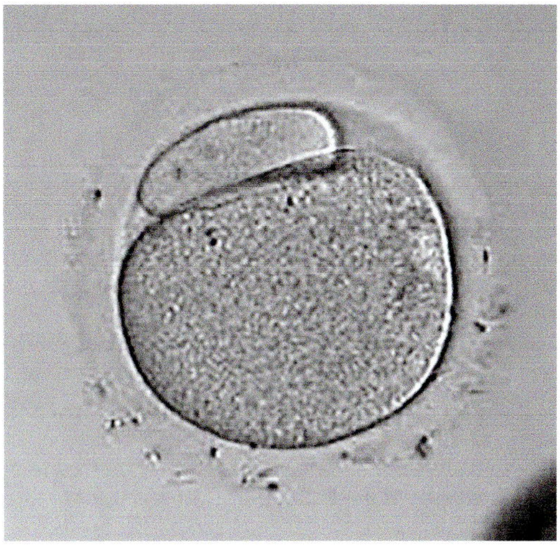

Fig. 8: Oocyte with a large polar body—abnormal oocyte.

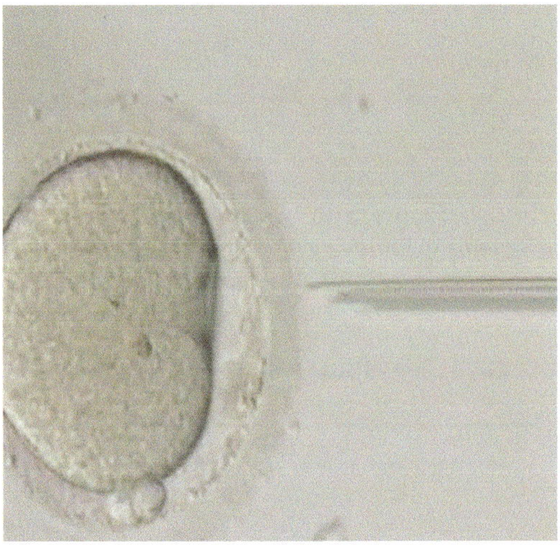

Fig. 9: Polar body at 6 o'clock position seen on intracytoplasmic sperm injection.

- Do not use oocytes with large polar bodies **(Fig. 8)**.
- Morphologically normal and motile sperms are used.
- Polar body should be at 6 o'clock or 12 o'clock position **(Fig. 9)**.

Prior to injection, oolemma rupture is confirmed. During ICSI, temperature and pH are maintained. After ICSI, fertilization is checked at 16–18 hours **(Fig. 10)**.

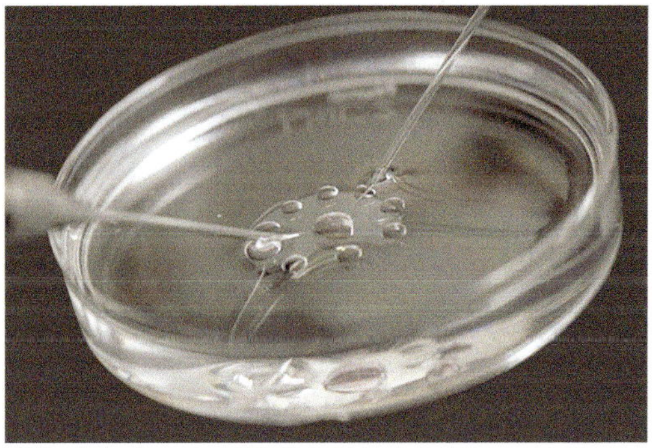

Fig. 10: Prepared intracytoplasmic sperm injection dish.

The clinical outcome does not differ between IVF and ICSI.

ASSESSMENT OF FERTILIZATION

- Two polar bodies with centrally located two juxtaposed pronuclei **(Fig. 11)**
- The fertilized embryo is divided into two equal cells with a distinct membrane in between.
- Cumulus cells are not removed in conventional IVF earlier but are removed at this stage. Fertilized oocytes are transferred into new Petri dishes pre-equilibrated with culture media.

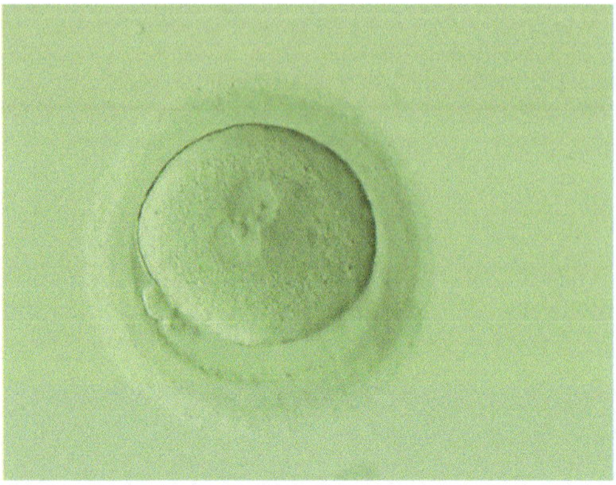

Fig. 11: Two polar bodies with centrally located two juxtaposed pronuclei in the fertilized ovum.

Zygotes are scored based on **(Fig. 12)**:

- *Pronuclei*: Size and symmetry
- *Nucleoli*: Size, number, equality, distribution
- Cytoplasm

The 2010 Istanbul consensus on zygote/pronuclei scoring is as follows. The consensus scoring system for pronuclei is given in **Table 1**.[1]

For optimum embryo culture conditions:

- Minimal fluctuations of temperature and pH
- pH, temperature, and osmolality changes can be minimized by oil overlay.
- One may use sequential or single-step media.
- Use low oxygen concentration for blastocyst culture **(Fig. 13)**.

Embryo grading is to be done for cleavage-stage embryos (Day 2–3 of insemination) based on **(Table 2)**:

- Blastomere regularity
- Cell/blastomere number or cleavage rate
- Fragmentation
- Multinucleation

Blastocyst can also be graded according to **(Tables 3 and 4)**:

- Stage of development

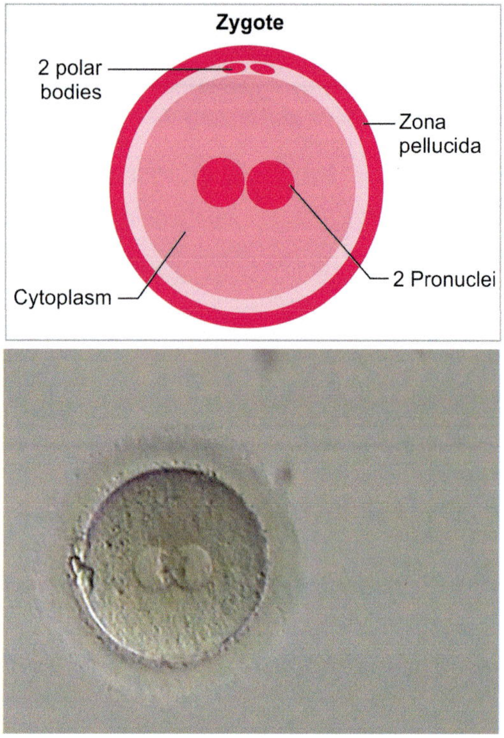

Fig. 12: Zygote with two polar bodies and two pronuclei on the diagram and in embryologic picture.

TABLE 1: Consensus scoring system for pronuclei.

Category	*Rating*	*Description*
1	Symmetrical	Equivalent to Z1 and Z2 category
2	Nonsymmetrical	Other arrangements, including peripherally sited pronuclei
3	Abnormal	Pronuclei with 0 or 1 nucleolar precursor body

- Inner cell mass (ICM)
- Trophoectoderm (TE)

Timing of observation of fertilized oocytes and embryo is given in **Table 5 and Figure 14**.

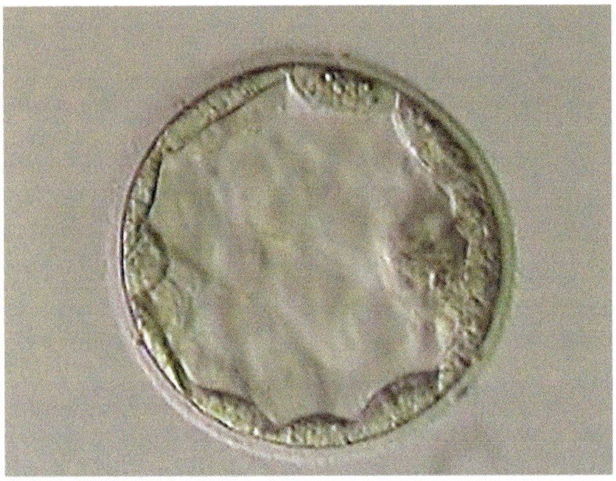

Fig. 13: Blastocyst.

TABLE 2: Cleavage-stage embryo grading.

Category	*Grading*	*Description*
1	Good	• <10% fragmentation • Stage-specific cell size • No multinucleation
2	Fair	• 10–25% fragmentation • Stage-specific cell size for majority of cells • No evidence of multinucleation
3	Poor	• Severe fragmentation (>25%) • Cell size not stage-specific • Evidence of multinucleation

TABLE 3: Blastocyst grading according to the stage of development.

Stage	*Development*
1	Early
2	Blastocyst
3	Expanded
4	Hatched/hatching

TABLE 4: Blastocyst grading according to inner cell mass and trophectoderm.

Category	*Grade*	*Rating*	*Description*
Inner cell mass	A	Good	Prominent, easily discernible, many cells compacted, and tightly adhered together
	B	Fair	Easily discernible, with many cells, loosely grouped
	C	Poor	Difficult to discern, few cells
Tropho-ectoderm	A	Good	Many cells forming a cohesive epithelium
	B	Fair	Few cells forming a loose epithelium
	C	Poor	Very few cells

TABLE 5: Embryo development at different embryo age after IVF.

Type of observation	*Timing (hours post-insemination)*	*Expected stage of development*
Fertilization check	17 ± 1	Pronuclear stage
Syngamy check	23 ± 1	Expect 50% to be in syngamy (up to 20% may be at the two-cell stage)
Early cleavage check	26 ± 1 hour post-ICSI	Two-cell stage
	28 ± 1 hour post-IVF	
Day 2 embryo assessment	44 ± 1	Four-cell stage
Day 3 embryo assessment	68 ± 1	Eight-cell stage
Day 4 embryo assessment	92 ± 2	Morula
Day 5 embryo assessment	116 ± 2	Blastocyst

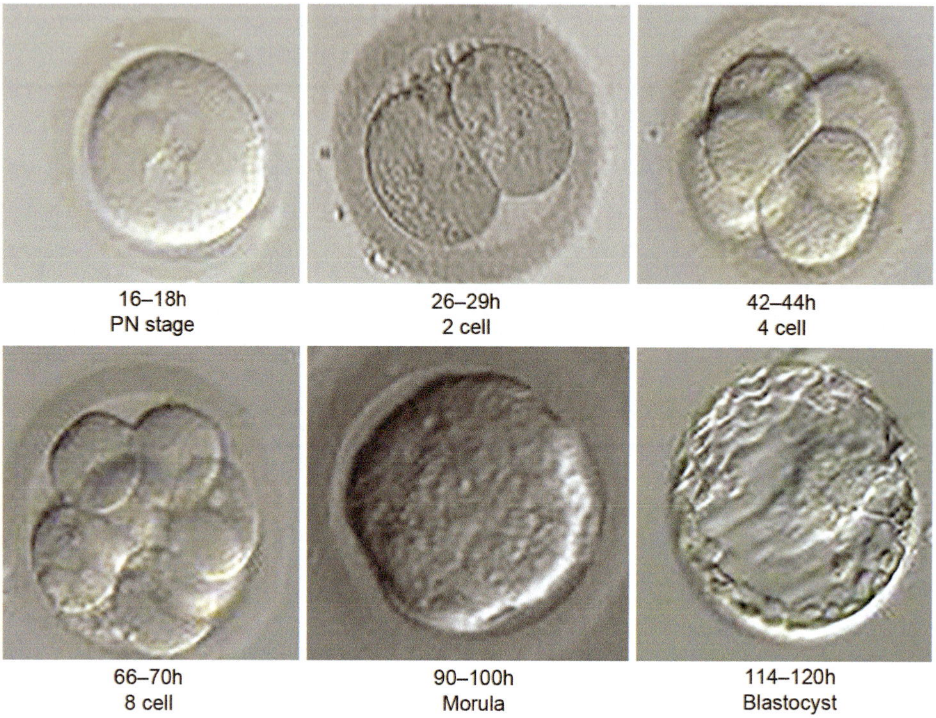

Fig. 14: Embryo at different duration after fertilization.

Embryo selection for transfer depends on:

- Number of embryos available
- Quality of the embryos
- Developmental stage of the embryos

Embryology has a big impact on the results of assisted reproductive technology (ART). Clinicians must be aware of the expected results and it is essential that they keep a close watch on the laboratory conditions, yield of ova, fertilization rates, blastocyst rates, and pregnancy rates per transfer.

CARRY HOME MESSAGE

- Basic knowledge of embryology is essential for every gynecologist.
- Confirm the checklist of preparations before oocyte retrieval procedure.
- Exposure to oocytes should be minimum.
- Check fertilization at 16–18 hours.
- For ICSI only M2 oocytes are used.
- Embryo grading closely correlates with clinical pregnancy rate.

REFERENCE

1. Alpha Scientists in Reproductive Medicine and ESHRE Special Interest Group of Embryology. The Istanbul consensus workshop on embryo assessment: proceedings of an expert meeting. Hum Reprod. 2011;26(6):1270-83.

34 Chapter

Evaluation of Subfertile Male

INTRODUCTION

Male factor is partially or completely responsible for infertility in 50% of couples. So evaluation of male for infertility is as important as evaluation of female. Because of the invention of intracytoplasmic sperm injection (ICSI), the research on male infertility has been stopped but now it has been realized that research on cause and medical management is very important for the management of male infertility. If semen analysis of a male is normal, then further investigations in case of infertility are not required unless there is a specific complaint.

HISTORY-TAKING

History-taking is extremely important for counseling and treatment of a patient.

- *Age*: The offsprings of males more than 40 years of age have a higher possibility of developing autism and schizophrenia.
- *Sexual history*: Coital frequency is elicited from the patient. Intercourse twice or thrice a week gives a good pregnancy rate. Penetration of sperm is for 6 days prior to ovulation. After ovulation, sexual relation does not increase the pregnancy rate. Erection or ejaculatory disorders can be diagnosed from history or the use of a lubricant must be asked for specifically.
- *Environmental agents*: There are many environmental factors that can decrease the sperm count. Hence, a detailed history of the profession should be taken and proper counseling should be done with the patient.
- *Surgery*: History of surgery should be asked for. Surgery for undescended testis, hernia, or varicocele has a great influence on the sperm count.
- *Onset of puberty*: Detailed history of onset of puberty is elicited. Delayed puberty or early puberty has influence on infertility.
- *Infection*: History of orchitis or history of filarial infection should be asked for and details of the treatment taken.
- *Personal habits*: History of alcohol, tobacco, coffee, and anabolic steroids should be asked in detail.
- *Drugs*: Whether the patient is taking any drug, e.g., antihypertensive or antidepressant, should be asked.
- *Chemotherapy or radiotherapy*: History of chemotherapy or radiotherapy, if the patient has taken, has a bad impact on semen parameters.
- *Systemic diseases*: Diabetes, hypertension, and other systemic diseases have influence on sperm count.

PHYSICAL EXAMINATION

General Examination

- *Rule out inadequate virilization*:
  - Klinefelter syndrome
  - Hypogonadism
  - Kallmann syndrome

- *Systemic diseases*:
  - Diabetes
  - Chronic alcoholism
  - Hypertension

Local Examination

- *Scrotum*:
  - Skin—thick in filariasis
  - Size—hydrocele, hernia
- *Testis*:
  - Position—ectopic testis
  - Size—reduced in testicular failure, measured by an orchidometer. It is 15 mL (4.5 × 2.5 cm).
- *Penis*: See for meatus
- *Epididymis*: See for consistency to rule out tuberculosis and other infections. It may be increased in presence of the cyst
- *Vas deferens*: Look out for the presence of vas deferens.
- Per rectal examination should be done for seminal vesicle and prostatic enlargement.
- Look out for varicocele and find out its grade:

  Grade I: Palpable with Valsalva maneuver

  Grade II: Palpable without Valsalva maneuver

  Grade III: Detected by visual impression

  Ultrasound helps to arrive at the correct diagnosis if physical examination is inconclusive. Most of the studies show improvement of semen parameters within 3–6 months. Clinically palpable varicocele should be operated whenever semen parameters are abnormal. Simple identification of varicocele and its treatment alter the course of a couple's fertility treatment toward a safer, less invasive, less expensive, and natural pregnancy.

Surgery for Varicocele

- Surgery
- Percutaneous embolization technique

Surgery

- *Nonmicrosurgical*: Retroperitoneal, laparoscopic
- *Low microsurgical approach*: Inguinal, subinguinal

  The latter has a lower recurrence rate.

SEMEN ANALYSIS

The parameters for normal semen according to the 2010 World Health Organization (WHO) criteria are given in **Table 1**.

The 2010 criteria differ from the previous criteria published in 1992.

Semen should be examined 2 weeks and 2 months apart after 3–4 days of abstinence or two semen analysis 1 month apart if first one is abnormal. Any major illness or medication is excluded in the last 3 months. This may lead to an azoospermic, teratozoospermic, asthenospermic, or oligozoospermic sample. It is considered better to report total sperms per ejaculate rather than sperm concentration per milliliter as this is a reflection of the average

TABLE 1: Normal semen parameters and their values according to the 2010 WHO criteria.

Seminal parameters	*Lower reference value*
Volume	1.5 mL
pH	7.2
Concentration	15 million/mL
Total number of sperms	39 million/ejaculate
Motility	40% total 32% progressive
Vitality	58% sperms alive/ ejaculate
Morphology	4% normal shape

testicular sperm production and what is available at the site of fertilization in the female reproductive tract. Conception increases with total ejaculate up to 140 millions/mL.

Motility: Agglutination is to be checked and antisperm antibodies (ASA) should be asked for, particularly in patients of unexplained infertility. For ICSI, ASA testing is not required.

In the new edition for motility, the percentage of motile spermatozoa and proportion of motile spermatozoa are assessed irrespective of speed. The presence of substantial forward progressive motility indicates no severe infection or inflammatory reaction. Motility is reported as three grades: progressive, nonprogressive, and immotile.

Progressive motility of 32% and total motility of 40% are considered normal **(Table 2)**.

SPERM MORPHOLOGY

According to the WHO criteria for normal sperm morphology **(Table 2)**:

- *1987*: 50% normal sperms
- *1992*: 30% normal sperms
- *1999*: 14% normal sperms
- *2010*: 4% normal sperms

Morphology is the most important predictor for fertilization in in-vitro fertilization (IVF) following conventional insemination.

- *Head*:
  - Smooth oval configuration
  - Length 5–6 μm
  - Diameter 2.5–3.5 μm
  - Acrosome: Must constitute 40–70% of head
- *Mid piece*:
  - Slender, axially attached
  - <1 μm wide and 1.5 × head length
  - No cytoplasmic droplets larger than 50% of the head size
- *Tail*:
  - Single, unbroken, straight, without kinks/coils
  - Approximately 45 μm in length
- A: Good fertilization with >14% normal sperms—IVF
- B: Very poor fertilization with <4 % normal sperms—ICSI
- Good correlation between sperm morphology and sperm functional tests such as zona pellucida binding assays and zona-free hamster-oocyte penetration assay.[1]
- Poor morphology also correlates with abnormal sperm calcium influx and an abnormal acrosome reaction.[2]
- CASA (computer-assisted semen analysis) is labor-intensive, expensive and laboratory-based method of semen analysis. Recently even automated smartphone-based diagnostic methods have also been developed.[3] Other sophisticated sperm function tests are cumbersome, expensive and impractical.

TABLE 2: Difference in normal semen parameters between 1999 and 2010 WHO criteria.

Seminal parameter	*WHO 1999*	*WHO 2010*
Volume	2 mL	1.5 mL
Concentration	20×10^6/mL	15×10^6/mL
Progressive motility	50%	32%
Morphology	15%	4%
Millions of progressive motility	20	7.2 (12)

ENDOCRINOLOGY

Investigations

- Serum follicle-stimulating hormone (FSH)
- Serum luteinizing hormone (LH)

- Serum testosterone
- Serum prolactin
- Thyroxine (T4), thyroid-stimulating hormone (TSH)
- Dehydroepiandrosterone sulfate (DHEA-S)
- Estradiol
- 17-hydroxyprogesterone (17-OHP)
- Cortisol

FSH, LH, and testosterone are the three main hormones to be assessed.

- *High FSH, high LH, and normal testosterone*: This indicates primary testicular failure. These patients have azoospermia and are advised microdissection testicular sperm extraction (mTESE) or artificial insemination by donor (AID) or adoption.
- *High FSH, normal LH, normal testosterone*: This also indicated primary testicular failure which may be due to inhibin deficiency also. The options for these patients are mTESE or AID or adoption. Exceptional cases may have varicocele and varicocele ligation may improve count.
- *Low FSH, low LH, and low testosterone*: This is because of hypogonadotropic hypogonadism. Rule out prolactinoma in these cases.
- *Normal FSH, normal LH, and normal testosterone*: This may be due to obstruction. Rule out retrograde ejaculation or germ cell failure. The most common cause is qualitative failure. The bioactivity of the hormones FSH and LH is poor, but immunoactivity that we assess by the enzyme-linked immunosorbent assay (ELISA) test is normal. This can be diagnosed by monoclonal antibody testing. But exogenous FSH and hCG can be supplemented in these cases and this may help spermatogenesis. This supplementation is suggested by Professor Ishidori from Sweden.
- *High testosterone, high LH, and normal FSH*: This is due to partial testosterone resistance. There is increased E2/T ratio which causes gynecomastia. There is oligo-astheno-teratozoospermia. The patient is taken for assisted reproductive technology (ART) as usually count does not improve by medical management.
- *Serum prolactin*: Increase in prolactin decreases libido. There is no gynecomastia or galactorrhea. It reduces the testosterone level. The most common reason is pituitary tumor. The patient presents with oligozoospermia.
- *Thyroid dysfunction*: Hyper- or hypothyroidism can cause oligozoospermia. Increased TSH can cause hyperprolactinemia. Autoimmune thyroiditis is very common. Treat the condition for oligozoospermia.
- *Adrenal dysfunction*: Infertility may be the only presenting symptom. There may be increased DHEA-S causing increase in the prolactin level. Some patients may show signs and symptoms of adrenal insufficiency. The signs and symptoms of feminization and soft testis may be seen. Rule out family history of congenital adrenal hyperplasia (CAH).

ULTRASONOGRAPHY

Systemic and logical evaluation by ultrasound helps us to distinguish between correctable and noncorrectable abnormalities.

- Scrotal ultrasound
- Transrectal ultrasound
- Penile Doppler

Scrotal Ultrasound

Testis appears homogenous, echogenic, and ovoid. These are bilaterally symmetrical. The volume of both testes is 12–15 mL. There is an echogenic line in the testis, known as mediastinum testis. A decrease in size indicates spermatogenic dysfunction but it decreases as age advances.

Epididymis is homogeneous and mildly hyperechogenic to testis. It is coma shaped on the lateral aspect of testis. It is 10–12 mm in diameter and it has body and tail.

Ultrasound can diagnose abnormalities such as testicular atrophy, cryptorchidism, neoplasm, orchitis, testicular infarcts, testicular trauma, and torsion.

Atrophy of testis: It may occur following inflammation, ischemia, trauma, torsion, cirrhosis, estrogen therapy, hypopituitary disorders, and aging. It is seen in Klinefelter syndrome, Y microdeletion in chromosome, and cryptorchidism. On ultrasound, it is seen as a small, hypoechoic testis with localized area of altered echogenicity. On color Doppler, flow is decreased. In most of the cases, epididymis is normal.

Varicocele and Ultrasound (Table 3)

It is most common on the left side (85%). In 5% of cases, it is bilateral. Only right-side varicocele is secondary to enlarged liver, hydronephrosis, abdominal tumors, or after 40 years of age. It is diagnosed by seeing dilatation of veins in pampiniform plexus in the spermatic cord and causes reversal of blood flow in internal spermatic and cremasteric veins **(Figs. 1A to C)**. It is seen in up to 40% of men with infertility but it is most common in secondary infertility (up to 70%). Semen parameters improve in more than 50% of men after surgery.

TABLE 3: Varicocoele grading by ultrasound.

Grade	*B-mode*	*Doppler*
Grade 1	Vessels > 2.5 mm in inguinal region only	Inguinal reflux for 2–3 seconds on Valsalva
Grade 2	Supratesticular vessels >3 mm	Supratesticular reflux on Valsalva for >3 seconds
Grade 3	Supra and peritesticular vessel dilatation >3 mm	Reflux in these vessels on Valsalva for >3 seconds
Grade 4	Peritesticular vessel dilatation with further dilatation on Valsalva, testicular hypotrophy	Reflux at rest which may or may not increase during Valsalva
Grade 5	Peritesticular vessel dilatation does not increase on Valsalva	Reflux that increases on Valsalva with filling of intratesticular vessels also

Transrectal Ultrasound

This is required to see prostate, seminal vesicles, vas deferens, and ejaculatory ducts. In a patient of azoospermia, semen volume is <1 mL and FSH is normal, Transrectal ultrasound (TRUS) should always be done to rule out ejaculatory duct obstruction.

Genetic Testing

- Male infertility and chromosomal aberration
- Male infertility with gene defect

CHROMOSOMAL ABNORMALITIES

ASRM (American Society for Reproductive Medicine) and AUA (American Urological Association) recommend karyotyping for assessment of Y microdeletion in all cases of azoospermia or count less than 5 million. In cases with bilateral absence of vas deferens, cystic fibrosis transmembrane conductance regulator (CFTR) should be tested. ESHRE has extended further indications for chromosomal testing in cases with recurrent pregnancy loss, malformations, and mental retardation.

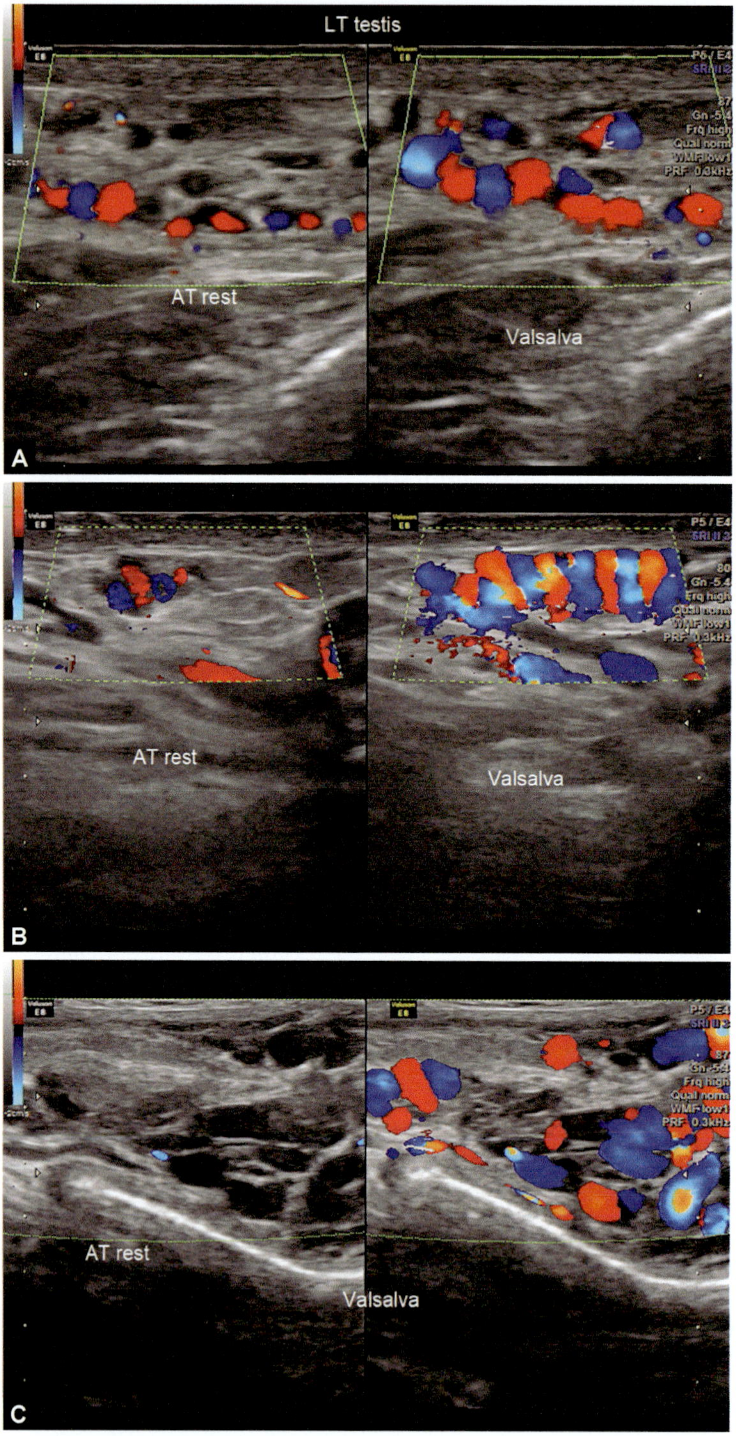

Figs. 1A to C: B-mode and color Doppler images showing grade 1 (A), grade 2 (B), and grade 3 (C) varicocoele.

Chromosomal abnormalities may be: (1) numerical and (2) structural.

Structural abnormality may have deletion, duplication, inversion, or translocation (multiple).

Numerical abnormalities include:

- Klinefelter syndrome
- XYY syndrome
- Noonan syndrome
- Chromosomal translocation

Structural abnormality includes Y chromosomal microdeletion (YCMD).

Y chromosomal microdeletion can be on the long arm of Y chromosome at the azoospermia factor (AZF) zone.

AZFa: Sertoli cell syndrome

AZFb: Complete absence of spermatid and sperms

AZFc: In 50% of cases sperms can be found in ejaculate but in others these can be retrieved by TESE.

Y chromosomal microdeletion is found in 5% of oligospermic males and in 14% of azoospermia males. Counseling is done with the couple that Y microdeletion might get transmitted to offspring if the sperms of the oligospermic male with Y microdeletion, are used. Some infertile men harbor *DAZ* deletion in germ line tissue and not in somatic cells and so it is not detected in peripheral blood tissue.

So Y microdeletion and karyotyping should be done in all patients of oligo-azoospermia with elevated FSH or testicular atrophy or in patients with impaired sperm production.

GENETIC ABNORMALITIES

In these cases, male infertility is because of a single gene defect. It is inherited as autosomal (dominant or recessive) or X-linked disease. The global incidence is $10/10^8$. These are also known as Mendelian disorders.

ABNORMALITIES

- Kallmann syndrome
- Congenital adrenal hyperplasia
- Prader–Willi syndrome
- Bardet–Biedl syndrome
- Hemochromatosis
- Cerebellar ataxia and hypogonadism
- Idiopathic hypogonadotropic hypogonadism
- Immobile ciliary syndrome
- Autosomal dominant polycystic kidney
- Cystic fibrosis transmembrane mutations
- Androgen receptor gene mutations
- Myotonic dystrophy
- Usher syndrome
- Beta thalassemia
- Sickle cell anemia
- *SRY* gene defect
- 5-alpha reductase deficiency
- Mixed gonadal dysgenesis

SPECIAL SEMEN TESTS

These tests are cumbersome, costly, time consuming, and not widely available. With invention of ICSI, the significance of all these tests has decreased.

- Sperm mucous penetration test—intrauterine insemination (IUI)
- Sperm membrane integrity test for prediction of IVF and ICSI success—hypo-osmotic swelling (HOS)
- Sperm acrosome reaction test—when abnormal, do ICSI or counsel for AID
- Sperm penetration test—IVF or ICSI
- Hemizona and zona binding test—ICSI
- Sperm nucleus integrity test
- ASA test—IUI/IVF/ICSI/AID

Despite the development of a wide assortment of tests and procedures designated to evaluate attachment to zona, penetration of oocyte membrane, or release of acrosome enzymes, we do not have a reliable validated test for sperm function.

The results of sperm function tests are not correlated with strict sperm morphology criteria, the most commonly accepted prediction of fertilization.

DNA FRAGMENTATION

This is:

- Due to apoptosis
- During spermatogenesis
- Due to oxidative stress

It has a negative impact on pregnancy by IUI or ART but an equal number of reports deny them. When DNA fragmentation is high in ejaculate, the results of ICSI are better with testicular sperm than with ejaculated sperm as it has lower zona fragmentation.[4]

Density-functional theory (DFT):

- Sperm chromatin structure assay (SCSA)
- TUNEL (terminal deoxynucleotidyl transferase dUTP nick end labeling) test
- Comet test

Routine use of all these tests is not justified as screening test or for primary diagnosis.

Treatment of DNA Fragmentation

- Antioxidants
- Varicocele repair
- Testicular sperms

DNA fragmentation of <30% gives a good pregnancy rate.

CARRY HOME MESSAGE

- Semen analysis is the gold standard for primary diagnosis of infertile male.
- Serum FSH will further guide for further diagnosis and management.
- Karyotyping and Y microdeletion should be done in all cases of oligospermia, azoospermia, RPL and with history of malformed child.
- Ultrasound is done to diagnose varicocele and to diagnose obstructive causes of azoospermia.
- Sperm function tests are not done routinely.
- DNA fragmentation test as primary diagnostic test or screening is not justified.

REFERENCES

1. Oehinger S, Mahony M, Ozgür K, Kolm P, Kruger T, Franken D. Clinical significance of human sperm-zona pellucida binding. Fertil Steril. 1997;67;1121-7.
2. Toner JP, Mossad H, Grow DR, Morshedi M, Swanson RJ, Oehninger S. Andrologia. 1995;27:143.
3. Agarwal A, Panner Selvam MK, Sharma R, Master K, Sharma A, Gupta S, et al. Home sperm testing device versus laboratory sperm quality analyzer: comparison of motile sperm concentration. Fertil Steril. 2018; 110(7):1277-84.
4. Esteves AC, Roque M, Bradley CK, Garrido N. Reproductive outcomes of testicular versus ejaculated sperm for intracytoplasmic sperm injection among men with high levels of DNA fragmentation in semen: systematic review and meta-analysis. Fertil Steril. 2017;108(3);456-67.

35

Chapter

Medical Management of Male Infertility

INTRODUCTION

Male factor is partially or completely responsible for infertility in at least 40–50% of all infertility cases. But in today's era of in vitro fertilization (IVF) and intracytoplasmic sperm injection (ICSI), very little importance is given to its medical management. In India, majority of our patients cannot afford multiple attempts of IVF. They may with all difficulties manage one cycle, the success rate of which is barely 25–35%. If the amount that costs for one IVF/ICSI cycle is instead used for medical management of oligozoospermia, it will improve the sperm count permanently. This can give better pregnancy rates than a single IVF/ICSI cycle; moreover, this can also give spontaneous pregnancies in the future also. This is the reason why we insist on the medical management of male subfertility as an important treatment option for couples with male factor infertility.

PREVENTIVE MEASURES

Preventive measures must be discussed with the patients before starting the treatment.

Smoking, Caffeine, and Alcohol

Bad effects of smoking and alcohol are person-specific and affect a lot who have abnormal sperm parameters. Smoking causes much more damage to patients with varicocele rather than in a normal male. It is essential, therefore, to advise patients to stop smoking and alcohol.

Occupational and Environmental Hazards

Many chemicals and particularly heavy metals damage spermatogenesis. Lead toxicity is well known. Environmental toxins and pesticides also play a major role in decreasing sperm count. Increased scrotal temperature also alters sperm parameters.

Drugs

Many drugs such as antopsychotic drugs, antidepressants, antibiotics, steroids, etc., also reduce the sperm count.

Mobiles and Computers

Because of high-frequency shortwave and generation of heat, these equipment can decrease the sperm count and motility.

CRITERIA FOR MEDICAL MANAGEMENT IN MALE INFERTILITY

Semen analysis is still the gold standard for further evaluation and management of an infertile male.

As shown in *Chapter 34, Tables 1 and 2,* the parameters for normal semen analysis have changed and with only 15 million/mL count, 30% motility, and >4% normal sperms, spontaneous conceptions can occur. The whole motto of medical management of a subfertile male is not to increase the sperm count 5–10 times or to achieve excellent semen parameters. The motto is to increase the count by a few million, so that ICSI can be converted to IVF, IVF to intrauterine insemination (IUI), and perhaps IUI into natural conception.

This case study about medical management of male infertility which is an eye-opener. It shows the importance and success of medical treatment of an infertile male and must be thought of before using high-end techniques for conception or after having failures with high-end assisted reproductive technology (ART)—IVF-ICSI.

Case Study

- An industrialist—9 years of infertility
- Semen count—3 million
- Seven IVF-ICSI failures
- Husband treated medically [follicle-stimulating hormone (FSH) + human chorionic gonadotropin (hCG)] (Professor Ishidori's regimen)
- Count increased to 22 million
- Conceived naturally—baby boy
- Spontaneously conceived and delivered another baby boy after 2.5 years

TREATMENT OPTIONS

- Specific therapy
- Empiric therapy

Specific Therapy

There is a definite cause of infertility and specific therapy should be given, which will be highly effective. This means that the treatment is based on the cause of infertility.

Hypogonadotropic Hypogonadism

Estrogen is low because of low FSH and luteinizing hormone (LH). This is common in congenital Kallmann syndrome associated with anosmia, deafness, renal abnormalities, and cleft palate.

It may also be associated with trauma, tumor, panhypopituitarism, isolated gonadotropin deficiency, etc.

This can be treated by:

- Clomiphene citrate (CC)
- Gonadotropins

Clomiphene citrate: It was a customary teaching that CC does not work in hypogonadotropic hypogonadism (HH), but there are several recent papers that suggest that CC is very useful for spermatogenesis.[1] It is useful in nonobstructive azoospermia (NOA) and HH.

The recommended dose is 25–75 mg on alternate days. The dose titration is done by morning serum testosterone estimation which should be between 6,000 and 8,000 ng/dL. This treatment is given for 3–9 months. In the same study, 64.3% of patients showed sperms in ejaculate with a mean density of 3.8 million/mL. In the rest of the patients, sperms could be retrieved from the testis.[1]

Gonadotropins: In these patients, FSH and LH are very low and have to be supplied from outside. For initiation of spermatogenesis, testosterone is very useful. So, hCG in a dose of 2,000–3,000 IU twice a week or 5,000 IU every fifth day is given for 6–8 weeks till the testosterone level comes to normal. Then, human menopausal gonadotropin (hMG)/urinary follicle-stimulating hormone (uFSH)/recombinant follicle-stimulating hormone (rFSH) 75 IU is added thrice a week. hCG is continued once a week, but the dose may be adjusted if gynecomastia occurs.[2] We have found excellent results with this regimen like other studies.[3] Gonadotropin-releasing hormone (GnRH) is not available in our country, but it is a good alternative to hCG-hMG/FSH regimen in HH. It is of no use in patients with disturbed spermatogenesis and high FSH. In about 40% of the patients, spermatogenesis starts. Normally, it takes 6–9 months[4] after FSH/hCG treatment for the sperm parameters to improve.

Hyperprolactinemia

In male, the most common cause of increased prolactin is macroadenoma and it is to be surgically removed. Diagnosis is suspected with the history of loss of libido and pressure effects on optic chiasma and is confirmed by MRI.[5] Macroadenoma is usually >1 cm and serum prolactin level is >200 ng/mL.

But surgery should not be done for microadenoma. The prolactin level is between 100 and 200 µg/mL in these cases, and bromocriptine or cabergoline is the treatment. Cabergoline is given 0.5–2 mg in doses divided twice a week to maintain prolactin levels between 10 and 15 µg/mL. Cabergoline is found to be better than bromocriptine.

Genital Tract Infections

Chlamydia is the most common infection and should be treated with doxycycline. In resistant cases, semen culture is done and treated accordingly. If there is prostatic infection, the quinolone group of drugs is given. But treating the infection does not necessarily improve the conception rates.

Disorders of Ejaculation

This has not been elaborated here as these are best to be managed by an andrologist. Patients with retrograde ejaculation can be treated medically or by IUI.

Immunological Causes

Nowadays, immunological causes in abnormal semen parameters are treated with IUI only. No steroids are given.

Isolated Testosterone Deficiency

It is treated with hCG 2,000 IU twice a week.

Congenital Adrenal Hyperplasia

This is treated with glucocorticoids—dexamethasone 0.5 mg at bedtime.

Empiric Therapy

Empiric therapy is the treatment prior to final diagnosis, based on clinical concepts or theories without proven efficacy. About 25% of cases of male infertility have idiopathic infertility. Empiric therapy is the only available form of treatment for them.[6,7] All proven drugs used now have been tried earlier as empiric drugs because when a new drug is tried, there is no evidence base. Clinical trials are ahead of all evidence-based medicine and this explains the place of empiric therapy in male infertility. Most empirical therapies are based on the theory that increasing the concentration of circulating testosterone and/or FSH will improve testicular function, especially spermatogenesis.

Clomiphene Citrate

This is the cheapest available drug. It has been mentioned in the Textbook on Infertility written by Insler that only a subgroup of patients are improved by CC therapy, but we do not know who all are in this subgroup and therefore this cheap, fairly safe drug can be tried in all patients. It is given 25–50 mg for 25 days for 3–6 months.[8] This could achieve a pregnancy rate of 40% in a group of 32 subfertile men. Men with partial androgen resistance and mild HH are the best candidates to respond to this therapy.[9] Follow-up is done every month. The dose setting should be such that it should increase FSH and testosterone should be normal with drug.

A study by Hussein et al. suggested considering a course of CC prior to sperm retrieval in patients with NOA.[1]

Human Chorionic Gonadotropin

Human chorionic gonadotropin in a dose of 2,500–5,000 IU twice a week is a very useful regimen in a patient with idiopathic oligozoospermia. This increases the testosterone level. Intratesticular testosterone is 100 times higher than serum level. So, exogenous hCG should be given rather than testosterone. The Leydig cells of the testis can respond positively to exogenous hCG and produce more amount of testosterone even under hypogonadotropic conditions. This suppresses endogenous gonadotropin levels by negative feedback. hCG-based hormonal therapy prior to a second micro-testicular sperm extraction (TESE) attempt is effective in men with hypospermatogenesis.[10] Even before the era of ICSI, we have very often used this drug with excellent results. We still use this drug for mild-to-moderate oligozoospermia **(Box 1)**.

This drug is very useful after varicocele ligation. The first reported studies showed 60% improvement in semen parameters.[11,12] Patients with relative androgen deficiency are more benefited.[13]

Follicle-stimulating Hormone + Human Chorionic Gonadotropin

This is a very useful combination for idiopathic normogonadotropic oligozoospermia.[14] The argument in favor of this therapy by Professor Ishidori (Sweden) is that these are the patients who have inadequate gonadotropin activity. Here, radioimmunoassay (RIA) results are normal but the bioactivity is low. This bioactivity can be assessed by monoclonal antibody testing, but is not easily available. To compensate for this deficient bioactivity, exogenous FSH and hCG are given for 3–6 months.[15] To our experience this regimen has proved to be very useful for idiopathic oligozoospermia. The case report described earlier in this chapter indicates the efficacy of this regimen.

Box 1: Mild, moderate, and severe oligozoospermia.

- *Normal count*: >15 million/mL or 30 million/ejaculate
- *Mild oligozoospermia*: 10–15 million/mL
- *Moderate oligozoospermia*: 5–10 million/mL
- *Severe oligozoospermia*: <5 million/mL

The treatment protocol is:
- hMG/rFSH 75–150 IU thrice a week
- Human chorionic gonadotropin 5,000 IU once a week

For maturation arrest at the spermatid level, only FSH can be given for completion of spermatogenesis.[16] FSH therapy improves fertilization after ICSI.

A significant reduction in sperm aneuploidy levels has been detected after varicocele repair[17] and in men treated with rFSH.[18]

Androgen

Testosterone has no role in improving spermatogenesis. Formerly, rebound therapy was given which is discarded because it causes permanent azoospermia in some patients. Testosterone is not a useful drug.[19,20]

Tamoxifen + Testosterone Undecanoate

The World Health Organization (WHO) recommends treatment with antiestrogens—tamoxifen for idiopathic oligozoospermia when motility and morphology are not significantly affected.[21] When serum FSH is not elevated, tamoxifen is given 20 mg/day.

When testosterone undecanoate 120 mg is combined with 20 mg tamoxifen, there is significant improvement in semen quality and an increase in pregnancy rate.

Pregnancy rates increased from 10.3 to 33% as described in one study.[22] So combination is more useful than only tamoxifen.

Zinc

Zinc is very useful in low testosterone levels with zinc deficiency. The recommended dose is 120–220 mg twice a day for 3 months. It improves the function of accessory glands. It helps in the exploration of immature cells. It helps in improving oligozoospermia as well as motility and maturation of spermatozoa.[23,24]

Ketotifen

Ketotifen inhibits histamine release from mast cells. It helps in blood-testis barrier dysfunction. The dose is 1 mg BD for 3–6 months.[25] It has incompatibility with alcohol.[26] The pregnancy rate in one study was 28.6% versus 0%.[27]

Antiserotonin Agents

Cyproheptadine hydrochloric acid (HCl) 4 mg TDS for 90 days can be given in two courses. It improves sperm count and motility in 33–50% of cases. The mechanism of action is that it reduces uptake of serotonin which reduces testicular damage.[28]

Captopril

Captopril is an angiotensin-converting enzyme (ACE) inhibitor. It inhibits kininase II and prevents degradation of kininogens to kinins. It is given in a dose of 50 mg/day for 3 months. It is contraindicated in presence of inflammation.[29]

Tissue Hormones

Pancreatic kallikrein converts kininogens to kinins which helps in cell proliferation. It helps in oligoasthenoteratozoospermia (OAT). It is given in a dose of 600 mg/day for 3–12 months,[30] but cumulative results are not promising.[31]

Anti-inflammatory Drugs

Chlamydia infection is very common in patients having male factor as a cause of infertility. It is extremely difficult to diagnose infection in the genital tract and is very expensive also. Instead, one course of doxycycline 100 mg BD for 14 days is cost-effective as the incidence of infection has been quoted between 28 and 91%. It prevents occlusion of passage and local immunity is improved. Tetracycline and metronidazole are very effective, but antibiotic therapy does not necessarily improve conception rates.[32]

Indomethacin

Prostaglandins have an inhibitory effect on testicular steroidogenesis. Indomethacin and ketoprofen raise FSH, LH, and testosterone. Indomethacin 25 mg TDS increases sperm count and motility.[33] It is inexpensive and nontoxic and should be tried. Diclofenac 50 mg is recommended for 3–6 months.[32]

Aromatase Inhibitors

Teslac (testolactone) is tried for improving sperm count and motility. It is given 50–100 mg twice daily. It prevents aromatization to estrogen. So, patients having low testosterone/estradiol (E2) are potential candidates to improve with this drug. It should be considered for obese patients and those with elevated E2 levels. Anastrozole is a very potent drug and is used in a dose of 1 mg/day.[34-36] Letrozole can be used as 2.5 mg/day dose. It is documented to improve sperm count and motility

Autocrine-paracrine Mechanism

Insulin-like growth factor 1 (IGF-1), IGF-2, epidermal growth factor (EGF), and transforming growth factor (TGF) are potent stimulants for spermatogenesis. So, FSH + growth factors can improve spermatogenesis. Corticotropin-releasing factor-β (CRF-β) endorphins are inhibitors of spermatogenesis. Naltrexone is the drug which prevents CRF-β endorphin system. So, FSH + Naltrexone can improve spermatogenesis.

Antioxidants

The definitive role of reactive oxygen species (ROS) testing in the diagnostic situation remains to be established, although detrimental effects of ROS on the male reproductive system are now well established.[37,38]

Therefore, systematic treatment of men with antioxidants has received great interest in recent years and it seems to have some clinical benefit, though the story remains somewhat confused.[39]

8-hydroxy-2′-deoxyguanosine, a biomarker of oxidative deoxyribonucleic acid (DNA) damage, highly correlated with sperm DNA fragmentation, in human sperm DNA. It has significant value in predicting the chance of a clinical pregnancy after IUI but not ICSI in ART.[40] Supplementing antioxidants (vitamins C, E, and folate) and micronutrients (zinc) can also be helpful in producing sperms with less DNA damage in an older man as well.[41]

Antioxidants are more useful as a follow-up or complementary treatment to conventional treatment of varicocele, antibiotic treatment for infection, or anti-estrogenic treatment for idiopathic oligozoospermia.[21] It has also been suggested that patients with asthenozoospermia should be advised to adhere to a diet rich in fruits, vegetables, poultry, skim milk, and seafoods and low in processed meat and sweets.[42]

According to Lipshultz, high doses of antioxidants have theoretical adverse effects and should be used in low or moderate doses. With exception of patients with specific vitamin deficiency, the efficacy of any vitamin therapy in normal men is questionable.

ANTIOXIDANTS

Antioxidants reduce sperms' oxidative stress and increase motility in asthenozoospermic patients, but it is yet unclear whether this improvement translates to higher full-term pregnancy rates.[43] Protective effects on DNA damage are most pronounced in the elderly people **(Table 1)**. DFI is negatively correlated to density, viability and morphology of the sperms. It increases the risk of early abortion. Couples under ART have lower live birth rate when DFI is high. But when ICSI is performed, though the effect of DFI is not seen, the live birth rate does not improve. Therefore, routine testing for DFI in assessment of male infertility is not justified. It is done only in selected group of patients. High DNA fragmentation is seen in idiopathic and male factor infertility and in those who have had difficulty in conceiving even after ART. Oxidative stress is increased in all these patients with high DFI. Increase in oxidative stress gives abnormal sperms.

Vitamin E

Vitamin E has a protective effect on lipid peroxidation in sperm membrane by ROS.

TABLE 1: Antioxidants used for oligoasthenospermia.

Tocopherol (vitamin E)	Glutathione
Ascorbic acid (vitamin C)	Arginine
Vitamin B_{12}	Carnitines
Folic acid	Coenzyme Q
Pentoxifylline	Vitamin D
Selenium	Lycopene

It increases sperm motility and increases the fertilization rate in IVF.[44] Vitamin E improves the motility of spermatozoa. The recommended dose is 300–600 mg daily for 6–12 weeks. Vitamin E improves sperm–oocyte fusion. So, it is included in certain media preparations. The addition of vitamin E in media reduces the damaging effect of configuration during sperm preparation.[45] Astaxanthin is a carotenoid extracted from the algae *Haematococcus pluvialis*. The potency of this antioxidant is much higher as a singlet molecular oxygen quencher compared with vitamin E.[46] A positive effect of astaxanthin on sperm parameters and fertility is seen in a study by Comhaire et al.[47] A pregnancy rate of 23% was achieved as compared to 3.6% in control group because of better fusion and increase in linear progression motility.

Vitamin C

Low levels of vitamin C lead to infertility due to disturbed sperm functions. Vitamin C improves sperm quality. The dose is 1,000 mg daily.[48]

Vitamin B_{12}

This is very useful for the synthesis of DNA and ribonucleic acid (RNA). It is useful for oligospermia and asthenospermia. The recommended dose is 1,000–1,500 µg/day for 6 months.[49]

Folic Acid

This is an addictive drug and along with other drugs, it helps to improve sperm functions. The dose required is 5 mg/day.[50]

Pentoxifylline

It improves microcirculation. The dose required is 1.2 mg/day for 3–6 months. It improves sperm count and motility.[31,51]

But there are various reports that indicate that pentoxifylline, sildenafil, and other methylxanthines when administered systematically give no response.[52] Sildenafil prior to semen collection may result in increased motility.[53]

Selenium

It is an antioxidant as well as an anti-inflammatory agent. It is concentrated in the male reproductive tract. Its highest concentration is in prostate and improves motility. The dose required is 225 µg/day. It is found that only 50% of patients improve as far as motility is concerned.[54]

Glutathione

It has a positive effect on sperm motility and is given in a dose of 600 mg intramuscular (IM) daily. Daily injections are cumbersome and therefore this treatment has not gained popularity.[55]

Arginine

It improves sperm motility and the recommended dose is 4 g/day.

L-carnitine and L-acetylcarnitine

L-carnitine (LC) brings acetyl-CoA into mitochondria. So, its role is important in sperm cell metabolism. The concentration of LC is highest in epididymal fluid (2,000 times higher) which is available to sperm cells. LC protects cell membrane and DNA against damage by ROS. A combination of LC and L-acetylcarnitine (LAC) is more effective in improving sperm motility than individually in patients with lower baseline levels.[56] LC and LAC are useful in idiopathic OAT and low-grade varicoceles. It is also useful in patients with prostate-vesiculo-epididymitis after treatment with nonsteroidal anti-inflammatory drug (NSAID).[57,58]

L-carnitine 1 g BD + LAC 500 mg BD + cinnoxicam 30 mg every 4 days showed a significant reduction in aneuploid sperms and improved ICSI pregnancies and live births in severe OAT patients.[59] The fact is that LC is not essential as it is synthesized in the body. The exogenous source is nonvegetarian food. Deficiency occurs in patients with hemodialysis, but there are several papers giving a controversial opinion regarding its role as an antioxidant. It has a selective role in oligoasthenozoospermia.[60]

We must remember that the positive effect of the drug does not last for a long time after therapy. So, during the treatment for fertility, the drug is to be continued. We cannot prescribe the drug and wait for the results. Simultaneous superovulation with IUI or ART is a must.

Total oxyradical scavenging capacity (TOSC) assays differentiate different forms of ROS and its role for specific antioxidants. So, in the future, we will be able to decide which antioxidant is required for a particular patient.

Coenzyme Q10

It is the component of the mitochondrial respiratory chain. It has a very important role in energy metabolism. It is biosynthesized in testis and has a protective role as an antioxidant for cell membranes and lipoprotein. The natural source of coenzyme Q10 (CoQ10) is broccoli, spinach, soybean oil, palm oil, vitamins, and minerals that act as cofactors for producing CoQ10.

It is available as 50–100-mg soft gel capsules that have almost 100% absorption. Therapeutic application of CoQ10 for 6 months increases its reduced form ubiquinol which improves the kinetic property of sperm cells.[61]

A reduced CoQ10 level is found in seminal plasma and sperm cells in an infertile man with idiopathic oligospermia and varicocele associated with oligoasthenospermia.

There is strong support as antioxidant by an indirect medium, but there is no conclusion for improved pregnancy rates by this therapy. Like LC, its beneficial effect also does not last long.

Vitamin D

Lately, Vitamin D receptors are found in testis with vitamin D metabolizing enzymes also. These enzymes are also found in epididymis and mature sperms.[62] Vitamin D can also be positively associated with testosterone and free androgen index and negatively with sex hormone-binding globulin (SHBG).[63] Still, another study has shown that 1,25-dihydroxyvitamin D3 [1,25-$(OH)_2D3$] increases intracellular calcium concentration and sperm motility and induces the acrosome reaction in mature spermatozoa. Vitamin D levels in serum were positively associated with sperm motility.[64] Combined treatment with taurine, cysteine, and glutathione statistically significantly ameliorated the reduction in sperm motility during in vitro manipulation of human sperm.[65] Though other studies do not show that low vitamin D is a risk factor for poor semen quality in a population of young healthy men.[66]

Note: We must remember that we should prescribe the drug only in full therapeutic dose, otherwise it will not be useful. The combinations of drugs available in the market should be fully studied well and should be prescribed to appropriate patients. Haphazard prescriptions simply add cost to the patients. Select the combo preparation that has three to four drugs in therapeutic dose.

Lycopene and Carotenoids

Improvement in sperm motility has been found with a higher intake of carotenoids, beta-carotene, and lutein, and improved sperm morphology is found with a high intake of lycopene.

- Lycopene—tomatoes
- Beta-carotene—carrots, lettuce, and spinach
- Lutein—spinach and lettuce

Omega-3 Fatty Acids

A positive effect on spermatogenesis is seen with an increased intake of omega-3 fatty acids in the form of diet and supplements rich in nuts and fish. It protects against environmental toxins and slows down the aging process.

Miscellaneous Methods

- *Acupuncture*: Though some workers have tried and documented improvement in males with oligozoospermia and azoospermia with acupuncture therapy. Large and reliable studies are yet to be documented.
- *Traditional Chinese herbal medicine*:
  - Ginseng—improves testosterone and sperm count
  - Astragalus
  - Sarsaparilla

  These drugs do not have research defining risks and benefits so they should be used with caution.
- *Diet*: The higher intake of processed meat and sweets is associated with a risk of asthenospermia while a high intake of fruits, vegetables, poultry, skim milk, and seafood is associated with a low risk. Preconceptional counseling for diet should be done, with the couple wishing conception.

DOSAGE OF DRUGS

- Clomiphene citrate 25–50 mg/day
- Human chorionic gonadotropin 2,000–5,000 IU twice a week
- FSH 75 IU thrice a week + hCG 5,000 IU twice a week
- Tamoxifen 40 mg + testosterone undecanoate 120 mg daily
- Zinc 100–2,000 mg BD
- Ketotifen 1 mg BD
- Cyproheptadine HCl 4 mg TDS
- Captopril 50 mg daily
- Pancreatic kallikrein 600 mg daily
- Indomethacin 25 mg TDS
- Anastrozole 1 mg daily—this is especially useful in patients with low testosterone levels. By preventing aromatization, it increases testosterone and sperm production.[67]

DOSAGE OF ANTIOXIDANTS

- *Vitamin E*: 300–600 mg daily
- *Vitamin C*: 1,000 mg daily
- *Vitamin B_{12}*: 1,000–1,500 µg daily
- *Folic acid*: 5 mg daily
- *Pentoxifylline*: 1–2 mg daily
- *Selenium*: 225 µg daily
- *Glutathione*: 600 mg IM daily
- *Arginine*: 4 g daily
- *LC + LAC*: 3 g daily
- *Coenzyme Q10*: 100 mg BD

Varicocele correction is to be offered to patients with a palpable lesion with one or more abnormal semen parameters.[68] Though some workers have tried a documented improvement in males with oligozoospermia and azoospermia with acupuncture therapy, large and reliable studies are yet to be documented.[69]

CARRY HOME MESSAGE

- HH can be successfully treated with hCG + FSH.
- Clomiphene, letrozole, hCG, and gonadotropins given for 3 months to oligospermic patients can give very good results in idiopathic infertility.
- Tamoxifen with testosterone undecanoate gives good results in male infertility.
- Zinc and vitamin E are useful to improve sperm motility.
- Antioxidants should be given in therapeutic doses only.
- By improving the count, IVF can be converted into IUI and IUI can be converted to natural cycle conception.

REFERENCES

1. Hussein A, Ozgok Y, Ross L, Niederberger C. Clomiphene administration for cases of nonobstructive azoospermia: a multicentre study. J Androl. 2005;26:787-91.
2. Sigman M, Jarow JP. Male infertility. In: Walsh PC, Retik AB, Vaughan ED, Wein AJ (Eds). Campbell's Urology, 8th edition. St. Louis: Saunders; 2002. pp. 1475-531.
3. Whitcomb RW, Crowley WF. Male hypogonadotropic hypogonadism. Endocrinol Metab Clin North Am. 1993;22:125-43.
4. Büchter D, Behre HM, Kliesch S, Nieschlag E. Pulsatile GnRH or human chorionic gonadotropin/human menopausal gonadotropin as effective treatment for men with hypogonadotropic hypogonadism: a review of 42 cases. Eur J Endocrinol. 1998;139:298-303.
5. Gillam MP, Molitch ME, Lombardi G, Coloa A. Advances in the treatment of prolactinoma. Endocr Rev. 2006;27:485-534.
6. Dubin L, Amelar RD. Etiologic factors in 1294 consecutive cases of male infertility. Fertil Steril. 1971;22:469-74.
7. Greenberg SH, Lipshultz LI, Wein AJ. Experience with 425 subfertile male patients. J Urol. 1978;119:507-10.
8. Paulson DF, Hammond CB, de Vere White R, Wiebe RH. Clomiphene citrate: pharmacologic treatment of hypofertile male. Urology. 1977;9:419-21.
9. Akin JW. The use of clomiphene citrate in the treatment of azoospermia secondary to incomplete androgen resistance. Fertil Steril. 1993;59:223-7.
10. Shiraishi K, Ohmi C, Shimabukuro T, Matsuyama H. Human chorionic gonadotropin treatment prior to microdissection testicular sperm extraction in non-obstructive azoospermia. Hum Reprod. 2012;27:331-9.
11. Glass SJ, Holland HM. Treatment of oligospermia with large doses of human chorionic gonadotropin. Fertil Steril. 1963;14:500-6.
12. Mehan DJ, Chehval MJ. Human chorionic gonadotropin in the treatment of the infertile man. J Urol. 1982;128:60-3.
13. Lunenfield B, Mor A, Mani M. Treatment of male infertility. I. Human gonadotropins. Fertil Steril. 1967;18:581-92.
14. Glezerman M, Lunenfield B. Hormontherapie mannlicher Fertilitäts storingen. In: Kaden R, Lubke F, Schirren C (Eds). Fortschritte der Fertilitats forschung III. Berlin: Grosse; 2007. p. 17.
15. Acosta AA, Khalifa E, Oehninger S. Pure human follicle-stimulating hormone has a role in the treatment of severe male infertility by assisted reproduction: Norfolk's total experience. Hum Reprod. 1992;7:1067-72.
16. Schwarzstein L, Aparicio NJ, Schally AV. D-tryptophan-6-leutinizing hormone-releasing hormone in the treatment of normogonadotropic oligoasthenozoospermia. Int J Androl. 1982;5:172-8.
17. Baccetti BM, Bruni E, Capitani S, Collodel G, Mancini S, Piomboni P, et al. Studies on varicocele III: ultrastructural sperm evaluation and 18, X and Y aneuploidies. J Androl. 2006;27:94-101.
18. Piomboni P, Serafini F, Gambera L, Musacchio C, Collodel G, Morgante G, et al. Sperm aneuploidies after human recombinant follicle stimulating hormone therapy in infertile males. Reprod Biomed Online. 2009;18:622-9.
19. Charny CW. The use of androgens for human spermatogenesis. Fertil Steril. 1959;10:557-70.
20. Charny CW, Gordon JA. Testosterone rebound therapy: a neglected modality. Fertil Steril. 1978;29:64-8.

21. Rowe PJ, Comhaire FH, Hargreave TB, Mahmoud AM, World Health Organization. WHO Manual for the Standardized Investigation, Diagnosis and Management of the Infertile Male. Cambridge: Cambridge University Press; 2000. p. 91.
22. Adamopoules DA, Pappa A, Billa E, Nicopoulou S, Koukkou E, Michopoulos J. Effectiveness of combined tamoxifen citrate and testosterone undecanoate treatment in men with idiopathic oligozoospermia. Fertil Steril. 2003;80:914-20.
23. Ebisch IM, Pierik FH, De Jong FH, Thomas CM, Steegers-Theunissen RP. Does folic acid and zinc sulphate intervention affect endocrine parameters and sperm characteristics in men? Int J Androl. 2006;29:339-45.
24. Wong WY, Merkus HM, Thomas CM, Menkveld R, Zielhuis GA, Steegers-Theunissen RP. Effects of folic acid and zinc sulphate in male factor subfertility: a double-blind, randomized, placebo-controlled trial. Fertil Steril. 2002;77:491-3.
25. Matsuki S, Sasagawa I, Suzuki Y, Yazawa H, Tateno T, Hashimoto T, et al. The use of ebastine, a mast cell blocker, for treatment of oligozoospermia. Arch Androl. 2000; 44:129-32.
26. Schill WB, Schneider J, Ring J. The use of ketotifen, a mast cell blocker, for treatment of oligo- and asthenozoospermia. Andrologia. 1986;18:570-3.
27. Yamamoto M, Hibi H, Miyake K. New treatment of idiopathic severe oligozoospermia with mast cell blocker: results of single-blind study. Fertil Steril. 1995;64: 1221-3.
28. Schill WB, Michalopoulos M. Treatment of male fertility disturbances. Current concepts. Drugs. 1984;28:263-80.
29. Schill WB, Parsch EM, Miska W. Inhibition of angiotensin-converting enzyme: a new concept of medical treatment of male infertility? Fertil Steril. 1994;61:1123-8.
30. Kamidono S, Hazama M, Matsumoto O, Takasa KI, Tomioka O, Ishigami J. Kallikrein and male subfertility: usefulness of high-unit kallikrein tablet. Andrologia. 1981;13:108-20.
31. Keck C, Behre HM, Jockenhovel F, Nieschlag E. Ineffectiveness of kallikrein in treatment of idiopathic male infertility: a double-blind, randomized, placebo-controlled trial. Hum Reprod. 1994;9:325-9.
32. Haidl G. Management strategies for male factor infertility. Drugs. 2002;62:1741-53.
33. Barkay J, Harpaz-Kerpel S, Ben-Ezra S, Gordon S, Zuckerman H. The prostaglandin inhibitor effect of anti-inflammatory drugs in the therapy of male infertility. Fertil Steril. 1984;42:406-11.
34. Schlegel PN, Raman JD. Aromatase inhibitors for male infertility. J Urol. 2002;167:624-9.
35. Pavlovich CP, King P, Goldstein M, Schlegel PN. Evidence of a treatable endocrinopathy in infertile men. J Urol. 2001;165:837-41.
36. Raman JD, Schlegel PN. Aromatase inhibitors for male infertility. J Urol. 2002;167:624-9.
37. Saleh RA, Agarwal A. Oxidative stress and male infertility: from research bench to clinical practice. J Androl. 2002;23:737-52.
38. Agarwal A, Saleh RA, Bedaiwy MA. Role of reactive oxygen species in the pathophysiology of human reproduction. Fertil Steril. 2003;79:829-43.
39. Agarwal A. Role of antioxidants in treatment of male infertility: an overview of the literature. Reprod Biomed Online. 2004;8:616-27.
40. Thomson LK, Zieschang JA, Clark AM. Oxidative DNA damage in sperm has a negative impact on clinical pregnancy rate in intrauterine insemination but not in intracytoplasmic sperm injection cycles. Fertil Steril. 2011;96:843-7.
41. Schmid TE, Eskenazi B, Marchetti F, Young S, Weldon RH, Baumgartner A, et al. Micronutrients intake is associated with improved sperm DNA quality in older men. Fertil Steril. 2012;98:1130-7.
42. Elsamian G, Amirjannati N, Rashidkhani B, Sadeghi MR, Hekmatdoost A. Intake of food groups and idiopathic asthenozoospermia: a case-control study. Hum Reprod. 2012;27: 3328-36.
43. Gharagozloo P, Aitken RJ. The role of sperm oxidative stress in male infertility and the significance of oral antioxidant therapy. Hum Reprod. 2011;26:1628-40.

44. Geva E, Bartoov B, Zabludovsky N, Lessing JB, Geva LL, Amit A. The effect of antioxidant treatment on human spermatozoa and fertilization rate in an in vitro fertilization program. Fertil Steril. 1996;66:430-4.
45. Keskes-Ammar L, Feki-Chakroun N, Rebai T, Sahnoun Z, Ghozzi H, Hammami S, et al. Sperm oxidative stress and the effect of an oral vitamin E and selenium supplement on semen quality in infertile male. Arch Androl. 2003;49:83-94.
46. Di Mascio P, Devasagayam TP, Kaiser S, Sies H. Carotenoids, tocopherols and thiols as biological singlet molecular oxygen quenchers. Biochem Soc Trans. 1990;18:1054-6.
47. Comhaire FH, Garem YE, Mahmoud A, Eertmans F, Schoonjans F. Combined conventional/antioxidant "astaxanthin" treatment for male infertility: a double-blind randomized trial. Asian J Androl. 2005;7:257-62.
48. Dawson EB, Harris WA, Teter MC, Powell LC. Effect of ascorbic acid supplementation on the sperm quality of smokers. Fertil Steril. 1992;58:1034-9.
49. Sandler B, Faragher N. Treatment of oligozoospermia with vitamin B_{12}. Infertility. 1984; 7:133-2.
50. Ebisch IMW, van Heerde WL, Thomas CMG, van der Put N, Wong WY, Steegers-Theunissen RPM. C677T methylenetetrahydrofolate reductase polymorphism interferes with the effects of folic acid and zinc sulphate on sperm concentration. Fertil Steril. 2003;80:1190-4.
51. Schill WB. Therapy of idiopathic astheno- and oligozoospermia with pentoxifylline. Fortschr Med. 1982;100:696-700.
52. Burger M, Sikka SC, Bivalacqua TJ, Lamb DJ, Hellstrom WJ. The effect of sildenafil on human sperm motion and function from normal and infertile men. Int J Impot Res. 2000;12:229-34.
53. du Plessis SS, de Jongh PS, Franken DR. Effect of acute in vivo sildenafil and in vitro 8-bromo-cGMP treatments on semen parameters and sperm function. Fertil Steril. 2004;81:1026-33.
54. Scott R, MacPherson A, Yates RW, Hussain B, Dixon J. The effect of oral selenium supplementation on human sperm motility. Br J Urol. 1998;82:76-80.
55. Lenzi A, Culasso F, Gandini L, Lombardo F, Dondero F. Placebo-controlled, double-blind, cross-over trial of glutathione therapy in male infertility. Hum Reprod. 1993;8:1657-62.
56. Lenzi A, Sgrò P, Salacone P, Paoli D, Gilio B, Lombardo F, et al. A placebo-controlled double-blind randomized trial of the use of combined L-carnitine and L-acetyl-carnitine treatment in men with asthenozoospermia. Fertil Steril. 2004;6:1578-84.
57. Cavallini G, Ferraretti AP, Gianaroli L, Biagiotti G, Vitali G. Cinnoxicam and L-carnitine/acetyl-L-carnitine treatment for idiopathic and varicocele-associated oligoasthenospermia. J Androl. 2004;25: 761-70.
58. Vicari E, La Vignera S, Calogero AE. Antioxidant treatment with carnitines is effective in infertile patients with prostatovesiculoepididymitis and elevated seminal leukocyte concentrations after treatment with nonsteroidal anti-inflammatory compounds. Fertil Steril. 2002; 78:1203-8.
59. Cavallini G, Magli MC, Crippa A, Ferraretti AP, Gianaroli L. Reduction in sperm aneuploidy levels in severe oligoasthenoteratospermic patients after medical therapy: a preliminary report. Asian J Androl. 2012;14:591-8.
60. Lenzi A, Lombardo F, Sgrò P, Salacone P, Caponecchia L, Dondero F, et al. Use of carnitine therapy in selected cases of male factor infertility: a double-blind crossover trial. Fertil Steril. 2003;79:292-300.
61. Balercia G, Buldreghini E, Vignini A, Tiano L, Paggi F, Amoroso S, et al. Coenzyme Q10 treatment in infertile men with idiopathic asthenozoospermia: a placebo-controlled, double-blind randomized trial. Fertil Steril. 2009;91:1785-92.
62. Jensen MB, Nielsen JE, Jørgensen A, Rajpert-De Meyts E, Kristensen DM, Jørgensen N, et al. Vitamin D receptor and vitamin D metabolizing enzymes are

expressed in the human male reproductive tract. Hum Reprod. 2010;25:1303-11.
63. Wehr E, Pilz S, Boehm BO, Marz W, Obermayer-Pietsch B. Association of vitamin D status with serum androgen levels in men. Clin Endocrinol (Oxf). 2010;73:243-8.
64. Bloomberg JM, Bjerrum PJ, Jessen TE, Nielson JE, Joenson UN, Oleson IA, et al. Vitamin D is positively associated with sperm motility and increases intracellular calcium in human spermatozoa. Hum Reprod. 2011;26:1307-17.
65. Yun JI, Gong SP, Song YH, Lee ST. Effects of combined antioxidant supplementation on human sperm motility and morphology during sperm manipulation in vitro. Fertil Steril. 2013;100:373-8.
66. Ramlau-Hansen CH, Moeller UK, Bonde JP, Oslen J, Thulstrup AM. Are serum levels of vitamin D associated with semen quality? Results from a cross-sectional study in young healthy men. Fertil Steril. 2011;95:1000-4.
67. Schlegel PN. Aromatase inhibitors for male infertility. Fertil Steril. 2012;98:1359-62.
68. Sharlip ID, Jarow JP, Belkar AM, Lipshultz LI, Sigman M, Thomas AJ, et al. Best practice policies for male infertility. Fertil Steril. 2002;77:873-82.
69. Senior K. Acupuncture: Can it take the pain away? Mol Med Today. 1996;2:150-3.

Chapter 36

Management of Azoospermia

INTRODUCTION

The prevalence of azoospermia in men is very rare, about 1% only, but in infertile men, the incidence is as high as 10–15%.[1]

Azoospermia indicates that no sperm is identified in the pellet after centrifugation in two separate samples.

Analyzing medical history, physical examination, laboratory investigations, and imaging are very important for the diagnosis and management of azoospermia.

DIAGNOSIS OF AZOOSPERMIA

Azoospermia is classified as:

- Pretesticular
- Testicular
- Post-testicular

Pretesticular

- Pretesticular includes endocrine abnormalities having an adverse effect on spermatogenesis. It is secondary testicular failure.
  - Hypogonadotropic hypogonadism
  - Kallmann syndrome
  - Craniopharyngioma
- *Pituitary*: Trauma, ablation, adenoma, meningitis, and isolated follicle-stimulating hormone (FSH) deficiency
- *Drugs*: Anabolic steroids and testosterone injections

Testicular

Testicular causes of azoospermia are called primary testicular failure. Here disorders of spermatogenesis are extrinsic to the testis. They are normally having nonobstructive azoospermia (NOA).

- *Congenital*: Cryptorchidism, Klinefelter syndrome, myotonic dystrophy, sex chromosome aneuploidy, Y microdeletion and anorchia, maturation arrest, Sertoli cell syndrome. Hypospermatogenesis may cause NOA.
- *Acquired*: Mumps orchitis, torsion, castration
- *Iatrogenic*: Radiotherapy, chemotherapy

Post-testicular

It may be because of ductal obstruction [obstructive azoospermia (OA)] or ejaculatory dysfunction. Retrograde ejaculation may also cause azoospermia.

- *Congenital*:
  - Congenital bilateral absence of vas deferens (CBAVD)
  - Cystic fibrosis
  - Mullerian prostate cyst
- *Acquired*: It is due to blockage because of injection, e.g., gonorrhea, chlamydia, tuberculosis, schistosomiasis.
- *Iatrogenic*: Vasectomy, herniorrhaphy, hydrocele repair, renal transplant.
- *Ejaculatory dysfunction*: It may be because of spinal cord injury or neurological damage.

In clinical practice, it is classified as NOA and OA. NOA is further divided into central NOA and testicular NOA.

EVALUATION OF AZOOSPERMIA

- History
- Physical examination[2]
- *Laboratory investigations*: Serum FSH (S. FSH) and serum testosterone (S. testosterone) first. FSH is considered abnormal if it is >7.6 mIU/mL.

Then add serum luteinizing hormone (S. LH), free testosterone, estradiol, and prolactin.

Obstructive Azoospermia (Flowchart 1)

These patients usually show a normal testicular size and normal FSH and normal spermatogenesis.

- Low ejaculate
- Normal ejaculate

Low Ejaculate Volume (<1.5 mL) with Normal FSH and Normal Testicular Volume

Its causes are:

- *Collection error*: Spillage or 2–3 days of abstinence

Flowchart 1: Management of infertile males based on semen volume.

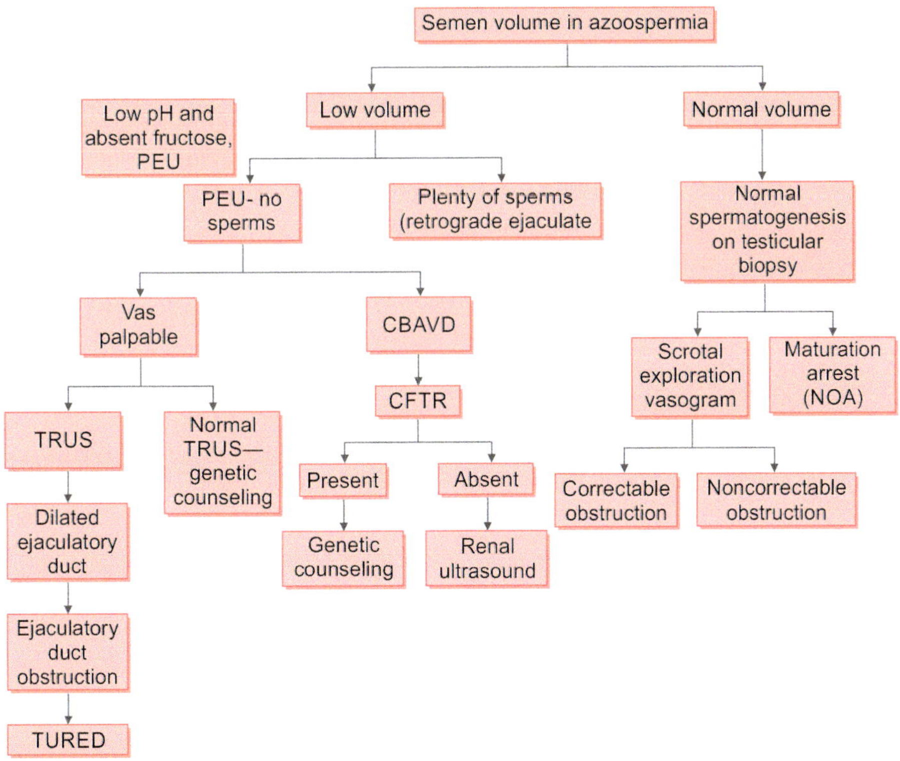

(CBAVD: congenital bilateral absence of vas deferens; CFTR: cystic fibrosis transmembrane conductance regulator; NOA: nonobstructive azoospermia; PEU: postejaculate urinalysis; TRUS; transrectal ultrasound; TURED; transurethral resection of the ejaculatory ducts)

- Retrograde ejaculation [postejaculate urine (PEU) analysis]. If retrograde ejaculation is present, millions of sperms can be seen in PEU.
- *Block at seminal vesicle or ejaculatory ducts*: In these cases vas is palpable, there is no retrograde ejaculation, and pH is <7.2. Then transrectal ultrasound (TRUS) is done to evaluate dilatation of seminal vesicles and ejaculatory ducts. Ejaculatory duct obstruction (EDO) can be easily diagnosed as it presents with the absence of fructose in semen and pH is <7.2 as the secretions of seminal vesicles are alkaline. Ultrasound diagnosis is based on dilated ejaculatory ducts, dilated seminal vesicles (>1.5 cm in diameter), and midline cyst for all cases of EDO. But a normal seminal vesicle size does not exclude EDO.

CBAVD: It is diagnosed by physical examination of the scrotum. In these cases also, the semen volume is low. About 10–15% of patients with CBAVD have unilateral renal agenesis not associated with cystic fibrosis. Cystic fibrosis transmembrane conductance regulator (CFTR) mutations may be explained by different genetic mutations that lead to anomalies in the Wolffian duct with a subsequent anomaly in the seminal vesicle, vas deferens, and epididymis.[3] In these patients, renal agenesis with genital abnormalities is found with no CFTR.

In patients with unilateral vas agenesis, segmental atresia of vas or seminal vesicle will be seen on the contralateral side in TRUS. Unilateral renal agenesis will be seen in approximately 25% of patients.

For patients with renal anomalies with unilateral or bilateral vas agenesis, the incidence of CFTR mutation is the same as the general population and so testing for mutation is not done. Females should be tested as a carrier.

Normal Ejaculate Volume with Azoospermia

In these cases, S. FSH and testicular volume are most determining factors and a testicular biopsy would be useful. Marked elevation of FSH and reduced testicular volume suggests NOA.

Testicular biopsy or aspiration can be taken:

- At the time of intracytoplasmic sperm injection (ICSI)
- Before stimulation of the female partner

The advantage of testicular aspiration or biopsy at the time of ICSI is that tissues can be sent for histopathological examination.

Normal testicular biopsy or aspirate indicates obstruction at someplace. It may be because of iatrogenic vasal injury during vasectomy, hernia repair, or pelvic surgery. It is mostly due to bilateral epididymal obstruction and it is treated by surgical exploration. Obstruction in the vas or ejaculatory duct may be diagnosed by vasography. But it can cause scarring and is better avoided.

During microsurgery of epididymal obstruction, sperms should be stored if assisted reproductive technology (ART) is planned for the future.

Few patients of azoospermia with normal semen volume may have maturation arrest on testicular biopsy and they have NOA and exploration is avoided.

S. FSH is related more to the number of spermatogonia and less to the number of spermatids or sperm count.[4] So high FSH means a lesser number of spermatogonia due to Sertoli cell syndrome. Hence, normal FSH with NOA is maturation arrest and high FSH indicates Sertoli cell-only syndrome.

Nonobstructive Azoospermia

- Clinical history
- Physical examination
- History of androgens or anabolic steroids

Investigations **(Flowchart 2)**:

- S. FSH
- S. LH
- S. testosterone
- S. prolactin
- CT scan of brain for pituitary tumor
- Scrotal Doppler for varicocele
- Karyotyping
- Y microdeletion

Patients have raised FSH and normal ejaculate volume so they do not require testicular biopsy. They often have bilateral testicular atrophy due to primary or secondary testicular failure. The exception is that men with maturation arrest will have a normal testicular size and FSH.

- Low gonadotropin and bilateral testicular atrophy:
  - It suggests hypogonadotropic hypogonadism. This is due to the hypothalamic disorder, e.g., Kallmann syndrome.
  - Pituitary disorders (congenital and acquired)
  - Functional and nonfunctional tumors associated with low gonadotropins. Because of low gonadotropins, testicular stimulation is absent. It may be because of exogenous testosterone or anabolic steroids. In this case, testosterone will be high with low gonadotropins. If testosterone is low, it is recently discontinued exogenous androgens. So in all patients of hypogonadotropic hypogonadism, inquire for the history of exogenous androgens or steroids.

Medical therapy for hypogonadotropic hypogonadism and primary testicular failure:

- In these cases, testosterone level is low and the testosterone to estradiol ratio is low. Treatment with aromatase inhibitor letrozole has been successful in getting sperms in ejaculate.[5]
- Treatment with clomiphene citrate is also very useful and sperm retrieval is successful for ICSI. For those who do not respond, human chorionic gonadotropin (hCG)

Flowchart 2: Management of infertile males based on serum follicle-stimulating hormone levels.

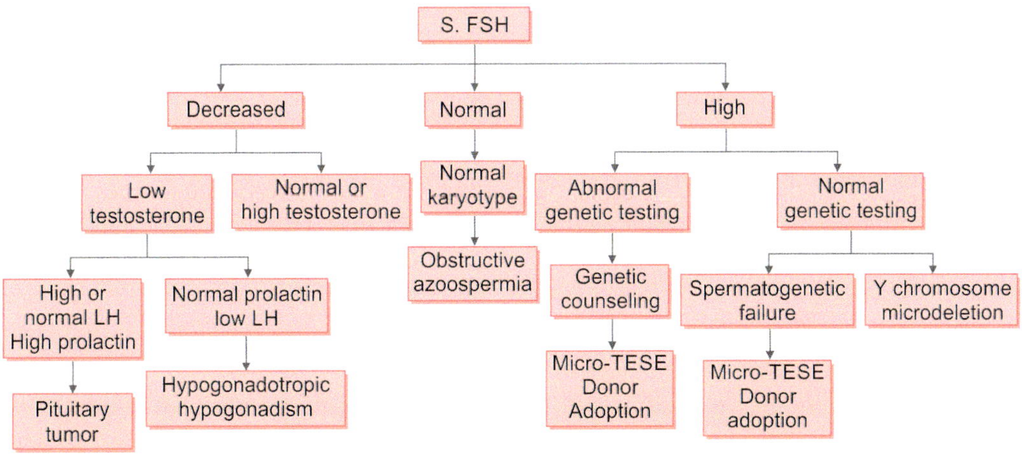

(LH: luteinizing hormone; Micro-TESE: microdissection testicular sperm extraction; S. FSH: serum follicle-stimulating hormone)

can be given twice or thrice a week in a dosage of 2,000–30,00 IU with human menopausal gonadotropin (HMG)/FSH thrice a week. This regimen is given for 3–6 months.[6]

- *Hypogonadotropic hypogonadism is one of the most medically treated causes of NOA*:
  - Gonadotropin-releasing hormone agonist (GnRHa) therapy. Pulsatile 5–20 μg/2 hourly via infusion pump rather than intravenously or intramuscularly. It is given for 12–24 months and has shown a 77% success rate.[7] It is very useful in patients with hypospermatogenesis.
  - hCG followed by hCG with HMG
- S. prolactin
  Brain imaging for prolactinoma
- *Unilateral or bilateral varicocoele*:[8] In these cases, FSH is elevated. Sperm can be seen in ejaculate in 10–40% of the patients after surgery, even if it does not appear in ejaculate. Good sperm cohort is achieved in biopsy after 3 months of retrieval.[9]
  It is not useful in Sertoli cell-only syndrome or maturation arrest. It is very useful in patients with hypospermatogenesis.

GENETIC TESTING

In cases of male infertility, 50% have genetic abnormality. In genetic abnormality, the two most common abnormalities are: (1) chromosomal abnormalities and (2) Y chromosome microdeletion.

Chromosomal Abnormalities

In almost 7% of cases of azoospermia, karyotype detects a genetic abnormality. Defects may be deletion of the entire chromosomes or a portion of chromosome or translocations and inversions are common. Sex chromosome aneuploidy, e.g., Klinefelter syndrome (47XXY), is very common amongst chromosomal abnormalities. These have NOA, with low/normal testosterone levels. So androgen deficiency causes osteoporosis, decreased muscle mass, diabetes, etc. These patients have an increased risk of thromboembolism, male breast cancer, and extragonadal germ cell cancers. So genetic counseling is mandatory. hCG is given in the dose of 3,000 IU, two to three times a week followed by FSH thrice a week. It may be continued for 6–12 months.[10]

Structural abnormalities in autosomes such as inversion and translocations are common. They may not leave azoospermia, but recurrent pregnancy loss (RPL) and chromosomal and congenital defects are common and thus, genetic counseling is a must.

Y Chromosome Microdeletion

It is diagnosed by the polymerase chain reaction (PCR) technique. Y chromosomal microdeletion occurs in the long arm of the Y chromosome. It has azoospermia factors AZFa, AZFb, and AZFc. Deletions of these locations are responsible for spermatogenesis dysfunction. It is found in 10–15% of azoospermic or severe oligospermic patients.[11]

Men with a deletion in AZFc may have sperm in ejaculate or sperms that can be retrieved after conventional or microsurgical testicular sperm extraction, i.e., conventional testicular sperm extraction (cTESE) or microdissection testicular sperm extraction (mTESE). However, deletions involving AZFa and AZFb predict a very poor prognosis of sperm retrieval and it should not be attempted in these patients.[12] Genetic counseling should be done before ICSI in AZFc deletion that offspring may be severely oligospermic or azoospermic.

Atypical Y chromosome microdeletion may be detected in rare cases.

Silber et al. showed that at least—four to six spermatids or spermatozoa are required in seminiferous tubules for sperms to reach ejaculate except for OA which has 15–35.[13]

INDICATIONS OF TESTICULAR BIOPSY OR ASPIRATION

When there is uncertainty whether it is NOA or OA, then a biopsy or sperm aspiration, called TESE or testicular sperm aspiration (TESA), respectively, is performed. This is done particularly in patients of azoospermia with a normal testicular size, with normal volume of testis, presence of one vas and normal FSH, with normal semen volume. It can differentiate hypospermatogenesis, i.e., only Sertoli cell or maturation arrest.

In patients with OA, diagnostic biopsy and surgical reconstruction are not required. Surgical reconstruction should be taken directly. Testicular atrophy with high FSH has NOA and biopsy should not be done.

The average spermatid count per tubule is the prediction of sperm count in the ejaculate. When spermatids are present, one will get some sperms in some tubules.

Sperms do not come in ejaculate unless there is a minimum concentration of spermatozoa because of the spill-over phenomenon.[13]

MANAGEMENT OF OBSTRUCTIVE AZOOSPERMIA

Obstruction may be at vas, epididymis, or ejaculatory ducts.

- Congenital—CBAVD, epididymal obstruction
- Acquired—Vasectomy, infection, trauma, iatrogenic injury

Microsurgical reconstruction

- Vasovasostomy at the scrotal or inguinal region for vasal obstruction due to vasectomy or vasal injury due to hernia or hydrocele repair
- *Vasoepididymostomy*: It is for idiopathic epididymal obstruction.
  Ideally, reversal is done when one detects sperms or sperm heads or only sperm heads are seen. Surgery is not done if no sperms are detected or if there is a thick and creamy discharge. Semen analysis is done after 1 month and then every 3 months till pregnancy is achieved.
  Microsurgical reconstruction depends on the age of the female. With young age, the results are better. Microsurgery is more cost-effective than ART.
- Transurethral resection for EDO

Sperm Retrieval Technique

This is done when postvasectomy obstruction, CBAVD, EDO, and unreconstructable causes of OA are present and thus most of the times ICSI is required rather than IVF or IUI.

Sperms retrieved from epididymis or testis have the same results. Results of frozen and fresh sperms retrieved also have the same results. These are comparable to ejaculated sperms also.[14]

Procedures on Epididymis

- *Percutaneous epididymal sperm aspiration (PESA)*: This is done without microsurgery. It is done under local anesthesia. 20 mL syringe is attached to butterfly needle and is inserted into the caput of epididymis after fixing it between the forefinger and thumb. With gentle suction, the pressure needle is withdrawn till sufficient fluid is aspirated. Sperms in this fluid can be used for ART.
- *Microsurgical epididymal sperm aspiration (MESA)*: When sperms cannot be retrieved by PESA, MESA can be performed. It is done under general anesthesia. Epididymal incision or

micropuncture is done for individual tubules. An operating microscope is used to identify individual tubule. Puncture sites are closed or cauterized. The best quality of sperms can be achieved near the testicular end of epididymis.

Procedures on Testis

- *Open testicular biopsy*: One tunical incision is necessary to obtain sufficient tissue and sperm. Testicular blood supply should not be damaged. This method is particularly useful when sperms cannot be retrieved from epididymis, and histopathological examination is possible. It can be done by conventional open biopsy or microsurgical open biopsy.
- *Percutaneous TESA*: A needle is inserted in the testicular long axis and repeatedly redirected with gentle pressure and is aspirated. This disrupts the tubules and when sufficient negative pressure is built, sperms can be obtained and tissues from testis will come out and will be sufficient to aspirate the sperms.
- *Percutaneous testicular biopsy (Per C Biopsy)*: It is done under local anesthesia with a 14 gauge biopsy gun. It is done to get a small cylindrical piece of testicular tissue. Multiple pieces can be taken.
- *Needle aspiration biopsy (NAB)*: This is done with an 18 gauge needle. This is done under local anesthesia with an 18 gauge scalp vein needle. It is introduced in the testis and suction is applied with a 10cc syringe with up and down movements done repeatedly. The procedure is repeated after rotating the needle 180° to cut the tissues. The needle is taken out by pulling the tubing and some testicular tissue will come out along with it. It is grasped near the skin and a sufficient length of tubules is pulled out. The needle is then flushed out for some more tissues. This is a simple, nonsurgical quick method and gives more tissue than PESA.
- Conventional testicular sperm extraction (cTESE)
- *Microdissection sperm extraction*: Even in only Sertoli cell-only syndrome or maturation arrest, few sperms can be retrieved.

  Both dilation and evacuation are used for NOA. In mTESE, seminiferous tubules with the largest diameter are dissected under magnification. mTESE retrieves more sperms than cTESE.[15] In general, mTESE is superior to cTESE and cTESE is superior to TESA. The testosterone level falls acutely after TESE but returns to 95% of the baseline after complete healing.[16]

But the recent paper by Majzoub et al. in 2021, say that TESA may be a suitable alternative to micro-TESE in selected NOA patients presenting with an average testis size >7.75 mL and serum FSH level < 8.5 IU/L.[17]

This is very useful information where expense and/or expertise availability is a problem.

Testicular sperm has lower level of DNA fragmentation than ejaculated sperms. So testicular sperms are taken for ICSI rather than ejaculated sperms in patients with high DNA fragmentation.[18]

CARRY HOME MESSAGE

- Correct diagnosis can improve the results of azoospermia.
- NOA maybe because of hypospermatogenesis which is treatable with ICSI.
- The results of OA are very good.
- S. FSH and semen volume can lead to a perfect diagnosis.
- Ultrasound helps to pinpoint the diagnosis.
- Medical management can help in NOA.
- AFZc deletion in Y chromosome microdeletion can have a good prognosis.
- Surgical treatment is a good option in OA.
- Micro-Tese can help in patients with raised FSH.

REFERENCES

1. Jarow JP, Espeland MA, Lipshultz LI. Evaluation of the azoospermic patient. J Urol. 1989;142(1):62-5.
2. Practice committee of the American Society for Reproductive Medicine. Diagnostic evaluation of the infertile male: a committee opinion. Fertil Steril. 2015;103(3):e18-25.
3. Mesrobian HG, Rushton HG, Bulas D. Unilateral renal agenesis may result from in utero regression of multicystic renal dysplasia. J Urol. 1993;150:793-4.
4. Ron EIR, Strassburger D, Friedler S, Komarovski D, Bern O, Soffer Y, et al. Extended sperm preparation: an alternative to testicular sperm extraction in nonobstructive azoospermia. Hum Reprod. 1997;12(6):1222-6.
5. Cavallini G, Beretta G, Biagiotti G. Preliminary study of letrozole use for improving spermatogenesis in non-obstructive azoospermia patients with normal serum FSH. Asian J Androl. 2011;13:895-7.
6. Hussein A, Ozgak Y, Ross L, Rao P, Neiderberger C. Optimization od spermatogenesis regulating hormones in patients with nonobstructive azoospermia and its impact on sperm retrieval: a multicentric study. BJU Int. 2013;111:E110-4.
7. Pitteloud N, Hayes FJ, Dwyer A, Boepple PA, Lee H, Crowley WF. Predictors of outcome of long term GnRH therapy in men with idiopathic hypogonadotropic hypogonadism. J Clin Endocrinol Metab. 2002;87:4128-36.
8. Shiraizi K, Oza S, Matsuyama H. Predictive factors for sperm recovery after varicocelectomy in men with nonobstructive azoospermia. J Urol. 2017;197(2):485-90.
9. Inci K, Hascicek M, Kara O, Dikmen AV, Gurgan T, Ergen A. Sperm retrieval and intracytoplasmic sperm injection in men with nonobstructive azoospermia and treated and untreated varicocoele. J Urol. 2009;182(4):1500-5.
10. Bhasin S. Approach to the infertile man. J Clin Endocrinol Metab. 2007;92:1995-2004.
11. Pryor JL, Kent-First M, Muallem A, Van Bergen Ah, Noiten WE, Meisner L, Roberts KP. Microdeletions in the Y chromosome of infertile men. N Engl J Med. 1997;336(8):534-9.
12. Hopps CV, Mielnik A, Goldstein M, Palermo GD, Rosenwaks Z, Schiegel PN. Detection of sperm in men with Y chromosome microdeletions of the AZFa, AZFb and AZFc regions. Hum Reprod. 2003;18(8):1660-5.
13. Silber SJ, Nagy Z, Devroey P, Tournaye H, Van Steirteghem AC. Distribution of spermatogenesis in the testicles of azoospermic men: the presence or absence of spermatids in the testes of men with germinal failure. Hum Reprod. 1997;12(7):2422-28. [Erratum in: Hum Reprod. 1998;13(3):780; Comment in: Hum Reprod. 1998;13(7):2034-35.]
14. Oldereid NB, Hanevik HI, Bakkevig I, Romundstad LB, Magnus O, Hazekamp J, et al. Pregnancy outcome according to male diagnosis after ICSI with non-ejaculated sperm compared with ejaculated sperm controls. Reprod Biomed Online. 2014;29:417-23.
15. Deruyver Y, Vanderschueren D, Van der Az F. Outcome of microdissection TESE compared with conventional TESE in non-obstructive azoospermia: a systematic review. Andrology. 2014;2:20-4.
16. Ramasamy R, Yagan N, Schlegel PN. Structural and functional changes to the testis after conventional versus microdissection testicular sperm extraction. Urology. 2005;65:1190-4.
17. Majzoub A, Arafa M, Khalafalia K, Alsaid S, Burjaq H, Albader M, et al. Predictive model to estimate the chances of successful sperm retrieval by testicular sperm aspiriation in patients with nonobstructive azoospermia. Fertil Steril. 2021;115(2):373-81.
18. Esteves SC, Roque M, Bradley CK, Garrido N. Reproductive outcomes of testicular versus ejaculated sperm for intracytoplasmic sperm injection among men with high levels of DNA fragmentation in semen: systematic review and meta-analysis. Fertil Steril. 2017;108(3):456-66.

Index

Page numbers followed by *b* refer to box, *f* refer to figure, *fc* refer to flowchart, and *t* refer to table.

R

S

T